THIRD EDITION

STUDENT SUCCESS
FOR HEALTHCARE
PROFESSIONALS

SIMPLIFIED

Laurie Kelly McCorry, PhD

Dean of Science, Engineering, and Mathematics
Bunker Hill Community College
Boston, Massachusetts

Jeff Mason, MFA

Lecturer, College of Communication
Boston University
Boston, Massachusetts

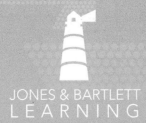

JONES & BARTLETT
LEARNING

World Headquarters
Jones & Bartlett Learning
5 Wall Street
Burlington, MA 01803
978-443-5000
info@jblearning.com
www.jblearning.com

Jones & Bartlett Learning books and products are available through most bookstores and online booksellers. To contact Jones & Bartlett Learning directly, call 800-832-0034, fax 978-443-8000, or visit our website, www.jblearning.com.

20598-5

Production Credits

VP, Product Management: Amanda Martin
Director of Product Management: Cathy L. Esperti
Product Coordinator: Elena Sorrentino
Senior Project Specialist: Alex Schab
Senior Digital Project Specialist: Angela Dooley
Director of Marketing: Andrea DeFronzo
VP, Manufacturing and Inventory Control: Therese Connell
Composition & Project Management: Absolute Service Inc.

Cover Design: Kristin E. Parker
Senior Media Development Editor: Troy Liston
Rights Specialist: Rebecca Damon
Cover Image (Title Page): © SEAN GLADWELL/ Getty Images
Printing and Binding: LSC Communications
Cover Printing: LSC Communications

Library of Congress Cataloging-in-Publication Data

Names: McCorry, Laurie Kelly, 1959- author. | Mason, Jeff, 1961- author. | Lochhaas, Thomas A. LWW's student success for health professionals made incredibly easy.
Title: Student success for healthcare professionals simplified / Laurie Kelly McCorry, Jeff Mason.
Description: Third edition. | Burlington, MA : Jones & Bartlett Learning, [2021] | Preceded by LWW's student success for health professionals made incredibly easy. Second edition / Tom Lochhaas, contributing writer. Baltimore, MD : Lippincott Williams & Wilkins, 2011, ©2012. | Includes bibliographical references and index.
Identifiers: LCCN 2019045746 | ISBN 9781975114459 (paperback)
Subjects: MESH: Health Personnel--education | Education, Professional--methods | Academic Success | Test Taking Skills | Professionalism | Vocational Guidance
Classification: LCC R690 | NLM W 18 | DDC 610.69--dc23
LC record available at https://lccn.loc.gov/2019045746

6048

Printed in the United States of America
24 23 22   10 9 8 7 6 5 4 3

Dedication

To our students

PREFACE

As teachers with a combined 50 years of classroom and laboratory experience with future healthcare professionals, we take the need for students to be academically and professionally prepared to succeed in their chosen careers seriously. The health professions students who fill our classes today are increasingly diverse and more often nontraditional students. Many are the first generation in their families to ever attend college. Many already have children of their own to support. Many have served in the armed services for extended periods of time. Many already have significant work experience behind them and are seeking career changes. Most of them work more than 25 hours a week while going to school full-time.

Their lives are complex, complicated, and filled with responsibilities, and yet, they are entering on a course of study that can at times be grueling. They will have lectures and labs to attend, clinical rotations or internships to complete, and long days and nights of studying. However, our experience over the years tells us that these students find their health professions educations just as rewarding as they are challenging.

Student Success for Healthcare Professionals Simplified helps students meet the demands and challenges of their studies by providing strategies for success in the classroom, the lab, the library, and the internship site as well as sound advice and guidance for maintaining their emotional and physical well-being. Along the way, the text provides hundreds of helpful tips and examples for everything from effective note-taking to healthier eating habits to reading and research skills to exercise and sleep routines.

In addition to a major reworking of the existing text, the third edition of *Student Success for Healthcare Professionals Simplified* includes four new chapters:

Chapter 8, "Medical Math for the Healthcare Professional"

Chapter 11, "Fundamental Writing Skills for the Healthcare Professional"

Chapter 14, "Succeeding in Your Future as a Healthcare Professional"

Chapter 15, "The Professionalism of the Healthcare Professional"

Student Success for Healthcare Professionals Simplified is organized into three main sections outlining the principles underlying student success, the skills and habits students develop to achieve success, and the strategies students use to step into productive careers as members of a healthcare team. The text is a rich source of wise counsel that students can return to again and again throughout their programs of study, long after the conclusion of the course in which they first encounter it.

CONTENTS

Part 2
SHARPENING YOUR SKILLS 81

Part 3
ENTERING A HEALTHCARE PROFESSION   233

PART 1

PRINCIPLES OF STUDENT SUCCESS

NOTES FOR PART 1

1

Focusing on Success

OBJECTIVES

- Understand your reasons for wanting to continue your education.
- Describe some obstacles that might limit your success as a student.
- Understand why a positive attitude matters for success.
- Stay motivated and focused on your studies.
- Know the importance of goals.
- Differentiate between short- and long-term goals.
- Set goals for yourself and make a plan of action to accomplish them.
- Describe the three traits of good academic character.

By opening the pages of this book, you have taken a big first step toward your goal of continuing your education. In fact, you have already shown that you are motivated to succeed as a student.

The decision to continue your education may not have been an easy one to make. Maybe you have not always had positive experiences with school. Or maybe you are worried about whether you will have the time, energy, or money to stick with it. These concerns are normal—they are also shared by many of your classmates. By using the strategies explained in this chapter, you can gain confidence and sharpen your focus on your studies.

In this chapter, you will take the first steps toward becoming a successful health-care student. You will think about why you are here—the dreams you have dreamt, the courage you have shown, the choices you have made, and the obstacles you have faced. You will learn about what motivates you and about how to keep a positive attitude and maintain focus. Most important, you will learn how to set and achieve your goals while following other tips that will help you succeed in school. Finally, you will also learn the importance of maintaining a good academic character.

Why You Are Here

You may have just graduated from high school, or perhaps, you are returning to school after several years to start a new career. Regardless of your age or experience, you need to think about your reasons for going to school. These reasons are the source of your motivation during those late night study sessions if you become tired and discouraged. Yes, even the best of students get tired and discouraged sometimes. And those are the times when it is most important to remember why you wanted to do this in the first place.

Taking a few minutes to be completely honest with yourself and really think about why you are here will give you a sense of purpose. A purpose that is personal

Other Members of Your Class

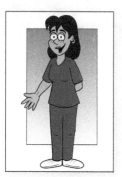

Amalia Torres
19 years old, Latina, female.
Amalia is the first member of her family to attend college. She aspires to a career in health care and has chosen a medical assisting program. She has no children, lives at home with her family, and doesn't have to work while going to school.

Michael Adams
31 years old, white, male.
Michael is an army veteran who was deployed twice to Afghanistan. He wants to pursue a career in health care as a radiology technician. Single, he lives with roommates and works evenings and weekends as an emergency medical technician (EMT).

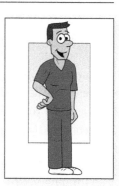

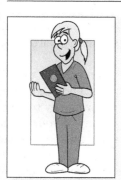

Jenna Pokaski
25 years old, white, female.
Jenna and her daughter, Maddie, live at home with Jenna's parents. While working weekends, she has enrolled in a physical therapist assistant program. She wants to set an excellent example for Maddie as well as provide her with a good future.

Devon Bradley
34 years old, black, male.
Devon has worked in facilities at Montgomery Hospital for the past 12 years. Married with two children, ages 5 and 7, Devon still works 30 hours a week while studying to become a surgical technologist.

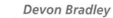

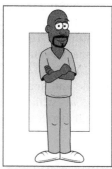

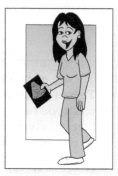

Thuy Nguyen
28 years old, Asian, female.
Thuy is returning to college after several years away to pursue a degree as an ultrasound technician. Single, she lives with three roommates and works evenings and weekends.

and important to you will help you set goals for yourself. With real and reachable goals, you will be more likely to succeed.

Student success means more than just passing your classes and earning your degree or program certificate. "Success," as we discuss the word throughout this text, also includes developing all the characteristics of a healthcare professional ready to practice in your chosen field.

What Motivates You?

What has led you to this point? Maybe you are interested in finding a career you truly enjoy. Or maybe, you would simply like to learn more about a subject that appeals to you. There are several reasons why people choose to continue their education.

- *You may want to improve your standard of living.* You may be the first in your family to attend college. The knowledge and skills you will learn in school will give you more career choices.
- *You may want to support your family.* You may come from a single-parent home or you may be a single parent yourself. The ability to provide for your loved ones is an important goal to pursue.
- *You may want to gain more self-confidence.* You may wish to continue your education to feel accomplished. Careers in health care provide both dignity and respect and are fulfilling work.

Whatever your dreams may be, they have brought you this far. Hold onto them and help yourself reach them by creating a plan for success.

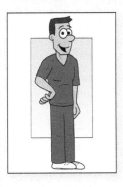

Michael's Motivation

At 31, Michael Adams feels that he wants to develop a solid career. He worked as a medic while in Afghanistan, and he now intends to take his education further. He believes that working as a radiology tech will allow him to work in health care with many different types of patients and move away from exclusively treating trauma.

Courage

It takes courage to pursue your dreams. You have already shown courage just by being here. Stepping into the unknown is never easy, but you have taken the first step. Right now, school may seem full of unknowns. If so, you should know that you are not alone—many students feel this way at first.

This text will answer questions you may have about school. You also will learn simple strategies to help you succeed as a student. Remember that it takes courage to do something you have never done before.

Choices

By choosing to continue your education, you are making your own path in life. You are showing real strength by making your own life choices and working hard for what you want. Just as you have made a decision to continue your education, you can choose to have a positive attitude and be a successful student as well.

Obstacles You May Face

You may find it easier to overcome obstacles when you are able to recognize them. You may already have overcome obstacles in getting this far.

ROLE PLAY Overcoming Obstacles	With a partner, take turns discussing the following questions. Ask each other follow-up questions and try to offer helpful suggestions.

- What has discouraged you in the past when you have considered continuing your education?
- How have people in your life helped or hurt your dream of going to school?
- What life experiences have influenced the way you see yourself?
- Do you foresee any obstacles in completing your education now?
- Do you feel confident you will be able to continue overcoming obstacles?
- Have you made a plan to overcome the obstacles you may face?

What are some of the conclusions you reached in your role play discussion? Recognizing the obstacles you have faced in the past can give you confidence to face future difficulties. Although it may not be fun to face challenges, you can benefit from your experiences.

This text will help you develop student success skills to overcome both personal and academic obstacles that may arise between now and graduation.

Ingredients for Success: Attitude and Motivation

Self-image affects your attitude and motivation. These two things are very important to your success as a student. If you feel good about yourself and have confidence, you will find it easier to develop a positive attitude and the motivation to learn.

Liking Yourself as a Student

Of all the factors that affect how well one does academically, attitude is probably the single most important. A positive attitude leads to motivation, and someone who is strongly motivated to succeed can overcome obstacles and succeed when others might give up or accept doing lower quality work. Your attitude toward education begins with your attitude toward yourself as a student. You may not have realized it yet, but you have become a new person. You are not just the same old person who happens now to be taking courses.

You may be feeling excited and enthusiastic, capable, and confident in your new life. However, if you are feeling any doubts, take comfort in knowing that you are not alone. A lot of new students worry that they are not good enough at school work or that they will not be able to keep up with all of the work assigned. Such worries can lead to fear of failure, which can lead to apathy.

An attitude that is less than positive, however, can hinder your motivation and ability to succeed. If you easily accept the possibility that you cannot succeed, that possibility can become a reality. This is called a "self-fulfilling prophecy," and psychologists have shown it happens often. For example, if you do not do well on a particular test, you might start thinking you are not very good with that class. Once you believe that, your studying will be less productive, your attitude will be less positive and enthusiastic, and you will set lower expectations for yourself. All these factors may lead to a lower score on the next test. If this happens, you will have made your own prophecy come true. However, if you tell yourself that you just weren't fully prepared for that first test but will do well on the next, your attitude and enthusiasm will contribute to more productive studying, and you will likely do quite well. If this happens, you will have made your positive prophecy come true.

If you sometimes have negative thoughts about being a student, think about why that is. You may be reacting to getting a low grade on some test. You may see other students who look as though they know what they are doing, and you worry that you do not know what you are doing. You can end up feeling out of place.

Some students also fall into a "victim mentality"—blaming their circumstances or other people if they are not successful. This is a kind of negative attitude that sets you up for failure. After all, if it is someone else's fault that things are difficult, then you can't expect to do well. Now that you are in school pursuing your education, you have the same opportunities as others and can succeed on your own abilities once you know how.

This text will help you learn the skills you need to succeed in your education—everything from how to study effectively, how to do better on tests, even how to read your textbooks more effectively.

Just remember that it all begins with a good attitude about yourself as a student. Remember your purpose—why you enrolled in your school or program to begin with—and stay enthusiastic.

The Attitude Adjustment

Your attitude often determine your performance in school. It is reflected in how much interest you take in your studies or how meaningful your work is to you. If you have a positive attitude about school, you will be better able to:

- figure out your responsibilities in the learning process
- set learning goals for yourself
- study for your classes in a more effective way
- improve your grades and performance as a student

What attitude do you currently have about learning? Find out by looking at some positive and negative examples of feelings about school. (See *Attitude Check* below.)

Motivation is related to attitude and is just as important. Motivation is what makes you want to accomplish a task. As a student, the right motivation can help you:

- get started on projects and assignments
- meet deadlines without last minute stress
- move closer to your goals
- keep working on tasks until you succeed

Attitude Check

Positive and Negative Attitudes toward Learning

When You Have a Positive Attitude, You Say:

- I'm good at studying. I focus well.
- I enjoy learning new things no matter what the subject may be.
- It is easy for me to learn new information.
- If the instructor doesn't tell me what to study, I'll develop my own studying strategy.
- I'm confident that I can learn and succeed.
- I have a support system of family, friends, and coworkers—and I rely on them often.
- I exercise my mind, as well as my body, on a regular basis.
- I consider myself an optimist.

When You Have a Negative Attitude, You Say:

- It is hard for me to study. I get distracted easily.
- I enjoy learning only about subjects that interest me.
- It is hard for me to process new information.
- If the instructor doesn't tell me what to study, I'm often lost.
- I'm doubtful about my ability to learn and succeed.
- I do not like to ask people for help, and I do not have a good support system.
- I'd rather watch TV than read a book, and I do not even have time to exercise.
- I consider myself a pessimist.

If you have more negative traits than positive, do not be discouraged. Recognizing a negative attitude is the first step toward changing it.

Making an Attitude Adjustment

There are many strategies you can use to develop a positive attitude. Here are just a few that have proven to work:

- *Talk positively to yourself.* We all have conversations with ourselves. You might not have been successful on a test and start saying to yourself, "I'm just not smart enough," or "That teacher is so hard—no one could pass that test." When we talk to ourselves this way, we can start believing what we're hearing, leading to the development of a negative attitude. Try instead to have upbeat conversations with yourself. Say, "I've been paying attention in class and doing my homework, and I just know I'm going to do well on that test!"
- *Spend time with positive people.* If the people you are hanging out with tend to complain a lot and blame others for their problems, you might want to make some changes. Try spending some time with other students who are happy with themselves as students. A positive attitude is contagious. You will also have more fun with people who are upbeat and enjoying life.

- *Overcome resistance to change.* You are no doubt very busy in your new life, and probably, many things have changed for you. Sometimes, we are slow to accept change and our attitude can become negative if we are always looking back. Consider instead your positive changes: the exciting and interesting people you are meeting, the valuable education you are getting that will lead to a bright future, and the challenges and stimulation you are feeling every day. Your first step in overcoming resistance to change will be to see yourself succeeding in your new life. Visualize yourself as a student taking control, enjoying classes, studying effectively, and earning good grades.

- *Overcome your fears.* One of the most common fears students have is a fear of failure. We all know we won't succeed at everything we try. The question becomes, what do you do about that? If you worry about failing, turn that worry around and use it in a positive way. If you worry, you may not do well on an upcoming exam; do not mope around and procrastinate. Instead, sit down and schedule your studying well ahead of time. Think of all the times you have succeeded. Tell yourself you will do it again now. With that attitude adjustment, you will more easily find you can.

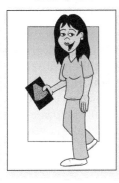

Thuy—A Strong Support System

The first time Thuy attended college, the experience was a bit overwhelming, and she had no real direction in terms of career goals. Now that she's a bit older, she has overcome her fear of committing to a career path. The college's department of admissions and then her academic advisor helped her to realize her potential to be successful in her chosen field of ultrasound technology.

Have a Strong Support System

As a student beginning a new education, you should surround yourself with people who support you and your goals. A strong support system helps you maintain a positive attitude, and a positive attitude will help you succeed in school.

Seek out support from people and resources such as:

- friends and family
- coworkers
- other students
- campus discussion groups
- instructors and tutors
- academic advisors
- student support services
- campus resources (libraries, computer labs, writing centers, etc.)

Be sure to discuss with your family and friends how your life is changing while you are in school. If you have young children, be sure to talk to them about these changes as well. Let your family and friends know that the new demands on your time aren't permanent and that you may need their help while you are in school.

Make these discussions positive and upbeat so that your family and friends feel good about how they are supporting your success as a student.

Uncertainty, Fear, Discouragement—Stop the Cycle

If you feel uncertain or fearful about school, you won't perform as well and then you will feel even more discouraged. This becomes a self-reinforcing cycle that can spiral further downward. By developing a positive attitude about learning, however, you can replace this with a cycle of self-confidence, strong performance, and success. Try the following:

- *Take responsibility for your education.* Do not simply rely on others to teach you. If a class becomes difficult, ask for help. Your instructor, a tutor, or a classmate may be able to explain difficult concepts.
- *Be an active learner.* Ask questions about things that interest you. Look for ways to expand your education beyond time spent in the classroom.
- *Decide what you want to learn from each course.* Evaluate what courses you enjoy most and, if you identify an area of difficulty, ask yourself why you find certain courses more difficulty than others. You may want to think about whether a particular degree or certificate program is right for you. (In Chapter 12, you will learn how to match your interests and abilities with the right healthcare career.)

Stress can be another cause of discouragement. When it seems like you have too much work to do and not enough time, stress can be overwhelming. Everyone experiences stress at one point or another. The good news is that there are many ways of handling stress. Choose a method that works best for you. How well you manage stress will determine how much it affects your performance as a student. When stress is managed well overall, small amounts of stress actually help you stay focused and complete tasks. Do not let stress control you. Instead, take control of stress. (Chapter 3 provides valuable tips for managing stress.)

Staying Motivated

To avoid discouragement, stay motivated. Use whatever motivates you to maintain focus on succeeding in school. Your motivation may come from within yourself (intrinsic) or from outside benefits (extrinsic). Although intrinsic motivation generally can be more powerful and longer lasting (because you really want to accomplish the task), extrinsic motivation is also a powerful force. Take the *Motivation Quiz* below to find out what motivates you to learn.

Motivation Quiz

1. I spend time studying for my courses because . . .
   a. I truly enjoy learning new information.
   b. I want to improve my grades and test scores.
2. I've chosen to go to school because . . .
   a. I want to excel at something.
   b. it will help me get a better job and a higher salary.

3. Going to school demonstrates to others that . . .
   a. I'm willing to take risks.
   b. I have an impressive résumé.
4. Learning new things . . .
   a. satisfies my curiosity.
   b. shows others I'm smart.
5. I'm continuing my education because . . .
   a. I'm very interested in the subjects I'm studying.
   b. I'm looking forward to future promotions in my career.

If you answered mostly a's, then you are intrinsically motivated. If you answered mostly b's, then you are extrinsically motivated. If you answered a combination of a's and b's, then you are motivated in many different ways.

ROLE PLAY **Intrinsic Versus Extrinsic Motivation**	With a partner, complete each of the statements 1 to 5 above with your own answers. Compare your responses. Try to determine whether your answer to each question indicates intrinsic or extrinsic motivation.

Understanding What Motivates You

To understand what motivates you to perform well in school, think about the tasks you accomplish outside school. Where does your motivation come from? For example, if you volunteer at a homeless shelter once a month, what motivates you? Do you help out because you feel good about yourself when you volunteer at the shelter? Do you like to talk with the people you meet there? Do you enjoy helping others?

Understanding what motivates you outside of school will help you determine what motivates you to do your school work. If you are intrinsically motivated, it may be enough to know that you accomplished a task—and that you are moving steadily toward your long-term goal. If you are extrinsically motivated, you may want to promise yourself a more concrete reward. The reward can range from having a nice snack after studying to enjoying a movie on the weekend. For a significant achievement—such as successfully completing the academic term—the reward can be larger, such as buying yourself a new laptop.

How to Stay Motivated

Suppose you have a lot of reading to do for a test tomorrow, and you have a paper due the next day. Maybe you are a little bored with one of your reading assignments. Maybe you would rather watch television or play a computer game. One of the interesting things about attitude is that it can change at almost any moment.

One of the characteristics of successful people is that they understand that interruptions will happen and plan ahead. Staying focused does not mean you become a boring person who does nothing but go to class and study all the time. You just need to plan ahead.

Planning ahead is the single best way to maintain focus and motivation. For example, do not wait until the night before an exam to start studying. If you know you have a major exam in 5 days, start by reviewing the material and deciding how many hours of study you will need. Then, schedule those hours spread over the next few days at times when you are most alert and least likely to be distracted. You should also allow for time to see friends, see a movie, or just relax, rewarding yourself for your successful studying.

When the exam comes, you will be relaxed. You will be in a good mood and feel confident. You will know the material, and you will do well. You stayed focused and planned well, and you even had some fun along the way. You have maintained a cycle of positive attitude and successful performance.

Planning is mostly a matter of managing your time well. The next chapter will look at specific ways to do that. Here are some other strategies for staying focused and motivated:

- *Remember why you are here.* If you are not feeling motivated, remind yourself why you are taking these classes. Remember the exciting career you are preparing for.
- *Walk the walk, and talk the talk.* Say it aloud—to yourself or a friend—with a positive attitude: "I'm going to study now for another hour before I take a break—and I'm getting an A on that test tomorrow!" It is amazing how saying something aloud helps you feel committed.
- *Remember your successes, even small successes.* As you begin a project or start studying for a test, think about your past success on a different project or test. Remember how good it feels to succeed.
- *Focus on the here and now.* For some people, looking ahead to goals, or to anything else, may lead to daydreaming that keeps them from focusing on what they need to do right now. Do not be too concerned about what you are doing tomorrow or next week or month.
- *Keep your world small.* If you just can't focus in on what you know you should be doing because the task seems too big and daunting (like sitting down to study for a final exam), break the task into smaller, manageable pieces. Do not start out thinking, "I need to study for the next 4 hours" (a plan that might feel depressing to many students), but think instead, "I'll spend the next 30 minutes going through my class notes from the last 3 weeks and figure out what topics I need to spend more time on." It is a lot easier to stay focused when you are sitting down for 30 minutes at a time.
- *Never try to multitask while studying.* You may think that you can monitor email and send text messages while studying, but in reality, these other activities lower the quality of your studying and lower your motivation.
- *Imitate successful people.* Does a friend always seem better able to stick with studying or work until he or she gets it done? What is he or she doing that you are not? *Visualize yourself* studying in the same way and getting that same high grade on the test or paper.
- *Reward yourself.* Give yourself a reward when you complete a significant task—but only when you are done. Some people stay focused better when there's a reward waiting.
- *Get the important things done first.* When you are not feeling motivated, it is easy to decide you need to do your laundry instead of studying. Although cleanliness is important, this is a form of procrastinating and trying to fool yourself into feeling you are accomplishing something by doing laundry. Stay focused!

Tips for Staying Motivated

- Keep your eye on your long-term goals to stay motivated with immediate tasks.
- Keep your priorities straight—but also save some time for fun.
- Keep the company of positive people; imitate successful people.
- Do not let past negative or less effective habits drag you down.
- Plan well ahead to avoid last minute pressures.
- Focus on your successes.
- Break large projects down into smaller tasks or stages.
- Reward yourself for completing significant tasks.
- Avoid multitasking.
- Network with other students; form a study group.

Bonus Benefits

While you motivate yourself to do well in school, you will be accomplishing other things along the way. These long-term rewards may include:

- the ability to apply your study skills to other areas of your life
- a greater understanding of the course material
- confidence and an improved self-image
- better grades and test scores
- stronger performance in classes in the future
- better options in terms of salary and career

The Balancing Act

You need to focus on your studies to do well in school. Worrying about money, your job, or other distractions can hurt your progress as a student. You should work to balance all aspects of your life.

If you need to balance going to school with working full- or part-time, have patience with yourself. You can take courses at a pace that fits your work schedule. You can learn time management strategies to create a manageable daily schedule that helps you maintain a good attitude and stay motivated. (You will learn about time management in Chapter 2.)

You also need to take care of yourself. You need to get enough rest, eat healthy food, and exercise regularly. The better care you take of yourself, the better you will be able to focus on reaching your goals.

Setting Goals That Are SMART

Goals help you avoid distractions. Goals keep you from procrastinating, losing your concentration, and losing your motivation in school.

Goals come in many shapes and sizes. They can be small or large, easy or hard, or short-term or long-term. Reaching your smaller goals will motivate you to keep reaching for your larger ones. Even completing a small task can give you a feeling of accomplishment. Overall, the more desirable a goal is, the more you will want to reach it.

Whatever kinds of goals you want to achieve, they should always be SMART goals. SMART is an acronym that means your goal is:

Specific. Your goal should be clear and specific. You should be able to say in one sentence what your goal is. "I want to earn a B+ on my Anatomy & Physiology (A & P) lab practical" is a specific goal.

Measurable. You should be able to measure—accurately and specifically—the success of your goal. For instance, a goal such as "I want to complete the 15 practice problems correctly before class on Friday" is easier to measure than "I want to be a good student this week."

Achievable. Your goal should be realistic. The goal of working hard every day over 4 weeks to write a passing 15-page research paper for sociology is more achievable—and realistic—than trying to write that same paper in a single all-nighter.

Relevant. Your goal should matter to you. The current goal of earning a passing grade in your A & P course is directly relevant to your larger goal of becoming a healthcare professional.

Time-sensitive. You should have a specific deadline by which you intend to accomplish your goal. The goal of raising your grade point average from 3.1 to 3.4—and making the Dean's List—by the end of the semester that has just started is a time-sensitive goal.

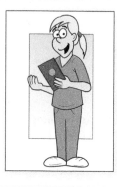

Jenna's Goals

Jenna's aunt Sarah is a physical therapist with her own local practice. Sarah is helping Jenna achieve her goal of becoming a physical therapist assistant. To do this, Jenna has had to learn that the goals she sets must be specific, measurable, achievable, relevant, and time-sensitive. As a future healthcare professional, what would your SMART goals be to succeed in your program?

Practice Setting Goals

Setting goals for yourself can take a little practice. Some people are natural planners and cannot help looking far ahead and setting goals. If you are like that, you may already feel comfortable setting goals and writing them down. But for those who like to dive right in and start "doing," goal-writing may at first feel frustrating and dull. But goal setting doesn't have to be complicated. Starting small will help you see how easy it is to write goals.

Begin by choosing goals that are simple and practical. By setting goals that are easily accomplished, you will pave the way for tackling larger goals in your future.

- An example of a good goal for right now might be to become familiar with your college's resources for helping students study. This goal is both simple and practical.
- An example of a bad goal would be promising to read your entire textbook before the first day of class. This is an unrealistic goal.

You should give yourself time by starting with smaller, more manageable goals. Once you have accomplished those, your goals can become more complex.

Long-Term Goals, Short-Term Goals, and Everything in Between

Goals can be divided into four main categories:

- Long-term (5 to 10 years away)
- Intermediate (3 to 5 years away)
- Short-term (6 months to 2 years away)
- Immediate (1 day, 1 week, or 1 month away)

Long-Term Goals

Long-term goals are often educational or career goals. These are things you hope to accomplish in the next 5 to 10 years. Such goals may include completing a new degree, reaching a specific job or career level, or even purchasing a first home.

Intermediate Goals

Intermediate goals are the next step after long-term goals. These goals are things you would like to accomplish in the next 3 to 5 years. If one of your long-term goals is to become a practicing medical assistant, your intermediate goals may include completing your education.

Short-Term Goals

Short-term goals will help you reach your intermediate goals. Short-term goals are usually 6 months to 2 years in the future. If your intermediate goals include obtaining a degree or certificate, it may be helpful to have several short-term goals each semester or term, such as to excel in certain courses of particular importance to your program.

Immediate Goals

Immediate goals are goals you want to accomplish today, this week, or this month. These goals are small tasks that can usually be completed quite quickly. Your immediate goals should help you reach a short-term goal. For example, suppose one of your short-term goals is to complete a lengthy research paper by the end of the semester. You can start by dividing the work into several smaller tasks that can be completed in a few hours or less. These tasks could include choosing a topic, doing the research, making an outline, and writing a paragraph or two at a time. By completing these smaller tasks (your immediate goals), you will accomplish your short-term goal.

Goal Writing Exercise

Writing down your goals will help you stay committed and focused on reaching them. Below is a form for writing out your goals. Keep in mind that writing down your goals doesn't make them permanent. You will be able to evaluate your progress and change your goals if necessary.

In addition, your long-term, intermediate, short-term, and immediate goals should all be linked together. For example, reading 20 pages of course

Continued

material today (your immediate goal) leads to getting a good grade in the course (short-term goal), which contributes to earning your degree or certificate (intermediate goal), which in turn leads to the opportunity to become a practicing healthcare professional (long-term goal).

Long-Term Goal (to be accomplished in the next 5 to 10 years):

_____

_____

_____

_____

Intermediate Goals (to be accomplished in the next 3 to 5 years):

1. _____

2. _____

Short-Term Goals (to be accomplished in the next 6 months to 2 years):

1. _____

2. _____

3. _____

Immediate Goals (to be accomplished today, this week, or this month):

1. _____

2. _____

3. _____

Double-check to make sure that each of your goals is SMART:

- **S**pecific
- **M**easurable
- **A**chievable
- **R**elevant
- **T**ime-sensitive

ROLE PLAY

Reaching Your (SMART) Short-Term Goals

With a partner, write down two of your short-term goals related to your education or professional life. Remember, short-term goals are goals you would like to accomplish over the next 6 months to 2 years. Explain the ways in which each of the goals is SMART. The numbered steps below can help you with this role play.

1. Write down your goal.
2. Set a reasonable deadline for your goal.
3. Think about possible obstacles to achieving your goal and how to avoid them.
4. Write down a step-by-step process to help you reach your goal— a plan of action.
5. Set reasonable deadlines for completing each step in the process.

If at First You Do Not Succeed, Revise and Try Again

Throughout the learning process, you may need to adjust your goals. Do not be afraid to make changes. Your goals are meant to serve *you*, not the other way around. They are not set in stone.

You may discover better ways of working toward your long-term goals. You may have to find creative ways of working around obstacles. You should be prepared to change short-term goals to help you achieve success.

Along the way, you may decide to work toward an entirely different long-term goal. You may even be attending school without a clear long-term goal in mind. Once you decide to pursue a particular career path, you may reevaluate and possibly change your previous goals. Do not be afraid to go back to the drawing board and change direction. Being excited about a long-term goal can be a great motivator.

Remember to Reward Yourself

Rewards will keep you motivated as you work toward your goals. Rewards can be large or small, as long as they are appropriate for the tasks completed. For example, if you do well on an exam for which you have been studying for the past 2 weeks, it may be appropriate to reward yourself with a nice dinner out with friends. A larger task deserves a large reward. However, it probably would not be appropriate to reward yourself with dinner out every time you complete a 20-minute assignment. Maybe taking 5 minutes to listen to a favorite song would be more appropriate. In other words, smaller tasks deserve rewards as well, provided that the rewards are smaller.

Peer Pressure and Penalties

Another way to stay motivated is to tell a friend about your goals. Having another person to hold you accountable will put more pressure on you to keep working hard. In this respect, peer pressure can be healthy. Just be sure to tell someone who supports your goals. Encouragement from others can be an excellent motivator.

An unproductive form of motivation is punishing yourself for not completing tasks. Punishment often has the opposite effect of motivation. It can discourage you and affect your attitude in a negative way. If you miss a goal by failing to complete a task, try adjusting your time line instead. (See *If at First You Do Not Succeed, Revise and Try Again.*) It is better to accomplish a goal a bit behind schedule than to become discouraged and give up on the goal altogether.

Will This Be on the Test?

Grades help students measure their progress toward meeting their goals. However, you should not put too much emphasis on grades. Although that is easier said than done, in the long run, learning should be the true goal. Focusing on learning will help you grasp new information and then correctly apply it to situations in the future. After all, you won't be a very effective healthcare professional if you do not learn the material in your courses!

Although grades should not be the primary focus of your learning experience, they can, of course, be great motivators. Achieving the grade you wanted on a big test for which you studied hard can help motivate you to study just as hard for the next one. Grades can also help you gauge your progress. You will feel great when you see yourself doing better and better. On the other hand, if you are not getting the grades you want, you will know you have to make some adjustments in your approach to your coursework.

To achieve your long-term goals, you may occasionally have to complete some school work that you do not enjoy very much or that doesn't seem relevant. Stay positive, even when you do not feel like completing these assignments. Although some tasks may seem dreary at times, you will always have the motivation if your main goal is to learn. Remember, if learning itself is a goal, you can more easily stay motivated to succeed.

Academic Character

This chapter's final topic is something you should be thinking about from your first day at school. You should be thinking about what kind of person you are as a student. You should think about what kind of character you will have in your future career.

The character you have as a student is the character you will have as a health-care professional. You are facing the challenges of your new career today—learning new information, dealing with associates (the classmates of today are the coworkers of tomorrow), and taking responsibility for your work and your decisions.

Working in health care is different from working in most other careers. You are entrusted with patients' personal information on a daily basis. One day, you might listen to very private concerns, examine people's bodies, or handle their financial information. You must take these responsibilities seriously. People share information in a healthcare setting that they would never share anywhere else. You may learn things about patients that their own families do not know about them. The trust your patients put in you is critically important, even sacred.

In school, you should develop the characteristics you will need to become a trusted healthcare professional. You should:

- *Be honest.* Be someone your instructors, patients, and colleagues can trust.
- *Avoid gossip.* Do not talk about other students, patients, or professional colleagues.
- *Be accountable.* Be accountable for what you do at school and work all day, every day.
- *Be responsible.* Be someone who never tries to get out of doing work.

Being Honest

You should be familiar with the term "academic honesty." This means that you are always doing your own work: no plagiarism from books or articles, no copying a classmate's work, and no cheating on tests or assignments.

Honesty and ethical behavior have critical importance in health care. How would you feel if your doctor or nurse had passed a final by cheating? Or plagiarized a final paper? Or had a lab partner who did all the work for him or her? You would think that doctor or nurse was not qualified to answer your health questions or treat you. You would be right. Doing your own work is never more important than when you are learning to care for someone's health. You *must* know the material—you won't be able to fake it in a professional setting.

Make a concrete commitment to honesty.

- Do your own work.
- Avoid plagiarizing. Make sure you understand ideas well enough to put them in your own words.
- Own up to work you have not done. If you are not prepared for a class or lab, admit it. Promise to make it up and that you will not let it happen again—and then do not let it happen again.

Even though you are honest, you may find that some of your classmates are not. Take a stand here, too.

- Expect the members of your study group to do their own work.
- Do not let anyone copy your work. Sharing notes is not the same as letting someone copy an assignment you completed. Notes are raw material, not finished work that uses ideas and analysis.
- Do not let classmates force you to cover for them if they have not done their work. You do not have to be confrontational, just firm.

Whenever you are in doubt about whether something you are doing is honest, think about it this way: Would you want your doctor or nurse to do what you are thinking of doing? If the answer is no, do not do it.

Avoiding Gossip

One of the biggest mistakes people working in a healthcare facility can make is gossiping about patient information. For example, suppose a coworker asks you a casual question about a patient. Even though it may seem like a harmless question, keep your lips sealed. Not only does sharing patient information violate the patient's privacy and the healthcare facility's policies, but such gossiping can also get you fired. (All healthcare professionals must follow the privacy regulations of the Health Insurance Portability and Accountability Act [HIPAA], about which you will learn more later.) You never know who is listening or where else that information might travel. Only share confidential information when it is required for providing care of the patient.

Even as a student, get in the habit of avoiding gossiping with other students. Although it may seem harmless to chat about other students, gossiping can be habit forming, and talking about others now will make it more difficult to avoid later in a professional environment. In addition to violating the privacy of others, gossip distracts people from focusing on the work at hand and can lead to conflict among healthcare staff.

Note that gossip and idle conversation about others extend also to your online presence in email and on websites like Facebook. Some students forget that even if they attempt to keep their personal information and images private online, this information can be shared or become public in other ways.

Being Accountable

Being accountable means you are able to explain your actions. You are held to certain standards. An employee, for instance, is accountable to a supervisor. As a student, you are accountable to:

- your instructor
- your classmates
- yourself

You have to be able to explain to your instructor the quality of your work, your attendance, and your attitude. This means, for example, owning up to whether you studied and explaining why you turned in an assignment late.

If you are working on a group project, you need to be able to tell the other group members about the work you have done toward the group goal—or why you didn't complete that work. You also need to be able to help everyone learn by participating in group discussions.

You are accountable to yourself in that you are working toward your own goals. If you are letting yourself down, you have to be able to admit it and then ask yourself why. You need to be honest in assessing your personal performance and behavior.

As a healthcare professional, you will be accountable to:

- your patients
- your supervisor
- your workplace

Helping patients is the reason why everyone at a clinic, doctor's office, or hospital is there. You are accountable to your patients.

When it comes to your supervisor, you will have to answer questions about the work you have done. For example, as medical assistant, you might have to answer questions such as:

- Did you file all the paperwork?
- Did you check every vital sign?
- Did you label all specimens?
- Did you write down symptoms correctly and pass them on to the nurse or doctor?

Most important, did you do all this correctly and on time?

Finally, you are accountable to your workplace—the healthcare facility where you work. Always work and act as though you might be called on to explain your actions.

The way to make accountability easy is to toe the line. Do what you are supposed to do when you are supposed to do it. Be focused on your work when you are at work. If you form that habit now while in school, all the tips you learn about prioritizing and scheduling will come to your rescue after you graduate.

Being Responsible

Personal responsibility is key in school, work, and life. At school, you need to be responsible for managing your time, completing your work, and doing your best. As a healthcare professional, you will be responsible for all those things and more—you will be responsible for caring for patients, too.

Here are some things to keep in mind about your responsibilities at school and later in your career:

- *You are responsible for your job.* You will have to answer when your job is not completed appropriately.
- *You are responsible for your time.* Manage your time well. Be able to account for it.
- *You are responsible for your property.* Make sure you have the materials and supplies you need to do your job. Make sure everything is where you need it, and clean up equipment and restock supplies after completing procedures.
- *You are responsible for security and privacy.* File sensitive patient information immediately and only share it with your supervisor.
- *You are responsible for being educated and informed.* Keep brushing up on your job skills. Read professional journals, talk with colleagues, and ask questions. Ask to sit in on specific procedures if you need improvement. Review your old textbooks and make sure you know what you are doing. Participate in continuing education activities such as professional presentations.
- *You are responsible for your actions.* Avoid the urge to blame someone else in a situation where your actions are being examined. Take responsibility for your

mistakes. It is much better than trying to lie or shift the blame. Your instructors, colleagues, and supervisors will respect you for being honest.

You are developing and enhancing these characteristics now while you are in school. Honesty, accountability, and responsibility are also the traits of a good student.

Chapter Summary

- One of the first steps toward student success is thinking about why you are interested in continuing your education.
- Learning to recognize and overcome obstacles will help you become a better student.
- A positive attitude and staying motivated are critical for achieving academic success. Work to develop a positive cycle of self-confidence and successful performance.
- Goals keep you from procrastinating, losing your concentration, or losing your motivation in school. Set goals for yourself so you can stay focused and organized.
- Short-term goals are usually set 6 months to 2 years in the future. These goals should help you reach your long-term goals or career goals. Your long-term goals represent the things you would like to accomplish in the next 5 to 10 years.
- When setting goals for yourself, make sure each goal is SMART.
- Develop a good academic character as a student that will serve you well also in your future career. Be honest, accountable, and responsible.

Review Questions

Objective Questions

1. The "S" in SMART stands for "Super." (True or False?)
2. Two types of motivation discussed in this chapter are _____ and _____.
3. Long-term goals have a time range of _____ years.
4. Revealing patient's name and medical history to your friends and family is a good way to demonstrate your good professional character. (True or False?)
5. "Being available to go out" on a Friday night is one of the primary traits of a good academic character. (True or False?)

Short-Answer Questions

1. List three reasons why people choose to continue their education.
2. Write three to five sentences about how people in your life have helped or hurt your goal of continuing your education.
3. List three groups of people or resources you could look to for support in your effort to be a successful student.
4. Explain the importance of a positive attitude for success in school.
5. List two strategies you can use to stay motivated.
6. What five characteristics should each of your SMART goals have?
7. List three examples of problems that can occur in health care if professionals were not honest, accountable, and responsible on the job.

Applications

1. Write out one short-term and one long-term goal you have. Then, on a separate piece of paper for each, list explicitly the ways in which each of these goals is SMART.
2. Ask a friend or family member who has already graduated from college what they remember as the most discouraging experience they had as a student. Talk about how they might have prevented that negative experience with a more positive attitude, more motivated studying, and the use of motivational strategies discussed in this chapter.

Fundamental Writing Skills

Chapter 11 of this text provides a thorough review of grammar, a basic overview of effective paragraph construction, a brief guide to APA formatting, and a brief explanation of electronic health records (EHR). You can work through the chapter over the course of the semester one section at a time, completing one of the nine sections along with each of the first nine chapters of the text. This step-by-step method will make completing the grammar section easier and less burdensome. At the conclusion of each exercise, you can check your comprehension in the accompanying online answer key.

You will find at the end of each of the first nine chapters a section number for one part of Chapter 11. The section number indicates the section and exercises you are to complete along with the chapter you have just read.

Section 11-1 in the writing skills chapter is the section you should complete at the end of Chapter 1. You can find this section on pages 197.

2

Getting Organized and Managing Your Time as a Healthcare Professional

OBJECTIVES

- Explain the importance of attending all classes.
- Explain the importance of using the class materials you receive.
- Explain the importance of your course syllabi.
- Describe strategies for using campus resources that can help you succeed.
- Describe effective time management strategies.
- Explain how to use a calendar, weekly planner, and a to-do list.
- Describe the symptoms of procrastination and explain how to keep on track.

Attending all your classes is necessary to succeed in school, but it is not sufficient to succeed. You must also be organized if you want to be successful. For example, the course documents you receive from professors—syllabi, course outlines, clinical plans—will let you know ahead of time what each course will cover and exactly which assignments or activities your professors consider most important. In this chapter, you'll learn how to use these course documents and campus resources to your advantage. You'll also learn how to organize your schedule and use your time efficiently. All of these skills will help you stay focused on what really matters for success.

Organizing for Classes

Attending all of your classes all of the time is essential if you want to succeed. But you must also ensure that all of your course materials are organized and that you are in control of your schedule.

Being There

Someone once said that 80% of success in life is just showing up. To some extent, this is true—true in that if you do not show up, you will have a 100% chance of failure. From the beginning to the end of the term, you'll want to attend every class. You have enrolled in your courses for a reason. Missing a class here and there will make it harder to achieve your goals. Attending every class should be a top priority.

Attendance from the first day is essential for several reasons. By attending, you will:

- get to know your instructors and other students
- take notes if your instructors lecture on the first day of class
- find out about helpful campus resources
- receive important handouts so you'll know what to expect during the semester

Although some students think that nothing important happens on the first class and may be tempted to skip, that's a dangerous way to start the term. It's true that some instructors use that first day to introduce students to the course and then let class out a few minutes early. But many instructors use the entire class time and start their lectures right away. They'll expect students to start taking notes on the first day. Missing the first class can put you behind before you even start.

Some students are also tempted to skip classes at the end of a term to spend extra time studying for final exams. But going to class should be your priority. Instructors often provide their own review of the course and tell you which items or ideas will be covered on the final exam. If you schedule your study time well and stick with your daily and weekly schedules, you'll have plenty of time to study *and* go to class.

Why Attendance Always Matters

Class time is important because it gives you a chance to see the material you're studying through the eyes of an expert—your professor. The professor goes over key points, provides analysis, and brings ideas to life in real-world applications. In class, you learn what is most important for succeeding in the course and for entering your new career.

Attending class means arriving on time—or even a few minutes early—and staying until your professor has concluded the class and dismissed everyone. The first 5 minutes of class are just as important as the middle of the lecture. During this time, your instructor might make important announcements. The last 5 minutes of class are equally critical because your instructor might take this time to summarize important information or answer questions about an assignment. If you have an instructor who is occasionally late, don't use this as an excuse to skip the first few minutes of class. Instead, make use of the extra time by bringing other assignments or notes to review until your instructor arrives.

Really think twice before you miss a class. Each time you miss class, you fall behind. Even if you keep up with the reading and other assignments, skipping a lecture or class discussion will cause you to miss out on an important part of the learning process. In class, the information from your assigned reading will be analyzed and used as a building block for new information you won't get from the textbook.

Class time offers information you can't get anywhere else. During class time, you will learn about the instructor's own experiences and opinions on what you read in the textbook. The instructor may also share journal articles that discuss what you've read and develop the reading's ideas further. Even if the instructor simply sticks to the textbook, you never know exactly how the in-class discussions with other students will develop that information. You may come across a new idea during discussion that you never would have thought of on your own. Although some students think that if they miss class they can still gain everything they need from borrowing another student's notes, they will still miss the value of class discussion and interaction with the instructor. More real learning goes on during this time than can ever be captured in notes.

Another important reason why you should attend every class is that your professor will notice if you skip a class or two. Professors quickly memorize faces, even in large survey courses. They know when you're absent. Even if the professor doesn't pick up on your absence at first, he or she will eventually notice, especially if you show up at office hours with a lot of basic questions that were answered during class. Even if attendance doesn't count in your course grade—and it often does—missing classes will affect your grade because you don't know the material, and you will also make a poor impression on your professor. Your attendance and engagement show everyone how seriously you take your education and demonstrate whether you have a true desire to start a new career. If you take your classes seriously, your professors will take you seriously.

If You *Must* Miss a Class

If you know you will have to miss a class, remember the following:

- You should ask your instructor if he or she teaches another section of the course that you might attend instead. Ask about any handouts or announcements.
- You should ask another student whose judgment you trust if you can copy his or her notes. Also ask if you can spend a few minutes with him or her after you've read the notes to go over things that may be unclear to you.
- You may not need to see your professor after missing a lecture class. Besides, no professor wants to give you 50 minutes of office time to repeat the lecture for you. But if you are having difficulty after the next class because of material you missed, be sure to stop in and see your professor and ask what you can do to get caught up.
- You should understand that the worst thing you can say to an instructor is "I missed class—did you talk about anything important?" This tells the instructor you don't consider class time important and that you're not taking responsibility for your own learning.

Using Class Materials

Although attending every class is an excellent beginning, being organized will help you make effective use of course materials. From the first day, your professors will give you various handouts in class or post them on your school's learning management system (LMS). These documents are critical for charting your path to success throughout the term.

Why All the Documents?

There's a reason instructors provide you with so many documents—either in paper or electronically on the LMS—at the beginning of the semester. They've spent the weeks before the first class planning every class session for the entire semester. They create a plan of the material they're going to teach and the order in which they will teach it. They're thinking about what you'll need to learn to be successful.

Among the course documents your professors may distribute or post online are:

- a syllabus
- a course schedule or course outline
- a course materials list
- study guides or lecture outlines
- practice exercises
- assignment instructions

These course documents make the learning process easier for you. You should understand the information they contain and how they all fit into the course plan.

Using the College's Learning Management System

Like many other schools, yours may require all professors to make their course content available on the school's LMS. Professors spend a great deal of time developing these course pages to help students get the most from their studies. Be sure you understand exactly how to use the LMS and how to access all course information through the LMS. Virtually, every LMS—whether it's Canvas, Blackboard, Moodle, or Brightspace—offers online tutorials that include narrated videos with step-by-step instructions on how to access content and complete necessary tasks. Be sure that you take advantage of these tutorials and be sure to ask questions when you need help.

Course Documents—Prepare for Your Classes

For the most effective learning, you need to come to class prepared. You can find out exactly what's coming next by reading—and using—your course syllabus and course outline. In fact, a quick review of these course documents at the beginning of the term can sometimes help you decide whether to add or drop a particular course. Look over the books and articles you'll be required to read. Consider how much time you'll have to spend in the lab. See how many exams you'll be taking and how much time you'll be expected to spend on homework. You may find that you've registered for too many demanding classes during the same term. If that's the case, you may want to talk to your advisor about your course load. You may need to consider rescheduling one of your courses for another semester.

The Course Syllabus

The course syllabus includes key information about your class. The syllabus tells you almost everything you need to know about the course and what the instructor expects of you. A typical syllabus includes:

- the instructor's name and contact information
- the course name, catalog number, and credit hours
- when and where the class meets
- the course objectives (what you will learn)
- the grading policy—how much tests, papers, daily participation, group work, and/or attendance contribute to your final grade

- information about whether the instructor will accept late assignments
- important policy information about academic integrity and disabilities services

Most professors will read through the syllabus in class on the first day and explain key points. Be prepared to highlight or mark these key points. This is an essential part of your first day because you will learn about what each professor considers most important. Some professors emphasize tests and papers, whereas others place value on participation in class. As your professor reviews the syllabus, you'll get an idea of what you need to do to succeed in the course. Listen carefully to the professor, and be sure to ask questions about anything you don't understand. As with all handouts you receive, keep your syllabus in a safe place you can quickly access.

ROLE PLAY **Understanding the Syllabus**	With a partner, examine the syllabus for this course. Can you identify all of the bulleted information in the above section? Does this information help you understand all you need to know to be successful in this course? Are any of your questions left unanswered by the syllabus?

Staying Organized

All of the content you receive from professors is important. Look through it all carefully, organize it, and don't lose any of it. Set up a binder or folder for each of your classes. Place your syllabus at the front of the binder or folder because you'll need to refer to it often. Then continue to file all the papers the instructor hands out in class. You don't want to misplace any of your course documents or leave them behind in class.

Course Grades

Successful students come prepared and have a plan. They think through what they have to do to do well in their classes. They access the grade book in the LMS to see what their current grades are, or, if the course is not using an LMS, learn to calculate what it's going to take to get the grade they want. This calculation often involves points or percentages.

However, many students find grades a source of confusion and frustration. They get their graded tests and assignments back but aren't sure what the numbers really mean in terms of their overall grade. This is an instance when the course syllabus can help you understand how to figure out where you stand grade-wise at any time during the semester. However, figuring out your grade can take some work. For now, keep in mind that the syllabus has the information you need to figure your up-to-the-minute grade. In Chapter 8, we'll take a closer look at how to calculate grades.

Class Schedule

Usually, a course outline, or schedule, is included with the syllabus and contains information about:

- what topics will be covered each day in class
- assignment due dates
- test and quiz dates

If the instructor has already organized the class schedule in calendar form and distributes it in paper, keep the schedule in your binder for easy reference. If the class schedule is just a list of dates, get out your calendar (which you'll learn to make later in this chapter) and carefully log the important dates. You might try using different colors, such as red for tests and blue for homework.

Course Materials List

The course materials list includes everything you'll need to participate in each class. This might include the following:

- *Textbooks.* If your school bookstore offers rental, used, or e-book versions of textbooks for sale, these can save you a lot of money—just make sure you obtain the right edition. Unless you must buy your books through your college's bookstore for financial aid reasons, you may also find less expensive copies elsewhere—just be sure to order early enough that you have your books before class starts. Some textbooks come with online access codes that your instructor may require you to use; if this is the case, you will need to buy an e-book or a new book. If you purchase your books before the first day of class, you will have a better idea of the material that will be covered in each course. Some schools offer used textbooks for sale at reduced prices. Because these books usually are sold on a first-come, first-serve basis, it pays to purchase your books early.
- *Workbooks.* These may come bundled with your textbook, or you may have to buy the workbook separately.
- *Photocopied readings.* Sometimes, an instructor makes handouts that he or she gives out in class. Other times, you'll need to retrieve handouts from the college's LMS, the campus library, or the resource center. Be sure you have the course materials list with you so you get the correct handouts.
- *Uniforms, stethoscopes, etc.* The course materials list, or your instructor, will specify where to purchase these items. Ask if there are stores or websites that offer special student discounts.

Sometimes an item on the list is recommended rather than required. Ask your instructor how important it is that you buy recommended items.

Getting Organized on Campus

However, attending class and organizing your course materials aren't enough to ensure your success. Your success as a student also depends on your knowing about and using other resources on campus.

College Catalogs, Credits, and Confusion

The college catalog is one of the most important documents you'll use in school. It describes all of the courses offered in your program as well as the requirements

Using Campus Resources— Amalia

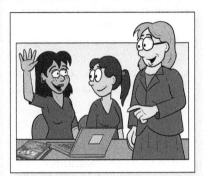

Amalia began taking classes a few months ago to become a medical assistant. Going to school and working as a server at a steakhouse near home kept her pretty busy. She thought about skipping the first day of class because she thought there wouldn't be much going on. She believed the professors usually just talk about unimportant stuff and let everyone out early on the first day. Besides, if she instead went to work that day, she would have an opportunity to earn overtime pay.

Amalia was conflicted about what to do, but ultimately decided to go to class, and she was so glad she did. The professor talked about many campus resources she hadn't even known existed. He gave the students usernames and passwords to access a free online tutoring system. Now, if Amalia needs to work at the steakhouse during a time when her study group is meeting, she can log on and talk to a tutor. This option never would have occurred to her if she hadn't gone to that first class. Being there on the first day has saved her a lot of time and trouble this semester.

for your degree or certificate program. It also helps you figure out when you will complete your education.

Your school may update the course catalog every year or every term. The most recent version will be available on your school's website. Know which version of the catalog applies to you and be sure to use it when planning your class schedule.

Tips for Scheduling Success

If you're attending a career or technical school, your course scheduling may be done for you. In other schools, though, you may be responsible for registering for courses and organizing your own schedule. The way you organize your class schedule can affect your success as a student. A well-organized schedule ensures that you will be able to devote enough time to each course. Here are a few tips for organizing a schedule that works for you.

- Schedule your classes evenly throughout the week. You can accomplish this by scheduling classes every day. Overloading your schedule to have class every other day can lead to unnecessary stress. Distributing your classes evenly throughout the week will keep you from becoming burnt out.
- Make allowances for difficult or challenging courses. You can do this by scheduling these courses when you are at your most focused. For example, schedule challenging classes in the mornings if you are a morning person or later if you're an afternoon person. Another way to get through difficult courses is to balance your

schedule for the term. Try to balance every difficult course with an easier one, if possible, so your schedule doesn't become overwhelming.

- Keep personal commitments in mind when scheduling classes. You may have to schedule your classes around work, family, and other obligations.
- Make informed decisions when choosing your professors. Certain courses may be offered by several different professors. When you have a choice, check with other students. If your school publishes student evaluations of professors, consult those. You want to have as much information as possible on each instructor's teaching style.

Get a Campus Map

The first step to becoming familiar with your campus is to locate a campus map. Maps may be found on the school's website or posted at different locations on campus. If your school has an information or student services office, the staff there can be helpful in answering questions about student parking and parking permits, if needed.

Each academic term, as you enroll in new courses in perhaps new locations, plan to arrive a few minutes early during the first week. Or, if possible, scout your classroom locations before the term starts so you know the route from the parking lot or bus stop and from class to class. New routines can be difficult to get used to. You can prevent unnecessary stress by giving yourself extra time to arrive at your classes.

Campus Resources

There are a lot of resources available on most campuses that you may not yet have heard about. Most schools provide a variety of free services to any student who seeks them out, although finding all of them can take some time. Bulletin boards crammed with flyers, advertising services, and events can all merge into a senseless blur.

Using your own initiative to find many free resources can be difficult and time-consuming but well worth the effort. Because so few students actually take the time to find all the resources available to them, an abundance of resources often waits for the person who does make the effort.

These resources and services can make a big difference in your student experience. Most are free for students or are already included in your tuition. Some of these services include the following:

- Tutoring
- Learning labs or tutorial centers
- Writing centers
- Computer labs
- Libraries
- Fitness centers
- Career placement services
- Counseling

Need help revising a paper? Visit the writing center. Need access to a computer to do research or work on a report? Visit the computer lab. The people working in these labs and resource centers are there to help. Take advantage of their advice and expertise.

Searching for Resources

If you're having trouble finding out about the resources offered by your school, you probably just need to know where to look. Here are some tips to get you started on your search.

- Visit your school's information or student services office and ask where you can find out about offerings such as free seminars, workshops, and learning labs.
- Ask your academic advisor to point you in the right direction. If you're struggling with a certain course, for example, your advisor may be able to suggest a possible tutor.
- Ask a librarian about resources available to students in the campus library. As a student, you may have access to specialized databases, videos, and professional journal articles.

ROLE PLAY

Campus Resources

With a partner, discuss campus resources you've used that you've found especially helpful. Are there any you are reluctant to use? Why? Explain why to your partner.

The Campus Library

Although you probably know where the library is located, you may need to learn how to use the unique services available there. Your campus library has a wealth of resources: online databases, videos, books, articles, and other supplemental materials. Find out if there's a free orientation tour on how to use the library so you know how to find everything you need. Knowing how to use the reference area of a library is invaluable, but you may need to ask for help to use it effectively. In Chapter 10, we will take a closer look at the all-important skill of information literacy.

Learning Labs

Libraries and learning labs are important campus resources. Most people know what a library is, but what's a learning lab? A learning lab is a place where students can go to meet with tutors or study groups, use campus computers, or use extra learning resources. These labs usually have very specialized learning materials in them. For example, there may be life-size plastic anatomical models to help you learn anatomy. Some will have computers to aid you in learning how to use certain software programs. Knowledgeable people who can help you make the most of these specialized resources usually staff campus locations.

Find out where your school's learning lab is located before you need it. Remember, your goal is to be prepared. This saves you the stress of hunting for these resources later when you may be pressed for time.

Campus Counseling Center

The campus counseling center is also a good place to investigate. These centers often sponsor free seminars on studying, how to stay healthy, and how to manage stress. These can be great places to pick up information to share with your network.

Human Resources

Don't think of resources only as offices and special rooms or buildings. The most valuable resources for heightening your learning are the people you see in your classrooms: your instructor and other students.

In later chapters, we'll talk about networking with students and forming study groups. Study groups can facilitate some of the most enjoyable—as well as most effective—ways to learn. You'll also be learning more about how to successfully interact with your professors. You should now start thinking of your instructors as your most valuable resources.

Help From Your Professor

In addition to being available by phone or email, almost all professors have regular office hours when they are available to meet with students one-on-one. You can go to your professor's office and talk over anything you need help with. Find out when the office hours are (they should be on the syllabus) and write them in your schedule.

Keep in mind that office hours are for everyone in the class, so your professor will have limited time to help you. If you feel as if you need more help, such as weekly extended one-on-one tutoring, consult your campus's learning lab or ask your professor to recommend a personal tutor.

There may be other options aside from meeting your professor in his or her office. Some professors may offer help by phone, email, or through virtual office hours via your college's LMS. Remember not to assume that you can call your instructor at any time or that you can call as often as you want. Your instructor's time should be respected and shared equally with other members of the class. Be sure to call only during the appointed times.

If you send an email, you may not get an answer immediately. Most instructors will tell you what their response time is for email. Ask your instructor about this if he or she doesn't include the information in the syllabus.

Disabilities Support Services

Students often have special physical, mental, and learning needs. These needs can include:

- physical disabilities
- mental disabilities
- learning disabilities

Schools across the United States are required to have resources to help meet these additional needs. For students with particular needs or disabilities, specially trained staff at the school can arrange for individual accommodations in the classroom. For example, students with hearing impairments may be able to apply for sign language interpreters to assist them. Students who have learning disabilities can work with their academic counselors to find extra teaching and learning aids.

If you believe you need special assistance in school, find the disabilities support services office to learn more about the resources available on your campus. If you aren't sure, set up a meeting with your advisor right away to find out where on campus the resources are.

Time Management—Organizing Your Time

A full-time student spends about 15 hours a week in the classroom and 2 hours of time preparing for each hour of class work. That's about 45 hours a week either spent in class or preparing for class. On top of these responsibilities, many students also devote time to their jobs, families, and other activities, along with time for exercise and socializing with friends.

This is one of the things virtually all students agree on—there's not enough time in the day for everything you want to do. But you can't "manufacture" time, nor can you "save" it for later. You only have so much time, so you have to learn to use it as well as possible. You need to be organized in your approach to time—this is called time management.

Time management is really a set of skills. These skills are worth learning because you can use them in your future career and throughout life. The better you manage your time, the less stress you'll feel, the more you'll get done, and the more time you'll feel that you have for doing things you enjoy.

Here are some of the characteristics of successful time management:

- Knowing how much time you should spend studying
- Knowing how to increase your studying time if needed
- Knowing the times of day you are at your best and most focused
- Using effective study strategies
- Scheduling study activities in realistic segments
- Using calendars to plan ahead and set priorities
- Staying motivated to follow your plan and avoiding procrastination

Where Does the Time Go?

We all have the same 24 hours a day, but some people just seem to have more time than others. How does that happen? Two different students might have identical amounts of homework in the same classes, work the same number of hours a week, and sleep and exercise in identical amounts, but one feels rushed and always behind in his studies, whereas the other feels calm and always has enough time to do a good job. What's the difference between them? Which type are you?

Chances are, these two students have different attitudes toward time. One may be more aware of time than the other—and therefore may be better able to manage it. Time management starts with being aware of where your time goes. Most people, in fact, cannot account for how they spend all their time.

Accounting for and learning to manage your time is so important for success as a student that it's worth spending some of your valuable time learning to better understand time. The following exercises and activities will give you a clearer idea where your own time goes. Step 1 is to see if you know how you actually spend your time day after day.

Step 2 in your time analysis is to actually track your time for a few days and see where you *really* spend your time. This may seem like a lot of work, but it only takes a minute or two a day. The self-knowledge most people gain from this activity is well worth the effort and can pay off through all your time in school.

Make copies of the *Daily Time Log* (page 37). Carry it with you and every so often fill in what you have been doing in 15-minute increments. Do this for several days and then add up the times for the different categories of activities in the

Making Time Work—Devon

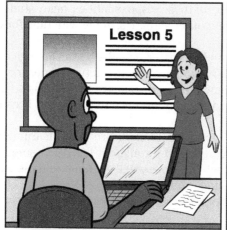

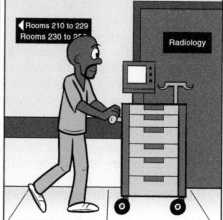

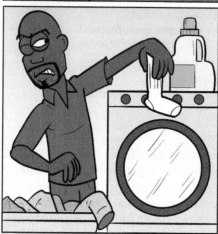

Devon Bradley is 34 years old and has two children, Daycia and Derek. Devon works almost full-time in facilities at Montgomery Hospital and goes to school Monday through Friday. His goal is to eventually become a surgical technologist. In a typical week, he spends 30 hours at the hospital; 45 hours doing school-related work; and many unaccounted for hours making dinner, helping with homework, and doing laundry. He doesn't have a lot of flexibility in his life or schedule. Managing time efficiently is the key to his success.

exercise on page 35. How does your actual time use compare with your earlier estimates? What have you learned about yourself?

Many students are surprised that they spend a lot more time than they thought just hanging out with friends—or spending time on Instagram, Facebook, Snapchat, Twitter, or any of the many other things people do. You can learn to use some of this time to your advantage. When you begin using a calendar or planner to schedule your study time the same way you plan ahead to attend class, you'll be on your way to efficient time management.

Time Management Strategies That Work

Because you don't have unlimited time, you want to efficiently use the time that you do have for your studies. This approach promotes academic success while

Where Does Your Time Go?

See if you can account for a week of your time. For each of the categories listed, make your best estimate of how many hours you spend. (For categories that are about the same every day, just estimate for 1 day and multiply by 7 for that line.)

Category of Activity	Number of Hours per Week
Sleeping	_____
Eating and preparing food	_____
Bathing, personal hygiene, etc.	_____
Working, volunteer service, internship	_____
Chores, cleaning, errands, shopping, etc.	_____
Attending class	_____
Studying, reading textbooks, researching (outside class)	_____
Transportation to work and/or school	_____
Organized activities: clubs, church services, etc.	_____
Casual time with friends (include TV, video games, etc.)	_____
Attending entertainments (movies, parties, etc.)	_____
Time alone with TV, video games, online activities, etc.	_____
Exercise, sports activities	_____
Reading for fun, other solitary interests	_____
Talking on phone, email, Facebook, etc.	_____
Other—specify: _____	_____
Other—specify: _____	_____

Now get out your calculator and total up all your estimated hours. Is your number larger or smaller than 168, the number of actual hours in a week? If your estimate is higher, go back through your list and adjust your numbers to be more realistic. If your estimated hours total to less than 168, do not make any changes. Instead, ask yourself this question: *Where does the time go?* We'll analyze it to find out!

still providing enough time to enjoy life with friends, family, and other activities. Try these strategies:

- *Prepare to be successful.* While you are planning ahead for studying, think yourself into the right mood as well. Fight off any negative thoughts by focusing on the positive. "When I get these chapters read tonight, I'll be ahead in studying for the next test, and I'll also have plenty of time tomorrow to do X." *Visualize* yourself studying well.

- *Use your best time of day.* Different tasks require different mental skills. Maybe you can focus best on reading later in the day after you've burned off restless energy with some exercise. Maybe you can write a class paper more successfully earlier in the day when you still have a lot of energy. Some kinds of studying you may be able to start first thing in the morning as you wake, whereas others need your most alert moments at another time.

- *Break up large projects into small pieces.* Whether it's writing a paper for class, studying for a final exam, or reading a long assignment or a whole book, students often feel daunted at the beginning of a large project. That leads to a tendency to put it off. It's usually easier to get going if you break it up into stages that you schedule at separate times—and then begin with the first section that requires only an hour or two.

- *Do most important studying first.* When two or more separate things require your attention, do the more crucial one first. If something interrupts your work and you don't complete everything you planned to do, you'll suffer less if the most crucial work has been done.

- *If you have trouble getting started, do an easier task first.* Similar to large tasks, complex or difficult ones can be daunting. If you really can't get going, switch to an easier task you can accomplish quickly. That will give you momentum, and often, you feel more confident tackling the difficult task after being successful in the first one.

- *If you're really floundering, talk to someone.* A problem getting going on a project or large assignment may be the result of not really understanding what you should be doing. Talk with your instructor or another student in the class. Usually, this will help you get back on track.

- *Take a break.* We all need breaks to help us concentrate without becoming fatigued and burned out. As a general rule, a short break every hour or so is effective in helping recharge your study energy. Get up and move around to get your blood flowing, clear your thoughts, and work off any stress that's building up.

- *Use unscheduled times to work ahead.* If you have a few minutes waiting for the bus, start a reading assignment, or flip through the chapter to get a sense of what you'll be reading later. Either way, you'll be better prepared when you reach your scheduled reading time and will likely need less time. Use other down time during the day and you may be amazed how much studying you can get done in casual times.

- *Keep your momentum.* Remember to prevent distractions that will only slow you down. Save checking for texts or messages, for example, until your scheduled break time.

- *Reward yourself.* It's not easy to sit still for hours of studying or work on a special project. When you successfully complete the task, you should feel good about yourself and the reward of a (healthy) snack or a quick video game or social media activity—whatever you enjoy doing—can help you feel even better about your successful use of time.

- *Just say no.* Tell others nearby when you're studying to reduce the chances of being interrupted. If an interruption happens, it helps to have your "no" prepared in advance: "No, I have to be ready for this test" or "That's a great idea, but let's do it tomorrow—I just can't today."
- *Have a life.* Never schedule your day or week so full of work and study that you have no time at all for yourself, your family and friends, your larger life. Without a personal life, even the most dedicated student will suffer in a way that can negatively impact studies.
- *Use a calendar planner and daily to-do list.* We'll look at these time management tools in the next section.

Daily Time Log

AM		**PM**	
5:00	_____	5:00	_____
5:15	_____	5:15	_____
5:30	_____	5:30	_____
5:45	_____	5:45	_____
6:00	_____	6:00	_____
6:15	_____	6:15	_____
6:30	_____	6:30	_____
6:45	_____	6:45	_____
7:00	_____	7:00	_____
7:15	_____	7:15	_____
7:30	_____	7:30	_____
7:45	_____	7:45	_____
8:00	_____	8:00	_____
8:15	_____	8:15	_____
8:30	_____	8:30	_____
8:45	_____	8:45	_____
9:00	_____	9:00	_____
9:15	_____	9:15	_____
9:30	_____	9:30	_____
9:45	_____	9:45	_____
10:00	_____	10:00	_____
10:15	_____	10:15	_____
10:30	_____	10:30	_____
10:45	_____	10:45	_____
11:00	_____	11:00	_____

Continued

11:15 _____	11:15 _____
11:30 _____	11:30 _____
11:45 _____	11:45 _____
AM	**PM**
12:00 _____	12:00 _____
12:15 _____	12:15 _____
12:30 _____	12:30 _____
12:45 _____	12:45 _____
1:00 _____	1:00 _____
1:15 _____	1:15 _____
1:30 _____	1:30 _____
1:45 _____	1:45 _____
2:00 _____	2:00 _____
2:15 _____	2:15 _____
2:30 _____	2:30 _____
2:45 _____	2:45 _____
3:00 _____	3:00 _____
3:15 _____	3:15 _____
3:30 _____	3:30 _____
3:45 _____	3:45 _____
4:00 _____	4:00 _____
4:15 _____	4:15 _____
4:30 _____	4:30 _____
4:45 _____	4:45 _____

Calendars

People who manage their time well aren't just successful students—they're successful people. They take all areas of their busy lives into account and give each task the right amount of time and attention. The one tool successful people swear by is their personal calendar or schedule.

Using a calendar can seem like a negative to some people. When they see those days fill up on the page or screen, they feel trapped and overwhelmed. How will they get it all done? A calendar is powerful; it shows you exactly what you're doing each day and how busy you really are. But this is a good thing. Being able to see each week or month at a glance will show you days where you're trying to do too many things at once. A calendar shows you places where your time stretches too thin and emptier places where you can move some of those tasks.

Most important, though, is that a calendar helps you to be prepared. If something unexpected comes up, you can consult your calendar and immediately determine how that emergency is going to affect you. A calendar will keep you on track and help you remember important dates. Developing a personal schedule goes a long way toward fulfilling your time management goals.

As a student, you need to do both short- and long-range planning. You'll need certain items to make this possible:

- A yearly calendar that you keep at home. This can be a paper calendar or an electronic version.
- A small weekly planner that you carry with you, adding new items as you hear about them. This also can be either paper or on your smartphone. You can add new information to your yearly calendar and check for any conflicts.
- A daily to-do list. You'll fill this list with items from your yearly calendar and/or your weekly planner.

You might choose to use an all-in-one organizer. Electronic organizers can store large amounts of information, yet they're small enough to carry with you wherever you go. Just be sure to keep a copy of all your information in a cloud-based platform, such as Google Calendar. You can also find printable weekly and daily planner pages on the web resource available via the access code that comes with every NEW text purchase.

What to Schedule on Your Calendar—and Why

Don't think of your calendar or planner as only an academic planner. Although it is that, it also has to include everything important in your life—academic, professional, and personal—in order to work well. You need to include many important things to keep your schedule organized and avoid time conflicts. The calendar won't do its job for you if you mark next Tuesday's test but not your doctor's appointment scheduled for the same time. Put your whole life—work, school, home—on your calendar.

Due Dates and Deadlines

Due dates and deadlines are very important and are usually stated in each course syllabus. Turning in work on time helps you stay on schedule and keep up with the rest of the class. Although some instructors have special policies allowing for work to be turned in late, many do not. Make a habit of turning things in when work is due.

Tests and Quizzes

Test and quiz dates should also be marked on your calendar. Carve out blocks of time to study beginning several days before each test. If you don't reserve time for studying, the opportunity to prepare could slip away from you. Prioritize your study time by scheduling it during a time of day when your mind is sharp.

Of course, you also have to prioritize attendance on test days. If there is absolutely no way you can be in class on a test day (due to a family emergency, illness, or other circumstance beyond your control), let your instructor know as soon as possible and ask if the exam can be made up. Many instructors will not allow this, but if yours will, do whatever you can to make it up on the day provided.

Projects and Group Work

When it comes to projects and group work, the scheduling isn't only up to you. As soon as you're assigned to a group, get together with your group members and block out times to work on the project. Start with the project due date and your instructor's recommendations of how much time you'll need to complete the work. Set aside times to work individually and times to get together.

It's tempting to leave this until later—why schedule time weeks in advance? But it's very hard to find one time when three or more people can get together. You and your classmates all have busy schedules. You'll have to prioritize your group work by getting out your calendars and determining a work/study schedule. That way, if someone tries to cancel, you can all remind that person that the date was agreed on long ago and should be honored.

You'll also have more team spirit if you're working together according to a reasonable plan rather than trying to cram in meetings with each other at the last minute or to assign work via email.

Homework

Homework usually includes writing or reading assignments. Some students don't take homework seriously enough to include it in their calendar planner—they may think they'll just get to it eventually. But homework is actually a very important part of student success.

Written assignments show your instructor how well you understand the material. They show how much work you've finished and whether you know exactly what you're doing. Reading assignments don't give the instructor immediate feedback on your performance, but most instructors consider reading to be just as important as written work. You might see questions about reading assignments on quizzes or tests. Your instructor may base class discussions on the assigned readings. If your instructor relies on class discussions, be sure to complete the reading so you'll be prepared to participate.

When planning your weekly schedule, try to estimate how long it will take you to complete each homework assignment. This will be easier to do as you become more familiar with your instructors and your coursework, but at first, it's probably a good idea to add 30 minutes to your estimate. For example, if you think it should take you an hour to complete a homework assignment, schedule an hour and a half, just in case it takes longer. If you find it really does take you just an hour, you'll have 30 minutes to review, get started on something else, or take a well-deserved break.

Often, you will have homework based on an assigned reading or lab work. Try to get into the habit of doing the homework soon after the reading or lab work is done, when it's still fresh in your mind. The old saying, "Don't put off until tomorrow what you can do today," is never truer than in the context of homework.

Field Trips

Field trips are invaluable opportunities to visit your future workplace, but they also can wreak havoc on your schedule. Do everything you can to make these trips. Your instructor will probably clarify whether it is important for you to attend. Put field trip dates into your calendar so you can prepare for them in advance. You might need to:

- arrange childcare if you have young children
- take the necessary time off work
- ask your spouse or a friend to pitch in and help with any other responsibilities you may have on those days

Also, be aware that you may run late getting back from the field trip, so try to schedule some extra time for delays.

Study Days

If your school schedules special reading or study days into each semester or term, plan to make use of these. Add these dates to your calendar well in advance. This will help you keep the days free as you schedule your other events and commitments. Try to avoid the urge to use your study days for any purpose other than studying!

Other Responsibilities

Like most students, you probably have family, work, or other responsibilities outside of school. Sometimes, you might have to put off doing homework because of a more pressing obligation. This is understandable and, when this happens, it's okay to adjust your schedule. The key is to stay balanced. When you postpone working on a homework assignment because of another responsibility, be sure to make time in your schedule to complete the assignment before it's due.

Take Time Off

Whenever you can, try to create free time for yourself. You have to plan breaks if you want to avoid burnout—the fatigue, boredom, and stress that can make life miserable. A break can mean many things—switching from one task to another, getting together with classmates to discuss a group project, or moving from one subject to another.

You can also avoid burnout by keeping your daily schedule flexible. Be realistic when you're planning. If your calendar shows you have 3 days to complete an assignment, avoid trying to cram it all into 1 day. If you schedule commitments too tightly, you might not complete them on time (or at all), which can leave you feeling discouraged.

Holidays

Holidays are times to relax and have fun, so make sure you do just that. It's tempting to put off coursework when you're busy, thinking, "I'll do that during vacation week." But vacation week often means your family is home, you're traveling, you're working to earn some extra money, or you're getting together with friends. You won't want to spend that time trying to get work done—or failing to get it done. Block off holiday time and keep it free of any school obligations. You'll need that time to rest so you can come back refreshed and ready to get back to your schoolwork.

Add/Drop Dates

You can avoid having to add or drop courses after the start of a semester by preparing properly before registration. Before you register for a course, gather as much information as you can. Meet with your academic advisor to determine the appropriateness of each course you plan to take. This way, you can avoid registering for courses you don't need. You'll also want to make sure you won't be taking several very demanding courses at the same time.

Even if you do everything right, you can occasionally run into snags after the semester begins. Maybe after attending your first few math classes, you find that it takes you a lot longer than you thought to complete the homework. It becomes clear that you won't have enough time this semester to devote to the class. For this type of situation, there is a solution—the drop/add period. During specific drop/add dates at the beginning of each semester or term, you can drop or add a course from your schedule without being penalized for it. Mark these dates on your calendar just in case this happens.

Keep in mind, however, that you need to be considerate of your fellow students. Often, there are students on waiting lists who need to take certain courses for their degree or certificate programs. Avoid using the drop/add period as a time to "test drive" courses. You may be taking a spot that someone else absolutely needs. Instead, plan ahead before you register and avoid the stressful drop/add shuffle altogether.

Last Day of Class

The last day of class is another important date to mark on your calendar. This date sometimes occurs several days before the start of exams. Although you should attend each class period during the term, being present on the last day before exams is particularly important. Professors often review material that will appear on the exams and answer questions during this last class. You need to be there.

Registration Dates for Next Semester

Approaching the end of one semester or term means it's time to prepare for the next. Mark registration dates on your calendar and give yourself enough time to prepare before registration begins. You might need to research certain courses or set up an appointment with your academic advisor to make sure you're on track for your degree or certificate plan. Remember, if you prepare properly before registration, you can avoid the drop/add hassle after the next semester or term begins.

It's also important to be prepared so you can register as early as possible. Required courses often fill up quickly. If you wait too long, you might not get into a course you need. Stay ahead of the game by going in on the first day of registration and getting your classes.

Managing Time by the Year

As mentioned above, you should keep a long-range yearly calendar as well as a weekly planner. You can use a traditional paper or an online calendar. Use this calendar to record:

- class times
- midterm and final exam dates
- due dates for papers and other projects
- deadlines for completing each phase of lengthy projects
- test dates
- your instructors' office hours
- important extracurricular and recreational events
- deadlines for drop/add
- holidays, school vacations, and social commitments

Get Yourself Off to a Good Start

You'll probably notice right away that the beginning of each school term is a very busy and important time. During the first few weeks of a term, the professor forms an opinion about what kind of student you are. Are you organized? Do you ask good questions? Do you know what you're supposed to do? Do you complete your work on time? Is your work done correctly? This kind of informal evaluation can help or hurt you. You'll want to be very organized from the start so you develop a good reputation as a student. Think of the beginning of each semester or term as a fresh start.

Finish Strong

In school, you need to start *and* finish each semester with the same amount of hard work and dedication. The end of the term is important because you'll be running out of time to catch up if you've fallen behind in your work. Avoid letting your strong start from the beginning of the semester go to waste. Look at your calendar well ahead of time and try to clear less important events from the last few weeks of class so you can focus on final project and exams.

Managing Time by the Week

Keeping a weekly planner helps you tackle the things listed on your long-term calendar, 1 week at a time. At the beginning of each week, you can plan for the tasks that are scheduled for that week. Here are some guidelines to follow as you create your weekly calendar.

- List regularly scheduled events and tasks first (such as class times, meal times, and the time you'll spend at work).
- Try to schedule time before each class for a brief review of your notes and to prepare for that day's lecture.
- When possible, allow yourself a few minutes after each class to review and organize your notes. Summarizing is a great—and quick—way to review the material you just covered.
- Use your time efficiently by grouping similar activities together.
- Make it a habit to complete assignments before they're due. This way, you'll be able to turn in your work on time even if you come across snags in your schedule.
- Plan to study for 50 to 90 minutes at a stretch and be sure to allow yourself 15-minute breaks between study sessions.
- Base your study time on how many hours of class time you have each week. It's safe to estimate 2 hours of study time for every hour you spend in class.

Today's Date:	Monday, Sept. 21st
8:00 AM	A&P Class—homework due
8:30 AM	Try to read A&P ch6 in free time
9:00 AM	
9:30 AM	
10:00 AM	
10:30 AM	Lab—don't forget the worksheets!
11:00 AM	
11:30 AM	
12:00 PM	Lunch at Student Union—meet study group
12:30 PM	for math at 12:15
1:00 PM	Review for math quiz
1:30 PM	
2:00 PM	Start planning topic for English paper
2:30 PM	Prof. Jones office hours 2–3 if questions?
3:00 PM	Math class—important quiz today!!
3:30 PM	(chaps 1–4)
4:00 PM	
4:30 PM	
5:00 PM	5:20 bus to work—grab a snack
5:30 PM	
6:00 PM	
6:30 PM	Work
7:00 PM	
7:30 PM	
8:00 PM	Finish A&P reading
8:30 PM	
9:00 PM	Start outline for Eng. paper—if time?
9:30 PM	
NOTES:	Email Mom when I get chance
	Need new printer cartridge

Sample planner page.

- If possible, study at the same time every day. Choose a time when you're awake and alert.
- Use gaps in your schedule (such as time between classes) as study time. This way, you'll get more work done during the day and you'll have time to relax or do other things in the evenings.
- Schedule at least 1 hour per week to review how you will need to prepare for each class period.
- Be flexible by leaving some time unscheduled.

Different Forms for Different Folks

A wide variety of planners and calendars are available for purchase, or you can download them from the Internet if you want to make your own. Is it better to have a separate page for every day—or a week spread over a two-page spread? How should the time slots be broken down? This is all up to you. You'll soon find out what system works best for you.

It's usually best, however, to start out having *more* room on the page per day rather than less. If you don't have room enough to write down everything and to cross out items and add new ones when things change, then the planner can't do its job well, and you may forget something important. The sample daily calendar page shown on page 43 is just one student's preferred way of doing it, but it works well for this student. See what works best for you.

Plan Ahead

It's best to create your weekly calendar on Sunday before the week begins. Looking at the week ahead will help you spot any conflicts before they occur, so you can reschedule tasks as necessary. Being able to view the coming week at a glance will also give you a chance to see how busy each day will be. Try to spread out your activities so each day is just as manageable as the next. You won't want to overload your schedule on Monday only to become burned out by Tuesday.

As you plan out your week, be realistic about the amount of time you estimate for each activity. In scheduling time for your commute to and from school, for instance, you should consider things such as the time of day and amount of traffic. If it takes longer to get to school in the mornings than it does to get home in the evenings, be sure to allow yourself enough time as you create your weekly schedule.

Other activities you should include in your weekly schedule are:

- homework assignments
- papers due
- upcoming quizzes and tests
- assigned readings

Managing Time With a Daily To-Do List

Even though you have a weekly calendar with key information for each day, it's still a good idea to have a to-do list for the next day's activities. This gives you a plan for the new day. Every night, check your weekly calendar and record the next day's activities on an index card, small sheet of paper, or electronic device. Include things such as homework, study time, errands, and other tasks that are specific to that day—all the personal and academic tasks you need to accomplish that day. The tasks on your list should be specific and you should be able to accomplish them in the time you have. Include little things not on your calendar that you still need to do, such as paying a bill before it becomes overdue, buying groceries, or asking a friend to borrow a book—whatever you don't want to forget.

Keep in mind that you can switch certain items around as the day goes on if doing this will make your day more efficient. The point is to get everything done, regardless of the order in which you wrote the items down. Allowing yourself some flexibility will keep you from becoming stressed.

It's also important to reward yourself for accomplishing everything on your to-do list. Cross off each item after you've completed it. This will give you a visual record of your success. Giving yourself 5 minutes of free time for each large task you finish is another good way to reward yourself—and to make sure you don't overdo it.

Or try this: Each day you complete everything on your to-do list, put a certain amount of money into a jar. At the end of the month, use the money to treat yourself. This works better than setting up punishments. Recognize achievement and use days you don't get everything done as opportunities to look at your schedule and to see what changes might make your days more efficient.

TO DO TODAY:

• Study for anatomy test
• Anatomy test
• Read 20 pages for lab practical
• Study group
• Start research for lab assignment
• Laundry

Sample planner page.

Priorities

A big part of keeping a schedule involves managing priorities. Should you read an assigned chapter in your English textbook tonight or study for the anatomy and physiology test tomorrow? Both are important—both need to be done. But which is the priority right now? Setting priorities is important to your success as a student. You'll need to set priorities for tasks, class attendance, and homework.

As you'll learn in coming chapters, it's better to start early on big projects (studying for an exam, writing a paper, etc.) and spread out the work over time. Use your weekly calendar to schedule things well ahead of due dates to ensure you have plenty of less stressful time to work ahead. Even though you may have that A & P test tomorrow, you ideally might have already studied enough for it and, instead of trying to cram tonight, you can do your English reading more leisurely and get to bed early.

It's all a matter of setting priorities and planning ahead.

Making Progress

When you have several tasks with the same deadline, it's tempting to switch back and forth from one task to another. This feels like progress on all the tasks—they're all moving ahead. However, you're probably losing valuable time. When you switch from one task to another, you lose momentum. Your brain has to switch gears and begin thinking about a new project, a process of removing something psychologists call "attention residue." When you return to the first task, you often have to backtrack by finding out where you left off and what other steps need to be completed to finish the task.

In an Hour or Less

If you have an hour or less to work, your priority should be completing a single task as opposed to inching forward on several tasks. Here are a couple reasons why it's better to focus on completing one task when you're short on time.

- Completing an activity on your daily to-do list will give you a sense of satisfaction. Once you've crossed an item off your list, you'll have one less task to worry about completing.

- Completing a task moves you closer toward your goals. Think about it this way: Your instructors won't give you credit for simply working on a homework assignment, but they *will* give you credit if you complete the assignment correctly and on time.

Those Marathon Projects

In the case of long-term projects, however, it's sometimes necessary to switch from one task to another. You can't expect to complete a 10-page research paper in one sitting. If you interrupt work on a long-term project to work on something else, write a few notes on the long-term project before you take a break from it. Your notes could include:

- the goal of the task
- a list of questions you need to answer
- the next step you need to complete

In this manner, when you come back to the long-term project, you'll be ready to get to work right away. Also, remember to keep all the materials you need for that project in one place so you don't have to spend time looking for them.

Procrastination Pitfalls

Procrastination is the enemy of time management. Procrastination is so common that we tend to fall into its trap easily, thinking it's not so bad to put things off. But procrastination is just a fancy word for wasting time, and you know that wasting time harms your success as a student. It leads to missed opportunities, poor performance, low self-esteem, and heavy stress.

When you procrastinate, you spend your time worrying instead of working. The task you postponed starts to weigh heavily on your mind. You imagine how hard it will be and you start to dread it—but this doesn't have to be the case. There are several steps you can take to recognize procrastination and put a stop to it.

Prioritize

One habit that leads to procrastination is failing to prioritize your tasks correctly. Putting low-priority (nonurgent) tasks ahead of high-priority (urgent) tasks is all too common. There are many familiar excuses for avoiding important work, such as:

- I'm not in the mood. I have to wait until I'm in the mood or I won't do well.
- I feel like taking a break to celebrate finishing one chapter. I'll read the second chapter after that.
- I'll do it tomorrow.
- I've got plenty of time—there's no rush.
- I don't know where to start.
- I like working under pressure.
- I need to do other things first or I won't be able to concentrate.

What's the thinking behind all these excuses? Often it's a lack of confidence. You might think the task is going to be too hard. You worry about being able to do it right. You fear it will take forever. You read every bit of material you can to prepare for the project—buying time before you have to begin. When you're worried about the outcome of a project, it's hard to find the motivation to get started.

Now's the time to shake off the lack of confidence that wastes your valuable time. First, remember who you are: a motivated, efficient student dedicated to your education and your future career. Then, remember why you're doing the project—to get the information and experience you'll need in your new career. Last, remember that nothing is as hard as it seems. You just have to start. The sooner you start, the sooner you'll be done.

Here are some ways to get started on that big project right away.

- Do a little bit at a time.
- Juggle your deadlines.
- Set realistic goals.
- Stay focused.
- Be confident about your decisions.
- Keep your goals in mind.

A Little at a Time

Try spending just 5 minutes on the project you've been dreading and putting off. Once you start, you'll probably find that you can keep working beyond 5 minutes.

Juggling Deadlines

Occasionally, the problem is having several deadlines in the same week. It's tempting to do the easier projects first, leaving time for the hardest one at the end of the week. But it would be wise to clear the most difficult project out of the way first. With the pressure off, you'll be able to relax a bit and work on the smaller projects.

If the projects are equally large, try parceling out the work. Set apart small tasks that can be done quickly for each project. Once you have those small tasks out of the way, you can focus all your energy on one project first and then the other. Completing several small tasks gives you confidence and gets you closer to being done.

Keep It Real

What if the problem is you have an unrealistic goal? Some students don't start projects in time because they set standards that are too high (by accepting nothing less than 100% or vowing to do something better and faster than everyone else in the class). Then, they're afraid they won't live up to those high standards. Or they won't stop working until they feel the project is perfect, which causes them to miss the deadline.

What is the solution? Weigh the consequences of handing in what you think is an imperfect project against the consequences of handing it in late or not at all. A passing grade for an imperfect assignment is better than a zero for not handing it in at all.

Be Confident About Your Decisions

Uncertainty leads to indecisiveness, which usually ends in procrastination. For example, if you're not sure which topic to choose for a project, it becomes easier to put off starting the project. When this happens, remind yourself that you have to be decisive to become a successful student. Have confidence in yourself. The next time you're feeling lost and having a hard time choosing a topic, use these tips to help you get started.

- Brainstorm for ideas with other students.
- Ask your instructor for suggestions.
- Research several topics that might interest you.

Keep Your Goals in Focus

Remember the long- and short-term goals you wrote down in Chapter 1? By keeping these goals in mind, you'll have an easier time staying on track and avoiding procrastination. When you're thinking about your goals, an assignment becomes more than just another task to get through. It becomes your ticket to reaching your short-term goal of passing the course. And passing the course moves you closer toward your long-term goal of eventually becoming a licensed healthcare professional.

By focusing on your goals, you can give yourself the motivation you need to complete assignments that you might otherwise put off. Review your goals whenever you feel the urge to procrastinate. Looking at your goals is also a good way to get back on track if you notice that you're putting too much energy into one assignment at the expense of other projects and commitments. Your goals will help you stay balanced and moving forward to greater success. Finally, keep your goals SMART.

Stay Focused

Where there's distraction, there's procrastination. Your mind will seek out distractions to avoid starting a project. You have to fight it. Work on the project in a quiet area that is free from distractions. If you're in the kitchen, you might eat or do dishes as opposed to working. If you're in the living room, you might be distracted by the TV.

Another good way to avoid distractions is to make sure you have all the materials you need before sitting down to begin a project. You can disrupt your train of thought if you're constantly getting up to find another resource. Even small interruptions can cause you to lose momentum. Instead, gather your materials before you get started and then prepare to focus.

Chapter Summary

- Make it a habit to attend all your classes. You'll be a much better student.
- Use the course documents provided by your instructor to find out what to expect in each course you take.
- Investigate what campus resources are available to you, including your instructors and other students, to help you achieve success.
- Organize your time by creating yearly, weekly, and daily schedules.
- Schedule your time well for efficient and effective studying.
- Avoid procrastination by dividing large projects into several smaller tasks and setting realistic goals to focus on. Focus isn't something you have, it's something you do. In other words, you can learn to stay focused.

Review Questions

Objective Questions

1. Attending class on the first day isn't as important as most other days during the term. (True or False?)
2. If your professor is in his or her office, you can walk right in with a question, even outside of office hours. (True or False?)
3. The _____ is a place on campus where you can find help from a tutor.
4. The online platform where materials for your course are located is called _____.
5. If you believe you may have a learning disability, you should keep it a secret from everyone at your new college. (True or False?)

Short-Answer Questions

1. What can happen if you get in the habit of skipping classes?
2. How can your syllabus help you be successful in a course?
3. What items do you need to put into your yearly schedule?
4. Name several techniques for controlling your procrastination tendencies.

Applications

1. Planning Exercise: Work with others as a group to create a long-term calendar for a student taking the course for which you are now reading this text. Plan out the entire school term by referring to the syllabus or class schedule for information on:

   - class times
   - midterm and final exam dates
   - due dates for papers and other projects
   - deadlines for completing each phase of lengthy projects
   - test dates
   - the instructor's office hours
   - deadlines for drop/add
   - holidays and school vacations

Fundamental Writing Skills

The section in the writing skills chapter you should complete at the end of Chapter 2 is Section 11-2. You can find this section on pages 203-207.

3

Maintaining Your Health and Well-Being

OBJECTIVES

- Understand how your health and well-being contribute to your success as a student.
- Evaluate and manage your symptoms of stress.
- Apply the principles of exercise, good nutrition, and sufficient rest to staying healthy.
- Know how to stay safe and avoid harmful substances.
- Create and use a budget for financial stability.

When you are in school, you don't need to put your life on hold. You still feel stress, or not, and you are healthy and happy—or not. If anything, health and well-being are even more important when in school than at other times. You are likely to be stressed by a complicated life with many pressures, and your studies may add to them.

For these reasons, it is critical to pay attention to your own health and well-being while being a student. Stress can make you unhealthy, but good physical and mental health can reduce stress. Your overall well-being involves not only managing stress but also optimizing your exercise, nutrition, and rest—the keys to good physical health—as well as maintaining personal safety and managing your finances. Paying attention to all of these dimensions of your life will contribute much to your success as a student.

Stress

The word *stress* usually carries a negative connotation. In the context of this discussion, stress is defined as a state of mental or emotional strain resulting from adverse or very demanding circumstances.

As you have probably experienced, stress can cause physical and emotional tension and has also been linked to illness. These are all negative effects. However, there are different types of stress and different reactions to stress. How you choose to manage stress can determine whether you have positive or negative reactions to it.

Eustress Versus Distress

The two main types of stress are the following:

- *Eustress.* This type of stress causes positive reactions and can be helpful. Low levels often motivate people to complete tasks, meet deadlines, and solve problems. You may encounter this type of stress every day. It can stimulate you to accomplish your day-to-day tasks.

- *Distress.* This type of stress causes negative reactions. High levels often cause people to overreact. Distress can cause you to feel nervous and unfocused and can impair your ability to complete your tasks.

Symptoms of Stress

Identifying the symptoms of stress can help you manage it more easily. Recognizing stress at an early stage can help you keep short-term symptoms from becoming prolonged symptoms.

Some of the short-term symptoms may include the following:

- Faster, shallow breaths
- A faster heartbeat
- Tightening of muscles in your shoulders, forehead, and the back of your neck
- Cold and clammy hands and feet
- A feeling of "butterflies" in your stomach
- Physical illness such as diarrhea, vomiting, or frequent urination
- Dry mouth
- Trembling of your hands and knees

These short-term symptoms are similar for most people. They are also easily recognizable. Short-term symptoms stop occurring once you remove yourself from the stressful situation. For example, you may experience short-term symptoms of stress immediately before giving a speech in class. After your speech, however, your heart rate will return to normal and your palms will no longer feel sweaty.

Prolonged stress can have more damaging effects over time.

- Your immune system begins to break down because of lost white blood cells, and you may become sick more easily and more often.
- Free fatty acids are released into your bloodstream, which can clog arteries and eventually lead to a heart attack or stroke.
- Your risk for developing many different diseases may increase.

The symptoms of stress are not always physical. Stress also can affect your mental and emotional well-being. Psychological symptoms include:

- losing your ability to think clearly or remember things
- having difficulty solving problems
- experiencing anxiety or fear
- losing your ability to sleep through the night
- changing your eating habits—either eating significantly less or more than usual
- worrying
- becoming easily exhausted

With all these effects, it should be clear that stress can really get in the way of academic success. Fortunately, you can learn to take control of stress before it begins to affect you seriously.

Taking Control of Stress

Just as there are different types of stress, there are different ways of dealing with it. Several healthy ways of managing stress include the following:

- Setting priorities
- Simplifying your life
- Learning to relax

- Thinking positively
- Gaining the support of others
- Maintaining a healthy body

Setting Priorities

Setting priorities means determining which commitments or tasks are necessary and which are not. Priorities help you manage your time wisely. By determining which activities are most important, you can avoid the stress that comes with trying to do everything. On a given day, your schedule may include attending class, studying, working, spending time with family or friends, and exercising or enjoying other hobbies. As you look at each task on your to-do list, ask yourself, "Is it absolutely necessary to get this task done today, or would it just be nice to get it done today?" Move the absolutely necessary tasks to the top of your list. After—and only after—those tasks have been accomplished, consider tackling the other items. If you're unable to complete all the tasks on your list, don't be discouraged. Instead, feel good about everything you did manage to accomplish that day.

Urgency Versus Emergency

Another way to reduce stress is to adjust your schedule to fit your needs. If you have too many responsibilities that you aren't able to manage, try to give yourself more time. You may be surprised to see how many false deadlines you impose on yourself.

For example, if your coursework becomes overwhelming, consider taking fewer courses during the next semester. It would be better to graduate a few months later than to become overly stressed, break down, and be unable to finish your degree or certification at all.

You can also avoid unnecessary stress by being able to tell the difference between an emergency and an urgency. When you feel stressed, divide your tasks into three separate groups:

- *Emergencies.* A task is an emergency if it absolutely must be done immediately. For example, taking an injured pet to the veterinarian is an emergency.
- *Urgencies.* A task is urgent if it is important but does not need to be dealt with immediately. For example, taking a pet in for its shots is urgent and should be done as soon as you have time.
- *Nonurgencies.* If a task is neither an emergency nor an urgency, it is a nonurgency. For example, whereas it is important to care for your pet, giving your healthy dog a bath is nonurgent.

If you have tasks that don't fit into any of the three groups, remove them from your list. They are not important and should be accomplished only if and when you have extra time.

Simplify Your Life

Because time is often short and most students have complex lives, simplifying your daily life can be another good way to avoid stress. The following strategies can help you simplify.

- Try to do all your errands in one place at one time. Going to several different locations may help you save money, but getting everything done at the same location saves you valuable time and energy.
- Don't watch TV every day.
- Let your voice mail take messages for you.

- Stop attending functions you don't enjoy if they are not required.
- Avoid optional activities if they take up valuable time, such as chatting with your coworkers after work.
- Learn to say "no" when you have too much to do. Practice saying "no" to at least one request or invitation every week.
- Take time for relaxing when the job's done.

Keep It Simple

With a partner, discuss your weekly routines. What can each of you do to simplify your lives? Which of your activities would be considered urgent and which would be nonurgent?

Relax Inside and Out

When you are stressed, your body reacts as if it's being attacked. Both your brain and the rest of your nervous system become overactive. You can help back off from this reaction and reduce the stress you feel by learning to relax your body and your mind.

Try relaxation and stress management techniques such as massage, yoga, and meditation. Exercise is another relaxation technique. When you're sweating on a treadmill or pushing up a hill on your bike, exercise may not seem so relaxing. But after you finish your exercise session, you'll feel stronger, calmer, and more positive.

Don't Forget to Breathe

The next time you feel tense, try following this simple relaxation exercise.

- Relax the muscles in your neck and shoulders.
- Slowly lower your head forward.
- Gently roll your head to the right and pause for 3 seconds.
- Gently roll your head to the left and pause for 3 seconds.
- Slowly roll your head down toward the center of your chest and pause for 3 seconds.
- Switch sides and repeat, moving from left to right this time.

Mind Over Matter

Stress can be caused or intensified by negative thoughts, such as worrying about school work or personal issues. To combat this stress, train your mind to focus on the positive. Try not to dwell on the stress you are facing; instead, acknowledge it and then move on to a solution. Focus on the goals you want to achieve and imagine how you will be successful. For example, you could start by acknowledging to yourself or a close friend that you are stressed about an upcoming test or the piles of paperwork waiting for you at work. Then, you could move on to a solution by making time to study thoroughly or by setting aside lower priority tasks.

Remember that imagining worst-case scenarios can lead to anxiety and stress. Worrying is rarely productive. On the other hand, if you spend your time thinking about success, you will stay motivated to achieve it.

It is also important to spend time with people who can help reinforce your positive thinking. Family, friends, classmates, and others can help you stay positive and remind you that people care about you no matter what. Other positive classmates can remind you that you are all in this together.

If you are unable to ignore your negative thoughts, try this meditation exercise.

- Find a quiet place and sit or lie down comfortably with your eyes closed.
- Begin to inhale slowly and exhale fully.
- As you exhale, imagine that you are expelling the stress and negative thoughts from your body.
- As you inhale, imagine that you are replacing the negative thoughts with encouraging, positive thoughts.
- Slowly inhale and exhale until you feel the tension and stress fading away.

Think Positively

If you want to succeed, you should think like a person who expects success. Some ways to train your mind to think positively include the following:

- Say something positive every time you have a negative thought. You may want to repeat an inspiring quote or a line from a song whenever your mind strays toward the negative. Gradually, you will overcome your anxiety.
- Get excited about upcoming projects and events. Imagine being successful in specific situations.
- Repeat positive mantras: "I *can* do this. I can *do* this."
- Be prepared. Have a "Plan B" in case obstacles arise.
- Learn from your mistakes. You don't have to do everything perfectly as long as you learn something.
- Think of tests and exams as ways to demonstrate what you have learned. Don't get discouraged for not remembering everything. Completing an exam should make you feel proud and accomplished, not worried and inadequate.

Be Positive—Amalia

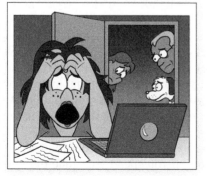

Amalia has done a good job of preparing for tomorrow's lab practical, but she still feels very anxious about the actual process of taking the practical. Having never taken one before, she doesn't know what to expect and is on the verge of panic. Her parents, never having gone to college, aren't really able to help her. What would you say to her?

Support Systems

There will be times when you will need to depend on others for support. Having a network of supportive friends or family members will help you deal with stress. People in your network of support may include:

- family members
- friends
- coworkers
- other students and classmates
- members of a religious group to which you belong
- people who share your interests in sports or hobbies

Discussing your problems or frustrations with others can help alleviate stress. People in your support system may be able to give advice or offer new perspectives. Surrounding yourself with people who care about you will encourage you to reach your goals.

ROLE PLAY

Controlling Stress

With a partner, discuss the symptoms you experience when stressed and the strategies that work for you to control it.

A Healthy Body Means a Happier You

As you are entering a healthcare career, you probably already know much about why good health is important. Taking good care of your body helps prevent many serious illnesses—and it also helps you handle stress more easily. Furthermore, you'll be able to succeed in school more readily if you're healthy.

Four keys to good health are:

- regular exercise
- a healthy diet
- sufficient sleep and rest
- avoidance of harmful substances

Exercise

Exercising is an important way to keep your energy level up and help you feel good about yourself. Aerobic activities, such as running, swimming, or cycling, strengthen your heart and offer many other benefits as well. People who exercise aerobically:

- are less likely to get sick
- have more energy and mental alertness
- are less stressed and tense
- sleep better
- maintain an appropriate weight more easily
- improve their self-esteem

Choose an activity you truly enjoy. If you try to force yourself to do something you dislike, you won't be motivated to exercise on a regular basis. Another way to stay motivated is to exercise with a friend or in a group. Many working people, for example, exercise during their lunch break. Exercise may seem like a luxury, but it's a necessity for fighting stress and maintaining good health. If you take good care of your body, you will be better able to keep up with your busy schedule.

For your body to receive the full benefits of exercise, you should work out at least three times a week for 20 to 30 minutes at a time. For even greater improvement, work your way up to exercising four to six times per week. Just remember to give yourself at least 1 day of rest each week.

Food = Fuel

Think of food as fuel. Eating breakfast every morning will prepare your body for the busy day ahead. You can give your body the energy it needs by eating healthy foods. This will prepare your body to deal with stress as well.

Food for Stress Control

Vitamin B, vitamin C, and folic acid all help your body handle stress. These nutrients can be found in citrus fruits and leafy green vegetables, among other foods. The next time you find yourself reaching for something sweet to lift your mood, try eating foods that contain tryptophan instead. This essential amino acid improves mood and sleep and can be found in foods such as:

- milk
- eggs
- poultry
- legumes
- nuts
- bananas

Food for Thought

Your brain needs nutrition to function properly. Eating right can give you the strength you need and help you stay alert throughout the day.

Part of healthy eating also means having a balanced diet of vegetables, fruits, grains, and low-fat proteins. It's important to cut back on things like sugar, salt, saturated fat, and caffeine. Several cups of coffee each morning may seem like the best way to wake up and get moving, but caffeine can cause tension and anxiety. As a result, you may find it harder to deal with stress. If you are looking for an energy boost, try healthier options, such as eating nutritious foods, exercising regularly, and getting enough rest.

The key to keeping your body and mind in top working condition is to have a well-balanced diet. Electrolytes, such as potassium, calcium, and magnesium, improve your physical and mental performance. Consider incorporating foods that contain these nutrients into your healthy eating plan.

Potassium is needed for the daily function of cells, tissues, and organs, especially muscle. Good sources of potassium include:

- fish, such as salmon, cod, flounder, and sardines
- vegetables, such as broccoli, peas, lima beans, tomatoes, and potatoes (with their skins)
- leafy green vegetables, such as spinach and parsley
- citrus fruits
- other fruits, such as bananas, apples, and dried apricots

Calcium is needed for bones, teeth, and muscle function. Good sources of calcium include:

- milk
- yogurt
- cheese

- soybeans
- some vegetables, such as collard greens and spinach

Magnesium helps to regulate muscle and nerve function as well as blood sugar levels and blood pressure. Good sources of magnesium include:

- some fish, such as halibut
- dry roasted nuts, such as almonds, cashews, and peanuts
- soybeans
- spinach
- whole grains
- potatoes (with their skins)

Eating for Health

Eating right can be simple. Just remember these basic guidelines.

- Include different types of food in your diet each day, such as vegetables, fruit, grains, and low-fat proteins.
- Check nutrition labels and look for foods low in saturated fat and cholesterol.
- Try to limit your intake of sugar, salt, and oils.
- Eat or drink caffeinated food or beverages in moderation.
- Drink plenty of water and avoid drinking too much alcohol.
- Balance the number of calories you eat each day with the amount of physical activity you do.

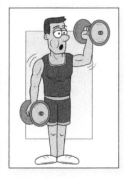

Exercise and Diet—Michael

After discharge from the army, Michael remained committed to exercising regularly and eating a healthy diet. After going to the gym, Michael and his classmate Bill went to Bill's apartment for dinner. On the way, they stop at a grocery store to buy food.

Prepare a menu for them. What should they eat to be at their best for an exam in Anatomy and Physiology first thing tomorrow morning?

Getting Enough Rest

Rest is also an important key to maintaining a healthy body. When you are well rested, you can complete tasks more efficiently. In contrast, feeling tired can increase the amount of stress you feel, which can wear your body down even more. Take cues from your body—when you feel tired, make sure you give yourself enough time to rest.

According to the National Institutes of Health, most adults need 8 hours of sleep each night. However, what if you're still unable to get a good night's rest even when you go to bed at a reasonable hour? Other things may be affecting your sleep.

- *Caffeine.* Depending on how much caffeine you consume on a regular basis, it may be affecting your body's ability to rest at the end of the day. Caffeine is a stimulant that can stay in your system for 6, or even up to 12, hours. Caffeine consumption later in the day may prevent your body from relaxing properly in the evening.

- *Nicotine.* Nicotine is a stimulant as well. If you are a heavy smoker, you may experience nicotine withdrawal during the night. Waking up multiple times can affect the quality of your sleep.
- *Alcohol.* Although having a glass or two of wine with dinner may make you feel drowsy, it can disturb your sleep later. Alcohol can cause you to wake up during the night. If you drink alcohol before going to sleep, you may wake up the next morning not feeling rested.
- *Food.* Eating foods that cause heartburn can affect your sleep. Not only does heartburn become worse after you lie down, it can also interrupt your sleep during the night. In addition, the amount of food you eat before falling asleep may affect the quality of your rest. Eating a large meal may make you uncomfortable and unable to sleep well. However, eating too little before bed also can make it hard to get a good night's rest.

On a positive note, a healthy diet and regular exercise can improve your ability to sleep. Making changes in those two areas may be all that's needed for you to start getting enough rest.

However, if you still have trouble sleeping, you may want to discuss it with your doctor. Getting good rest not only helps you manage stress, it is extremely important to your physical, emotional, and mental health as well.

Getting Enough Sleep

When you are tired, you're more likely to feel helpless, incapable, and defeated. Nothing sabotages a positive attitude like fatigue. Make sure you get 8 hours of sleep each night. That may seem like a lot—another luxury—but it's necessary for your emotional, mental, and physical health. Sleep is key to good performance in school, at work, and in life in general. While taking courses, you have been asking yourself to do more each day, so you will need to give your body the rest it needs. Getting enough rest will also help you do more in your job and make more of your career.

ROLE PLAY

Changing Your Diet

With a partner, discuss which foods you will try to consume more and which foods you will try to consume less.

Avoid Harmful Substances

"Substance" is the word health professionals use for many things people take into their bodies besides food. When people talk about substances, they often mean drugs—but alcohol and nicotine are also drugs and considered substances just as other drugs are.

Substances—any kind of drug—have effects on the body and mind. People use these substances for their effects. Some people use substances to try to alleviate stress. But many substances have negative effects, including being physically or psychologically addictive, and over time, they actually increase one's stress. What is important with any substance is to be aware of its effects on your health and on your life as a student and to make smart choices. Use of any substance to the extent that it has negative effects is substance abuse.

The most commonly abused substances are tobacco, alcohol, and prescription and illegal drugs:

- If you smoke now, planning and support can help you quit for good. You might begin by visiting websites such as https://smokefree.gov or https://www.lung.org /stop-smoking/i-want-to-quit. Before your quit day, take time to prepare for challenges. Know what to expect in the first days of being smoke free. Identify your reasons for quitting and plan how to ask for help if you need it. Some individuals use e-cigarettes to quit smoking tobacco cigarettes. However, there are still potential pitfalls. The nicotine in e-cigarettes is harmful for developing babies and can lead to addiction and harm brain development in children and young adults into their early 20s. These cigarettes may also contain heavy metals and cancer-causing chemicals.
- Alcohol is the most commonly used drug on most campuses. About a fourth of all students report academic problems resulting from alcohol, resulting in lower grades. Each year, more than 1,825 college students between the ages of 18 and 24 years die from alcohol-related injuries, almost 700,000 students in this same age range are assaulted by another student who has been drinking, and almost 100,000 students experience alcohol-related sexual assault or date rape.
- People use prescription and illegal drugs for the same reasons people use alcohol. They say they enjoy getting high. They may say a drug helps them relax, have fun, enjoy the company of others, or escape the pressures of being a student. Like other substances, many drugs have harmful effects on the body, affect one's judgment in ways that may increase the risks for injury, and involve serious legal consequences if the user is caught. If you have a problem using drugs, see a counselor at your campus health clinic for confidential help.

Enjoy Your Life

Don't let your busy life as a student prevent you from having a social life. Friendships and interactions with others help us all control stress—and just have fun. However, sometimes, students feel they are so busy with their studies and work that they should never take time out to enjoy the company of others.

School also offers the opportunity to meet many people you would likely not meet otherwise in life. Make the most of this opportunity as these social interactions may lead to several valuable benefits including the following:

- Friendships with people who understand you and with whom you can talk about your problems, joys, hopes, fears without worrying how they may react
- A growing understanding of diverse people, how they think, and what they feel, which will serve you well throughout your life and in your future career
- A heightened sense of your own identity, especially as you interact with others with different personalities and from different backgrounds

When you join study groups with other students, you get the best of both worlds: while enjoying the social interaction, you are also learning more and in more ways than when you study alone.

Staying Safe

Your health and well-being as a student involve one more thing: personal safety and security. Although most campuses are safe places, our world as a whole, unfortunately, is not always safe. Safety issues on college campuses include assault, date rape, and other violent crimes. By following a few common sense guidelines, you can stay safe both on and off campus.

- It is unwise to meet off campus with people you don't know very well, especially after dark. Go to parties with friends—and stay with them to avoid becoming separated. Because date rape drugs are sometimes added to drinks at parties, do not drink anything unless you know for certain it has not been tampered with.
- Do not give out your personal contact information (phone number, email address, etc.) until you have gotten to know a person well.
- Be cautious about what you post on social media.
- Be careful if your date is drinking heavily or using drugs.
- Stay in public places where there are other people. Do not invite a date to your home before your relationship is well established.
- If you are sexually active, be sure to practice safe sex. Remember that most birth control methods do not protect against sexually transmitted diseases.

ROLE PLAY **Staying Safe**	With a partner, discuss the strategies that you employ to stay safe on campus and in your community.

Financial Well-Being

One of the most common reasons for students to drop out of school before completing their program is financial: taking on too much debt. Tuition and the student loans to pay it can be crippling. However, by learning to budget and controlling your spending, you can avoid any more debt than is necessary to complete your education.

Get a Job

Most students work at least part-time. If you practice good time management (see Chapter 2), you should have enough time for both work and school. Some students with greater financial responsibilities can work full-time while taking part-time classes.

Your school may have an on-campus job office that will help you find a job if needed. The best jobs are those on or near campus, so you do not lose time commuting and can interact with the school community. Working around other students and professors helps you feel connected to your school work and may provide more satisfaction.

Spending Less

Recall the exercise in Chapter 2 where you estimated how you spend your time. When you actually monitored your time, you may have been surprised where much of it went. The same is true of money: most people really don't know where it all goes. See how much you know about your own spending habits with the activity *Where Does the Money Go?*

Where Does the Money Go?

Do your best to remember how much you have spent in the last 30 days in each of the following categories:

1. Coffee, soft drinks, bottled water $ _____
2. Fast food lunches, snacks, gum, candy, cookies, etc. $ _____
3. Social dining out with friends (lunch, dinner) $ _____
4. Movies, music concerts, sports events, night life $ _____
5. Cigarettes, smokeless tobacco $ _____
6. Beer, wine, liquor (stores, bars) $ _____
7. Lottery tickets $ _____
8. Music, DVDs, other personal entertainment $ _____
9. Mobile phone apps $ _____
10. Video or computer games, etc. $ _____
11. Gifts $ _____
12. Hobbies $ _____
13. Travel, day trips $ _____
14. Bank account fees, ATM withdrawal fees $ _____
15. Credit card finance charges $ _____

Now, add it all up: _____

Be honest with yourself: is this *really* all you spent on these items? Most of us tend to forget small daily purchases or underestimate how much we spend on them. Notice that this list does not include essential spending for things like room and board or an apartment, groceries, utilities, tuition and books, and so on. The greatest potential for cutting back on spending is to look at the optional things you spend your money on.

ROLE PLAY

Where Does the Money Go?

Complete the *Where Does the Money Go?* exercise in this chapter. With a partner, describe how you might change your habits to cut back in some areas to help minimize your debt.

Because most students cannot simply work more hours to provide a greater income, the better solution to avoiding debt is to learn to spend less. Helpful strategies include the following:

- Be aware of what you are spending. Write down everything you spend for a month to discover your habits.
- Use cash instead of a credit card for most purchases—you will pay more attention.
- Look for alternatives. Buying bottled water, for example, can costs hundreds of dollars a year. Carry your own refillable water bottle and save the money.
- Plan ahead to avoid impulse spending. If you have a healthy snack in your backpack, it's easier to avoid the vending machines when you're hungry on the way to class.

- Shop around, compare prices online, buy in bulk. Buy generic products instead of name brands.
- Stop to think a minute before spending. Often, this is all it takes to avoid budget-busting purchases. With larger purchases, postpone buying for a couple days. You may find you don't "need" it after all.
- Make and take along your own lunches instead of eating out on campus.
- Cancel cable TV and watch programs online for free.
- Use free campus and local Wi-Fi spots and cancel your home high-speed connection.
- Cancel your health club membership and use a free facility on campus or in the community.
- Avoid ATM fees by finding a machine on your card's network (or change banks); avoid checking account monthly fees by finding a bank with free checking.
- Get cash from an ATM only in small amounts so you never feel "rich."
- Look for free sources of entertainment instead of movies and concerts—most colleges have frequent free events.
- If you pay your own utility bills, make it a habit to conserve: Don't leave lights or your computer on all night.
- Use your study skills to avoid any risk of failing a class. Paying to retake a course is one of the quickest and most unfortunate ways to get in financial and, perhaps, academic trouble.

Managing a Budget

Most people do not use a budget to help manage their money—and most people in our society admit to frequent financial troubles. These two facts are clearly related.

How can you know if you can afford to buy a new laptop or cell phone right now? Can you afford to eat out tonight or should you go home and cook dinner? Should you take that weekend trip? Will you be tempted to spend the money because it is there in your checking account or because your credit card has not hit its limit yet? What about those textbooks you need to buy, or those groceries, or the utility bill that arrives tomorrow—will you have money for those things too?

Unless you keep a budget, you really can't know for sure. That seems so simple—but then again, *not* keeping a budget is why so many people have so many money problems. Using a budget is just like using a calendar to schedule your time: It keeps you on track. Managing a budget involves three steps:

1. Calculating all your monthly sources of income.
2. Calculating and analyzing all your monthly expenses.
3. Adjusting your budget (and lifestyle, if needed) to ensure the money isn't going out faster than it's coming in.

This may seem time-consuming the first time you create and use a budget, but this is time very well spent. Soon, it becomes an automatic, easy process.

Step 1: Calculate Your Income
Use Table 3-1 to account for all funds available to you on a monthly basis.

Step 2: Track Your Expenses
Tracking expenditures is more difficult than tracking income. Some fixed expenses (tuition, rent, etc.) you should already know, but until you have actually added up everything you spend money on for a typical month, it's hard to estimate how much

TABLE 3-1	MONTHLY INCOME AND FUNDS	

Source of Income/Funds	Amount in Dollars
Job income/salary (take-home amount)	_____
Funds from parents/family/others	_____
Monthly draw from savings	_____
Monthly draw from financial aid	_____
Monthly draw from student/other loans	_____
Other income source: _____	_____
Other income source: _____	_____
Other income source: _____	_____
Total Monthly Income	_____

you are really spending on cups of coffee or snacks between classes, groceries, entertainment, etc. You can start with the numbers you estimated earlier in *Where Does the Money Go?* Put these into the spaces in Table 3-2.

Note that there are *many* spending categories in Table 3-2. This is important because if you find you need to cut back your spending to stay on budget, you need to know *specifically* where you can make the cuts.

Step 3: Balance Your Budget

Now, compare your total monthly income with your total monthly expenditures. How balanced does your budget look at this point? Remember that you probably had to estimate several of your expenditures. You can't know for sure until you actually track your expenses for at least a month and have real numbers to work with.

If your expense total is significantly higher than your income total, then you will have to make adjustments. First, you need to make your budget work on paper. Go back through your expenditure list and see where you can eliminate items. Students cannot live like working professionals. There are many ways to spend less so that you can live within your budget. For example, if you discover that you have to increase what you spend for textbooks, you may choose to spend less on eating out—and subtract the amount from that category that you add to the textbook category. Get in the habit of thinking this way instead of reaching for a credit card when you don't have enough in your budget for something you want or need. This is a long-term strategy for controlling your financial life. A computer spreadsheet or financial program to track all your expenditures and manage your budget may facilitate this process.

School Loans, Grants, and More

Most schools offer financial aid. The federal government also offers several different types of aid. According to the U.S. Department of Education, millions of students receive some form of financial aid every year. Categories include the following:

- *Flexible payment plans.* Some schools allow students to make several smaller payments throughout the semester instead of paying one lump sum for tuition expenses.
- *Loans.* A loan is an amount of money given by a lender. Loans must be repaid within a certain period of time, usually with interest. The federal government, as well as private lenders (banks), offers several different types of student loans.

TABLE 3-2	MONTHLY EXPENDITURES	

Expenditures	Amount in Dollars
Tuition and fees (1/12 of annual)	_____
Textbooks and supplies (1/12 of annual)	_____
Housing: monthly mortgage, rent, or room and board	_____
Home repairs (estimated)	_____
Renter's insurance (1/12 of annual)	_____
Property tax (1/12 of annual)	_____
Average monthly utilities (electricity, water, gas, oil)	_____
Optional utilities (cell phone, Internet service, cable TV)	_____
Dependent care, babysitting	_____
Child support, alimony	_____
Groceries	_____
Meals and snacks out (including coffee, water, etc.)	_____
Personal expenses (toiletries, cosmetics, haircuts, etc.)	_____
Auto expenses (payments, gas, tolls) plus 1/12 of annual insurance premium—or public transportation costs	_____
Loan repayments, credit card payoff payments	_____
Health insurance (1/12 of annual)	_____
Prescriptions, medical expenses	_____
Entertainment (movies, concerts, nightlife, sporting events, purchases of CDs, DVDs, video games, etc.)	_____
Bank account fees, ATM withdrawal fees, credit card finance charges	_____
Travel, day trips	_____
Cigarettes, smokeless tobacco	_____
Beer, wine, liquor	_____
Gifts	_____
Hobbies	_____
Major purchases (computer, home furnishings) (1/12 of annual)	_____
Clothing, dry cleaning	_____
Memberships (health clubs, etc.)	_____
Pet food, veterinary bills, etc.	_____
Other expenditure: _____	_____
Other expenditure: _____	_____
Other expenditure: _____	_____
Other expenditure: _____	_____
Other expenditure: _____	_____
Total Monthly Expenses	_____

- *Grants and scholarships.* Unlike loans, grants and scholarships do not have to be paid back. The qualifications are often highly specific. There may be a grant or scholarship at your college or in your community that you qualify for.
- *Work-study programs.* Some schools participate in work-study programs by arranging part-time jobs for students with financial need.

Financial aid is available to most students. It is important to note that you should make an appointment with one of your school's financial aid advisors. An advisor can help determine which type of aid will work best for you. Never take out more loans than you really need for your education. Doing so could lead to a significant financial burden as you begin your new career.

Chapter Summary

- Control stress by setting priorities, simplifying your life, learning to relax, thinking positively, and maintaining social supports.
- Promote good health, reduce the risks of disease, and make it easier to succeed in school with regular exercise, good nutrition for physical and mental health, and plenty of sleep every night.
- Balance your school life with a social life that can contribute much to your well-being.
- Ensure you take steps to maintain your personal safety on and off campus.
- Use your personal budget to keep control over your finances and prevent debt that could stall your academic progress.

Review Questions

Objective Questions

1. The type of stress that causes positive reactions is referred to as _____.
2. Prolonged stress strengthens your immune system. (True or False?)
3. A task is _____ if it is important but does not need to be dealt with immediately.
4. Stress causes your nervous system to become overactive. (True or False?)
5. For your body to receive the full benefits of exercise, you should work out at least _____ times a week for _____ minutes at a time.
6. Vitamin B, vitamin C, and folic acid help your body handle stress. (True or False?)
7. A glass of wine will likely help you to sleep through the night. (True or False?)

Short-Answer Questions

1. Describe three specific stress reduction techniques that work for you as an individual.
2. Name four foods you will try to eat more of to improve your health and three dietary substances you will try to minimize in your meals. Explain why.
3. Describe the benefits of regular exercise.
4. Describe the benefits of creating and managing a budget.

Applications

1. Complete Tables 3-1 and 3-2. Make adjustments until you have a balanced budget.

Fundamental Writing Skills

The section in the writing skills chapter you should complete at the end of Chapter 3 is Section 11-3. You can find this section on pages 207-212.

4

Interacting With Others as a Healthcare Professional

OBJECTIVES

- Explain why you should get to know your instructors.
- Describe how participating in class contributes to your success as a student.
- List the benefits of networking with other students.
- Explain why you should participate in campus life.
- Explain why diversity is important.

Your success in school depends on more than simply sitting in classes, reading textbooks and doing homework, and completing assignments and tests. Education is an active learning process, and students learn most effectively through interacting with their professors and other students. This experience includes interacting one-on-one with your professor, participating in class discussions with the professor and other students, and networking with other students outside class. This chapter explains how to create a network that can benefit your studies while helping you share what you've learned with others. People in your network can be great resources of information, advice, and support. As you meet more people through all your educational experiences, you are also learning more about cultural diversity and gaining skills that will serve you well in your future as a healthcare professional (HCP).

Getting to Know Your Professors

From the first day of class, you should get to know your professors. At the start, you may wonder what your professors will be like. Will they be nice? Are they going to be fair? Will they present the material so you can understand it? Are you going to like and respect them? Are they going to like and respect you? As you listen and observe in class, you will begin to pick up on the instructor's personality, communication style, and perception of students.

Getting to know your professor will help you feel comfortable in the classroom more quickly. In turn, you will be able to concentrate on your studies sooner and more effectively.

Teaching Styles

Some professors like to share their philosophies about teaching. They'll also let you know how they prefer to run their classes.

- Some professors like a formal atmosphere in which they lecture and students raise their hands during a specified question-and-answer period.
- Others prefer a more informal environment in which there's open classroom discussion and students can interrupt at any time to ask questions.

Knowing your professor's teaching style gives you an advantage in the classroom. You'll learn to anticipate your instructor's next moves. This will help you study for exams, take effective notes, and participate in class. The sooner you can do this, the easier it will be to do well in the course.

Making a Good Impression

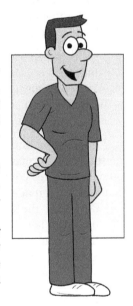

Getting to know your professors involves more than simply observing them. Keep in mind that they are observing you, too. You are making an impression whether you want to or not. You should want to make a good impression from the start by being attentive in class, participating in class discussions, and interacting with the professor.

An important first step is to introduce yourself to the professor early in the term, even on the first day of class. Although doing this may seem intimidating, this is a very important step toward becoming a successful student.

Most professors welcome opportunities to meet their students. They enjoy teaching, and they like to get to know their students. As soon as the professor learns your name and knows that you're serious about learning, you've taken an important step toward your success in the course.

Be Assertive

Try to introduce yourself in a manner that conveys confidence. Try saying something such as, "Hi, my name is Michael Adams. I'm taking this course for my Radiology Technician Degree. I'm really looking forward to a great semester. I'll see you at the next class." It's as simple as that.

You may want to plan ahead and practice what you're going to say. If you're especially nervous about this introduction, you might want to write down what you'd like to say and memorize it beforehand. When you approach the professor, relax by taking a slow, deep breath. Then, put on a friendly smile, make eye contact, and make your introduction. If you're comfortable offering a handshake, that would be appropriate, too.

If your professor didn't explain how to contact him or her outside of class, now is an ideal time to ask about that. Should you have any questions over the course of the semester, you'll need to know how to get in touch with your professor. Some professors prefer email. Others prefer a visit during their office hours or a phone call. Be sure to make a note of this information.

Making a Good First Impression

Some places, such as large lecture halls that hold hundreds of students, may not be the best places to introduce yourself after class. In these cases, consider seeking out the instructor during office hours to make your introduction. Your professor certainly will remember you and be impressed. Furthermore, in this more relaxed setting, the professor may engage you in conversation for a few minutes about your career plans or the class. You may walk away with some interesting insights and valuable information.

Instructor Conferences

You should try to have an individual conference with every instructor at least once during the semester or term. A student–teacher conference gives you the opportunity to ask questions about lecture content, learn about your instructor's expectations of students, or discuss any other important issues related to the course.

Here are a few tips to consider when scheduling a conference:

- Decide on a specific topic to discuss, such as your first test or a confusing concept from a recent lecture.
- Write down any questions you'd like to ask about that topic, putting your most important questions at the top of the list. After all, your instructor may have a limited amount of time to meet with you.

If you're organized and prepared for the meeting, you'll have a better chance of getting the information you need in that short period of time. Also, if the idea of a student–teacher conference makes you nervous, having questions already written out will put you at ease and help you stay focused.

By taking the initiative and meeting with your professor one-on-one, you'll demonstrate that you're engaged and concerned about your success as a student. You'll also gain a better understanding of your professor. This will help you to be aware of your instructor's expectations rather than blindly assuming you're doing well in the course.

Participating in Class

Participating in class—interacting with the instructor and other students as part of the group—is essential for being actively engaged in learning. Those who fail to participate, who sit passively in the classroom listening to others, are often not fully engaged. As a result, they may not learn as well as those who make the effort to speak up. This principle applies both in lecture and discussion classes as well as in laboratory classes.

Succeeding in Class

Here are several tactics you can use to join in and participate, helping to ensure your success in the classroom:

- Sit at the front of the room.
- Make sure you can see projection screens and in-class demonstrations.

- Make sure you can hear your instructor clearly.
- Ask questions of the instructor when appropriate.
- Answer questions the instructor asks the class.
- Respond to the comments of other students when invited by the instructor.

But Why Participate?

Remember that education is an *active* experience. You don't just passively receive knowledge and skills by sitting there like a stone. Participating in class is the best way to actively engage. Here are some of the benefits of participating:

- Research shows that students who actively engage by participating in class learn more—and thereby earn higher grades. One reason for this is that when you speak out in class and answer instructors' questions, you are more likely to remember the material than if you were passively listening to others speak.
- Paying close attention, thinking critically about what an instructor is saying, and making an effort to relate the lecture content can dramatically improve your enjoyment of the class and your impression of the professor. You also may discover your professor is much more interesting than you first thought.
- Asking the professor questions, answering the instructor's questions, and responding to other students' comments are all important ways to make a good impression on the professor. Then, in office hour visits and other interactions, the professor will remember you as an engaged student. This helps you form an effective relationship with the professor if you later need extra help or maybe even a mentor.
- Participating in class discussions is also a good way to start meeting other students. You may meet others with whom you can form a study group, from whom you can borrow notes if you miss a class, or with whom you can team up in a group project.

Sit in the Front Row

Most of us have been to school assemblies or conferences where there are rows of seats. The front of the room is where the speaker's chair or podium stands. As everyone files in to choose seats, not many people go straight to the front row to sit. Even when there is "standing room only," seats in the front row often stay empty. However, sitting up front in the classroom is actually very helpful.

Often, students would rather blend into the background. They don't want to be noticed by the professor or other students. Although you may have serious reservations about sitting at the front of the classroom, you'll find that sitting there is in your best interest.

If you believe that only the strongest students sit up front, you may be right. But they probably became strong students by choosing to sit up front, in addition to employing other strategies. Classroom success takes effort. Sitting in the front row is one way to demonstrate that you're willing to make that effort. Finally, you can more easily interact with the instructor when you sit up front.

When choosing a seat up front, be sure to find one that lets you hear the professor well. If you miss hearing important information in any class, your overall performance in the course can suffer.

Classrooms can often become quite noisy places, especially between tasks or when the professor is assigning new tasks—for instance, when he or she discusses clinical rotation assignments. This is a very exciting time in health professions classes. Often, before the professor can finish explaining all the details, students start talking among themselves. Some students begin asking the instructor questions while other students continue talking back and forth. The noise level rises. Unfortunately, this is when students either completely miss what the instructor is saying or hear it incorrectly and then misinformation can be passed from student to student.

By sitting near the instructor, however, you'll be more likely to hear over the noise. When you're able to hear clearly, you can be one of the informed students who leave class knowing exactly when and where you are supposed to go for your clinical assignment.

Steps to Better Class Participation

If you're one of those students who has always sat quietly in class, you may have to take active steps to start participating. The following are some tips to getting started.

When your instructor asks a question to the class:

- Raise your hand and make eye contact, but don't wave your hand all around trying to catch attention or call out.
- Be sure you have something to say before speaking. Take a moment to gather your thoughts, and if you're nervous, take a deep breath. Speak calmly and clearly.

When you want to ask the professor a question:

- Don't ever think your question is "stupid." If you have been paying attention in class and have done the reading and you still don't understand something, you have every right to ask. Many others in the class may have the same question.
- Ask at the appropriate time. Even if the instructor has said you can ask a question at any time, don't try to interrupt the instructor mid-sentence. Wait for a natural pause and a good moment to ask. However, unless the instructor has asked students to hold all questions until the end of class, don't let too much time go by or you may forget your question.
- Be sure what you're asking is a real question, not an admission that you weren't paying attention. If you drifted off during the first half of class, try not to ask a question about something that was already covered.
- Try to remain open-minded and show you really do want to learn. Try not to let your question sound like a complaint or disagreement. You may want to ask, "Why would so-and-so believe that? That's just crazy!" But take a moment to think about what you're feeling. It's more effective to say, "I don't understand what so-and-so is saying here. What evidence did he or she use to argue for that position?"
- Be sensitive to the needs of other students and try to avoid dominating a discussion.

When your instructor asks you a question directly:

- Be honest and admit it if you don't know the answer or are not sure. Don't try to fake understanding or make excuses. With a question that asks for an opinion, feel free to express your ideas openly. If you don't have an opinion yet, you should feel comfortable saying why.
- Organize your thoughts before answering. Instructors seldom want just a yes-or-no answer. Give your answer and then provide reasons for your position.

Student Participation Helps the Professor

By staying engaged and asking questions about the lecture, you'll also help your professor clear up any misunderstandings about the material. Other students might be confused about the same concepts that are confusing to you. The professor's answers to your questions may be helpful to your classmates as well.

Finally, by speaking up in class, you'll let your professor know how well you're grasping the material he or she is presenting. When the professor believes that students are keeping up with the pace of the class, he or she will know the teaching is effective. If students are not keeping up, the professor can make adjustments or present the material in a different way.

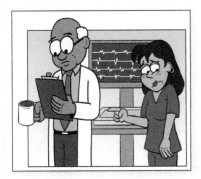

There Are No Stupid Questions—Amalia

Amalia is having trouble understanding how to read an EKG. Shy and unsure of herself, she's afraid to ask the professor a question about how to it. She's also afraid of holding up the class and perhaps appearing unprepared. If you were Amalia's lab partner, what could you say to help her feel more comfortable asking the question?

Networking With Other Students

Networking with other students is another important way to actively engage in your education. Networking should be an integral part of what you do—not only while you're in school but also later on in your healthcare career. In school, your network is an informal academic support system that you develop with some of your classmates.

So what exactly is networking? How does it differ from simply having friends?

Your Network

You've heard of television networks and computer networks. A network is an interconnected group or system. A television network is a group of local stations that shares the same programming. A computer network is a group of computers that shares information. A network can be big or small.

A network is also a group of people who choose to share information and expertise with one another. Usually, people network with others who share their interests or occupation. A network has several key features:

- It is voluntary—you choose to join and participate in a network.
- It is focused—you share information and expertise on a specific topic.
- It is respectful—members all treat each other with respect, sharing ideas and asking questions freely.

Sometimes, a network forms naturally. For example, your instructor might put you into a group in class. You might find this group stays together even after the course is over. But most often, networks have to be purposely created.

Why Network?

Networking is valuable for many reasons. Having a study group you can count on, getting tips for succeeding in a certain professor's course, and being able to borrow notes from someone when you can't get to class are all good reasons to network. As a student, networking gives you advantages you wouldn't have if you chose to keep to yourself.

Perhaps the most important reason to network is to give and receive support. Your peers at school probably understand better than anyone else the challenges you're facing. Members of your network can offer support by:

- listening to your ideas
- sharing ideas with you
- making study time more enjoyable
- helping you in difficult times

Networks provide support by bringing people with the same goals together to help each other. The more you give, the more you get, and the better you feel.

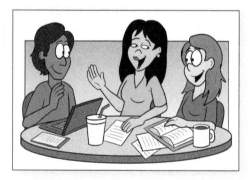

Unexpected Benefits of Networking—Thuy

At first, Thuy didn't like the idea of networking when she started taking courses. It was hard for her to meet new people, and she usually preferred to work on her own anyway.

However, when she started having trouble in her medical terminology course, she knew she had to ask for help. Her academic advisor suggested that she talk to some of her classmates and try to form a study group. This wasn't easy, but she introduced herself to a couple of the other women in her class, and the three of them started meeting regularly every week. Not only did her grades improve but she also ended up gaining two friends—something she hadn't expected at all.

Creating an Informal Network

Even if you're shy or not very good at meeting new people, you'll find that informal networking is fairly simple and painless. Begin by introducing yourself to students sitting near you in class. If a conversation ensues, good. If not, you can speak to them again at the next class.

After you've spoken to another student a few times, bring up the idea that the two of you could work together. Propose that the two of you periodically share or compare lecture notes. Mention that you think doing this might help both of you understand the material better. You also can offer to share your notes if your classmate ever has to miss a lecture. If you're willing to help someone else, that person may be willing to share information with you.

Because everyone's schedules are already full, you may at first have difficulty arranging a time to meet. You might suggest meeting in the campus library or student study lounge a few minutes before class once a week. Your new acquaintances might not take you up on your offer right away. If they don't like the idea of networking, they may not realize they're turning down an excellent opportunity. If the first student you talk to is not interested, don't take it personally. Just move on, meet other classmates, and try again.

Creating a More Formal Network

Creating a more formal network requires three things:

1. You have a reason for forming the network, which helps to keep the network focused. The reason may be to form a study group, for example. This study technique is discussed in more detail in Chapter 7.
2. You add value to the network. You can contribute information as well as consume it.
3. You have rules for participation.

Creating a network takes time, but it's worth the effort. If you develop a network of people you know and like, who can help you *and* learn from you, then you'll get the full benefit of this kind of interaction. Learning how to network successfully is very important for your future career as an HCP, when you'll need to keep up on the latest information and techniques.

The Members of Your Network

Begin by making a list of some classmates you'd like to include in your network. Choose two or three people from that list. Your network can grow over time, but it's best to start small. You'll find it's easier with a small group to get to know everyone and to arrange times to meet.

To narrow your list, think about the people you've included:

- How much time does each person have to spend?
- How might each person contribute?
- What are people's strengths and weaknesses?
- Have you ever worked together before?

Weaknesses don't necessarily disqualify someone—we all have them. But think about how that person will fit into the group.

Setting Up the Rules

Once you have your list, approach the people on it and suggest networking. The key here is to be clear about what you're proposing and to be respectful. If you want to have an informal network, in which members email or text when they have a question or something to contribute, explain that. If you want a formal network, in which members meet regularly—in addition to emailing, texting, or having one-on-one conversations—make that clear.

Remember to be open to the suggestions and constraints of others. If someone can't meet when you'd like but is very valuable to the network, be flexible so you can include that person. If someone doesn't have the time or simply doesn't want to be part of a formal network, graciously thank that person and look for someone else. That student can still be a personal, one-on-one source of information and sharing for you.

Using Your Network

Remember, networking means interaction. Everyone in the network contributes information *and* consumes it. That's what makes the network valuable: Everyone benefits from everyone else's knowledge and different ways of looking at things. When you network, you share what you know with others who do the same, creating something new in the combination of ideas. It's the sharing of ideas, or the dialogue, that makes a network successful.

Give Credit Where Credit Is Due

Information shared in a network is free. If something is shared in a network, all the members of the network should be allowed to use the information. But that doesn't mean you write down what someone else says and pass it off as your own opinion or knowledge. Always acknowledge the other members of your network. Be honest by saying your idea was inspired by someone in your network.

Stay Safe

Once your networking group is established, you're likely to have people's phone numbers and other personal information, such as email addresses or home addresses. Guard these carefully and don't share them with anyone without asking first. Furthermore, remember not to wear out your network with constant contact, especially with network members who are busy with their home lives and jobs.

When to Network

Informal networking goes on all the time—between classes, over lunch, and on the phone. Activate your formal network at specific times:

- *At the beginning of the semester.* Find out which students in your class have had this instructor before and what you should expect. Ask them for tips and advice about being successful in this class, but *never* ask for old tests and quizzes.
- *After class or lab sessions.* Talk about the ideas you had during class, find out what your classmates thought, and then debate and expand the conversation. Take notes of your conversations next to your lecture notes.
- *After a missed class.* Call on your network to fill you in, but remember not to lean on your network to do your work for you.

Network Online

You also can network online. This works well for a network that is spread out. For instance, if your cousin is an HCP in another state, you can include him or her in an online network. Just remember to be careful online. All the rules for face-to-face networks apply here. Only talk online with people you trust and don't invite strangers in without talking with the whole group first. Avoid giving out network members' email addresses. You should only share information online with people you know and trust.

Academic Advisors and Counselors

So far in this chapter, we've discussed the many benefits of interacting with both instructors and other students—and the value this has for your academic success and future career. But there are others, too, on campus with whom your interaction is very important, including those in administrative and counseling offices. Among these, the most important for students are academic advisors.

They Are Here to Help

A school's academic advisors are there to guide students. Advisors work with course catalogs and student problems every day. If you have a question about your program's requirements, or if you just need advice, your school's academic advisors are great resources. They can often provide you with information you won't find in the college catalog.

It's also important to establish a relationship with your academic advisors for the future. While most schools have career services offices that offer job placement services, your academic advisors may be important contacts to have in your network once you begin looking for a full-time position in your field.

Campus Life

The social world of your school is an important part of the total experience. Social relationships help make you feel more at home on campus and contribute to your happiness and success as a student. Take advantage of opportunities to meet new people and become involved in campus life.

- Leave the opportunity open for meeting new people. For example, don't follow the same routine with your meals on campus, but try to sit with different people so you can get to know them in a relaxed setting. Study in a common area or lounge where others may happen on you when you need to take a break or study with someone else.
- Stay open in your interests. Don't limit yourself just to past interests, or you'll miss many opportunities to make friendships that may start based on some other activity.
- On the other hand, don't try to get involved in everything going on around you. Overcommitting yourself to too many activities, or trying to join too many social groups, may cause you to spread yourself too thin. Remember, it's the quality, not the quantity, of your social interactions that matters.
- Let others see who you really are. How can others know they want to spend time interacting with you if they don't know who you are? Take the time to get to know them and to let them get to know you.
- Show some interest in others. Don't talk just about your interests—ask others about theirs. Show other students that you're interested, that you think they're worth spending time with, that you really do want to get to know them. You can easily show your feelings with casual comments like, "It was really fun studying together—I think we should do it again!"
- Once a friendship has started, be a good friend. Respect your friend for who he or she is and don't criticize that person or talk behind his or her back. Take the time to understand your friend when he or she is feeling sad, or frustrated, or just "needs a friend." Give emotional support when your friend needs it and accept his or her support as well when you need it.

Clubs and Organizations

Organized groups and activities offer a great way to enrich your social interactions on campus. But participating in organized activities requires some initiative—you can't be passive and expect these opportunities to come looking for you. A stimulating life on campus offers many benefits, including the following:

- Organized groups and activities facilitate your transition into your new life as a student.
- Organized groups and activities help you experience a much greater variety of social life. If you interact only with other students your own age with similar backgrounds, you'll miss out on the broader campus diversity: students who are older and may have a perspective you may otherwise miss, upperclassmen who can share much from their experience, and students of diverse heritage or culture whom you might not meet otherwise.
- Organized groups and activities help you gain new skills, whether technical, physical, intellectual, or social. Such skills may find their way into your résumé when you next seek a job, scholarship, or other future educational opportunity. Employers like to see well-rounded students with a range of proficiencies and experiences.
- Organized groups and activities are fun and a great way to relieve stress and stay healthy. As discussed in Chapter 3, exercise and physical activity are essential for health and well-being, and many organized activities offer a good way to keep moving.

Finding Activities You Like

There are many ways to learn about groups on your campus and opportunities for various activities. Start by browsing the school's website, where you're likely to find links to student clubs and organizations. Watch for club fairs, open houses, and similar activities on campus. Especially near the beginning of the year, an activity fair may include tables set up by many groups to provide students with information. Look for notices on bulletin boards around campus. Stop by the appropriate school office, such as the student affairs or student activities office or cultural center. Most schools attempt to provide information about all clubs and groups on campus.

Diversity

We live in an increasingly diverse society. In many parts of the country, Latinos comprise more than 50% of the population, and as of 2020, one in three Americans, and about half of all college students, is a person of color. But the word *diversity* refers to much more than racial and ethnic differences. Diversity refers to the great variety of human characteristics—ways that we are different even though we are all human and share more similarities than differences. These differences enrich humanity and all of us as individuals.

Experiencing diversity while in school brings many benefits both in the present and for the future:

- Experiencing diversity in school prepares you for the diversity you will encounter throughout your life. As an HCP, you will work with other professionals and patients who may be very different from you. Success in your future career will require you to understand and interact with people in new ways and with new skills. Experiencing diversity in school assists in this process.
- Research indicates that students learn more effectively in a diverse educational setting. Encountering new concepts, values, and behaviors leads to thinking in deeper, more complex, more creative ways. Studies have shown, for example, that students who experience racial and ethnic diversity in their classes are more engaged in active thinking processes and develop more intellectual and academic skills than others with limited experience of diversity.

- Experiencing diversity on campus is beneficial for all students as they have more fulfilling social relationships and report more satisfaction and involvement with their academic experience.
- Experiencing diversity helps break patterns of separateness and prejudice that have characterized American society throughout its history. Discrimination against others—whether by race, gender, age, sexual orientation, or anything else—is rooted in ignorance and sometimes the fear of people who are different. Getting to know people who are different is the first step in accepting those differences, furthering the goal of our society becoming free of all forms of prejudice and unfair treatment of people.
- Experiencing diversity makes us all better citizens in our democracy. When we can more effectively understand and consider the ideas and perspectives of others, we are better equipped to participate meaningfully in our society. This is especially important for those in healthcare careers.
- Experiencing diversity enhances self-awareness. We gain insights into our own thought processes, life experiences, and values as we learn from people whose backgrounds and experiences are different from our own.

What Is Cultural Diversity?

When people talk about cultural diversity, they are referring to the ways in which all people are similar to and different from each other. Racial classifications, ethnicity, gender, sexual orientation, religious affiliation, socioeconomic status, and age are all elements of cultural diversity.

It's natural to note differences between yourself and those around you. As you enter the world of health care, you should understand that, regardless of differences, you must treat everyone with equal care and respect. This means refusing to allow any preconceived ideas about others to affect the quality of your work. By openly accepting diversity, we can move closer toward appreciating the things that make people different and treating everyone with the same care and respect.

Cultural diversity is an especially important part of health care because of the genetic characteristics, cultural values, and belief systems that affect people's health. By knowing and understanding these cultural differences, you'll be able to provide better care.

Race and Ethnicity

The term *race* is typically based on a person's physical characteristics, such as skin color, facial features, hair texture, and body stature. *Ethnicity* is the concept of identifying with the traditions and values of a particular cultural group. Although the terms *ethnicity* and *race* are often used interchangeably, they refer to different aspects of a person's identity. An individual can be of one race, yet identify with a different ethnicity.

In health care, race is sometimes a factor in diagnosis and treatment because genetic traits are often more common in certain racial groups than in others. Likewise, ethnic values and traditions can also affect a patient's health and well-being.

Gender Roles

It's important to consider gender roles when interacting with others of a different background. In some cultures, for example, the male is considered the head of the household. In these cases, a male family member might speak for his female family members. In other cultures, women are the dominant family members. It's important that HCPs consider this when providing care. Gender roles may influence the way in which a patient prefers to be treated. Every patient has a different role in the family, and as an HCP you should be sensitive to the different needs and priorities of each.

Sexual Orientation

A person's sexual orientation is a personal matter—for you, your fellow students, and patients and coworkers with whom you will interact in the future. Again, you should not prejudge another person but accept all forms of diversity. In health care, there are times when sexual orientation may be an important issue, such as when addressing sexually transmitted diseases. Regardless of what information patients choose to reveal, it's important to avoid making judgments or assumptions about a patient's sexual orientation or lifestyle choices.

Religion

Everyone has freedom of religion in our society and all people's religious choices should be respected. In health care, patients' religious beliefs and values may affect how they wish to be treated by HCPs. For example, a person's religious affiliation can influence decisions about diet and nutrition, sexual lifestyle, and other health matters. As an HCP, you'll need to be sensitive to each patient's values and beliefs when providing care. You can do this by respecting the personal choices made by patients and adapting care to suit each patient's needs.

Socioeconomic Status

Socioeconomic status is yet another way in which people are different, and no one should be judged or discriminated against based on such differences. A person's socioeconomic status should not affect the kind of care and treatment that an HCP provides. Every patient, regardless of financial situation, should be given the best possible care and attention. Avoid stereotyping patients according to their level of education or how much money they make. Instead, focus on each patient as an individual worthy of your attention, respect, and sensitivity.

Age

Age is another of the many ways in which individuals differ. In health care, age is often important because the aging process affects the health of patients in different ways. Younger patients often have healthcare needs different from those of older patients. You'll need to be sensitive to patients' changing physical and emotional needs as they grow older. It's also essential that you avoid making assumptions about a patient based on age. It is important to remember that physical fitness and health can vary for different people at every age and stage in their lives.

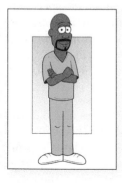

Fitting In—Devon

At 34, and with two children, Devon sometimes wondered whether he really fits in with the other students in his classes, most of whom were at least 10 years younger. However, he has come to discover that some of the younger students recognize that he has had valuable life experiences and therefore has much to offer. What are some ways diversity in the classroom positively impacts the learning experience? How do the diverse members of your class contribute in positive ways?

The Importance of Celebrating Diversity

Diversity is not something just to know in your head like a concept you've learned in school. Diversity is an essential part of the rich experience of humanity—something to be celebrated and embraced as part of being human. Don't think of diversity as something to be aware of just in your future healthcare profession as you work with patients. You'll grow as a person as you seek out diverse experiences now as a student and actively promote understanding of the many differences among us all.

Here are suggestions for what you can do to celebrate diversity, challenge old stereotypes, and promote a healthy multiculturalism on your campus and in your community:

- Acknowledge your own uniqueness, for you, too, are diverse.
- Consider your own (possibly unconscious) stereotypes so you can work to eliminate them.
- Don't try to ignore differences among people.
- Don't expect all individuals within any group to be alike.
- Don't apply any group generalizations to individuals.
- Take advantage of campus opportunities to increase your cultural awareness, such as cultural fairs and celebrations, concerts, and other programs.
- Take the initiative in social interactions with members of diverse populations.
- Work through any conflicts as in any other social interaction.
- Take a stand against prejudice and hate when you see them.

Chapter Summary

- Make a good first impression on your professors. Introduce yourself and plan a visit for an individual conference during office hours.
- Sit in the front of the room. Have a great seat with the best view and best sound. This sets you up for successful participation in class.
- Ask questions in class and answer those posed by your instructors. Active engagement in the process is the most effective way to learn.
- Network with other students to get ahead. Develop good study networks that will help you learn and support your academic goals.
- Networking is important because it allows you to share your ideas and learn from others. Networks also can be a source of support during the challenges you face as a student.
- Investigate campus organizations and activities to become part of the wider academic community while having fun and maintaining your health.
- Challenge yourself to more effectively understand and celebrate the differences among people. Never prejudge others who are different from you in any way.

Review Questions

Objective Questions

1. Sitting in the front row of the classroom is not a good idea because you won't be able to see all of the other students behind you. (True or False?)
2. You should understand from the start of any class that the professor is really only interested in the material and not the students. (True or False?)

3. A _____ is a group of people who choose to share information and expertise with one another.

4. In addition to speaking up in class and asking and answering questions, you should make time to visit the professor during his or her _____.

5. Experiencing diversity can help you learn more effectively and enjoy your education. (True or False?)

Short-Answer Questions

1. Why is it important to sit in the front of the classroom?

2. What is an example of a time when health professions classrooms become particularly noisy? Why is it essential to be able to hear your instructor at a time like this?

3. Give an example of how you might be making an impression on your instructors even when you may not be aware of it.

4. How would introducing yourself to your instructor help prepare you for future clinical experience?

5. List three benefits of developing both an informal and formal network with other students.

6. What are two challenges you might face when creating a network?

7. List at least six ways in which people may be different from each other.

8. Why should diversity be celebrated?

Applications

1. Networking Exercise: Talk with at least two fellow students at school about creating a network. Each of you will then come up with one other person you know and trust from one of your classes. Give yourselves a week to contact the other people. Then, meet as a group to see how you all get along. If everyone seems like compatible network members, decide on a place and time to meet regularly.

2. Campus Life Activity: Using the suggestions presented in this chapter to learn about campus organizations and activities at your school, find at least three in which you might be interested in participating. Using the school's website or other resources, investigate these three to learn more about what goes on in each. Discuss your findings with a partner.

Fundamental Writing Skills

The section in the writing skills chapter you should complete at the end of Chapter 4 is Section 11-4. You can find this section on pages 212-220.

PART 2

SHARPENING YOUR SKILLS

NOTES FOR PART 2

5

Making the Most of Your Learning Style as a Healthcare Professional

OBJECTIVES

- Describe the brain's role in learning.
- Identify your learning style and know how to make the most of it.
- Explain how critical thinking applies in healthcare settings.
- Describe Benjamin Bloom's six levels of cognitive learning.

Do you know there are different styles of learning? For example, you might absorb information better when you see it (as in a chart) than when you hear it (as in a lecture). Some people learn better when they can "do" the material, as in a lab experiment. Most classes are made up of students who have a variety of different learning styles. What works for one student might not work as well for the next.

This chapter discusses several major learning styles and how you can use your individual learning style, as well as other methods, to become a successful student. We'll also talk about the importance of critical thinking and how it relates to both learning and your future career.

Learning Styles

Your brain, and how it functions, is a contributing factor to the way you learn. By understanding how your brain works, you'll be on your way to understanding your particular learning style. And by being aware of your learning style, you'll discover ways you can learn more efficiently.

The Brain and Learning

The human brain weighs about 3 pounds. Although small, this organ functions as the control center for the entire body. It determines how a person thinks, feels, and acts. The brain is where all learning takes place.

Brain Zones

The three main areas of the brain include:

- the brain stem
- the cerebellum
- the cerebrum

Your Hardworking Brain

It's true that people use only a percentage of the brain's full capability. Even so, the human brain is responsible for an amazing number of functions, each of which takes place in specialized areas of the brain.

- Brain stem (lowest level of the brain; connects the brain with the spinal cord)
  - Involuntary functions and life-sustaining processes such as circulation, respiration, and digestion
- Cerebellum (between the brain stem and the cerebrum)
  - Balance and coordination of skilled voluntary movements
- Cerebrum (highest and most complex level of the brain; accounts for 80% of the brain's weight)
  - Voluntary initiation of movements
  - Sensory perception (sight, hearing, smell, touch, and taste)
  - Language
  - Personality, intellect, memory, emotional reactions, reasoning, and thinking
  - Thermoregulation

On a Cellular Level

There are two main types of cells in the brain:

- *Glial cells* provide structural and metabolic support for neurons.
- *Neurons* are cells specialized for transmitting information in the form of electrical signals. Neurons communicate extensively with other neurons in the brain. They also obtain sensory input and communicate with effector tissues, such as muscle and glands, in the peripheral parts of the body. Amazingly, electrical signals travel along the length of a neuron at a rate of 200 miles per hour (100 meters per second).

Making Connections

Each infant is born with a complete set of neurons. As a child learns, those neurons develop connections between themselves. Every time sensory cells are stimulated by outside forces, nerve impulses travel from one neuron to the next in the brain.

Every time you learn something new, the neurons in your brain begin sending messages in a certain pattern. If stimulation is repeated, it becomes easier for the same nerve impulses to travel from one neuron to the next. This is because patterns begin to form, and the neurons involved gain better connections between themselves. Your neurons "learn" these patterns and develop faster ways of communicating with each other. This is the foundation of memory or learning.

Losing Ground

Learning new information causes the number of connections between your neurons to increase. However, as soon as you stop learning new things, some of those connections begin to disappear. The solution to the problem is continued learning. You can rebuild those lost connections by relearning things you've forgotten.

What's Your Style?

Now that we have looked at how the brain functions, let's focus on learning styles. A learning style is an individual's preferred way to receive and process information during the learning process. One student may learn better by reading about a topic, whereas another student may learn better by hearing the instructor talk about the topic.

Three major learning styles are:

- visual
- auditory
- kinesthetic

It's likely that you prefer one particular learning style to the rest. There is no right or wrong style, no best or worst style—people simply learn in different ways. The key is to identify your own style and then use this knowledge to your advantage. Being aware of your learning strengths can help you improve your studying and test-taking skills. You'll also be better equipped to compensate for your weaknesses. By making your learning style work for you, you'll get more out of your courses. You'll have improved interaction with your instructors and other students. As an added benefit, you'll also more fully enjoy the learning process.

Visual Learners

Visual learners prefer to read about things or watch demonstrations. They like looking at charts, diagrams, and images. They like it quiet when they study. They may use arrows and circles when taking notes to visually show relationships of ideas or their importance.

If you're a visual learner, seek out all kinds of visual materials. These include the following:

- Textbooks
- Demonstrations (in class or on video)
- Handouts from your instructors
- Information on the Internet
- Lecture notes

Here are some study tips for visual learners:

- Sit near the front of the classroom.
- Pay close attention to visual presentations.
- Take notes using visual cues (circles, arrows, color highlighting, concept maps).
- Highlight in your textbook and jot margin notes.
- Make flashcards that include visual cues to help you remember key concepts.
- When studying, visualize things the instructor wrote on the board or included in a PowerPoint presentation.

Visual Learners—Amalia and Jenna

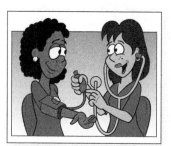

Amalia found the lecture on the theory behind taking a patient's blood pressure confusing. However, when her professor demonstrated how to perform this skill in the medical assisting lab, Amalia understood the concept more clearly.

Jenna was confused by the textbook description of how to assess gait. However, she immediately understood when she observed a demonstration in the physical therapist assistant lab.

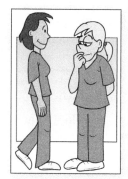

Auditory Learners

Auditory learners gain the most information when they hear about things. This includes listening to your instructor and other students as well as recorded presentations. If you learn best by listening, think of where you can find auditory information. Resources that may be helpful to you include the following:

- Class discussions
- Class lectures
- Question-and-answer sessions
- Reading aloud
- Recorded lectures or speeches (video or online)

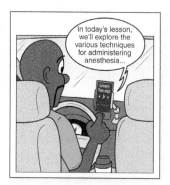

An Auditory Learner—Devon

Devon finds it helpful to tape lectures and listen to them a second time as he drives to work. The more times he hears the material, the more likely he is to remember it.

Here are some study tips for auditory learners:

- Choose a class seat where you can hear well without noisy distractions.
- Form a study group with others who prefer to talk over course topics.
- Read your notes and new material out loud when studying.
- Record key class lectures (with the instructor's permission) and review later as needed.
- Be sure to participate in class.

Kinesthetic Learners

Kinesthetic learners prefer to learn by doing. They like to move around and may have difficulty sitting still for long periods. They prefer a hands-on approach to learning. If it's easier for you to grasp information after putting it to use by actively doing something, you're a kinesthetic learner. Enhance your learning opportunities by trying the following:

- Seek out workshops and skills labs.
- Volunteer to perform in-class demonstrations.
- Attend field trips.
- Help out with group projects.
- Seek out internships or volunteer work in your field.
- Offer to tutor a classmate.

Here are some study tips for kinesthetic learners:

- Use interactive computer learning aids to engage with the subject.
- Study while physically moving; take frequent breaks to walk around; read assignments on a treadmill or exercise bike.

Kinesthetic Learners—Michael and Thuy

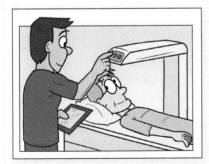

Michael grasped the basics of how to position a patient's elbow for an x-ray; however, he excelled in the radiology lab where he performed this skill.

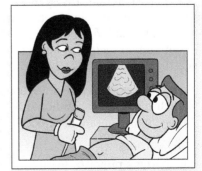

Thuy had trouble understanding the procedure when her professor described how to perform an abdominal ultrasound during the lecture. However, she better understood and performed well when she practiced this skill in the lab.

- Make flashcards frequently and sort them into groups to show relationships between ideas.
- If having difficulty sitting still, chew gum, walk around, or rock in a chair while reading or studying.
- Talk to a study partner while walking or jogging.
- Hold or play with an object such as a pencil or an eraser while studying.

Discovering Your Own Learning Style

From the preceding discussion, you probably already have a good idea about your own style. In reality, however, few people have purely only one learning style. You may favor one dominant approach, but likely you still learn through other styles also. To gain more insight for your preferences and receive tips to help you learn as fully as possible, take a few minutes to check out the learning styles assessment by accessing the following website: https://www.how-to-study.com /learning-style-assessment.

Your Learning Style

With a partner, discuss the strategies you use to help you learn. What kind of learner are you? How can you improve your strategies to further enhance your learning?

Students with different learning styles, or mixes of styles, will gain from different study and preparation techniques. It pays to find out what works best for you!

How Large Do You Think?

Another difference in how people learn and think involves the scope of thought. Some people just naturally think in large, abstract terms—thinking globally. Others naturally think more in terms of the details. As with the previous learning styles, understanding your own thinking and learning preferences can help maximize your learning in classes.

Global Learners

Global learners excel when they think about the "big picture." If you're a global learner, you may find that you enjoy learning how concepts are related to one another. Your favorite instructor may be one who gives plenty of analogies to show how the information is connected. Or you may prefer a class where the instructor lays out certain facts and helps students make conclusions about the material. If this is the case, try using the following tips to get the most out of your courses:

- Summarize your lecture notes and draw conclusions about the material.
- Sketch diagrams to show how different ideas come together to form the "big picture."
- Come up with questions about the topics covered in class.

Detail Learners

Detail learners prefer to learn new information in a logical pattern. For example, many people have had the experience of purchasing items labeled "some assembly required." If you're prone to looking at instruction manuals and following directions closely—as opposed to jumping right in and randomly trying to fit pieces together—you're probably a detail learner.

If you're a detail learner, you may do best in a class where the instructor follows a strict outline or explains processes in a step-by-step manner. Regardless of your instructor's teaching style, there are ways you can use your strengths to your advantage:

- Summarize your lecture notes with bulleted points.
- Draw diagrams to relate small pieces of information (details) to larger themes or ideas.
- Create a to-do list for yourself before you sit down to study.
- Write down questions as they come to mind during lectures or while reading.
- Think of examples you can use to illustrate particular details.

Critical Thinking and Learning

Closely related to learning skills are critical thinking skills. It's especially important for healthcare professionals to have solid critical thinking skills. When you think critically, you analyze information to form judgments about it. The information may be gathered from your observations, personal experience, reasoning, or communication. In your profession, you may be required to gather and analyze information and evaluate results on a daily basis. If you're able to think critically and make good judgments based on the information you can gather, you'll have a positive impact on your patients' health.

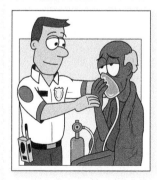

Critical Thinking Skills in the Workplace—Michael

As a medic in the army, Michael used his critical thinking skills every day when he assessed wounded soldiers and had to decide which injury was most serious and how to proceed. He uses these same critical thinking skills as an Emergency Medical Technician (EMT) while he is in school to become a radiology technician. With a partner, discuss what critical thinking skills you need in your current job. What critical thinking skills do you expect to need in your chosen healthcare profession?

Direct Yourself to Learning

Individuals who are successful in both school and the workplace have achieved their success by becoming self-directed learners. Being a self-directed learner means that you take responsibility for your own education, regardless of your preferred learning style. In the coming chapters, you'll learn more about different ways to accomplish this.

For example, if you're having a hard time understanding a particular concept in class, you can find other resources, ask your instructor for clarification, or meet with your study group. Although test scores are important, your main goal in school should be to learn the material. Being a self-directed learner means studying not only to do well on tests and quizzes but also to store information in your long-term memory. It means being able to apply that information to new situations once you become a practicing healthcare professional.

Likewise, successful professionals must be self-directed learners. Once you are no longer a student, you'll have to take even more responsibility for your own learning. This may mean keeping yourself up-to-date on the latest research by reading articles related to your field or requesting to observe a procedure you've been struggling to learn. In these cases, you should be aware of what you need to learn and how you can go about increasing your knowledge and improving your skills.

Regardless of your past experience as a student, you can achieve success now by becoming a self-directed learner. You have chosen to further your education because of your motivation toward a particular career goal. Contrary to how you may feel at first, you *can* control a great deal of what you learn and how your educational experience will unfold.

Learning is a process. By understanding how the process works, you can begin to develop the learning skills you'll use as a student and later in your professional career.

Bloom's Learning Levels (Bloom's Taxonomy)

Cognitive learning, closely related to critical thinking, occurs in several stages. Benjamin Bloom, a noted neuropsychologist, assigned the following names to these stages in the 1950s:

- Knowledge
- Comprehension
- Application
- Analysis
- Synthesis
- Evaluation

Although other psychologists have developed new theories about thinking since the 1950s, most theories are similar to Bloom's. In other theories, the stages may be named or ordered differently, but their descriptions remain relatively similar.

Knowledge

During the knowledge stage, you memorize information and repeat it word for word. At this point, you don't necessarily have to understand the information to memorize it. Some examples of things you may need to memorize are:

- formulas in a math class
- people's names, addresses, and phone numbers
- simple instructions, such as steps in a clinical skill (e.g., taking vital signs)

Comprehension

In the comprehension stage, you understand information enough to be able to restate it in your own words. If you take effective notes during class, your notes should reflect your comprehension. You can accomplish this by:

- drawing charts and diagrams
- summarizing and paraphrasing information

- describing how concepts are related
- explaining the material to someone else

Application

During this stage, you use the information you've memorized and comprehended to accomplish a task. Examples of application include:

- using a mathematical formula to solve a problem
- using a rule or principle to classify information
- successfully completing a project after receiving and following directions
- completing a lab assignment for a science class

Analysis

Analysis involves breaking information into parts to understand how those parts are organized and related to one another. For example, when you read an article in a magazine, you first look at the different pieces of information presented. An author may provide several anecdotes to illustrate a single main point. Then, you analyze the different pieces of information by thinking about how they are related. How does each anecdote relate to the author's theme or main point? What message is the author communicating?

Synthesis

In the synthesis stage, you put your analysis to use by developing a new idea. In a sense, you take parts of information and put them together in a different way to form a new concept. This stage of learning and thinking is more creative than the others. It includes:

- building on the pieces of information contained in your notes and writing a paper or presentation or solving a patient case study
- forming a plan for conducting a lab experiment

Evaluation

During the last stage in critical thinking, you evaluate information. This means you use other methods, such as comprehension and analysis, to determine whether information has value or relevance. Evaluation can include:

- determining which conclusions are supported by facts and research
- judging the value of a work of art or a piece of writing based on specific standards
- determining the value and relevance of information presented in a textbook, lecture, or class discussion

Be Critical

When reading your textbooks or other material, you shouldn't just passively receive the information but rather be an active reader. During active reading, it's important to be a critical reader. Now is the time to analyze the text and question the author. By asking questions about the text, you'll begin to think critically about the material. As a result, you'll improve your comprehension and remember more. You'll be better able to apply, analyze, and evaluate the information. Ask yourself:

- How would I apply this information if I were caring for a patient?
- How is this material related to what I've studied in the past?
- How does this information measure up to the information in other sources I've read? Does it support or contradict what I already know about the topic?

- Are there any inconsistencies?
- Does the author present an objective view of the material? Is the information based on assumptions, facts, experiences, or opinions?
- Do I agree with the author? Why or why not?
- On which topic would I like more information?

Chapter Summary

- Your brain plays a role in determining your learning style.
- Play to your strengths by identifying your learning style and being aware of how to enhance it.
- Enhance your learning and prepare for your future career by thinking critically about what you are learning.

Review Questions

Objective Questions

1. Three functions of the cerebrum include _____, _____, and _____.
2. Individuals who tend to be logical and analytical are considered "_____-brained."
3. Kinesthetic learners benefit from recording and listening to lectures. (True or False?)
4. Visual learners benefit from flash cards and handouts. (True or False?)
5. The comprehension level of Bloom's Taxonomy may involve summarizing and paraphrasing information. (True or False?)
6. Memorizing medical terminology definitions would occur at the _____ level of Bloom's Taxonomy.

Short-Answer Questions

1. Describe the benefits of knowing your own learning style preferences.
2. What types of resources or activities would be helpful to someone who is an auditory learner?
3. Write a definition for critical thinking in your own words.
4. Why do synthesis and evaluation learning skills come after knowledge and comprehension skills?

Applications

1. Take the learning styles assessment by accessing the following website: https://www.how-to-study.com/learning-style-assessment. How will these results affect how you study? How may they influence you at your clinical internship?
2. Partner with other students based on your learning style assessment results (visual, auditory, or kinesthetic). In your group, come up with an idea for an activity or project that would help students with your learning style understand the information in this chapter. Then, write three to five sentences explaining

how and why the activity or project would accommodate your learning style. Present your ideas to the other two groups in the class.

3. Review *Bloom's Learning Levels*. Draw a pyramid, set of stairs, skyscraper, or another image to illustrate Bloom's six levels of learning. Label each level and provide a practical example. For instance, a practical example for the lowest level of learning, knowledge, could be memorizing the definition of a key term and repeating it word for word. Apply these examples to your field of study.

Fundamental Writing Skills

The section in the writing skills chapter you should complete at the end of Chapter 5 is Section 11-5. You can find this section on pages 221-224.

6

Listening, Taking Notes, and Reading as a Healthcare Professional

OBJECTIVES

- Explain the importance of active listening techniques in the classroom.
- Describe different lecture styles and how to adjust to them.
- Discuss ways to improve your learning in the classroom.
- Explain the importance of effective note-taking in class.
- Describe a strategy for reading actively.
- Explain a note-taking outline.

Effective listening, note-taking, and reading are all essential if you want to succeed as a student. During lectures in college, you would be mistaken to think that your only responsibility is to sit quietly while your instructor speaks. This strategy might even have served you well in high school, but in college, you have the opportunity to do much more. By using the strategies discussed in this chapter, you'll be able to take charge of your own learning process. Once you're in control, nothing can stand in the way of learning new things and accomplishing your long-term goals.

Listening Skills

We discuss the importance of listening carefully throughout this text. You should practice and develop good listening skills throughout your time in college. These skills will play a big role in your success not only as a student but also as a healthcare professional. When miscommunication occurs in health care, the results can have negative consequences for patients. Failing to understand—or even hear about—assignments in school can, at the very least, result in frustration and poor grades that don't reflect your true ability.

A lot of valuable information is available in class from the first day forward. Because professors present most of that information verbally, you would do well to start sharpening your listening skills. Always be sure to listen closely instead of jumping to conclusions. Watch and listen for essential clues in the classroom. Ask questions if you don't hear something and write down as much as you can to help you remember what the professor said.

Active Listening

To become an active participant in your own learning process, try to keep your mind engaged instead of allowing yourself to sit back and relax while your professor lectures. Make an effort to listen actively. To better understand the material, think of questions to ask the professor. You can write your questions in your notes and refer back to them at the end of the lecture. If your instructor offers to answer questions toward the end of class, take the opportunity to ask then. If not, look up the answers on your own after class.

There may be times, however, when you'll have a question that can't wait until the end of the lecture. If you believe that your professor is moving too quickly, politely raise your hand and ask him or her to repeat or clarify a specific point. But keep in mind that you should do so only when you have prepared for the class properly beforehand—don't embarrass yourself by asking something you should already have known from doing assigned reading.

Stop, Look, and Listen

Active listening involves thinking about how you are listening and continually working to improve your listening skills. When you are listening actively in the classroom, you're doing more than simply hearing words. You're also deciphering main ideas, deciding what information is most important, and adjusting how you listen according to your professor's teaching style.

Whether you need to become an active listener or merely improve your active listening skills, all students can follow these guidelines:

- Avoid doing things that can distract you from listening.
- Identify main ideas.
- Pay attention to the speaker's transition cues.
- Mentally organize information as you hear it and devote your attention to material that seems more important.
- Take effective notes.

Poor Listening Strategies

There are several behaviors that could undermine your attempts to be an active listener. Make an effort to avoid:

- letting distractions interrupt your train of thought
- tuning out difficult material
- allowing your emotions to cloud your thinking
- assuming the material is boring
- concentrating on the speaker's quirks
- letting your mind wander
- pretending to listen
- listening only for facts and not ideas
- trying to write down every word in your notes

Identify Main Ideas

Identifying main ideas is a key element of active listening. Each lecture you hear will include main ideas, even though different speakers may present those ideas in different ways. Some of the approaches your professors may take are:

- introducing new topics
- summarizing main points

- listing or discussing a main idea's supporting details
- showing two sides of an argument or issue
- discussing causes and effects related to a main idea
- identifying a main idea's problems and solutions

Always Listen for Signal Words

Listening for signal words is another way to guide yourself through a lecture. These words are almost like a running commentary in the classroom. They let you know which direction your professor is headed.

Signal words can indicate transitions in a lecture. By paying attention to transitions, you'll be able to organize your thoughts and your notes as you listen actively. A few examples of signal words and phrases are the following:

- *Likewise.* This word indicates that the speaker is about to show how two concepts or examples are similar.
- *On the other hand.* When you hear this phrase or something similar, you know that the speaker is about to begin discussing a contrasting fact or opinion.
- *Therefore.* This word usually indicates that the speaker is about to present an effect in a cause-and-effect relationship or a logical conclusion.
- *Finally.* This word lets you know that the speaker is arriving at the end of a point or the end of the lecture.
- *To sum up.* This phrase indicates the preceding points are about to be pulled together for the main idea. Be sure to get this in your notes!

Always Try to Understand What Is Most Important

The ability to separate more important information from less important information is a skill all active listeners need. Professors often have similar ways of communicating important information. Some write key terms and concepts on the board as they lecture. Some use a PowerPoint or Prezi presentation with key points bulleted. Others distribute copies of lecture outlines at the beginning of class. By picking up on these clues, you'll have an easier time determining what information your instructor considers most important.

The following behaviors also can draw your attention to important material. Your instructor may:

- pause to allow students to write down information in their notes
- repeat facts or definitions
- emphasize certain information with tone of voice
- tell students directly what information is important (e.g., "Remember this for next Tuesday's test.")
- use gestures and facial expressions to draw attention to key information
- use visual aids, such as video, life-size plastic models, and information or images on projector screens
- have students turn to certain pages in the textbook

Your professors will not always say, "This information is important." They will more likely use their behavior to give you the clues you'll need to figure out on your own what is most important. One way to pick up on these clues is to listen closely. Pay attention not only to your professors' words but also to the tone and volume of their voices as well. Another way to notice clues about important material is to observe closely. Even if you are listening to every word your professor says, if your head is buried in your notebook the whole time, you might miss certain clues. Look up from your notes from time to time to observe your professor's actions.

Hand gestures and facial expressions can often indicate important information as clearly as words.

LISAN and Learn

One of the benefits of active listening is that it helps you take more effective class notes. You'll learn about different note-taking methods later in this chapter. In deciding what format to use when taking notes, make sure your note-taking method encourages active listening. The LISAN method of note-taking focuses on the following:

L *Lead instead of follow.* While listening, think about what your professor might say next.

I *Ideas.* Ask yourself what the main ideas of the lecture are.

S *Signal words.* Listen for signal words that indicate transitions in the lecture. In which direction is the lecture headed?

A *Actively listen.* Make sure your mind stays engaged. Ask questions or make a note to yourself to seek clarification for difficult concepts later.

N *Notes.* Write down main ideas, key terms, and all other important information. Be selective.

Listening Levels

Listening must reach a certain level before it is considered active. Consider the chart below to determine how well you listen in class. What level are you?

Level	Explanation
Reception	Hearing words without thinking about them
Attention	Passive listening; not making an effort to understand the information
Definition	Entering into active listening; attaching meaning to certain facts and details but not yet organizing the material in your head
Integration	Relating new information to your background knowledge and knowledge from previous classes
Interpretation	Putting information into your own words; paraphrasing
Implication	Thinking about how different pieces of information fit together; drawing conclusions
Application	Considering how the information applies to you personally; using it in new situations
Evaluation	Making judgments about the accuracy and relevance of the information

Remember that active listening is a learned skill. By following the directions in this chapter, you can learn to listen at a higher level. And once you know how to apply and evaluate information as you listen, you'll be that much further on your way to becoming a successful student.

Potential Listening Problems

Sometimes, the lecture can be difficult to follow because the professor is speaking either so fast that you have trouble keeping up or so slowly that your mind wanders. Either way, you can make the effort to gain the most from the class.

At Breakneck Speeds

What happens if the professor is moving through the material too quickly? If you're prepared for class and keeping up with your reading and still can't keep up with the lecture, you should speak up. When doing this, be specific. Avoid interrupting with a vague statement such as, "I don't understand." This kind of statement implies that you didn't prepare for class. Also, the professor won't know what information you need explained more fully. Instead, show your professor what part of the material you *did* understand by summarizing it in your own words. Then, ask a specific question. For example, you could say, "I understand that sterile technique means doing things to prevent contamination, like wearing sterile gloves and using sterile instruments. But could you explain the difference between sterile technique and aseptic technique? Are they the same?"

Occasionally, you may feel as if you're the only student in the class who isn't keeping up. You're not alone—many students have felt this way at one point or another. Continue to make an effort to listen more closely and continue taking notes, being careful to write down confusing terms or concepts. After class, look in your textbook or ask your instructor for clarification. This practice of writing down what you don't understand is also helpful if you meet regularly with a tutor. It gives you specific pieces of information to review.

At a Snail's Pace

Alternatively, you may encounter professors who present material at a much slower pace. If you allow yourself to become bored during these classes, your mind will begin to wander. To stay focused on the material, follow one of the guidelines below:

- Practice summarizing information in your head. By forcing your brain to think about putting ideas into your own words, you'll stay alert.
- Try to memorize definitions of key terms as your professor goes over them. Instead of simply reading the definitions or hearing about them, you'll be committing them to memory for future reference.
- Predict what information your professor will cover next. This causes you to consider how your professor thinks. You will gain a better understanding of what your professor expects students to know.

Make Adjustments

Occasionally, you'll have to make your own adjustments for an instructor who doesn't present information clearly. In such cases, you may have to think of examples, draw conclusions, or apply new information on your own. To do these things, you'll need to maintain active listening.

Here are several tips you can use to make sure you keep listening actively:

- Put your cell phone away.
- Remember your purpose for listening.
- Pay special attention to the beginning and end of the lecture, when your instructor might introduce and summarize key points.
- Take effective notes.

When an Instructor Moves Too Slowly—Devon

Devon had been excited to start his first semester of Anatomy and Physiology. By the second week, though, he noticed that the professor moved much more slowly through the lecture material than Devon expected. His mind began to wander in class, and he would think about parts of his life away from school—his kids, his wife, and his job at the hospital. In lab, he discovered that he had missed important elements of a few lectures because he hadn't been concentrating on the material. To counter this, Devon decided to try to anticipate what the professor might say next during lectures, and he found that this strategy helped him concentrate much more effectively on the material. His lab scores improved, as did his grades on quizzes.

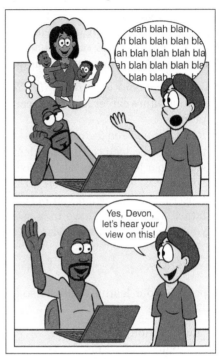

- Sit up straight to avoid feeling sleepy and to show your interest in the lecture.
- Make sure your eyes stay focused on the professor.
- Ignore external and internal distractions by concentrating on the instructor's words.
- Analyze the material.
- Listen for main points.
- Make a note of words or concepts you don't understand so you can look them up after class.
- Adjust to the pace of the lecture.

Learning in the Classroom

So far, we've discussed how to listen actively in the classroom. But much more goes on in the classroom than just the professor's spoken words. To be an active learner, you'll also use observational skills, your own thinking skills, note-taking skills, and much more—often all at the same time.

Different Teaching Styles

During your time in school, you will come across many different types of professors. One may seem disorganized and another doesn't seem to cover the material in your textbook. Some professors might not tell you exactly what you'll need to know for tests and quizzes. Although these situations may seem frustrating at first, you shouldn't use them as excuses to give up. To become a successful student, you'll need to learn to adjust to different teaching styles.

When faced with these difficult situations, you should use them as opportunities to engage in your own learning process. When you're an active participant, you can achieve goals rather than simply learning the required material. You can accomplish things such as the following:

- *Improving your learning skills.* You'll use these skills not only in school but also in your future career as a healthcare professional. Remember, learning is a lifelong process.
- *Recognizing how lecture content is organized.* Whether your professor follows the textbook, lectures independently of the text, or uses other media, you should shape your learning focus for each class.
- *Discovering how to measure up to your instructor's expectations.* This is also a useful skill for when you become a practicing healthcare professional. In the future, you may not have to answer to a professor, but you will want to know if you're meeting your supervisor's expectations.

Improve Your Learning Skills

Improving your learning skills also helps you succeed in the classroom. Learning skills include:

- memorization
- the ability to apply new knowledge
- interpretation of difficult material
- the ability to identify different teaching styles

You may find that a professor is not an ineffective or bad lecturer but rather one who presents material differently from your other professors. Or you may find that the material in a particular class requires a different style of teaching than you're used to. When this happens, look for clues to discover your professor's teaching style. Then, use your different learning skills to help you adapt to the class.

Memorize It

You'll probably find that a lot of memorization is required in your introductory courses, such as biology or anatomy and physiology. However, your professors may not always tell you which specific information to memorize. In these cases, look for clues to identify important information and commit it to memory.

For example, if your professor writes a new concept or a definition on the board, you should make an effort to memorize it. Likewise, if your professor distributes a handout depicting a diagram or a list of facts, it would be wise to remember that information as well. By learning to pay attention to your professor's cues early, you'll know what material to memorize before the first quiz or test.

Apply It

Some professors focus on getting students to consider how the course material will apply to their future careers. If this is your professor's goal, you'll do well in the course by showing that you can apply new knowledge. There are several ways in which your professor might encourage you to do this:

- If your professor gives many written assignments, be prepared to give examples of real-life applications in writing.
- If your professor has students work through case studies during class, expect to see similar case studies on tests.
- If your professor often calls students to the board to solve problems, be prepared to explain to the rest of the class how you would apply your new knowledge.

Interpret It

In advanced science and health courses, professors may ask students to interpret new information. This means you'll be expected to put ideas into your own words to show how well you understand the material. You'll recognize instructors who focus on interpretation by the fact that they often use class periods to ask questions and provide guidance on student responses. If your instructor uses this method, be sure to complete all assigned readings before class. Being prepared will allow you to participate in class discussions.

Know When to Make Adjustments

Watching for identify shifts in your instructor's teaching style keeps you alert and helps you follow along with the lecture. For example, the notes you take during a class discussion are different from the notes you take when your instructor gives you key terms and definitions to memorize. During a group discussion, you're focused more on ideas and the relationships between them. You won't be writing down everything said in that class. In contrast, when your professor gives you a definition to memorize, you'll need to either highlight the definition in your textbook or copy it word for word into your notes.

The next time your professor interrupts a class discussion to write an important date or key term on the board, you'll be able to identify the switch from an interpretive style of teaching to a memorization mode. You'll be able to adapt to this shift in teaching style by making that adjustment and recording the information from the board into your notes.

By listening actively, you'll soon become more familiar with your professors' behavior. Pay attention to patterns in the way your professors teach. One may tell students directly that a particular concept is important, whereas another may give less obvious clues, such as becoming animated or using gestures when explaining important points. Once you can recognize shifts in a professor's teaching style, you'll begin to get more out of each lecture.

Discover How Lecture Content Is Organized

The content in lectures can be organized in one of two ways:

1. *Text-dependent.* In lectures where the content is text-dependent, the material is presented very similarly to the way it's presented in your textbook.
2. *Text-independent.* In these lectures, professors cite resources other than the textbook when presenting the information they consider most important.

Regardless of how closely their lectures follow the text, many professors use media as well to help them present lecture content.

A Textbook Case

If an instructor often conducts text-dependent lectures, it's especially important that you complete the assigned reading before class. If you're familiar with the material already, you'll have an easier time following the lecture.

It's also important to bring your textbook to each class. As your professor talks about sections in the text, note important ideas in the margins of your book. Highlight any passages or definitions your instructor reads aloud. If your professor mentions that a particular section is unimportant or that you don't need to know the information it contains, cross it out.

Some students don't like to mark up their books by writing in the margins or highlighting sections of text. Students know that if they try to sell their books back to the college bookstore after the term, the bookstore will pay more for books that haven't been marked up. At first, this may sound like a good plan for the budget-conscious student. However, carefully consider whether not marking your textbooks is worth it. Being able to highlight and quickly refer back to important lecture points is likely well worth the few dollars difference. It's even better not to sell your textbooks back at all but instead to keep them and build a reference library to use later in your professional career.

Beyond the Text

For lectures in which the content is text-independent, the focus shifts from your textbook to your notes. It's important to take effective notes during these lectures because you won't be able to refer back to your textbook for information you missed. After class, review or outline your notes to make sure you understand the key points. To gain a better understanding of the information, you may want to discuss each lecture with a classmate. You can even take turns "teaching" each other the material, which will help you retain the information. You can also use supplementary material, such as online programs or articles from databases, to review concepts presented by your instructor.

Before you sit down to study any material, set study goals to remind yourself what information you need to learn. This is essential when dealing with content that doesn't appear in your textbook. You'll need to create your own learning objectives for the information in your lecture notes because the chapter objectives from your textbook may not apply.

A Media Frenzy

A third element that affects lecture content is the use of media. Handouts, video, PowerPoint or Prezi presentations, plastic models, and other media give students new ways of learning material. For example, a video might cause you to have an emotional response to a certain topic, whereas a plastic model might give you an opportunity to practice your clinical skills. With each form of media, you connect to the material in a different way. Often, this allows you to learn and understand more information than you would by simply hearing your instructor discuss it.

When dealing with media in the classroom, focus on two key questions. Ask yourself:

- Why is the instructor using this particular medium?
- How does this medium meet my learning needs?

For instance, suppose your instructor plays a YouTube video during class. If the segment is about a topic you've already covered, it can help you review necessary information. But if the segment introduces a new topic, it can meet your learning needs by providing you with background knowledge.

Making the Adjustment

If a speaker is hard to follow, make an adjustment by using the strategies listed in the chart.

If Your Instructor Doesn't . . .	You Should . . .
explain goals for the day's lecture	set goals yourself by referring to your textbook or syllabus
go over information covered in the previous lecture	review your lecture notes for a few minutes before each class
provide an introduction or summary at the beginning and end of a lecture	write a brief summary of each lecture after class
supply an outline of each lecture	review the assigned reading before class or outline your notes after the day's lecture
give students enough time to write notes before moving on to the next topic	politely ask your instructor to repeat or clarify information
speak in a clear, loud tone of voice	politely ask your instructor to speak louder, or move to a closer seat, as long as you don't disrupt the class
answer students' questions without being sarcastic or discouraging	avoid taking your instructor's remarks personally
stay on topic and instead begins talking about personal experiences	think about how the instructor's stories relate to the topic
explain the chapter and instead reads directly from the textbook	follow along by highlighting the text your instructor reads or outline or summarize the text in your notes
provide the main points of the lecture	reread your textbook after class and locate main points
clarify confusing information or provide examples	ask your instructor to provide an example or come up with an example on your own
write key terms and definitions on the chalkboard	look up key terms in a dictionary or in the glossary of your textbook

Participate in Class

Active learning includes fully engaging with the learning process while in the classroom. Participating in class by asking the instructor questions, answering questions the instructor poses to the class, and responding to the comments of other students all help you engage more fully in the process. Be sure to try the participation techniques you learned in Chapter 4 to stay active and involved in all your classes, rather than passive and uninvolved.

Seeing Is Believing

It may seem obvious, but being able to see in the classroom is critical to your success in the course. Make sure you have a clear view of the instructor and the front of the room. Pay special attention to where visual aids, such as projector screens, are located. Be sure to choose a seat with an unobstructed view of boards and screens. The instructor may write key terms or main ideas on the board during a lecture. Being able to see this information will be helpful as you take notes.

Charts and Models

Instructors often use anatomical charts and plastic lifelike models, particularly in health science courses, such as anatomy and physiology. For example, when you are learning about the human skeletal system, a full skeleton model may be used in class. Seeing the model up close will help you learn and remember the names of the bones more easily.

Skills Demonstrations

Skills demonstrations are common in many health professions classrooms. In fact, many health science classrooms are designed specifically for demonstrations and student practice sessions. It's especially important to scope out such a room and choose a seat nearest the location where the demonstrations are going to be given. This way, you'll be able to see everything being demonstrated.

In skills labs, students learn and practice new clinical skills, such as how to take a patient's blood pressure or count a pulse. During labs, you'll be asked to perform the skills your instructor has demonstrated. Having a clear view of in-class demonstrations will make it easier for you to learn new skills and perform them correctly.

Getting the Most out of Class

Listening in class, watching presentations, participating in discussions and asking questions, and taking notes are key ways to increase learning in the classroom, but they're not the only methods. To increase your learning potential, also pay close attention to:

- information presented in handouts
- key terms or ideas the instructor writes on the chalkboard
- any questions raised by classmates and your instructor's responses to those questions
- your own opinions and thoughts about material presented by your instructor
- material that isn't covered in the textbook
- your instructor's introductory and summary statements (given at the beginning and end of each lecture)

Remember that using your personal learning style can give you an advantage in the classroom, as discussed in Chapter 5. Being aware of *how* you learn can help you increase the amount of information you understand and remember. Try to use a variety of learning techniques both to accommodate your own learning style and to increase your skills with other styles as well. Follow the tips for your own style presented in Chapter 5. Not only will you begin to perform better academically but also you'll have better communication with your instructors.

Effective Note-Taking

Another way to get the most out of your classes is to take good notes. This is a good habit to develop from the first day of class and use during the rest of the course. One of the immediate benefits of note-taking is that it familiarizes you with your instructor's teaching style. Moreover, recent studies have shown that when students take notes, they retain more information with greater duration and accuracy. Without taking notes, however, students retain less of the information presented, and they do not retain it as long or as accurately.

Some Things to Consider: Writing Notes by Hand Versus Typing Notes on a Laptop

Recent research has also demonstrated that students who write their lecture notes by hand are more likely to effectively retain the information than students who type the same lecture on their laptops. Researchers have also noted that students using laptops are more likely to be connected to the school's Wi-Fi network and thus more susceptible to the distractions of the Internet, such as email, apps like Facebook and Instagram, or even online shopping.

Note-taking often involves listing main ideas and summarizing information in your own words. It keeps your brain engaged and helps you analyze information while your instructor is speaking.

- Notes provide you with memory cues to help you review and study the information covered during class. This can be critical when the time comes to prepare for tests and quizzes.
- Lecture notes show you what material the instructor considers important. The notes can help you gauge what information will appear on tests and quizzes.
- Taking notes helps you stay more focused during the lecture. You'll more easily become familiar with, and better understand new material.

This section discusses several methods all students can use to take effective notes.

Take Notes in Class

It may seem as if some students were born with the ability to take good notes—but note-taking is a learned skill. You can learn how to take effective notes by using the following guidelines:

- Use your own shorthand.
- Make sure your notes contain personal applications.
- Use a note-taking strategy that fits your style of learning and your professor's style of teaching.

- Organize your notes while taking them.
- Review your notes after class, correct any unclear writing, and write a summary of the class.

Shorthand Helps You Keep Up

Develop your own shorthand for taking notes. By abbreviating words and using symbols, you'll be able to keep up with a fast-paced lecture. To improve your speed in taking notes:

- Abbreviate commonly used words. For example, the abbreviation pt. can be used for the word *patient*. You can make up your own abbreviations. Just remember to use them consistently.
- Develop shorthand symbols for other common words. For example, the symbol → means "leads to" or "causes." The symbol > means "greater than."
- Leave out conjunctions (*or, and, but*) and prepositions (*of, in, for, on, to, with,* etc.) if they aren't needed to understand the idea.
- Take a moment to think before you jot down a note. This helps you focus on one thought and write it down quickly and concisely.
- Don't try to write down the instructor's exact words except with definitions or other precise wordings.
- Don't copy text directly out of the textbook. Instead, highlight the text in your book and refer to the appropriate page number in your notes.

Apply It

Be sure to include personal applications in your notes. Write down cues to help you link new information to your previous knowledge. This not only helps you maintain active listening but also helps you study the material later.

Using someone else's lecture notes should be a last resort. Copying notes doesn't allow you to analyze the material. For this reason, borrow notes only on the rare occasions when you are unable to attend a class. You'll have an easier time learning the information if you're present for each lecture and take notes yourself.

Note-Taking—What's Your Style?

Develop a note-taking style that works best for you. Following are some suggestions for personalizing your method of taking notes:

- Remember how to read your own shorthand by creating a key to keep in your notebook.
- Copy down information and diagrams that your instructor writes on the board.
- Write neatly so you can use your notes when studying for quizzes and tests.
- Leave space in your notes that you can fill in later with information from your textbook.
- Read over your notes after class and make any necessary corrections.
- Separate groups of ideas by skipping a line in your notes.
- Use a color-coding system to mark groups of ideas or to emphasize important terms and concepts.

Your note-taking style also should work well with how your instructor lectures. Your notes can be formatted in several different ways. Keep your instructor's teaching style in mind when choosing the best format for your notes:

- *Outline.* This format works well with instructors who follow strict outlines and give very organized lectures.

Use Symbols + Abbr.

The chart lists some common note-taking abbreviations and symbols. Speed your note-taking by using these shortcuts or coming up with your own.

Abbreviations		Symbols	
Abt	about	Ⓡ	right
b/c	because	Ⓛ	left
Dx	diagnose or diagnosis	↑	increase, increased, or increasing
e.g.	for example	↓	decrease, decreased, or decreasing
h/a	headache	→	leads to or causes
Hx	history	>	more than
Imp	important	<	less than
Incl.	including	Δ	change
Pt	patient	~	about, approximately
Px	physical	+	and, in addition
Rx	treat or treatment	#	pounds or number
s/e	side effects	*	important or stressed by instructor
s/s	signs and symptoms	p̄	after
w/	with	ā	before
w/o	without	—	negative
		c̄	with
		s̄	without

- *Asymmetrical columns.* If your instructor frequently gives reminders ("Remember this for the test on Tuesday.") or refers to your textbook during lectures ("Let's look at page 52."), this format may work best for you. See the following section "The Cornell Method of Note-Taking."
- *Compare/contrast.* This format works well with an instructor who often discusses two separate topics at the same time to show how the topics are similar and different.
- *Concept map.* This format works well with instructors who provide many anecdotes or examples of a single main idea but who don't necessarily follow a strict outline.

Another formatting tip is to leave space (2 inches or so) at the bottom of each page for a brief summary. Reviewing your notes and summarizing each page after class helps you process the information.

Formatting Your Notes

Below are a few examples of different note-taking formats.

Outline: This format helps you organize the information.

```
I Taking Notes
   a. Use shorthand
      1. abbr. words
      2. use symbols
   b. Organize notes
   c. Include personal
      applications
```

Asymmetrical columns: This format allows plenty of room for you to write comments, questions, or reminders next to your lecture notes.

```
Test on Tues. | Taking Notes
              | • use shorthand
              | ✓ abbr. words
              | ✓ use symbols
See pg. 52    |
              | • Organize notes
              | • Inc personal
              |   applications
```

Compare/contrast: This format gives you an easy way of looking at how two different concepts are alike and different.

```
Topic A              | Topic B
• create a key       | • Outline
• info and           | • Asymmetrical
  diagrams           |   columns
• neat               | • Compare/
  handwriting        |   contrast
• leave space        | • concept map
  for more           |
```

Concept map: This format allows you to show how several different anecdotes or examples are connected to a single main idea.

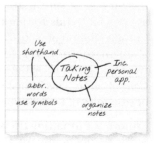

The Cornell Method of Note-Taking

The Cornell method was developed in the 1950s at Cornell University and is still recommended by many schools because of its usefulness and flexibility. It works well for taking notes, defining priorities, and studying.

The Cornell method uses four boxes: a header, two columns, and a footer. The header is a small box across the top of the page where you write the course name, the date of the class, and other identifying information. Beneath are two columns: a narrow one on the left and a wide notes column on the right. The wide column is used for notes in an outline, list, or concept map format. The left column is used for main ideas, key words, questions, and clarifications. Use the right column during class and the left both during the class and when reviewing your notes later. Use the box at the foot of the page to write a summary of the class. This helps you make sense of your notes during future studying. An example is shown at right.

Medical Terminology	Prof. Smith 9/21 pg 1
	Basic Word Parts I Root II Suffix III Prefix Root ~ Combining for + vowel (usually o)
Why Greek/ Latin? (goes back to old days)	from Greek or Latin eg. "cardio"=heart (cardio) then add suffix (or more than 1) to end of root+vowel (combining form) and (maybe) prefix at beginning
Any number of suffixes available?	Suffix (can be multiple) -usually written alone with hyphen -itis (inflammation) eg. "-logy" (study of) So: "cardiology"=study of heart
What about multiple prefixes?	card: +0 +logy (root) (added vowel) (suffix)

Once you learn basic word roots and common suffixes and prefixes, you can figure out lots of medical terms! (but still use a dictionary)

Using Index Cards

Some students like to take notes on index cards. Cards work well also with the Cornell method. Use the lined side of the card to write your notes in class. Use one card for each key concept or topic. Use the unlined side of the card for notes normally in the left column; after class, write key words, comments, or questions here. You can then use the cards as flash cards with questions on one side and answers on the other. Write a summary of the class on a separate card and keep it on the top of the deck.

A Cinematic Experience

You may need to use a slightly different approach when taking notes on a film, video segment, or PowerPoint presentation shown during class. Although the classroom may be dark, these are not good times to tune out or doze off.

If the room is too dark for you to take notes during a film, pay close attention and jot down a brief summary or a few key points after class. If the film or TV show moves too quickly and doesn't allow you enough time to take effective notes, consider watching it again. Often, instructors place these types of presentations on reserve in the campus library. Watching the film or looking at the slides a second time will give you a chance to write down any important information you missed during class.

Finding a Happy Medium

The amount of notes you take determines their effectiveness. Taking too few notes means you won't have enough material to jog your memory later. However, taking too many notes during class won't give you enough time to think about and process the information. So how do you know when enough is enough?

If your notes resemble a brief, disorganized list of facts, you're probably taking too few. In this case, focus on noting how those facts relate to one another. On the other hand, if your pen never leaves the page during class, you might be taking too many notes. Instead, work on writing down only the most important information. By finding a happy medium, your notes will become more effective.

A Note After Class

The most important thing to remember about your notes is to review them. Try to look over your notes within 24 hours after class. It's easier to make corrections and add to your notes while the lecture is still fresh in your mind. Reviewing your notes soon after you take them also helps you commit the information to memory.

Getting Organized

As we discussed in Chapter 2, organization is critical to your success as a student. It also makes a difference in the effectiveness of your notes. Your lecture notes can be an excellent study tool, but not if they're in a disorganized jumble of papers. Take the time, either during or after class, to organize your notes. You'll thank yourself later.

Academic Reading

Do you like to read? Maybe you've been out of school for a few years, but you still read newspapers, magazines, or novels? If you have been away from school for some time, it's likely that your reading has been casual. The sort of concentrated reading you will do in your textbooks is very different from that casual reading. For each hour in the classroom, you may spend 2 to 3 hours studying between classes and most of that will be reading. Reading assignments are much longer than in high school and much more difficult. Textbook authors often use many technical terms and cover complex material. Some textbooks are written in a style that may be much dryer than what you're used to.

For all these reasons, it's a good idea to think about *how* to read and develop habits to remember more about what you read. Even if you don't like to read, you can develop these skills, which will pay off in a big way.

Preparing for Class—the Need to Read

Even if you attend every lecture and participate in all classroom activities, you still need to prepare for class and read your course material. Reading is assigned by your instructor to help you understand concepts more fully.

In most courses, approximately 75% of the information you receive will be in the form of printed materials. This means reading is an important part of preparing for class. If you learn best by reading, here's your opportunity to take advantage of your learning strengths and put them to good use.

If you don't happen to be an eager reader, stay encouraged. Regardless of your personal learning style, all students can use the same methods to develop better reading skills and improve comprehension. Ways you can get more out of reading include:

- skimming for main ideas
- using active reading techniques
- reading chapter summaries to check your comprehension

The information in the following sections shows you how to become a more successful reader. Perhaps, you have avoided reading in the past whenever possible. Being aware of this quality in yourself is the first step toward improving on it. If you enjoy reading, the guidelines in this section helps you hone your preferred method of learning.

If you use these methods often enough, they'll become routine. Soon, you'll be able to read a chapter without consciously thinking about the different tasks involved in reading.

The Anatomy and Physiology of a Textbook

First, take out one of your textbooks and give it a good looking over. Textbooks generally have a number of elements in common, and thinking about these will help prepare you for getting the most out of your reading. Here are key elements in most textbooks:

- *Preface, introduction, or foreword.* This part of the book provides perspective about the author's point of view. This section may also guide you on how to use the textbook and its features. It may provide hints as to why your instructor selected the book for your course.
- *Author profile or biography.* This helps you understand what the author considers important.
- *Table of contents.* This is an outline of the entire book. It is very helpful in making links between the text and your course's objectives and syllabus.
- *Chapter preview, learning objectives.* These sections indicate what you should pay special attention to. Compare these objectives with the course objectives stated in the syllabus.
- *Chapter introduction.* Introductions are "must reads" because they give you a road map to the material you are about to read, directing you to notice what is truly important in the chapter or section.
- *Exercises, activities.* These features give you a great way to confirm your under-standing of the material. If you have trouble with them, you should go back and reread the section. They have the added benefit of improving your recall of the material.

- *Chapter summary, highlights, or review.* It is a good idea to read this section before reading the body of the chapter. It will help you strategize about where you should invest your reading effort. Answer review questions after reading the chapter to confirm your understanding of the material.
- *Photos, illustrations, graphics.* Many students are tempted to skip over graphic material. Don't! Take the time to read and understand all graphics. They increase your understanding, and because they engage different learning styles, they create different memory links to help you remember the material. Use your critical thinking skills to understand why each illustration is present and what it means.

Paying attention to these textbook elements before you begin a reading assignment helps set you up for a successful experience. Now you can begin the actual reading process.

The Steps of Effective Reading

With a newspaper or magazine, you probably just start reading from the top. Maybe you look over at a photo or illustration first, but generally, you just read from the start to the end. You could do it this way with a textbook, too, but you'd not learn nearly as well as you can using a more structured approach. Try using the following steps.

Start by Skimming

Before you begin reading a chapter, flip through the pages and skim the material first. Doing this will give you a chance to look at the general organization of the chapter and identify key points. The purpose of skimming is to get your brain ready to absorb more information during active reading. By taking the time to skim over the chapter first, you'll give your brain the time it needs to begin organizing information in your head. This means you'll be able to mentally file information as soon as you begin reading. Not only does skimming allow you to understand the material more quickly, it also helps you to remember more of what you read.

When skimming a chapter, follow these guidelines:

1. Look at the illustrations, graphs, charts, and tables. Read any captions.
2. Read the chapter introduction (usually located in the first paragraph).
3. Read the section headings throughout the chapter.
4. Take note of emphasized words in bold or italics as you flip through the pages.
5. Read the chapter summary (usually located in the closing paragraph).

Graphic elements, such as charts and tables, illustrate important concepts covered in the chapter. Often, graphics provide snapshot views of the same information it may take several pages of text to explain. If you glance at each graphic element while skimming a chapter, you'll give yourself a quick preview of the material.

Build a Solid Foundation

When preparing to read a difficult chapter, make sure you first have some background knowledge of the topics covered. When you have a good foundation of knowledge on which to build, you'll have an easier time understanding complex new ideas.

For example, suppose a dental assistant and an experienced radiology technician both read a section in a textbook on using contrast media in certain x-ray procedures. Which individual would be able to comprehend the material more quickly and easily? Although both people may have had some experience taking x-rays, the radiology technician is likely to have a better foundation of knowledge in this particular area. The technician's background and experience would give him or her an advantage over the dental assistant, who has not had the opportunity to work with contrast media. Even the technician's familiarity with the vocabulary used to describe such procedures would make it easier for him or her to read and understand the text.

As a student, how can you expand your foundation of knowledge? One way to give yourself some background information is to read an online or magazine article on the topic. Another way to prepare for reading a difficult chapter is to attend a lecture or seminar on a related topic. At the very least, you'd become familiar with the vocabulary used in the chapter. By the time you sat down to read your textbook, you would be able to focus your energy on trying to understand the concepts presented, rather than having to try to figure out what specific words mean.

Look at the Structure

Another tactic to use when skimming text is looking at how the chapter is organized. The chapter may be structured in several different ways:

- *Subject development or definition structure.* These paragraphs present a single concept and then list supporting details. Introductory paragraphs usually are structured this way.
- *Sequence structure.* These paragraphs usually include signal words, such as *first, second, next, then,* and *finally.* The information in these paragraphs is presented in sequential order. Numbered lists also fall into this category.
- *Compare and contrast structure.* These paragraphs discuss how two or more concepts are alike and different. Words that signal comparisons include *both, similarly, too,* and *also.* Contrasting statements may include the signal words *yet, but, however,* or *on the other hand.*
- *Cause-and-effect structure.* These paragraphs often include signal words or phrases, such as *cause, effect, due to, in order to, resulting from,* and *therefore.* These paragraphs explain how one idea or event results from another idea or event.

Once you identify how the chapter is organized, you'll be on your way to pinpointing the most important information. This will help you focus when the time comes to read the full chapter.

Now You Are Ready to Read

After you've skimmed the chapter, you can begin reading actively. Note that active reading goes beyond simply recognizing the words on each page. It includes using other tactics to aid your comprehension. To make sure you're reading actively, try putting some of the following guidelines into practice:

- Read aloud or at least in such a way that you can hear the words of the text in your head.
- Take notes or draw graphics as you read. (The Cornell note-taking method works well for reading also.)
- Write down any questions you have about confusing concepts or ideas.

- Think about how information in the chapter relates to important points outlined in the table of contents (or outlined at the beginning of the chapter).
- Make a note of any difficult sections you'd like to read a second time.

Stay Focused

Active reading requires concentration. Here are some basic guidelines to help you stay focused (Chapter 7 provides additional study tips):

- Read during the time of day you are most alert.
- Avoid trying to read too much at one time. When you start to feel your mind wandering, take a 5-minute break.
- Find a quiet place to read. Avoid distractions, such as watching TV, looking at your laptop or phone, or listening to loud music.
- Sit in a comfortable (but not too comfortable) chair in order to stay awake and alert while reading.
- Supply yourself with a healthy snack and water to avoid getting distracted by being hungry or thirsty.

Keeping What's Important

As you actively read each chapter, highlight important ideas or mark them with sticky notes. You can also make notes right in the margins. Just be careful not to mark too much text. If 90% of the material on every page is highlighted, it doesn't truly show which ideas are most important. But a chapter that is highlighted correctly is an excellent study tool. Being able to locate key ideas quickly will help you study more efficiently.

When deciding which text to highlight, think about what should be considered truly "important" material. Here are some guidelines:

- Highlight any information your instructor emphasizes in class. If your instructor considers a particular topic important, chances are that topic may appear on a test or quiz.
- Highlight portions of text that answer any questions you came up with while skimming the chapter.
- Look for and highlight topic sentences. These sentences generally include the main idea(s) in each paragraph.

Highlighting can help you find important information later, but keep in mind that it doesn't actually help you learn the material. To learn the information, spend a few extra minutes summarizing the text you highlighted in your own words. If you prefer, create a chart or diagram instead to illustrate key points. This helps you process the information and commit it to memory.

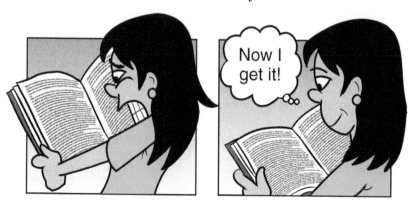

Learning to Highlight Only the Important Parts—Amalia

When her textbooks arrived from the online college bookstore, Amalia was eager to begin studying. She found a quiet place in the library each day and dedicated several hours to her work. While reading her texts, she held a yellow highlighter in her hand, intending to mark all of the important material immediately as she came to it. She marked and marked. However, in the second week when she tried to review a chapter she'd read the week before, she noticed that she highlighted virtually everything on every page. As a result, she had a difficult time knowing what was important and what wasn't. She decided to change her highlighting strategy. From then on, she would still hold a highlighter ready, but she would wait and read a whole paragraph or even a page first, and then she would go back through the section marking what was truly important. She soon found that when she went back to review, she could much more easily understand what material was most important.

Highlighting Text

By highlighting text and making notes in the margins of your textbook, you'll remember more of what you read. You'll also be able to locate key ideas later when studying for the next test or quiz. Keep these guidelines in mind as you read:

- Read the entire paragraph or section before highlighting any of it.
- Highlight portions of text that answer any questions you thought of while skimming the chapter.
- Look for items presented in sequential order and number them accordingly.
- Highlight key terms, names, dates, and places.
- Summarize main ideas in the margins.
- Insert a question mark next to confusing paragraphs or sentences. Write any questions or comments you may have in the margins.
- Mark any information your instructor considers important with a star or exclamation point.
- Highlight important information in the table of contents or create a list of the most important topics.

Make It Personal

Another way to make sure you're reading actively is to connect with the material on a personal level. By making the information more personal, you'll have an easier time remembering it. You can do this by the following:

- *Making associations.* For example, you might be able to remember an important date by associating it with the birthday of someone you know. (Chapter 7 discusses associations in more detail.)
- *Having an emotional response to the material.* Reacting to the information you read will make it more memorable.
- *Drawing pictures to illustrate different concepts.* A picture might be easier to remember than a paragraph of text.

Learn the Vocabulary

Reading actively also involves making sure you understand the vocabulary used to describe new concepts. You should always determine the meaning of an unfamiliar word before continuing your reading. In scientific texts especially, it's important to know the meaning of the technical terms used. Knowing the vocabulary makes your job of understanding the material much easier. For example, suppose you are reading a passage discussing what happens to the body during a myocardial infarction. Knowing that *myocardial infarction* is the medical term for "heart attack" would help you understand the passage more readily.

When you notice an unfamiliar word, first try to figure out its definition from context clues. Context clues can include other words or sentences that provide hints about the word's meaning, as well as root words, prefixes, and suffixes. If you're unable to determine the word's meaning from the context, look it up in a dictionary or glossary. Saying it aloud will help you remember it. Then make a note of the definition and pronunciation in the margin of your textbook or in your notes. If the word appears once in the chapter, it may appear again.

When skimming a chapter, you may notice many unfamiliar words. It may be helpful to look up all the definitions before you begin actively reading the text.

Read Chapter Summaries

In most textbooks, all chapters are formatted similarly. The chapter summary usually appears toward the end of the chapter in the form of a summary paragraph, bulleted statements, or review questions.

One of the last steps in active reading is reviewing the chapter summary. Read the chapter summary and refer back to the table of contents to make sure you understood the key points of the chapter. If there are sections you didn't understand, reread them or make a note to ask your instructor for clarification.

When rereading, try using a different method from what you used during your first active reading of the chapter. You can adjust the speed of your reading by reading a particular section more slowly, for example. Reading aloud is another method. When rereading text, make an effort to understand each sentence before continuing. Think about how each new concept you encounter relates to other information in the chapter.

Make a Plan for Your Reading

- *Pace yourself.* Unless it is very short, divide the assignment into smaller blocks rather than trying to read it all at once. If you have a week to do the assignment, for example, divide the work into five daily blocks, leaving an extra day for review.
- *Schedule your reading.* Try to read at the time of day when you are most alert.
- *Choose the right space.* Read in a quiet, well-lit space. Sit in a comfortable chair with good support. The library is an excellent option. Don't read in bed because that space is associated with sleeping.
- *Avoid distractions.* Active reading takes place in short-term memory. With every distraction, you lose continuity and have to restart. Multitasking—listening to music or texting while you read—makes for poor reading comprehension and makes the reading take much longer.

- *Prevent reading fatigue.* Give yourself a 5- to 10-minute break every hour. Put down the book, walk around, have a healthy snack, stretch, or do deep knee bends. You'll feel refreshed and be better able to stay focused.
- *Read more difficult assignments early* in your scheduled reading time when you are freshest.
- *Stay interested.* Actively go looking for answers that pop up in your mind as you read. Carry on a mental conversation with the author.

Use Your Reading Notes Before Class

Review your textbook and create a note-taking outline before each lecture. This familiarizes you with the material and helps to organize your notes. By locating key terms and main ideas beforehand, you'll provide yourself with a basic outline to follow and fill in during the lecture. In essence, your note-taking outline is your "road map" for the lecture. By using it, there's less chance of getting lost.

To determine which terms and concepts to include in your outline, follow these steps:

1. Look at the general layout of the chapter. Make a mental note of each section's length—longer sections will need more space in your outline.
2. Read the introductory paragraph. The first paragraph in a chapter often lists main ideas.
3. Review any graphs, charts, or diagrams.
4. Search for any bold or italic words. If a word or phrase is emphasized in the chapter, it should be included in your outline.
5. Look over passages you highlighted while reading, including margin notes, questions, and other notes.
6. Read the closing paragraph. The last paragraph in a chapter usually summarizes important information and draws conclusions.

During the lecture, fill in any gaps left in your outline. Add to it by including information from the lecture that is not provided by your textbook.

Chapter Summary

- Develop your active listening skills to get the most out of every class.
- Avoid behaviors that can interfere with active listening.
- When listening actively, identify main ideas and pay attention to signal words.
- Use techniques to compensate for different lecture styles and become an active participant in your own learning process.
- Learning involves several skills, including memorizing, applying, and interpreting new information.
- Develop a note-taking style that works for you. Keep your instructor's lecturing style in mind when deciding how to format your notes.
- Reading is a multipart process that includes skimming, active reading, and later reviewing and rereading.
- Give yourself a road map to follow during class by creating a note-taking outline.

Review Questions

Objective Questions

1. Actively texting an old friend during a Medical Office Procedures lecture is a form of active listening. (True or False?)
2. Students who write notes by hand during a lecture generally remember more of what was said than do students using laptops. (True or False?)
3. The best note-taking format for a lecture illustrating the similarities and differences of two topics is _____.
4. A good place to look for a course textbook's outline of topics covered is _____.

Short-Answer Questions

1. List at least five behaviors that could be interfering with your ability to listen actively in class.
2. How would you cope with an instructor who moves too slowly?
3. Which note-taking format would work best in a class where the instructor routinely gives a lot of anecdotes and examples to illustrate a single main idea?
4. What should you do with your class notes after you've written them in class?
5. What are at least three things you can do to make sure you're reading actively?

Applications

1. Group Exercise: Using a highlighter, read the first five pages of this chapter and highlight important passages following the guidelines given in this chapter. Then go back through these pages, looking only at what you have highlighted, and mark with a large penciled asterisk one key concept that would most likely be on a quiz covering this chapter. Finally, get together in groups of three or four students and compare what you have highlighted and marked with the asterisk. Talk about how you know what is most important here.
2. Analysis Exercise: Select a few pages of notes you took in one class session of a different course at any time *before* reading this chapter. Examine these notes to see how well they follow the guidelines suggested in the "Take Notes in Class" section of this chapter. What could you have done differently to improve the process of taking notes in class and the resulting notes?

Fundamental Writing Skills

The section in the writing skills chapter you should complete at the end of Chapter 6 is Section 11-6. You can find this section on pages 224-227.

7

Study Skills

OBJECTIVES

- Use course materials to focus on your study goals.
- Select and prepare a study space.
- Improve your concentration and memorization skills.
- Explore different study strategies to improve your efficiency.
- Build and use a study group effectively.
- Make use of supplemental study materials.
- Improve your study skills for math and science.

Much of your time as a student will be spent studying. Fortunately, there are many simple strategies you can use to make the most of your study time and the resources available to you. In this chapter, you'll learn how to study effectively, starting with selecting a study space and preparing yourself for studying. You'll learn tips for improving your concentration and long-term memory as well. Study strategies can help you make the most of your time to help ensure your success as a student. In addition, you'll learn how to form and work with a study group and how to use a textbook and other resources as you study. Finally, you'll learn some special study skills for math and science.

What Are You Going to Study?

Although it may seem obvious, you need a focus before starting to study. Are you studying a chapter to prepare for class? Studying for an upcoming test? Studying how to perform a certain healthcare procedure before you do it in the lab tomorrow? Start by considering your reasons for studying and setting your goals.

This step begins with materials your instructor has provided you, including:

- the syllabus
- study guides and lecture outlines
- practice exercises
- assignment instructions

Start With the Syllabus

Chapter 2 points out the importance and the use of the syllabus for each class. The syllabus gives you key information such as reading assignments, exam dates, and due dates for papers and other out-of-class work. Chapter 2 also discusses how to manage your time well by scheduling study periods well ahead of time to avoid last-minute "cramming," which is the least effective way to study. Your syllabus is your road map for starting to get organized for studying, but it's not your only resource.

Study Guides, Lecture Outlines, and PowerPoint Slides

Many instructors not only tell you what general topic you'll cover each day of class, but they may also provide an outline of each day's lecture for you. These outlines are often in the form of handouts with the PowerPoint slides for each class. You can use this outline as you prepare for class. It allows you to focus your reading and studying on the points listed in the outline. Keep these main ideas in mind as you read to help you prepare well for class. The slides are often incomplete so that you will need to take notes on them during the class. As a result, the PowerPoint handouts help to not only keep you organized but also require you to take notes in your own words. You'll find them very helpful when studying for tests.

Practice Exercises

Some instructors provide practice exercises for you. These may be on a handout or on the course website. Practice exercises are a great way to become proficient with the material. If your instructor goes to the trouble of giving you practice exercises for a chapter or section, you should assume that the material is particularly important to know and that it may be on a test. File these exercises in a safe place so you can use them later as you study. Save any completed exercises so you can check your work when you get graded tests back.

Assignment Instructions

Your instructor may give you a handout that tells you exactly how certain assignments are to be completed. These instructions can include things such as:

- style guides for papers and lab reports—details on how papers should be typed, how to format your citations and works cited page, what margins to use, etc.
- step-by-step walkthroughs—such as for clinical procedures; sometimes, many different procedures start with the same basic steps
- research tips—resources for finding information on the Internet or in the library

Remember to file your assignment instructions in your notebook under the correct tab.

Getting Organized to Study

Studying is much more efficient when you're organized. Organization is a key to your success not only as a health professions student but also as a healthcare professional. Being organized for studying simply makes the most efficient use of your time.

If you're already a very organized person, you may not need to make any changes in your system for keeping track of things. On the other hand, some of us are less than organized or even hopelessly disorganized. The following tips and suggestions are simple, easy to implement, and will help you improve your ability to organize.

Three-Ring Binders and Folders

The first step to getting organized is finding or making a place for everything. This means you'll need to find a place to keep the materials and supplies for each class you're taking. Many students find that the best organizational system uses three-ring binders (or twin-pocket folders with notebook fasteners) with tabbed dividers.

Dedicate one binder for each class. Keep all handouts, notes, charts—everything related to that class—together in that binder.

Labeled Dividers

Next, decide how you want to organize the material in each binder, using labeled tabbed dividers or a similar system. You may find it helpful to use the same set of divider names in each binder. This will minimize the time it takes to find things. Use a pen or colored permanent marker to label the tabs on the dividers. You can purchase tabbed dividers or make your own from card-stock paper. The following is an example of a typical set of divider names:

- Schedule
- Syllabus
- Handouts
- Assignments
- Notes

In this system, your class schedule is at the front. This helps you see at a glance what's going to be covered in the next class period. The syllabus needs to be accessible, too, because it contains other critical information. Every time you receive a new handout, place it behind the "Handouts" tab; do the same with assignments. The last section is for taking notes in class and during your reading. Keep a supply of new notebook paper behind this tab.

Organizing Your Notes

You may prefer to use a spiral notebook instead of loose-leaf paper for taking notes. Just be sure to keep the notebook with the appropriate binder for each class. To avoid confusion, use a separate notebook for each class.

Chapter 6 describes how to take good notes in class. After class, take a few minutes to organize your notes by following these simple steps:

- Record the date of the lecture.
- Number your pages.
- Write down reminders about upcoming assignments and due dates. Make sure the dates are written in your weekly planner.

The Backpack Black Hole

One final note about organization: Beware the backpack black hole. If you are in a rush after class, it may be tempting to gather your papers, shove them into your backpack, and forget about them. The only problem with this method is that when you need to review one of those papers several days or weeks later, you might not be able to find it. A lack of organization makes it easy for important papers to get lost. The backpack black hole occurs when things go in and are never seen again.

Studying 101

Studying seems simple: Get out your books and notes and study them. But what does it really mean to study? Studying involves:

- refreshing your memory
- taking in new information
- organizing, understanding, and memorizing data

It's no surprise that many students sit down to study and find themselves feeling overwhelmed by all that is required. To make things worse, any little distraction can throw a wrench in the works, keeping you from studying efficiently. That's why it's important to study the way that is right for you.

Select a Study Area

First, find a good place to study. Look for a location that is free of distractions. (See *How to Find a Distraction-Free Study Area*.) Make sure the area is large enough for you to arrange all your study materials. Think about any furniture you might need, such as a desk or large table.

Many students prefer to sit at a table when they study. This arrangement keeps them alert and focused while helping them keep their materials organized. They can put the study materials they're using on the table and keep materials they'll need later set aside. Other students feel more comfortable sitting on a sofa, with their study materials on a coffee table or spread out on the floor below. One place you may want to avoid studying is your bed, which may tempt you to take a nap.

How to Find a Distraction-Free Study Area

Think about two or three areas that might make good study spaces. Then choose the place that best addresses these questions:

- Is there enough light so I can read without straining my eyes?
- Is the temperature comfortable? If it isn't, can I change it?
- Are there a lot of other people in the same space who could interrupt me?
- Are there things in the space that will distract me from studying?
- Is there a TV or radio in the space that might be turned on?
- Is this space easy for me to get to on a regular basis?
- Will cooking odors come into this space, making me feel hungry and distracted?
- Is this space big enough so it won't get cluttered when I spread out all my materials?

Lighting

Make sure your study space has good lighting you can control. Light is very important. Too much will make your eyes hurt, whereas too little will make your eyes strain. The light should shine evenly over all your work and not directly into your eyes.

Temperature

You'll want to be comfortable when you study. Being too cold will distract you; it's difficult to take notes with cold fingers. Being too warm also can hurt your accuracy, speed, and mental sharpness and can make you sleepy. For good studying, the best temperature is between 65° F and 70° F (18° C to 21° C).

To make sure your study space is a comfortable temperature, test out a few spaces. Sit down and read or study for a half hour. Are you under an air-conditioning or heating vent that will make you too cold or too hot? Are you near a door that causes a draft whenever it's opened? These factors are out of your control and should disqualify a potential study space.

Surroundings

Your study space should be inviting. You should feel good about yourself when you're there. A pleasant space can make you more alert. Here are some tips for improving your study surroundings:

- The right kind of background music can promote relaxed alertness, which stimulates learning. It also may improve your recall. In theory, if you always study biology with Bach in the background, you'll remember biology facts when you hear Bach. Be careful with music that is too loud or distracting.
- Let your phone store voice mails and texts until a later time.
- Turn off the TV (or better yet, study in a room without a TV).
- Some people like white noise: a bubbling aquarium, quiet instrumental music, or even an electric fan. White noise blocks out other sounds without creating a distraction.

Comfort

Your brain is part of your body. If your body is uncomfortable, your brain has a harder time doing its work. When you're studying, you need your brain to focus on your work, not your aching back. You can stay comfortable by having good posture, avoiding eyestrain, moving around, and eating healthy snacks during long study sessions. (See *Fit for Studying*.)

Fit for Studying

Here are some ways to stay alert and be comfortable as you study:

- Sit up straight to keep your back and neck from getting stiff. It's worth the effort and it can become a habit if you stick with it. Sitting up straight also keeps you alert and helps you concentrate.
- Position your reading material at a 45-degree angle from your work surface at least 15 inches away from your eyes. If you're too close, your eyes can't focus properly. If you're too far away, you'll strain forward.
- Don't be afraid to get up and walk around every so often when you're studying. Stay in your study area, but try pacing around or performing simple stretching exercises. When you stand, 5% to 15% more blood flows to your brain. This means your brain gets more oxygen and is more stimulated.
- What about food? If you're going to study for more than an hour at a time, bring a healthy and easy snack. A bite to eat may also serve as a reward as you accomplish tasks and goals during your studying.

Getting Started

Sometimes, it's easier to find a good study space than to actually sit down in that space and study. Getting started can be the hardest part.

The first step in meeting that challenge is planning ahead. Decide which tasks you want to accomplish before you sit down to study and develop a plan for accomplishing those tasks. As mentioned previously, start with your syllabus and other course materials to get focused. The next step is breaking your big tasks down into smaller tasks. Several small tasks will be easier to accomplish than one big task. With each accomplishment, you'll become more confident, which will motivate you to keep going.

The Purpose of Studying

Before you start a study session, plan it out by asking yourself the following questions:

- What do I want to get out of this study time?
- What do I need to learn from the material?

Skim the material you need to study and decide how much of it you'll really need to dive deep into and how much you can cover with just a few notes. Not everything needs detailed attention. That way, you'll spend your time wisely and get more out of studying.

Timing

Choose your study time carefully. Try not to set aside time you usually spend eating or socializing for studying; you'll only think about what you're missing. This can be hard to do when you're a busy working student with a family. You might feel that you don't have any time when nothing else important is going on. But there probably are adjustments you can make to your daily routine. For example, if you usually spend 2 hours watching TV after dinner, try spending just 1 hour watching TV and use that other hour for studying.

Try to study when you are naturally more productive and awake. Some of us are morning people; others are night owls. If you tend to feel fresh and alert in the mornings, consider planning some of your study time then. If you're groggy and tired in the morning, but come alive when the sun goes down, evenings are probably the best time for you to study. Use your planner, as described in Chapter 2, to schedule your study sessions at your best times throughout the week.

Attainable Goals

Breaking up big tasks is part of setting attainable goals. When you set realistic goals, you set yourself up for success. By taking small steps toward your ultimate goal, you get moving, which is the most important thing.

For example, suppose you have a reading assignment that you don't feel like starting. Begin by telling yourself that you will read for just 5 minutes, so at least you can get some of the assignment done. After the first 5 minutes, tell yourself that you will keep reading for a few more minutes and keep repeating this cycle. Before you know it, you'll have read for a half hour or more and maybe even completed a good portion of the assignment.

Study Mode

Here are some more questions to ask yourself before and during study time to get your brain into study mode. These questions will help enhance your study time retention and later recall.

- Why is this information important?
- What does this information tell me about other topics?

- Is this information fact or opinion?
- What if I looked at this material in a different way?
- How can I compare and contrast different information?
- Does this material remind me of something else I've learned?

Concentration

We've already talked a little about the distractions that can interfere with your study time. External distractions, like noises or people walking by you, can cause you to lose your concentration. There are internal distractions as well, like hunger or anxiety, that can make studying difficult.

You can learn to improve your concentration skills so you can overcome those distractions. But it takes motivation to improve your concentration. You must want to learn the material in front of you. You have to know why it's important to your future career. Your desire to learn will help you stay focused on studying. In addition, you need to be awake, alert, and prepared to learn. Being alert the first time you study helps you avoid multiple review sessions.

As a bonus, improving your concentration during study time also helps you remember more material. This means you'll get better scores on tests, quizzes, and assignments.

Do You Have a Wandering Mind?

Some people seem to remember everything they see or hear. Other people cannot remember what they had for breakfast. Does your mind wander? To find out how well you pay attention, ask yourself the following questions. If you answer *yes* often, you may have a wandering mind that could use some concentration strategies.

- Do you forget the names of people you just met?
- Do you ask people to repeat themselves?
- Do you lose track of what's going on around you?
- Do you sometimes stare blankly at a page?
- Do you sometimes feel like you don't remember information you just read?

It's normal for your mind to wander occasionally. However, the most important thing is being aware of when this happens, so you can get back on track.

Prepare Your Mind and Body

First, you'll need to prepare your mind and body to concentrate. Strategies that may help you find your focus before you begin studying include the following:

- Take a walk for 5 to 10 minutes to clear your head and relax your body.
- Meditate for about 5 minutes. Sit quietly, perhaps in your study area with the lights off. Sit up straight and picture something still and peaceful. Breathe deeply and slowly.
- Try to avoid caffeine. Too much can cause you to become jumpy and make it harder to concentrate.

Concentrate

Next, work on improving your concentration as you study. You can do this by using some of the strategies discussed earlier in this chapter, such as avoiding distractions and setting realistic goals. Other good ways to improve your concentration include the following:

- Study during a time of day when you're awake and alert.
- Focus on one topic at a time.
- Keep your brain active by engaging in different activities, such as reading, taking notes, and spending time thinking.
- Take a short break every 45 minutes to 1 hour.

As with so many things, practice makes perfect when it comes to concentration. It might seem discouraging if you get distracted easily the first few times you study. But keep at it, and you'll train your brain to stay focused.

Improve Your Memory Skills

Information is stored in different ways in your brain. That's why it's easy to remember some events or people and hard to remember others. Memory isn't a sense; it's a skill you can develop and improve. By understanding how memory works, you can learn ways to improve it.

The Memorization Process

Why is it that you remember some things but forget others? It depends in large part on how your brain processes memories. The three stages of information processing are:

1. sensory memory
2. short-term memory
3. long-term memory

As you learn new material in school, your goal is to get the most important information into your long-term memory—and then to keep it there. That way, you'll be able to recall what you learned during tests and put your knowledge to use later when you're on the job. Let's look at how memories move through the three stages.

Sensory Memory

Information enters your brain as sensory input (sight, sound, smell, taste, touch) and is held on to for a fraction of a second. Sensory memory is not consciously controlled, as you subconsciously gather thousands of bits of information. In fact, this is much too much information to respond to or remember. Fortunately, your brain filters and selects things to pay attention to. For example, you ignore the feeling of your clothes on your body but respond to someone saying your name or to the instructor describing a clinical procedure. The information your brain selects depends largely on its importance to you and how you can link it to existing knowledge to make the new information meaningful. This attention and conscious perception is the first step of the memory process.

Short-Term Memory

Once you have selected meaningful information, it moves into short-term memory, which lasts for only a few seconds. Short-term memory is limited and can't hold much information. Research has shown that short-term memory can hold five to nine chunks of information, depending on how the information is grouped.

For example, you can remember the numbers 1-9-2-9-0-0-7 by grouping them: 1929 and 007. It can be easy to remember 1929 because it's a date, and 007 is famous from James Bond movies. This way, instead of trying to remember seven different numbers, you only have to recall two groups of information. Grouping makes space for more data in your short-term memory.

Break It Up

When you first learn something new, it's hard for your brain to group the information when it's not sure of relationships among the bits of material. You can make things easier on your brain by learning small chunks of information at a time, instead of trying for one large chunk all at once. Your brain can organize small amounts of information more easily.

Long-Term Memory

After information has entered short-term memory, your brain either forgets it or moves it to long-term memory, where it is organized and stored for long periods. How long depends on how completely the information is processed and how often you recall and use it. (See *Strengthening Long-Term Memories.*) There are many ways to help move information from short- to long-term memory, but the best way is to recall and use information immediately and often. The more often you think about or repeat a piece of information, the stronger it will be in your long-term memory. Unlike short-term memory, long-term memory has almost unlimited storage capacity.

Memory Retrieval

Memory retrieval is the process of getting information out of your long-term memory and returning it to your conscious mind. In other words, you are remembering something. There are two methods of retrieving memories:

- Recognition
- Recall

Recognition

Recognition is the association of something with something previously experienced and involves comparing new information with information stored in memory. Examples of this process include recognizing someone's face or answering true/false and multiple-choice questions on an exam.

Recall

Recall is the retrieval of information from memory without a cue and involves actively reconstructing the information by activating all of the neurons involved in storing the information. Examples of this process include remembering the items on your shopping list or answering essay questions on an exam.

Improving Memory

There are several strategies that you can use to improve your memory. These include the following:

- Selection
- Association
- Organization
- Rehearsal

Selection

Selection is when you single out the information you want to remember and identify the ways you want to process that information. We make conscious decisions about what is important all the time. For example, a professor may know the names of the students in his class, or a student knows the locations of each of her courses. This information has been selected by these individuals because it is important to them. They have made a conscious decision to remember it.

Strengthening Long-Term Memories

There are many ways to make sure important information gets into your long-term memory. Use the following tips while you're studying to help you identify and sort long-term memory information.

When working alone:

- Attach strong emotions to the material you're studying.
- Rewrite the material in your own words.
- Build a working model of the material you're studying; create an image of it that you can remember.
- Create a song about the material or put definitions to a familiar tune.
- Draw a picture or create a poster using intense colors.
- Repeat and review the material 10 minutes after you read it, 48 hours afterward, and 7 days afterward.
- Summarize the material in your own words in your notes.
- Immediately apply what you've learned to activities in your daily life.
- Use mnemonics and acronyms to organize the material.
- Write about the material in a journal.
- State key information out loud, as though you were lecturing to a group of people.

When working with others:

- Act out the material or role-play a situation related to the material being studied.
- Join a study group or other support group.
- Discuss the information with another student to gain an additional perspective and solidify the material in your mind.
- Make up and tell a story about the material.

Association

Association is a very powerful way of committing something to memory. It involves making an association between something you already know and the thing you're trying to learn.

For example, to remember information about a particular disease, try associating that information with someone you know who has the disease. This will provide a memory cue that helps you recall the information later.

Organization

During organization, you memorize information in an ordered way. For example, if it seems there are many steps involved in cardiopulmonary resuscitation (CPR), break the process down into smaller chunks made up of a few steps each. With repetition, you can push each chunk or group of steps into your long-term memory. Rewrite the steps, recite them out loud, or act them out. This will help you remember the steps more efficiently and move them into long-term memory.

Rehearsal

An athlete may practice a certain skill over and over to perfect his or her technique. Think of a tennis player serving the ball again and again, going through the same motions each time. You can use a similar method to improve your memory skills. Rehearsal involves repeatedly reviewing information you've learned over short periods of time.

Several short bursts of rehearsal are better than one long cram session. For instance, rehearse the steps for CPR for 5 minutes four times a day over 3 days rather than once for an hour. Challenge yourself to rehearse the steps at different times during the day, such as while on the bus ride home, while you're making dinner, or while you're in the shower. Rehearsing information moves it into your long-term memory.

Hunting Down a Memory

The next time you have trouble remembering something important, try these strategies to search for your lost memory:

1. Say or write down everything you can remember about the information you're seeking.
2. Try to recall events or information in a different order.
3. Recreate the learning environment or relive the event. Include sounds, smells, and details about the weather, objects, or people who were there. Try to recapture what you said, thought, or felt at the time.

Memory Retrieval

Information you process might not stay in your long-term memory if you don't use it regularly. It can also be forgotten if you are not interested in the information, if your purpose for learning is not strong, or if you have few or no connections between that memory and other information.

Show Your Interest

In general, the more you care about a topic, the stronger your memory of it will be. For example, if you know you have a quiz next week on a particular topic in anatomy class, you'll store information about that topic more successfully in your long-term memory.

Understand It

It is possible to memorize information without understanding it. Most of us know the lyrics to a favorite song, even if we might not have thought about what those words really mean. But you have to understand a concept to be able to remember and apply it. Try putting new concepts into your own words and explaining them to someone else. If you can make someone unfamiliar with the concept understand it, you've got it.

Process Information Deeply

The more deeply your brain processes a topic, the more solid your long-term memory of that topic becomes. Processing depth depends on how you process the information as well as your:

- background knowledge
- desire for learning
- intended use of the information
- level of concentration
- interest in the topic
- overall attitude

Use Study Strategies

There are many study strategies that can help you recall information later during tests and clinical exercises. We have already discussed a few of these strategies. Using a variety of study methods helps your brain take in and store the same information in different ways. This creates multiple pathways for your brain to use when you're trying to recall the information later. Train your brain by determining which study strategies work best for you.

Pay Attention

You can't remember something if you never learned it, and you can't learn something if you don't pay enough attention to it.

Practice

Practice and repetition are very similar to rehearsal. Practice not only helps you store information in your long-term memory but also helps you retrieve that information when you need it. Here's how you can apply the strategy of practice and repetition as you study:

- Repeat information out loud or in a group discussion.
- Write or diagram the same material several times.
- Read and then reread information silently.

Spaced Study

Spaced study is a method that allows you to alternate short study sessions with breaks. Study goals are set by time or task. For example, you could read for at least 15 minutes or read at least 10 pages at a time. After meeting your goal, you would take a short break and then move on to the next goal.

Spaced study works for several reasons:

- It gives immediate rewards for your hard work.
- It helps you complete manageable amounts of work.
- It helps you set deadlines so you can make efficient use of your study time.
- It keeps information moving into your long-term memory.
- It gives you study breaks to keep you sharp when you're studying complex subjects.

Make Associations

Always try to make links between familiar items and new information you want to remember. Once you establish them, these links become automatic. Each time you recall a familiar item, you also remember the information you associated with it. Involve as many senses as possible. Try to relate information to colors, textures, smells, and tastes.

Follow these steps to form associations as you study:

1. Select the information you want to remember. For example, suppose you want to remember information about osteoporosis, a condition that causes a person's bones to become brittle.
2. Next, create an association to the information. To remember facts about osteoporosis, you might associate that information with a person you know who has the condition. (Osteoporosis reminds me of Mary, who broke her hip. Osteoporosis → Mary → brittle bones.)

Acronyms and Acrostics

Acronyms and acrostics are handy for recalling information, too. Acronyms are created from the first letter of each item on a list. For example, *ASAP* is an acronym for the phrase "as soon as possible." The acronym *HOMES* helps people remember the Great Lakes:

H Huron
O Ontario
M Michigan
E Erie
S Superior

Acrostics are phrases or sentences that are created from the first letter of each item in a list. In health care, a well-known acrostic is one about the 12 cranial nerves: ***On Old Olympus's Towering Tops, A Finn and a Swedish Girl Viewed Some Hops.*** This stands for the olfactory, optic, oculomotor, trochlear, trigeminal, abducens, facial, sensorimotor, glossopharyngeal, vagus, spinal accessory, and hypoglossal nerves.

Acronyms and acrostics work in situations where it's hard to find a personal association for a piece of data. These strategies associate key information to a new but easily remembered word or phrase, improving your memory of the information.

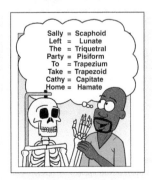

Wrist Bones—Devon

An adult human has 206 bones in his or her body. Each wrist has eight bones and Devon found that he needed help remembering them. He talked to his anatomy professor who told him about a memory-jogging phrase to remember the carpal bones in the order in which they are found. **S**ally **l**eft **t**he **p**arty **t**o **t**ake **C**athy **h**ome represents the scaphoid, lunate, triquetral, pisiform, trapezium, trapezoid, capitate, and hamate bones.

Put Information in Context

You can understand a piece of information more easily once you put it in a larger framework of understanding. For example, a small area on a street map makes more sense when you view the map in its entirety. Sometimes, it helps to see how the information you're studying fits into the bigger picture.

You can apply this practice to studying by learning more about a topic in general before focusing on a particular assignment. After you've gained some background knowledge of a certain topic, you'll be able to associate new information about that topic with what you already know. Your brain can then find a place for the new information in your memory.

Reduce Interference

Interference sometimes occurs when you're trying to remember two very similar pieces of information. Your brain must work harder to recognize the differences between the two pieces of information before you can commit both to memory.

For example, if you're trying to learn a lot of new terms and two of them are similar, you might have trouble remembering either of them. To reduce interference, try to relate each new term to information you already know. Your background knowledge will help you recognize the differences between the two terms, allowing you to store each as a separate memory.

If you need to study similar subjects one after the other, take a break between study sessions. Moving to a different study space or changing positions will reinforce the difference between the two subjects. Moving will allow you to associate one subject with one location and the next subject with the next location. This way, your brain can better organize the new information in your memory.

Create Lists

Lists are another well-known study aid. You can organize ideas by categories that they have in common. The point is that you create a classification system of some kind. Because items relate to each other within the system, you can rearrange and reorganize that information as needed to help your recall.

For example, suppose you're learning about different types of drugs in a pharmacology course. To help you study the material, you create lists of drugs according to what they're used for. Drugs used to treat diabetes are placed in one list, with drugs used to treat heart conditions in another, and so on.

Use Imagery

People often think visually—in images instead of words. Visual aids can help you recall familiar and unfamiliar information when you're studying. This is because images are stored differently than words in the brain. Adding meaningful doodles, colors, or symbols to your notes allows you to organize them visually by topic. When you use visual representations effectively, you'll remember more information with less effort.

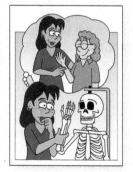

Visualize It—Amalia

Amalia, a medical assisting student, found that she just couldn't remember which is the radius and which is the ulna in the forearm. Then, she realized how she could use imagery to help her remember. She pictured herself taking a patient's radial pulse—the end of the radius is located right beneath that pulse. Now, when she has to remember the forearm bones, she pictures the patient's arm while taking a pulse, and this image helps her remember which bone is the radius.

Think in Pictures

Imagery helps you link concrete objects with images, like a picture of a tree with the word *tree*. It also links abstract concepts with symbols, like a heart shape for *love*. As you study, draw pictures or symbols to illustrate important concepts. These visual cues will give your brain yet another way to remember the information.

Use Color Coding

Colors can give meaning to the information you're studying as well. For example, you could use a variety of highlighters to color-code your lecture notes according to topic. You could also use color to indicate key points or to mark two or more related concepts in your textbook. Using color gives you a way to visually organize the material you're trying to learn and remember.

Improve Your Efficiency of Studying

There are many ways to improve your efficiency as you study. Most of these techniques focus on helping you restate material in your own words. These include *reciprocal teaching* and *metalearning*.

Reciprocal Teaching

Reciprocal teaching is a method that will help you:

- summarize the content of a passage
- ask one good question about the main point of a passage
- clarify difficult parts of a passage
- predict what information will come in the next passage

Reciprocal teaching starts when you and the instructor read a short passage silently. Then the instructor summarizes, questions, clarifies, and predicts based on the passage. Next, you read another passage, but this time you do the summarizing, questioning, clarifying, and predicting. The instructor may give you clues, guidance, and other encouragement to help you master this method.

You can use the reciprocal teaching method in your individual study time after you've learned to use it. You can also use it when studying with a classmate.

Metalearning

The prefix *meta-* means something that is aware of itself and refers to itself. Metalearning is a process in which you ask yourself questions to become aware of your own motives, understanding, challenges, and goals.

In metalearning, you ask yourself a series of questions:

- *Why am I reading or listening to this?* In the metalearning process, you briefly state your purpose for studying certain material. Your purpose and goals set the stage for your study time.
- *What's the basic content of this material?* Preview material before you read. For long or complex material, translate your preview into a chapter map or outline. You also might want to write what you know about the topic and what you'd like to know or think you will know once you're done studying.
- *What are the orientation questions?* Orientation questions give background information on a topic or concept by asking about definitions, examples, types, relationships, or comparisons. The purpose of using orientation questions is to see how many questions you can ask about the material and how many answers you can find.

- *What's really important in this material?* Identify information you should focus on, ignore, or just skim. As with planning ahead, this helps you figure out where to spend your time. If you can't decide whether something is important or whether it should be skimmed or ignored, assume it's important.
- *How would I put this information in my own words?* Putting things in your own words is called paraphrasing. Paraphrasing helps you understand concepts better and identify gaps in your learning right away. Make sure you can put unique terminology for each subject into your own words.
- *How can I draw the information?* Visual learners can get a lot out of drawing the information they're studying. Representing information in pictures is very useful for building understanding.
- *How does the information fit with what I already know?* If you already have a solid foundation of knowledge about a topic, you can learn new things about that topic more easily.

Effective Study Strategies

With a partner, discuss which of the strategies described in the preceding sections work well for you. Which strategies have you not yet tried that you think may be helpful?

Rest, Relax, and Eat Right

As you study, your brain needs time to sort information and store it in your memory. To do that, your brain needs rest. Have you ever had a busy day at work and then dreamt about doing the same tasks? That's no accident. During deep sleep, the brain keeps sorting and storing information, saving important information, and forgetting unimportant details. By getting enough rest and relaxation, your brain can take a break from processing information, allowing it to catch up. This is another important reason to study material on several different days as opposed to just the night before the test. The information is much more likely to be stored in long-term memory.

As Chapter 3 explains, what you eat also affects how your brain functions. A healthy, balanced diet gives you the energy and nutrition you need for studying.

Reward Yourself

After studying, reward yourself for a successful study session. The reward can be something small, such as allowing yourself to watch a TV show in the evening. The reward itself isn't as important as getting a good feeling about the work you've done—and a positive attitude toward studying, as you learned earlier in this chapter, will motivate you to keep at it.

Study Groups

Most of the study techniques we've discussed so far in this chapter are things you can use on your own to learn and remember information, but they also work well when you study with others in a group. Study groups also allow for additional ways of learning and can be one of the best ways for students to master their course material.

Study groups may be informal, like simply talking with a friend in the same class about an upcoming test or project that is due. More formal groups involving two or three others can be organized and scheduled for regular time. Both types of study groups can be very effective.

Study Groups—Informal or Formal?

Being part of a study group can help you learn and study course material. Even if your study group is not always able to answer your questions, teaching others can be a good way to learn. Explaining difficult concepts to someone else will help you review the information and get a firm grasp of important points. Going over course material with other students is an excellent way to help you understand it better and move it firmly into your long-term memory. This process can work in both informal and formal study groups.

Informal Study Groups

Students often get together before or after class to go over the material. These are informal groups where you are under no obligation to attend. When joining with others even in an informal group, however, you are expected to contribute to the discussion.

If you notice students gathering after class, hang around and see what they're talking about. If they're going over class material, introduce yourself and see if you can participate, too. Remember the discussion of networking in Chapter 4—studying with others is also a great way to build your network. Once you've discovered others in your class with whom you study well, consider making a more formal study group with them.

Formal Study Groups

A formal study group is more organized. Students in the same class purposefully decide to get together to study, usually periodically during the school term. It helps to have a scheduled time to study together in a formal group rather than having to depend on casually finding someone in the class to talk with.

Review the section in Chapter 4 on networking with other students for suggestions on how to form a formal study group.

Building a Study Group

A formal study group doesn't just happen—you and other students have to put in a little effort to get it started and keep it on track. You'll need to consider a few issues to build an effective group:

- How many students in the group?
- How and when to schedule meetings?
- Where to meet?
- How to ensure everyone participates fairly?

Study Group Size

It's easier to stay on task when everyone in the group is interested in the same thing—studying. If the group becomes too large (more than four or five members), it can be broken down into smaller groups. Meeting with a smaller number of people makes it easier to review all the necessary material and answer each other's questions.

Scheduling Meetings

It's great to have a regularly scheduled time for a study group—a time when everyone comes prepared to discuss a certain topic. Meeting regularly to go over materials helps you all come up with new ideas and approaches.

It can be hard to find a time when busy people can meet. Do the best you can to come up with a regular meeting time, such as every week or every 2 weeks. If evenings are best, meet then. If two half-hour meetings a week are better for everyone's schedule than one hour-long meeting per week, go with two half-hour meetings.

Online Meetings

If you are unable to find a time to meet in person, you can create an online group site or message board. Each member of the group can visit the group site and contribute to it whenever he or she is free. You can create a group on various websites where members log in and talk via instant message boards. Be vigilant about keeping passwords strictly within the network for safety's sake. You'll want to avoid having strangers posting on your site.

Where to Meet

There are many places for a study group to meet. Many students find it easiest to meet on campus in a common area or in a library discussion room. If your regular meeting time falls during the school day, this may be the best option for you.

Meeting off campus may work better if your meeting time falls after classes have ended for the day. It also may work better for members who are not on campus (professionals in the workplace or students at another campus). In this case, meet at a centrally located coffee shop or take turns hosting the group at your homes. Be sure you know each member in your group well before you agree to meet somewhere or invite him or her to your home.

Keeping the Group Focused

When it comes to study groups, remember the four Cs. A successful study group will have members who are:

- committed—interested in learning the material
- contributors—willing to share their knowledge
- compatible—able to overlook differences and focus on studying together
- considerate—willing to arrive at meetings on time

To have productive meetings, your group might choose to designate a "timekeeper." This person keeps everyone moving along at a good pace so your group will be sure to cover the necessary material during each session.

You might also need to designate a "gatekeeper." This person makes sure the group stays focused on appropriate topics. When people start to discuss things unrelated to the course material, that person can remind everyone to stay focused.

It's everyone's responsibility to prepare before meeting with the group. You should be familiar with the material you'll be studying together, even if you have questions about it. Your questions may be helpful to the rest of the group. Make sure you can explain other concepts in your own words. Successful study groups have a give-and-take. If the group answers your questions about one concept, you may be able to return the favor by explaining another idea to the rest of the group.

Contributing

Students in an effective study group listen to every member because every member has something valuable to say. Even though not everyone is an expert or has 20 years of experience, all students should study hard, make the most of what they do know, and want to learn more.

In an effective study group, all members share their ideas and information. No one should be worried that what he or she says will be taken out of context or used to try to gain an unfair advantage. No one should try to gain from other people's experiences without sharing his or her own. In a good group, everyone contributes fairly and benefits equally.

Study Group Members

A study group should be made up of people you like and respect. A study session should be stress free and can sometimes include informal conversation. You should be able to laugh, share funny stories, and confide your doubts and worries without being concerned that the whole school will find out about your conversations later. Be sure to have the same respect for the other members of your network. If someone mentions any personal matter in the group, avoid the urge to gossip. Keep personal information private. This is an exceptionally good practice for future healthcare professionals.

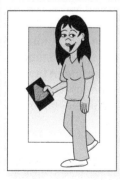

Study Group—Thuy

Thuy, an ultrasound technician student, had returned to college after several years away. She was concerned that she had "forgotten" how to study. When studying alone, she found her mind wandering, thinking about other things. She needed help from others to keep her focused and able to study efficiently. She joined a group of classmates that met each day after lab. The group was not only beneficial, it was enjoyable.

More Resources for Studying

We have discussed how you and your study group can use your textbook, class notes, and materials from your instructor when studying. In addition, there's a whole world of supplemental materials out there to help you learn. Never discount the value of using additional materials when studying, even when not assigned or required by the instructor.

Using Supplemental Materials

Using supplemental material is another way to accommodate your personal learning style. If you have a hard time learning information from a lecture or a textbook, it's especially helpful to supplement your education. When the same information is presented to you in a variety of ways, you'll learn more and have better recall of important points. You may also use supplemental material as a way of finding out more about an interesting topic covered in one of your classes. Whatever your reason may be, making use of supplemental material gives you an advantage as a student.

Your textbook may include a website with features for finding supplemental materials. Browse the text materials near the front of the book for information about resources available for students.

Software and Online Resources

There are many kinds of educational software that you may find helpful. Such software may be available with a textbook, at a computer lab at your school or library, or online. Types of software that are particularly beneficial to students include:

- practice exercises
- tutorials
- simulations
- assessments
- video and audio podcasts

Software such as this may be included with your textbook. Some commercially available software may also be helpful, depending on your particular field of study. You can also find printable weekly and daily planner pages on the web resource available via the access code that comes with every NEW text purchase. Aside from requiring an Internet connection, supplementary material on the Web is often, in practical terms, indistinguishable from software running on your own computer.

Practice

Some online software provides practice exercises. These may be in the form of quizzes you can take or problems you can solve. Their purpose is to help students learn and remember facts and vocabulary. They can also aid in your understanding of how different concepts are related. The more you practice, the more you'll be required to use your new knowledge. This increases your ability to remember and comprehend the material in your textbook.

Tutorials

If you find yourself lost even after attending lectures and getting clarification from your instructor, tutorial software or websites can help. These are designed to teach concepts. Although they may include brief quizzes to assess your level of knowledge, the main focus is instruction. The material may be presented in several different formats, making use of text, images, audio, and video. They may also be interactive, with content covered depending on student responses.

Simulations

Simulations are another type of educational software or Web application. Simulations are computerized versions of real-life experiences. They are interactive and often require decision making on the part of the student. Health profession students can use these programs to learn or hone their clinical skills. The beauty of simulations is that they are forgiving of mistakes made during the learning process.

After all, it's better to make a mistake while caring for a simulated patient than to make one while caring for an actual patient.

Assessment

Assessment software can be beneficial to students and instructors alike. On one hand, computerized testing helps students determine their level of knowledge. As a student, being aware of how much you know can help you set goals for yourself. It allows you to focus on what you have yet to learn. On the other hand, assessments can also be helpful to instructors. Once they can determine their students' progress, they can adjust their curricula appropriately.

Podcasts

Instructors at some schools video or audio tape their lectures and make these available for students as podcasts that can be played on a computer or smartphone. If your school produces podcasts, your instructor will tell you about this. Because a recording cannot capture the full experience of attending class, don't consider a podcast a replacement for attending class—but it can be a helpful review when needed.

In addition, educational podcasts are available online or through "iTunes U." You do not need a smartphone to view these videos or listen to audios; programs on many subjects are available to everyone through the free iTunes program or the learning management system (LMS) of individual schools. For example, if you are having difficulty understanding the anatomy of a particular organ or body system, dozens of video podcasts are available to help walk you through this information. Podcasts from other schools do not replace your textbook, of course, and may contain more or less detail than you need to understand for your course, but when used as supplementary material, they can enrich your understanding.

Online

As discussed in detail in Chapter 10, you can find a wealth of supplemental material online for any course you're taking.

- Make sure websites are trustworthy. Websites that end in .gov or .edu generally contain reliable information.
- Make sure any website you use is accurate (up-to-date and unbiased). Personal websites, like blogs, may have a lot of information, but there is no guarantee that the information is accurate.
- Only use websites that are free. Never give out your own personal information to use a website.
- If possible, get a list of reliable websites from your instructor.
- Textbook publishers usually have websites where you can find lots of resources to help you study.

Other Resources for Studying

With a partner, discuss which of the resources described in the preceding sections work well for you. Which resources have you not yet tried that you think may be helpful?

Study Skills for Math and Science

Many people have something we call "math anxiety" or feel apprehensive about taking science courses. Perhaps the world of numbers and science seems strange and alien to them, or maybe they had a bad experience with a math or science class when they were younger. It can be hard to overcome this anxiety, especially in a society where this anxiety is accepted as normal and understandable.

However, overcoming this anxiety is essential. Math is used in daily life, and math classes are unavoidable when you're in school. Most healthcare careers also require some familiarity with the sciences, particularly those involving the human body. You'll want to be able to approach these classes with confidence and a fresh attitude.

The Importance of Math

Many people struggle through high school math, hoping or assuming they'll never need to use it later in life. But math is all around you. Healthcare professionals need to be competent in math to perform many tasks:

- Measuring solutions
- Figuring dosages
- Converting pounds to kilograms for weights
- Creating department budgets
- Scheduling staff assignments
- Handling patients' claims and bills

Math Myths

One of the reasons it's hard to overcome math anxiety is that people believe things about math that just aren't true. Let's look at some of the most common math myths and how to shake them.

Succeeding at Math

People think of math as much harder than other topics, a kind of mystery where numbers are a foreign language. Sometimes, students are told they just can't do math and should leave it alone.

Are you a problem solver? Are you driven to succeed? If your answer is yes, then you probably have greater math aptitude than you think. Math is all about solving problems. All you have to learn is the language of math—numbers—and you can start solving math problems.

Understand Math to Learn It

A calculator is just a tool to do math problems faster. A calculator might be able to multiply more easily than you can, but it can't tell you what the x stands for in an algebra equation or why an x is used in that problem in the first place. It can't explain what a square root is or how it's used in real life.

Think of your calculator as a tool to help you perform basics like addition, subtraction, multiplication, and division faster and with fewer errors. However, your calculator can only take you so far. Therefore, the successful healthcare student needs to learn how math really works.

In fact, math is used in everyday life, even though you may not always see it or realize it. For instance, learning how to make conversions between different systems of measurement will help you calculate proper medication dosages for patients. Learning about other math concepts will allow you to create budgets at work and at home and complete many other vital tasks. Basic math is needed to balance your checkbook, understand a mortgage payment or interest on a car loan, and cope with many day-to-day aspects of life.

Success in Math Class

Some students dread math class. Somehow, they have the feeling they're supposed to know the material already. They're embarrassed to admit they don't understand a problem or a concept. But a math class is where you *learn math*. If there's any place in the world where you can put your math fears on the table and conquer them, it's math class. Some resources that will make math class a success for you include the following.

Talk to Your Instructor

Many students are embarrassed to tell their instructor they don't understand something. But your instructor is there to help you. If you hide the fact that you don't understand something, your instructor can't help you. If you let your instructor know, you can get the help you need.

Use Your Textbook

Most math textbooks have plenty of practice questions, either at the end of each chapter or grouped together in the back of the book. Use these practice questions. Working through them helps you see some of the underlying patterns of a concept or technique and helps get you in the swing of using certain functions or solutions. Never skip over math questions or problems because it's likely the next material you'll need to understand will build on what you're reading and doing now. If you skip over something that doesn't seem clear, the problem will only grow worse.

Tutoring

There are people other than your instructor who can help you with math. You can find mentors at school or in your own family. Tutors are usually available. Ask your instructor or check bulletin boards in the math department and student centers; you'll probably find many ads posted that offer tutoring services. Some may even be free. There are also interactive online tutoring sites. Finally, a math study group can be a huge help.

Write It All Down

Do each step of a math problem on paper, not in your head. Even if you know the formula well, write down each step. It helps you focus and gets your mind in the problem-solving groove. Just like a great musician still practices scales each day, you should write down even basic steps. It can also help you find careless errors in your work.

Read Carefully

Get in the habit of reading very carefully when you go through a math problem. Most errors occur when you misread a problem. Read through each problem out loud so that each part of it makes sense to you. Sometimes, you might think you see "add" when the symbol actually says "divide"; talking through the problem helps eliminate these kinds of errors.

Solve More Problems

Students sometimes think that the assigned materials are the only ones they should use. But supplementary materials can give you fresh examples and practice problems. These extra materials can be very valuable. Before you invest in one, make sure it has a lot of examples and step-by-step instructions. It should include proofs or derivations for the formulas it uses. Remember, different authors might use different notation systems, so be sure to familiarize yourself with them.

Preparing for Math Class

Math is sequential—every concept builds on a previous concept. If you miss one step, the next one won't make sense to you. That's why it's important to go to every class and set aside time each day to go over what you've learned. Here are the basics to review daily:

- Vocabulary
- Basic formulas
- Working cooperatively
- Testing yourself

Vocabulary

Like many subjects, math has a specialized vocabulary. If you don't know the most common math terms, you'll have trouble with problems you could otherwise solve. Make a list of key words and study them. This list can include words emphasized by your instructor or your textbook as well as words you find you have trouble remembering.

Treat math like a foreign language; you learn a language by picking out vocabulary words and memorizing them. You have to know how to pronounce vocabulary words, what they mean, and when they are used.

Basic Formulas

Like vocabulary, math formulas form the basis for solving math problems. It's valuable to understand why a formula works the way it does. It's especially important to memorize basic formulas because these are the formulas you'll use most often.

Teamwork

Many instructors have come to realize the benefits of letting students work with a partner. Once you find a good partner, you can help each other solve problems. A partner can bring you the following:

- *Another point of view.* This helps you see more possibilities, thus improving your learning.
- *Increased personal accountability.* If a partner is depending on you to help him or her study and learn, you will take that responsibility seriously.

- *An audience.* If you can explain a concept to your partner, you can explain it to the instructor on a test.
- *Praise and encouragement.* You and your partner will support each other and provide positive feedback, helping to create confidence.

Even if your instructor does not pair you with a partner, remember that you can set up your own study group to go over the math you're learning in class. Often, it's easiest to learn how to apply formulas when talking them through with other students. Just make sure you really understand the concepts. If you let others do your thinking for you, you'll have trouble with future math problems that build on the understanding of these formulas.

Studying Science

Much of the preceding discussion of math and studying math is also true of the sciences. In fact, many people have the same anxiety or apprehensions about science as they do about math, and understanding many of the sciences requires understanding mathematical formulas.

Try to apply all the same principles when studying for your science courses. Most important, don't be afraid to ask your instructor questions.

If you feel frustrated reading scientific information or texts, take a moment and remind yourself that health care is largely based on science. To understand how illness can be prevented or treated, we need to understand how the body works, beginning with basic biology. To understand how to take x-ray exposures and process images, we need to understand the basic physics of x-ray beams and their interaction with matter. Even to understand medical terminology, we need to feel comfortable with scientific language. Although you may not immediately see the value of something scientific you are studying, rest assured that as you enter your chosen healthcare career, that knowledge will have a big payoff because you will better understand the reasons for actions you take on the job. The more you understand the scientific side of health care, the more deeply involved you'll feel in your work—and the happier you'll be with your career choice.

Chapter Summary

- Set goals for each study session to give yourself a game plan to follow and to make the most efficient use of your study time.
- Get organized. Organize your school papers (notes, syllabi, schedule, etc.) for quick and easy access.
- Consider the lighting, temperature, and surroundings when choosing a study space.
- Get more out of studying by using strategies to improve your concentration and memory.
- Use different study methods, such as repeating information, taking short breaks, and using acronyms or acrostics.
- Rest, exercise, and proper nutrition will give you the energy you need to stay alert and focused as you study.
- Develop effective study groups that will help you learn and support your academic goals.
- Use supplemental material to increase your learning.

Review Questions

Objective Questions

1. Breaking up one large task or assignment into several smaller ones is typically less daunting and easier to complete. (True or False?)
2. Avoiding breaks during studying helps to maintain your concentration. (True or False?)
3. Short-term memory lasts for a fraction of a second. (True or False?)
4. Selection involves the process of consciously deciding what is important to remember. (True or False?)
5. A very powerful strategy for committing something to memory involves making an _____ between something you already know and the thing you're trying to learn.
6. CNA is an _____ for certified nurse assistant.
7. The brain continues to process information and store it in long-term memory during sleep. (True or False?)

Short-Answer Questions

1. What are at least two tips for getting organized?
2. Describe at least three different study strategies.
3. What are four characteristics that members of a successful study group should have?
4. How does assessment software benefit students and instructors?
5. Explain why it's not a good idea to expect a calculator to do all of your math for you.

Applications

1. Study Space Checklist: Make a list of the characteristics you find most important for a study space. Then locate at least two places that meet your criteria—your principal study area and a backup when the first is not available for any reason.
2. Getting Organized Checklist: Compose a checklist of things to do in order to organize your paperwork for each class.
3. Study Group Planning: Choose one of your classes and look around at the other students in the room. Based on what you have observed about them from how they interact in the classroom, select three students you'd ideally like to have in your study group. (If you haven't already formed a group for that class, talk to these students soon to see if they're interested.)

Fundamental Writing Skills

The section in the writing skills chapter you should complete at the end of Chapter 7 is Section 11-7. You can find this section on pages 228-230.

8

Medical Math for the Healthcare Professional

OBJECTIVES

- Describe how strong math skills are important in the health professions.
- Apply the order of operations in math.
- Understand the importance of vital signs and their normal ranges.
- Calculate body mass index.
- Know how to use military time.
- Understand how angles and degrees are used by healthcare professionals.
- Distinguish between the three measuring systems.
- Understand how ratios and proportions are used in the administration of medication.

Healthcare professionals (HCPs) need to be competent in math to perform a variety of tasks. Examples of areas where math is used in health care include:

- vital signs
- body mass index (BMI)
- time conversion
- angles and degrees
- conversions between measuring systems
- calculating medical dosages
- statistics
- radiography and sonography
- surgical technology
- anesthesia in the operating room
- staff scheduling
- billing and record keeping
- many other calculations

HCPs routinely use addition, fractions, ratios, algebraic equations, and other math skills to deliver the correct amount of medication to their patients or to monitor changes in a patient's health in disciplines including nursing, medical assisting, radiography, sonography, phlebotomy, and physical therapy. HCPs must obtain reliable data and accurate calculations to prevent, diagnose, and treat medical problems.

Order of Operations in Math

Many math formulas used by HCPs in their daily routines may be complicated and contain several steps. Even when using a calculator, the HCP needs to know which step is calculated first, second, third, etc. The order of operations in math is the order in which we add, subtract, multiply, or divide to solve a problem. A mnemonic often used to remember to the correct order is **p**lease **e**xcuse **m**y **d**ear **A**unt **S**ally.

1. Parentheses
2. Exponents
3. Multiplication/division (from left to right, as found in the problem)
4. Addition/subtraction (from left to right, as found in the problem)

Consider the following example: $(11 - 5)^2 \times 2 - 3 + 1$

1. Parentheses: $6^2 \times 2 - 3 + 1$
2. Exponent: $36 \times 2 - 3 + 1$
3. Multiplication: $72 - 3 + 1$
4. Subtraction: $69 + 1$
5. Addition: 70

Order of Operations in Math

The formula used to convert body temperature measured in degrees Fahrenheit into degrees Celsius is $(° F - 32) \times 5/9 = ° C$. With a partner, convert $101° F$ into $° C$.

Vital Signs

Vital signs are a group of the most important measurements that assess the general physical health of the patient and the status of the body's vital functions. The normal ranges for a patient's vital signs vary with age, weight, gender, fitness level, and overall health. HCPs must understand how these measurements are obtained and what they mean. Four of the most important vital signs and their normal ranges are the following:

- Pulse or heart rate (HR) (beats per minute): Average adult range is 50 to 80 beats per minute, typically taken at the wrist (radial artery).
- Blood pressure (BP) (millimeters of mercury or mm Hg): Average adult range is 110 to 120 mm Hg systolic (during the heartbeat) and 70 to 80 mm Hg diastolic (between beats).
- Respiratory rate (RR) (breaths per minute): indicator of acidotic states; average adult range is 12 to 20 breaths per minute.
- Body temperature (BT) (degrees Fahrenheit or ° F): indicator of infection or inflammation, which cause a fever; average adult range is 98° to 100° F.

HCPs must know the units of measurement for each of these signs and how to read the instruments that measure them. For example, on BP gauges, each large line represents 10 mm Hg and each small line represents 2 mm Hg.

Another example involves a fast and easy method for obtaining a patient's HR. The HCP could count the HR for 15 seconds then multiply by 4 to calculate beats per minute.

Body Mass Index

BMI is a useful measure of overweight and obesity. This index is calculated from height and weight. As such, it is a good estimate of body fat and a good gauge of a patient's risk for certain diseases including heart disease, hypertension (high BP), type 2 diabetes, gallstones, breathing problems, and certain cancers. The equation used to calculate BMI is the patient's weight in pounds, times 704.7, divided by the square of the patient's height in inches.

$$BMI = \text{weight (pounds)} \times 704.7 / \text{height (inches)}^2$$

A normal BMI is less than 25. Overweight is between 25 and 29.9, and a BMI greater than 30 is considered obese.

For example, the calculation of BMI for a woman who weighs 152 lb and is 5 ft 8 in in height is:

$$BMI = 152 \times 704.7 / (68)^2$$
$$BMI = 152 \times 704.7 / 4624$$
$$BMI = 23.16$$

As you can see from this calculation, this patient's BMI is in the normal range, which reduces her risk for the adverse conditions listed earlier.

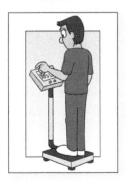

Body Mass Index—Michael

As mentioned in Chapter 3, Michael is very serious about physical fitness and works out at the gym regularly. He is 6 ft 2 in tall and weighs 175 lb. With a partner, calculate Michael's BMI. How do you interpret this value?

Time Conversion

Most healthcare institutions use military time in medical documents to prevent confusion between AM and PM times. To convert an AM time to military time, simply remove the colon between the hour and minutes. If the hour is less than 10, add a zero before the hour (e.g., 6:15 AM is 0615 in military time). To convert a PM time to military time, add 12 to the hour (e.g., 8:30 PM becomes 2030 in military time). Midnight (12:00 AM) is 0000 in military time and noon (12:00 PM) is 1200.

Military Time

With a partner, convert the following AM and PM times into military time: 7:00 AM, 10:30 AM, 3:45 PM, and 12:05 AM.

Angles and Degrees

Angles are measured according to the relative size of the gap between a line and a reference plane—a flat area that is either real or imaginary. This distance is measured by degrees, units of measurement that represent 1/360th part of a circle. Degrees are represented by a degree sign (°) placed after the number. Angles are used in several areas of health care:

- Medical assistants, phlebotomists, medical laboratory scientists, nurses, dialysis technicians, and paramedics must insert a needle into a patient's vein at the proper angle.
  - Venipuncture is the process of obtaining intravenous (IV) access for the administration of fluids to the body or for withdrawing blood for testing. The superficial veins of the arm are typically used. These include, in order of preference, the median cubital vein, the cephalic vein, and the basilica vein. The angle at which the needle is inserted is usually 30 degrees or less. This helps to ensure that the needle is going into the vein along the vein's length as opposed to going through the vein from top to bottom.
- Physical therapist assistants (PTAs) evaluate patients' joint movements.
  - Range of motion (ROM) is the movement of a joint to the extent possible without causing pain. Injury or surgery may have a negative impact on a patient's flexibility or ROM. In this case, the PTA would have to assist the patient with exercises to restore the patient's ROM to normal levels. Imagine a patient who is instructed to start with one arm against his or her side. This would be the reference angle or 0 degrees. The patient is then instructed to raise that same arm so that it extends straight out from the shoulder while keeping the elbow straight. This is the 90-degree angle. The higher the patient can raise his or her arm past the level of the shoulder, the greater the ROM.

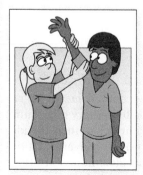

Range of Motion—Jenna

As a physical therapist assistant student, Jenna practices ROM activities with her lab partner. With your own partner, consider the patient in the preceding paragraph. How far would the patient have to raise his or her arm to achieve a 45-degree angle? A 180-degree angle?

Measuring Systems

The three commonly used systems of measurement are the following:

- Household system: used by people at home (e.g., when following directions for a recipe)
- Apothecary system: a system even older than the metric system, only rarely used by pharmacists
- Metric system: most commonly used by HCPs, pharmaceutical companies, and scientists

Most Americans think in terms of household or apothecary measurement: pounds, ounces, Fahrenheit temperature, and inches. Measurements in medicine are based on the metric system, which is more accurate than the household system and is based on multiples of 10.

- Weight: Pounds must be converted to kilograms (lb/2.2 = kg).
- Liquid volume: ounces to cubic centimeters or milliliters (oz/0.0338 = ml)
- Temperature: Fahrenheit to Celsius ([° F − 32] × 5/9 = ° C)
- Length or height: inches to centimeters (2.54 × in = cm)

Conversions

With a partner, calculate the following:

- A female patient who weighs 120 lb into kilograms
- A patient's urine output of 16 oz into milliliters
- A patient's body temperature of 104° F into Celsius
- A male patient with a height of 5 ft 10 in into centimeters

Calculating Dosages

When a pharmacy dispenses a medication to you personally, the dosage is already measured. However, as an HCP working with patients, the measuring may be your job. Decimal points and zeros are critically important on medication orders and administration records. When you read a drug order, study it closely. If a dose does not sound right, it is possible that the decimal point was left out or put in the wrong place. For example, an order that calls for ".5 mg lorazepam by mouth" may be misread as "5 mg of lorazepam." The correct way for this order to be written is to use a zero as a place holder to the left of the decimal point. The order would then be written as "0.5 mg lorazepam by mouth." This greatly reduces the possibility of making a medication error.

Ratios and Proportions

HCPs use ratios and proportions when administering medication. For example, pills may come in doses that are smaller or larger than what is ordered. Consider the case where the medication order is "750 mg every 4 hours as needed for pain." However, the tablets from the pharmacy are 250 mg each. The HCP will need to calculate the number of pills to administer. In this example, the desired dose is divided by the available dose or 750 mg/250 mg. Therefore, three pills will need to be administered to achieve the desired dose of 750 mg.

Some medications are calculated based on patient's weight so HCPs need to use the formula milligram drug per kilogram weight (mg drug/kg weight). A patient's weight is often known only in pounds. Therefore, the patient's weight is converted from pounds into kilograms. Then the number of milligrams/kilogram (mg/kg) can be determined.

HCPs use ratios and proportions in other ways as well. For example, white blood cell counts are generally reported as a numerical value between 4 and 10. For example, a count of 7.2 really means that there are 7,200 white blood cells in each milliliter of blood. White blood cell counts are indicators of infection or cancer of the blood, such as leukemia. Another example involves creatinine levels in the blood, a common index to measure kidney function. Creatinine levels in a blood sample are reported as X mg/dl (deciliter) of blood. The average adult range is 0.5 to 1.2 mg/dl. A level of 1.3 or greater could indicate impaired kidney function.

Using Syringes

Syringes contain markings to indicate volume and are marked in units of milliliters. Syringes are read by identifying the number that is at the *end* of the rubber stopper. Consider the following example. The HCP has an order to administer 4 mg of Valium to a patient. The liquid form of this medication is in a vial labeled 10 mg/2 ml. What volume of drug is withdrawn from the vial? Once again, the desired dose is divided by the available dose and the order of operations is applied:

- 4 mg/(10 mg/2 ml)
- Parentheses: 4 mg/5 mg/ml
- Division: 0.8 ml of drug withdrawn from the vial

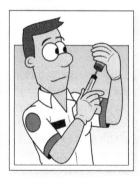

Liquid Medication—Michael

As an Emergency Medical Technician (EMT), Michael delivers liquid medication to patients often. With your own partner, calculate the volume of liquid medication to be withdrawn from a vial in order to administer 7.5 mg of drug. The vial is labeled 5 mg/ml.

Calculating Intravenous Drip Rates

The majority of IV bags include instructions to give the patient a particular amount of IV fluid over a certain number of hours. Large bags of IV fluids contain 1,000 cc (or ml). When an IV medicine must be given without an electric pump, the HCP must calculate the correct number of drops per minute to administer. For example, the patient's order may be to give 1,000 cc every 8 hours.

Another example may involve a small bag of antibiotic medicine with an instruction to give 500 mg over 30 minutes. In each case, the HCP would need to calculate the proper drip rate.

Statistics

HCPs often discuss statistics with patients. Examples include the outcomes of treatments such as medication or surgery, the prevalence of certain diseases in particular populations, or the occurrence of side effects. These statistics help patients make informed decisions about their care.

Medical Imaging

Students in radiography and sonography technician programs take a course covering topics in physics that are of special significance in medical imaging. Specific areas include:

- Newton's laws and the concepts of mass, force, energy, work, and power
- heat and its production and transfer
- the physics of wave motion
- general concepts of modern physics including Einstein's energy equation and the Heisenberg Principle

  Students in cardiac ultrasound programs need to understand the following:

- Bernoulli's equation, which relates pressure and the velocity of blood flow and is used to evaluate valvular heart disease, such as valvular stenosis (abnormal narrowing of the valve opening)
- Continuity equation, which relates the cross-sectional area of heart valves or blood vessels with the velocity of blood flow

Finally, radiography and sonography technicians need to be able to read dimensions, both two-dimensional for x-rays and three-dimensional for computed tomography (CT) scans, in order to correctly interpret the images of the inside of a patient's body.

Surgical Technologists

Some surgeries involve implants and prostheses, which require the placement of rods, plates, and screws. Surgical technologists use their math skills to understand the measurements involved with these procedures.

As with nursing students, surgical technology students must have an understanding of pharmacology and the calculations involved in the administration of medications.

Anesthesia in the Operating Room

HCPs responsible for anesthesia use math to prepare safe solutions and the correct levels of oxygen for surgical patients. They must consider factors such as the patient's weight, the desired drug or solution dosages, and the amount of dilution needed so that the active chemical is not too strong. Once again, the ability to understand and use ratios and proportions is required.

Other Needs for Math Skills in Health Care

There are many other examples of the need for solid math skills in the healthcare professions. A few include the following:

- An HCP with a supervisory position is likely to be involved with staff scheduling. Depending on the number of employees involved, calculating the number of hours each employee works and ensuring adequate unit coverage could become quite complicated and needs to be accurately completed.
- Billing and record keeping require math skills as well as organizational skills.
- The HCP may need to calculate the fluid intake and output of a patient. This would involve adding up every cc of fluid taken in by any route and the amount voided or otherwise released from the body.
- A patient's doctor may need to know the number of calories the patient has consumed in a day.
- The HCP may need to calculate a patient's ovulation date or expected date of confinement, also referred to as the due date in pregnancy.

An HCP may need to calculate a patient's glycemic index, which is a measure of the effect that carbohydrates have on blood glucose levels. An understanding of these values is important in the management of diabetes.

Chapter Summary

- HCPs across the disciplines routinely use a variety of math skills to carry out their jobs and care for their patients.
- Ratios and proportions are commonly used by HCPs, particularly in calculating dosages and in monitoring changes in a patient's health.

Review Questions

Objective Questions

1. 6:1 is a _____.
2. The most common system of measurement used in health care is the _____.
3. A/an _____ is a measured amount of medication given at specific intervals of time.
4. The distance between a line and a reference plane in an angle is measured in _____.

Short-Answer Questions

1. Why are basic math skills important for HCPs even if they normally use calculators?
2. Describe how HCPs use their math skills in three different areas of health care.

Applications

1. Calculate your BMI. What range do you fall in?
2. Atenolol is prescribed for many conditions including high BP. The initial dose used to treat hypertension is one 50-mg tablet once per day. Anne returned to

her doctor after taking this dose for 4 weeks. Because her BP remained high, the physician increased her dose to 100 mg per day. However, Anne had refilled her prescription for the lower dosage yesterday. She has 29 tablets left in the vial.

    a. How many of the lower strength tablets should Anne take each day to achieve the new higher dose?

    b. For how many days can she do this until she runs out of tablets and has to fill the prescription for the 100-mg tablets?

3. Sit in a chair and face forward. Proceed by turning your head to the left as far as possible without pain. Estimate your range of motion in degrees. Was it <90 degrees, 90 degrees, or >90 degrees? How would you describe your flexibility?

Fundamental Writing Skills

The section in the writing skills chapter you should complete at the end of Chapter 8 is Section 11-8. You can find this section on pages 230-232.

9

Test-Taking Skills

- Understand and fight test anxiety.
- Prepare and study for tests.
- Use different strategies to do well on objective, subjective, and other forms of tests.
- Know how to calculate grades.
- Apply concepts to certification or licensure exams.

Does anyone you know love taking tests? Probably not. Tests are something all students face, and tests cause almost everyone anxiety. In this chapter, you will find out how to plan and prepare for tests so you can improve your test-taking abilities and feel more confident. You will also learn about special skills for managing test anxiety. Tips and guidelines are presented for math tests and special exams such as those required for certification or licensure in many healthcare careers.

Health and Stress Management

Doing well on a test starts with how well you take care of your mind and your body. Studying is certainly key to your success, but how you care for your health and how you manage stress are very important, too.

The following is a quick review of what Chapter 3 describes about caring for your body for maximum functioning and low stress:

- Regular exercise can lower stress, keep you fit and looking good, and make you feel better mentally and physically.
- Sometimes rest is more important than completing every task on your daily to-do list.
- A balanced and nutritious diet is important for your health and managing stress.
- Breathing and relaxation techniques or yoga can help release tension.

Chapter 3 also explains that your mind needs recharging. The following is a review of some of the techniques you can use:

- *Keep negative thoughts under control.* Use positive imagery to move your mind toward your goals and away from your fears.
- *Calm your body to calm your mind.* When you have negative thoughts, use body-calming techniques (such as those discussed in Chapter 3) to enter a more calm and relaxed state of mind.
- *Visualize yourself achieving your goals and overcoming obstacles.* Think about how you feel when you visualize these things and remember that feeling when negativity rears its head.

- *Build a social support network.* Family, friends, classmates, coworkers, and people who share your interests are all good choices for a social support network. They give you an outlet for discussing your problems with people who care for you and want to help.

Test Anxiety

Recall the definition of *eustress*—good, or healthy, levels of stress. But most of us are more familiar with *distress*—high, unhealthy levels of stress. Most students experience some stress at test time, but for some, increased stress at test time interferes with their ability to think. They know the material. They've studied hard and effectively. But they just get so tense at test time that they can't put down the right answers. The way to beat test anxiety is to first recognize it and then prepare to fight it.

Avoid Mental Blocks

The most common test anxiety experience is a mental block. Although many students experience some level of this, students with severe test anxiety might read a test question over and over and never take in its meaning. Other symptoms of severe mental block include:

- doing poorly on a test after proving you know the material during class and in study groups
- feeling sweaty, shaky, or physically ill before and during a test
- obsessing over how well you're doing compared with other students
- thinking about how to get out of finishing the test, such as by faking an illness

If you're so overwhelmed with test anxiety that you can't do well on tests—even when you've attended every class, studied hard, and proven that you know the material—talk to your instructor about it. Your instructor might have another solution you haven't thought of. Alternately, ask a peer tutor or friend to "test" you with questions you haven't seen and a set time limit for completing the work. Taking practice tests beforehand can help you ease into the real thing.

Recognize Test Anxiety

You have read about what goes wrong for anxious students. But a little anxiety can be a good thing. Slight anxiety can improve your focus and mental sharpness. It keeps you from feeling complacent and helps you stay motivated to study. If you consistently feel nervous and distracted, however, test anxiety is probably taking over.

Test anxiety may produce many effects before and during a test, including:

- freezing up, when your brain doesn't take in the meaning of questions or you have to read questions over and over to understand them
- panicking about tough questions or about time running out before you're done

- worrying about the grade you will receive
- becoming easily distracted, daydreaming, or thinking about how you could escape taking the test
- feeling nervous about your ability to do well or about how you will do compared to others
- having physical symptoms of stress, such as sweating, nausea, muscle tension, and headaches
- feeling like you're not interested in the topic or you don't care how well you do on the test

Prepare to Fight Anxiety

The key to staying on top of anxiety for most successful students is using a combination of techniques to prepare for tests. This section discusses tips and guidelines all students can use. Remember that you need to prepare your mind and body. Keeping this balance will help you overcome your test anxiety and do your best.

Study Well

Studying well is the best preparation for a test—and the best cure for test anxiety. Studying can give you a sense of accomplishment that boosts your self-confidence. When you know the material backward and forward, you won't feel as nervous going into the test.

Relax Your Mind

Relaxation, along with other stress-reduction techniques, can help lessen test anxiety. When your body is relaxed, your mind is free to absorb new information. Try using breathing exercises or meditation to clear your mind.

Think Positively

Test anxiety can result from low self-esteem. Focus on being positive about tests. Say to yourself, "I've studied hard and I know this material. I can do this." Being prepared and having a positive attitude often lead to success.

Give Yourself a Break

If you start to feel anxious during a test, consider doing something to break the tension, such as putting down your pencil, closing your eyes, and taking a few slow deep breaths. If your shoulders are hunched, make a conscious effort to lower them and relax. If the instructor allows, you might even get up and sharpen your pencil or ask a question. Sometimes you can feel anxiety because you're physically tired and need a break.

Get Adequate Rest

Rest and relaxation are great fatigue fighters. You can do more when you feel rested and relaxed than when you're tired. Try using these tips before your next test:

- Get enough sleep—at least 7 to 8 hours at a time.
- Change activities from time to time.
- Exercise on a regular basis.
- Relax by allowing yourself breaks for TV, music, friends, or light reading.

Sit Up Straight

Your posture matters when you're studying or taking a test. If you're sitting in an uncomfortable position, it stresses your muscles. This stress is communicated to your brain, which in turn creates anxiety. Slouching can hurt your back and make you feel tired. Sit up straight and allow your concentration to return.

Eat Well

Good nutrition keeps you healthy. It also can improve your study habits and test-taking skills. Class time, work time, and study time often conflict with meal times. To counter this, avoid skipping meals and eat nutritious snacks between sessions.

Stay on Schedule

When a test approaches, try to maintain a normal routine. If you typically take a walk before dinner, avoid skipping your walk to study. If you usually sleep 8 hours a night, avoid the urge to cram until 2:00 am. Breaking good habits will only contribute to your mental and physical stress.

Defeat Test Anxiety

Here's a checklist of things to do the next time you're feeling nervous about a test.

Before the test:
- Talk to your instructor and classmates about what the test will cover.
- Use the study skills you learned in Chapter 7. Develop a method that works for you.
- Divide your study time over several days instead of trying to review everything the night before the test. Use the time management skills you learned in Chapter 2.
- When studying, use all your resources, including your textbook, lecture notes, and completed homework assignments.
- Create 3 × 5 inch cards for all key concepts or formulas that might appear on the test. Use the flash cards to practice and test your memory.
- Take a practice test. Find a room that's free of distractions and give yourself a specific amount of time to complete the test.
- Try to avoid studying right before taking the test. Put your notes away and take some time to relax.
- Arrive 5 minutes early so you will be ready when the instructor begins the test. Just don't arrive too early—sitting in an empty classroom or listening to other students' nervous chattering might make you feel anxious.

During the test:
- Break the tension. If your instructor allows it, get up to ask a question, sharpen your pencil, or get a drink.
- Focus on tensing and relaxing muscles in different parts of your body, such as your neck and shoulders. Then close your eyes and take a few deep breaths.
- Calm your nerves by putting the test into perspective. Life will go on after the test is over. Remember that doing your best is sufficient.
- Think of something calm and soothing when you feel test anxiety getting the best of you.

Preparing and Planning Ahead

When it comes to test taking, preparation is important. Knowing *what* you need to do *before* you have to do it gives you time to work out the best *way* to do it.

Know What Will Be Covered

You can't study well for a test if you don't know what kind of test it will be. If you know what kind of test to expect, you can put your study time to good use. Objective tests, such as short answer, sentence completion, multiple choice, matching, and true or false, in large part require you to remember facts and details and to recognize related material. Essay and oral tests require you to make good arguments about general topics and to support your arguments with critical details.

Test Format

You should always attend class, but it's especially important leading up to a test. Your instructor will probably explain the format of the test during class time. If not, visit your instructor during office hours and ask these questions:

- Will the test be comprehensive or will it cover select material only (like a few chapters)?
- Approximately how many questions will there be?
- How will the questions be weighted? For example, will multiple choice questions be worth 5 points each, whereas essays will be worth 20 points?
- How much will this test count toward my final grade?
- What materials will I need? A calculator? Scrap paper?

Learn From the Past

If you've already taken tests in the course or attended another course given by the same instructor, you probably have some idea of what the upcoming test will be like. For example, you might know that the instructor focuses on details rather than principles or sometimes uses trick questions.

If it's your first test for a particular course or instructor, however, you can still do a little extra preparation. Ask your instructor if practice tests or exams from the past are available for students to study. But remember, although past tests can give you an idea of what the upcoming test may be like, you are unlikely to see the same questions on this test.

Learn From the Class

Think about how you've learned things in class so far. Which topics has the instructor spent the most time discussing? Have you focused on details or large concepts in class discussions? Some instructors offer review sessions before the test. If your instructor does this, be there and be prepared. Plan ahead of time for the review session by writing down the questions you'd like to ask.

Plan Ahead

Thorough preparation short-circuits anxiety. This includes knowing the dates on which tests are scheduled and studying accordingly. The class schedule likely lists test dates and other deadlines. Put those test dates in your planning calendar. If your instructor didn't provide a class schedule at the beginning of the term, ask about approximate dates of tests.

Create a Game Plan

First, create an organized study plan. For example, you could set aside some time to study each day for a week before the test. Studying every day keeps the material fresh in your mind. Give yourself enough time to review your lecture notes, study materials, and old tests (if possible) several times. Choose a good place to study. Consider your study group; you can ask each other questions of the sort likely to appear on the test. Commit to studying and you'll be as prepared as possible for the test.

You might already review your notes after each class, which is good practice. But remember that it's not enough before a test. You'll need more intense review. In some classes, you may even have unannounced pop quizzes in between tests. In those cases, you'll be glad you spent extra time studying.

The Trouble With Cramming

The trouble with cramming is that it doesn't work. You simply can't cram data into your brain and have it stick. Most of the information disappears in a few hours. Furthermore, by the time you sit down to take the test, your brain is so tired that it can't retrieve most of the data it did manage to retain. As a result, you "blank out" and are unable to answer questions you might otherwise have easily answered.

Study Efficiently

When you have a test coming up and you feel unprepared for it, the best thing to do is stay calm and focused. Double-check with your instructor or a classmate about the format of the test. Use your textbook to create a master study outline. Focus on chapter headings, summaries, highlighted words, formulas, definitions, and the first and last sentences of every paragraph. Write key points and an outline of each chapter on notebook paper.

When you're done outlining in this way, review your class notes and handouts. Make some "must-know" flash cards for what you feel is the most important information. Flip through the flash cards until you're too tired to continue. Make sure to wake up at least 1 hour before the test to review your outline and flip through the flash cards again.

Include All Course Materials

Remember to bring the necessary materials to your study session. Before you begin studying, gather your review materials, textbooks, and notes. Look for information about the main terms, facts, concepts, themes, problems, questions, and issues that were covered in those materials. It's especially handy to compare the way your textbook covers an idea or concept with how your instructor covered it in class.

When you're studying for a test, it's not a good use of your time to try to reread entire chapters of your textbook. Instead, armed with your knowledge about what kinds of questions will be asked and which topics will be covered, use your textbook's index and glossary to look up just those topics. Find definitions of key terms in the glossary and look for important details in handouts and other supplementary material. Make lists of definitions and rehearse them.

Make a Study Sheet

Summarize your notes on one piece of paper. Review this study sheet, then place it face down and try to recreate your notes from memory. Think about where each topic was placed on the page. That way, when you encounter a certain topic on the test, you can flash back to your notes page and actually "see" the information.

Equations and Graphs

For math or science tests, practice your skills by rewriting equations and graphs. Solve sample problems and write out formulas. If you have trouble with certain formulas or graphs, make a separate sheet for the difficult ones and review it during gaps in your schedule throughout the day.

Main Terms

For short-answer tests, go through your textbook or lecture notes and make a list of important terms. Then add the definitions and think of an example of each term that you could use in a short answer.

Practice Essay Questions

For an essay test, prepare by doing a practice run. First, look at previous assignments and tests to see how essay questions are worded. Then, choose a topic from the material you're studying now and develop an essay question. Finally, write an answer for your essay question, giving yourself as much time as you'll have during your upcoming test. (See "Subjective Tests" for tips on how to develop a good essay.)

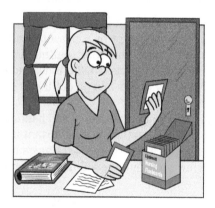

Test Preparation—Jenna

Jenna is dedicated to her studies and reviews her class notes every night. She even prepares flash cards to review whenever she has a few moments. The night before a test, Jenna has her daughter, Maddie, watch a movie with her parents. This way, she can continue preparing for the test without interruption. With a partner, discuss your most effective strategies to use when preparing for a test.

Practice Tests

Practice tests help you recognize the topics you struggle with most, which focuses your studying. To make a practice test, look at your study sheet and turn it into a series of questions. Then, answer the questions as if you are really taking a test. Sit in a quiet room and give yourself a certain amount of time to work. You may feel less anxiety when you take the real test if it feels familiar.

After you complete the practice test, use your study resources to check your answers. Spend extra time studying the questions you answered incorrectly.

Test Day

On the day of the test, there are several things you can do to make sure you are prepared:

- *Rest.* You need at least 7 to 8 hours of sleep the night before a test.
- *Eat small meals.* Breakfast is the most important—just avoid eating too much, or you'll feel sleepy.

- *Avoid excess caffeine.* You don't want to be jittery.
- *Exercise.* Even a short exercise session will help you feel mentally and physically invigorated.
- *Have your test materials ready to go.* Do this the night before so you won't waste time frantically searching for something on test day. Include all written materials, notes, pens, erasers, pencils, calculators, and whatever else is allowed or required.
- *Arrive on time.* Make sure you wear a watch. Not only will this help you avoid being late or having to rush to be on time but also during the test you can track how much time is left. It's best to arrive 5 minutes early so you can be seated and ready by the time the test begins.
- *Pay attention to the test instructions.* Do this before you rush right to the questions. Read or listen to directions, such as "copy the question" or "show your work." Then, skim the test. Jot a few notes that bring bits of information to mind. By reviewing questions quickly in advance, your brain can work on answers to longer questions while you complete shorter questions.
- *Budget test time efficiently.* After you skim the test, think about how to budget your time. Think about how much time you have to finish the test, the total number of questions, the type and difficulty of each question, and the point value of each. If you start to lag during the test, don't stress. You can recover by adjusting your schedule.

Test-Taking Strategies

You'll take many kinds of tests during your student career, each of which requires unique strategies. There are objective tests, such as multiple choice and true or false, and subjective tests, such as essays. There are vocabulary, reading comprehension, open-book, take-home, oral, and standardized tests as well.

You've probably seen some of these test types before. You might even have an idea of which kinds of tests you find easier or more difficult. No matter where your strengths or weaknesses lie, all students can use the same basic tips to improve their test-taking skills.

Bloom's Taxonomy and Question Types

Before we look at different types of test questions that are commonly used, it's helpful to understand how instructors think about tests—and what it is they're actually testing. The system developed by Benjamin Bloom to explain different cognitive levels or ways of thinking has shaped how many educators think about what and how they want their students to learn. This is called Bloom's Taxonomy of the Cognitive Domain or sometimes Bloom's learning levels. The six learning levels are described in Chapter 5:

- Knowledge
- Comprehension
- Application
- Analysis
- Synthesis
- Evaluation

As you prepare for a test in any course, it helps to think also about these levels. Your primary consideration involves the learning activities on which your course focuses and what kinds of test questions may be used to assess your mastery of that learning.

For example, let's say you have been learning how to take patients' vital signs—to take a temperature, measure blood pressure, and so on. Your instructor has emphasized that accuracy is the most important aspect of performing these skills. You need to perform each step in each procedure correctly. As described in Chapter 5, this learning is primarily in the first two levels of Bloom's Taxonomy: knowledge and comprehension. You have to remember exactly what steps to follow, for example, in using blood pressure equipment. You also need to understand what you are doing—the comprehension level—in order to do your job well. You can expect, therefore, that a test that includes this topic will likely include knowledge and comprehension types of questions. As noted in Chapter 5, this means not only recalling pertinent information and facts but also being able to describe in your own words information such as how to measure blood pressure.

Although knowledge and comprehension may be most important for this learning, the next level in the taxonomy is likely also important: application. This is because as you learned the steps for how to take blood pressure, you also learned you may need to vary the equipment or process in different situations. Can you explain *why* to use a different blood pressure cuff for a child or an adult with a large arm—and how the readings you obtain may be inaccurate if you do not? Because the application learning level is also important for this topic, it's likely the test may include questions such as this.

Remember that the three highest learning levels—analysis, synthesis, and evaluation—are involved in critical thinking. In these levels, it's not enough just to remember how to do something, why, and how to apply it in a new situation. Instead, you're expected to think more deeply about the issues involved. For example, you take a patient's temperature and find it normal, but an hour later, it is 3° F higher. Do you evaluate that fact as meaningful? Do you just record the information as you've been taught and go on about your work, or do you decide this is a significant change you should report immediately to a physician or nurse in case the patient's condition is rapidly declining? Why, or why not?

As you begin to prepare for any test, review in your memory how your instructor talked about the information you have been learning. This will help you determine whether the test may focus more on memory and comprehension or higher level thinking such as application, analysis, and evaluation—or perhaps both. This will also help you know what kinds of test questions to expect.

For example, objective test questions such as multiple choice and true or false are usually used for memory and comprehension. Test questions focusing on high-level understanding may include objective questions as well but are also likely to include short-answer and essay questions.

Objective Tests

Typically, there is only one right answer for each question on an objective test. The point is to test your recall of facts. Most standardized tests are objective, with one or more of these types of questions:

- Multiple choice
- True or false
- Short answer
- Sentence completion
- Problem solving

When taking an objective test, first look over the entire test to see how many questions there are. Try to answer them in order, but if you hit a difficult one, move on to the next. Just make sure you mark any tough questions so you remember to come back to them. You can go back to the hard questions you marked when you've reached the end of the test and have extra time. Working on the easier questions first may help you answer the hard ones, as information from other questions might spark memories and prompt you to remember the answers.

How to Decipher Multiple-Choice Questions

There are certain guidelines to follow on a multiple-choice test:

- Read each question carefully. Phrases like *except, not,* and *all of the following* provide important clues to the correct answer.
- Try to answer each question before you look at the answer choices. Then, try to match your answer to one of the choices. Even if you feel you have a match at choice one, read the rest of the choices to see if there's an even closer match.
- Use a process of elimination to narrow your answer choices. Some answers are clearly wrong. Cross them out and focus on the ones that might be correct.
- Try not to get bogged down and spend an excessive amount of time when answering each question. You won't have time to go back and answer truly hard questions if you take too long checking and double-checking the ones you think you answered correctly.

The *Best* Answer

Sometimes, test instructions tell you to choose the "best" answer. That means more than one answer choice may technically be correct, but only one choice fully answers the question. You have to prioritize the answers to determine which best answers the question.

When you're prioritizing answer choices, use well-known theories or principles. For a question that asks what you would do first, for example, think of Maslow's hierarchy of needs. This theory says that although all needs seem important, they can be ranked. Needs at the bottom of the rankings can be dropped. In a well-written test, all answer choices seem plausible. No single choice stands out as obviously wrong. To apply Maslow's hierarchy to tests, you have to try and rank the choices. Look for a clue in the question that makes one answer better than the others. Sometimes, questions and answers are taken word for word from your textbook or lecture notes. If you recognize familiar words or phrases in only one of the options, that option is likely the right answer.

Be alert for "attractive distracters," or words that look like the correct answer but aren't. For instance, if *ileum* is the correct answer on an anatomy test, *ilium* might be included as another answer choice.

True or False?

In general, true or false questions are meant to see if you recognize when simple facts and details are misrepresented. Most true or false statements are straightforward and are based on key words or phrases from your textbook or lectures.

Always decide whether the statement is completely true before you mark it as true. If it is only partly true, then the statement should be marked false. Statements containing extreme words can be tricky. Watch out for words such as:

- all
- always
- never
- none
- only

Short Answer

Short-answer questions usually ask for one or two specific sentences, such as writing a definition or giving a formula. When you're taking a short-answer test, quickly scan the test items to organize them in three categories:

- Answers I know without hesitation
- Answers I can get if I think for a moment
- Answers I really don't know

Answer the questions you know first and then move on to the questions that need a little thought. Once you're rolling and feeling confident, go for the tougher questions.

Note that most short-answer questions are objective questions with only one correct answer. In some cases, however, a short-answer question may be subjective, allowing you to demonstrate your understanding through a variety of possible answers. Either way, make sure your answer is clearly and concisely stated.

Filling in the Blanks

Sentence completion or fill-in-the-blank questions usually ask you to supply an exact word or phrase from memory. Sometimes, you can use the length and number of blanks as a clue to the best answer. Many instructors will indicate whether they expect one word, two, or a phrase by using longer and shorter blanks. Make sure your answer is consistent with the grammar of the sentence, as well. For example, if the question reads, "The medical term for heart muscle is _____ muscle," the answer should be *cardiac*, not *cardio* or *cardium*.

If you're really in doubt, go ahead and guess—you may receive partial credit.

Many times, the question itself will give clues to the right answer. For instance, a date may help you narrow the scope of answers by providing a historical point of reference. Suppose you think a scientific discovery might have been made by either Anton van Leeuwenhoek or Louis Pasteur and the date given is 1870. The right answer would have to be Pasteur because van Leeuwenhoek died in 1723.

Problem-Solving Tests

Problem-solving tests are most often found in subjects dealing with numbers and equations, such as math and science. With a problem-solving test, read through all the problems first before answering any of them. Underline keywords in the directions and important data in the questions. Make notes next to any questions that bring thoughts or data points to mind. Then, go back and begin to fully answer the questions.

Questions to Answer First

Students often think they should start with the hardest problems so they can be sure those problems will be completed. They believe they can rush through the easy questions at the end. It's actually better to start with the easy questions because they warm up your brain and build your confidence. Additionally, rushing to complete easy questions at the end can lead to careless mistakes and omissions.

Moving On

If you have trouble solving a problem, move on. When you come back to that problem, take advantage of the fact that you've been working on something different and you may look at the old problem in a new way. Will any of the strategies or formulas you used on other problems work? There's usually more than one way to solve a problem. If the strategy you started with isn't working, try something else.

Show Your Work

Show your work by including each step needed to solve a problem. If you make a mistake, the instructor will be able to see where you got off track and may give you partial credit. When you write down all your work, you can also check it yourself before you turn in the test. Checking your work helps you make sure you haven't made any careless errors or forgotten anything.

Subjective Tests

In a subjective or essay test, there's no single right answer. Instead, you are graded on how well you demonstrate your understanding of the material. Essay tests require more thought and planning. Follow these steps for successfully completing essay tests:

- Read all the directions, underlining important words and phrases.
- Read all the questions, even if you're not required to answer them all. Jot down facts and thoughts for each question.
- Estimate how long you think you'll need to answer each question.
- Choose the questions you want to answer, when given a choice.
- Outline each answer.
- Write the answers.
- Review and proofread your answers.

Read the Questions Carefully

When you read all the directions in a test first, you reduce your chance of losing points by not following them. For example, the directions may ask you to provide three supporting facts for your statement. If you skip over that part of the directions, you might provide only one or two facts. When you're reading through the directions, underline the key points so you can refer to them with a glance as you write.

Preview the Questions

Next, read through each question and make notes about any ideas or facts that come to mind. You can include things like formulas, names, dates, and your impressions. You'll need this information later as you create an outline. This step also helps you choose which questions to answer because it gives you an idea of how much you know about each topic.

Plan Your Time

The next step is estimating how long it will take to answer each question. Consider things like the number of questions and how many points each question is worth. If one question is worth half the test grade, for example, plan to spend half your time answering it. Factor in things like the time you'll need to organize an outline, write the essay, and proofread your work.

Organize an Outline

When you begin making an outline, start with your thesis statement. Choose a title that reflects your thesis and write it at the top of your paper. That way, you can use your title and thesis statement to guide your writing and keep it on track.

Content and organization typically count for most of the points on an essay test. The five-paragraph format is a good way to organize your information. (See *Five-Paragraph Format.*) If you run out of time and can't finish your essay, you can at least turn in your outline to let your instructor know that time was the problem, not comprehension.

Five-Paragraph Format

The five-paragraph format is an easy-to-follow structure for stating and supporting an opinion. It's a great way to get started on your essay, and it also helps you finish writing by taking the guesswork out of where to go next.

1. *Introduction.* Briefly outline your opinion and the facts you will use to support it.
2. *First point.* State your first point and include one to two supporting facts.
3. *Second point.* State your second point and include one to two supporting facts.
4. *Third point.* State your third point and include one to two supporting facts.
5. *Conclusion.* Pull together the three main points in a summary.

Note, however, that there's nothing magic about the number *three* for your key points. If you have only two main points to make, don't make up some third thing just to have three in the body of your essay—that would weaken your essay overall. Similarly, if you have a fourth key point to make, don't leave it out just because you think you *must* have five paragraphs. In other words, your essay should reflect what you actually have to say on the subject.

Follow Your Outline

When you are writing your essay, adhere to your outline to avoid wasting time. Your thesis statement should be a clear, but brief, answer to the essay question. In your introduction, explain what the remaining paragraphs in your essay will discuss. The essay question may ask you to "explain a cause-and-effect relationship" or "summarize key ideas." Be sure to follow directions here.

Each paragraph in the body of the essay should make one point and support it with facts. This will help you be clear in your writing. There's no need to develop long, winding arguments. Go straight from point A to point B and give the facts that led you there. Avoid making several points in one paragraph or bringing in facts that don't really apply to your point or that you'll use later. Each paragraph should have a topic sentence that flows from your thesis statement. Write simple, direct sentences that follow one another logically.

In the conclusion, restate your thesis and then refer to the points you've made that prove it. Use the conclusion to draw your ideas together.

When you're done writing, go back and read the question you've answered and the directions again. Make sure you've answered the question fully. Then review your essay for grammar errors and make sure your handwriting is legible. Make corrections where necessary.

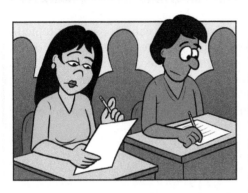

Essay Test—Thuy

It took some practice, but now, Thuy does very well on essay tests. She begins by writing an outline on a separate sheet of paper, leaving space between the sections. Then she writes one sentence that provides a fact to back up her point under each section in the outline. After that, she goes back and writes one more sentence with a fact under each section. She continues to fill in the outline until it is complete and then she copies it onto her test paper.

Essay Quick Check

After completing an essay, check your work. Ask yourself these questions regarding the following three elements of your essay:

Content:
- Did I adhere to my thesis statement?
- Did I support each point I made?
- Did I use examples?
- Did I distinguish fact from opinion?
- Did I mention any exceptions to my general statements?

Organization:
- Did I open with my thesis statement?
- Does the thesis statement answer the question?
- Did I follow my outline?
- Does my conclusion pull together all my points?

Writing mechanics:
- Does every sentence make a clear point?
- Did I use all words correctly?
- Are spelling, grammar, punctuation, and sentence structure all correct?
- Is my work neat and my handwriting legible?

Other Types of Tests

Other types of tests include the following:

- *Vocabulary.* These tests assess your ability to remember the meaning of a word and to use it correctly. They're used in foreign language courses or fields with specialized terminology such as medical terminology.
- *Reading comprehension.* These tests require you to read a passage and answer questions about its content.
- *Open-book and take-home.* You're usually allowed to use any materials you want when taking these kinds of tests. Critical thinking is more important than a good memory here. However, there's less slack given for making factual errors.
- *Oral.* Speaking clearly and fluently is key here. If you can choose your topic in advance, do so and prepare like you were going to write an essay, with a thesis statement and outline. Try to make three points supported by facts.
- *Standardized.* The Graduate Record Examination (GRE) and Scholastic Assessment Test (SAT) are two examples of standardized tests. They are used for placement and admissions. Most tests required for certification or licensure in a healthcare career (discussed later in this chapter) are also standardized tests.

Learn From Your Mistakes

Reviewing your test after it has been graded can help you learn where you got off track and what you need to go over before the next test. When you get a corrected test back, ask yourself:

- Was there one concept or problem that tripped me up?
- How would I sum up the instructor's comments?
- Did I prepare adequately? How should I prepare differently next time?
- Did I make any careless mistakes? How can I avoid them next time?
- What can I learn from my mistakes?

Tests give you an opportunity to evaluate how well you're doing in a course. Many instructors review tests with the entire class. One final test-taking strategy is to review your own test when it's given back to you. Try to learn from the comments your instructor made. If you have questions, make an appointment to see the instructor during office hours.

Remember, it's never good to argue with an instructor about your grade in class. But if you have questions or believe the instructor made an error in grading, approach the instructor privately outside of class. Be sure to present your concerns in a respectful way.

Succeeding on Math Tests

Many students are especially anxious about math tests. With good study habits and advance preparation, math tests should not be any more difficult than other types of tests.

Math questions generally fall into one of two categories: number questions and word problems. Both types involve solving problems and using math principles. Several strategies can be used to approach either type of test.

Practice Tests

Take some practice tests to prepare for test day. Many textbooks include practice questions. You also can find many websites that offer practice tests. Take the test without looking at the answers and then grade yourself. You'll be glad you took practice tests when you sit down for your actual exam—they build your confidence and get you used to performing under test conditions.

Number Problems

Here are a few simple steps that can help you increase your likelihood of success when taking a number problem test:

- *Work carefully and deliberately.* You can sabotage yourself by being careless or working too fast. Thorough work is required. Write carefully, perform the calculations in reverse to check your answer, keep numbers in straight columns, and copy accurately.
- *Write out all steps.* Sometimes, students feel that showing all their work is childish. But it's a good practice at any age. If you write out your work, you can catch errors in it more easily.
- *Estimate first.* Try to estimate the answer to a problem before you start working. Then, solve the problem without referring to the estimate. When you finish your calculations, compare your answer with the estimate to see how close they are. If they're not close, you may have made a mistake in your calculations—a decimal point in the wrong place, an extra zero, etc.
- *Make sure your calculations use all the information given in the problem.* There's rarely unnecessary data given in a math problem. Most of the time, each piece of data is essential to solving the problem.
- *Read each question twice.* After you think you have the right answer, read the question again. Use a mental checklist. Did you show your work? Did you answer in the correct units? Did you answer all parts of the question? Does your answer make sense? If your answers are yes, you're on the right track.
- *Be persistent.* Everyone gets stuck sometimes. There are ways you can get yourself moving again. Round fractions up to whole numbers to put a problem into simpler form. Try to figure out what information you think you're missing. What doesn't make sense? Where do you lose track? If all else fails, move on to other questions and come back to the tougher ones later.

Avoiding Careless Mistakes

Careless mistakes result when students speed through problems. To avoid these mistakes and increase your accuracy, follow these tips:

- Write your numbers carefully so your sevens don't look like ones or fours and your eights don't look like sixes or zeroes.
- Whether you're doing simple or elaborate calculations, keep your digits in straight columns. You don't want numbers in the tens column being counted in the hundreds column.
- If you copy a problem onto another page, double-check to make sure you copied it accurately. You'd be surprised how often you can overlook a silly mistake—like writing a subtraction sign instead of a division sign—and not even realize it.

Word Problems

Word problems have a bad reputation for being difficult. However, word problems simply put numbers in a nonnumber context. There are some things you can do to make word problems more approachable:

- Look at the big picture.
- Plan well.
- Use strategies for dealing with difficult word problems.
- Learn from past mistakes with similar problems.

The Big Picture

When you're facing a test that includes word problems, look over the whole test first. As you read each problem, jot down notes in the margin about how you might solve it.

Work on the easiest problems first. Those are the problems where the solutions you should use are easy to identify. Solving easy problems first warms up your brain and builds confidence.

Plan Well

Consider planning for the test as you would plan time for a study session. Allow more time for problems worth more points. Budget time at the end of the test to review and to go back to difficult problems.

Those tough problems can derail your planning, but it doesn't have to be that way. Stay calm. Try not to give in to panic or feeling overwhelmed. There are several strategies you can use to solve tough problems:

- Mark keywords and numbers, which can narrow the problem down to its essential elements.
- Sketch a diagram of the problem to make it more comprehensible.
- List all the formulas you think are relevant and decide which to use first.
- Think about similar practice problems and how you solved them.
- Guess at a reasonable answer if other strategies fail and then check it. If you can't work out the problem to get to your answer, you may think of another solution.

Learn From Your Mistakes

After the test is over and you get it back from the instructor, read through the comments and suggestions. Try to avoid making assumptions about why you missed certain problems. Assumptions like "I just can't do math" or "It's just too hard" are unhelpful and counterproductive. Instead, ask yourself these questions:

- Did I make careless mistakes?
- Did I misread questions?
- Did I miss the same kind of problem repeatedly?
- Did I remember formulas incorrectly or incompletely?
- Did I run out of time?
- Did I practice enough, or did I skimp on practice problems?
- Did I let my anxiety get the best of me, making me miss problems I really know how to solve?

Based on your answers to these questions, you can identify ways to improve your performance on future tests.

Calculating Grades

One of the reasons many students are anxious about tests is that they generally contribute heavily to the grade for the whole course. It's important, therefore, to understand how much any given quiz or test counts toward your grade and to be able to calculate your current grade status regardless of which systems your instructor may use. Calculating your grade involves looking at what activities—tests, quizzes, homework, papers, etc.—earn points and how much each counts toward your final grade. Your syllabus usually provides this information.

In the following section, we'll describe how to calculate grades for point systems, averages, and weighted grade systems.

Understanding Grades

Your instructor might assign points or percentage values to each activity on the syllabus. If your instructor uses a point-based system, the easiest way to determine your grade is to convert the points to percentages. For example, if you take a test and receive a score of 40 out of 50 possible points (40/50), you can convert this score to a percentage to figure out your grade on the test. When figuring out percentages, remember to divide the number of points you received by the total number of possible points. A score of 40/50 equals 80%.

At any point during a semester or term, you also should be able to figure out your overall grade in a course. Let's say your syllabus lists the following information:

- Five quizzes—worth 40 points each
- Test 1—worth 100 points
- Test 2—worth 200 points

So far, the class has taken one quiz and Test 1, for a total of 140 possible points (40 + 100 = 140). After adding up the points you received on the quiz and test, you find that you have a total of 120 out of 140 possible points (120/140). Based on this information, you can figure out your overall percentage grade.

$$120 \div 140 = 85.7\%$$

If you keep track of your quiz and test scores (as well as any other graded activities) throughout the term, you'll be able to determine your overall grade in a course at any time. Knowing your grade in each course can help you gauge whether you're on target to meet your goals. Also, by keeping tabs on your grades, you can react early if they begin to slip. You may realize that you need to put in more study time, meet with your instructor, or visit the tutoring center. But if you wait until the end of the semester to figure out your overall grade in a course, it may be too late to improve it.

Averages

Now let's look at a grading system based on *averages*. Suppose your instructor says that the average of six test grades will be your final grade in the course. By the middle of the term, the class has taken three tests. For example, if your test grades were 78%, 91%, and 95%, what would your overall grade be so far? Follow these simple steps to determine your average grade:

1. First, add your three test scores (78 + 91 + 95 = 264).
2. Then, divide the total by the number of tests you've taken so far (264 ÷ 3 = 88).

This means your grade in the course would be 88%.

Weighting

In some cases, each activity listed on a syllabus is *weighted*, or assigned a certain percentage of the final grade. This means some activities will affect your final grade more than others, as shown below:

- Five quizzes—each is worth 10% of your final grade
- Test 1—worth 20% of your final grade
- Test 2—worth 30% of your final grade

Let's analyze these percentages. At first glance, it looks like the quizzes are not worth as much as Test 1 or Test 2. But look more closely; the syllabus says that *each* quiz is worth 10% of your final grade, which means:

$$5 \text{ quizzes} \times 10\% = 50\%$$

Therefore, the quizzes will make up 50% or half of your final grade.

Projects, Papers, and Homework

Many instructors also include activities such as projects, papers, homework, and participation in a student's final grade. Let's look at a scenario with several weighted activities:

- Four quizzes—each is worth 5% of your final grade
- Test 1—worth 10% of your final grade
- Test 2—worth 20% of your final grade
- Group project—worth 5% of your final grade
- Homework—worth 5% of your final grade
- Attendance and participation make up the rest of your grade.

Now, which is most important? You might think the quizzes or tests are more important to your final grade than your attendance and participation. Look more closely:

- Quizzes are 20% of your final grade (4 quizzes × 5% = 20%).
- The tests together equal 30% of your grade (10% + 20% = 30%).
- The group project plus homework equal 10% of your grade (5% + 5% = 10%).

That leaves 40% for your attendance and participation—the largest percentage of all.

Calculating Your Grade

So how do you figure out your grade in a course where the activities are weighted? Let's determine a student's grade based on the following syllabus information:

- Quizzes—average of six quizzes is worth 15% of your final grade
- Test 1—worth 25% of your final grade
- Test 2—worth 60% of your final grade

Suppose a student averaged all her quizzes for a score of 70%. On Test 1, her grade was 80% and on Test 2, she received a score of 90%. How can we determine her final grade in the course if the activities are all weighted differently?

1. First, take all three scores and multiply each by the appropriate percentage, as listed on the syllabus. This will give each score the correct weight.

   Quizzes—70(0.15) = 10.5
   Test 1—80(0.25) = 20
   Test 2—90(0.60) = 54

2. Next, add the three products you came up with in step 1.

   10.5 + 20 + 54 = 84.5

3. The sum is the student's overall grade in the course: 84.5%.

Grading Scales

It's no use knowing how many points you earned or what your grade averages were if you're unable to translate that information into a letter grade. Here's a sample grading scale from a syllabus:

97–100 = A+
94–96 = A
90–93 = A−
86–89 = B+
83–85 = B
80–82 = B−
76–79 = C+
73–75 = C
70–72 = C−
66–69 = D+
63–65 = D
60–62 = D−
59 and under = F

For example, if a student received an overall grade of 84.5% in a course, that would translate to a B.

Many schools use the 4.0 system to calculate student grade point averages (GPAs). To do this, they assign point values to each student's letter grades. Here's a sample list based on the 4.0 system:

A = 4.0
A− = 3.7
B+ = 3.3
B = 3.0
B− = 2.7
C+ = 2.3
C = 2.0
C− = 1.7
D+ = 1.3
D = 1.0
D− = 0.7
F = 0.0

Let's calculate the GPA of a student who has completed one semester. Suppose this student took four 3-credit courses during his first semester. His overall grades were A, B+, A, and C−. What would his GPA be?

1. First, list the point values assigned to each of the letter grades the student received.

   A = 4.0
   B+ = 3.3
   A+ = 4.0
   C− = 1.7

2. Next, find the average of the four point values.

$$4.0 + 3.3 + 4.0 + 1.7 = 13.0$$
$$13.0 \div 4 = 3.25$$

3. The average is the student's GPA: 3.25 (which, rounded to the nearest decimal point, comes to 3.3).

Keep in mind that the 4.0 system varies from school to school. For example, certain courses may be weighted more than others. You can talk to your academic advisor if you have questions about the system your school uses.

The End of the Semester

Suppose you are nearing the end of the semester and you just have one more biology test to take. You'd really like to reach your goal of getting a B in the course, but you're not sure if that's possible. What grade would you have to get on the last test in order to get a B in the course?

1. First, look at the syllabus to see how much each graded activity is worth. For example, suppose your syllabus lists this information:
   - Five quizzes—average of 5 quizzes is worth 20% of your final grade
   - Test 1—worth 30% of your final grade
   - Test 2—worth 50% of your final grade

2. Next, list your scores for each activity. Let x stand for the score of your last test because you haven't taken it yet. For the sake of this example, we'll use the following scores:
   Quizzes—70%
   Test 1—75%
   Test 2—x

3. Then, take all three scores and multiply each by the appropriate percentage, as listed on the syllabus. This will give each score the correct weight.
   Quizzes—70(0.20) = 14
   Test 1—75(0.30) = 22.5
   Test 2—x(0.50) = $0.5x$

4. Now, add the three products you came up with and make the sum equal to 80, as below. (This will be a basic algebraic equation used to find the value of x.) The value of x is the percentage grade you will need to get on the test in order to receive a B (or at least 80%) in the course.

$$14 + 22.5 + 0.5x = 80$$
$$36.5 + 0.5x = 80$$
$$36.5 + 0.5x - 36.5 = 80 - 36.5$$
$$0.5x = 43.5$$
$$0.5x \div 0.5 = 43.5 \div 0.5$$
$$x = 87$$

5. And you have your answer. In order to receive a B in the course, you would have to score at least 87% on the last test.

Grade Calculation Practice

At the midpoint in a semester, suppose a student has received the following scores:

- Quizzes—8/10, 6/10, 9/10, 10/10
- Homework assignments—5/5, 4/5, 3/5, 5/5
- Research paper—139/150
- Midterm exam—184/200

Based on the information above, calculate the following percentages (check your answers in the Appendix):

Question 1. What is the student's average quiz grade?
Question 2. What is the student's average homework grade?
Question 3. What percentage grade did the student receive on the research paper?
Question 4. What percentage grade did the student receive on the midterm exam?
Question 5. If each activity is weighted equally, what is the student's overall grade in the course so far?

Certification and Licensure Exams

After you complete your educational program, to enter many healthcare careers, you may be required to take a licensure examination. This is a test mandated by state law to ensure you are prepared to practice in your field. Such a licensure examination is used in most professions, such as a law school graduate having to pass the bar exam before practicing law.

Certification may also be required or optional for you, depending on your chosen health career and your state. In most healthcare careers in which certification is available but voluntary, it is still a good idea to become certified because this usually makes it easier to find the kind of job you want and to advance within your career. Certification, like licensure, requires an examination after completing your educational program. Certification is usually controlled by a professional association.

Because there are a multitude of specific health careers with their own legal requirements for licensure (which may vary by state) and different associations controlling certification, it is impossible to tell you *exactly* what to expect from these exams in your specific field. But you can easily find out yourself, and we can generalize about most licensure and certification exams. Follow these guidelines:

- Don't wait until you're almost finished with school before thinking about an upcoming licensure or certification exam. You should find out at the start of your program what the certification requirements are for your profession. Start by asking an instructor about what exam(s) you will need or want to take.
- Visit the website of your state's licensing agency and the professional association that administers the certification exam. Print out the basic information and highlight things like when the exam is given, when and how to register for the exam, what the exam covers, and the type of questions on the exam.
- Pay special attention to the test itself and the testing situation. Most such exams are multiple choice, and some are given only on computers at the test site.
- Plan a study schedule well in advance of the exam, reviewing your educational materials related to topics you can expect on the exam. Use the study strategies described earlier in this chapter and in Chapter 7.
- Prepare for the type of test as described earlier in this chapter, such as how to perform best on multiple-choice tests.
- Practice exams (and often review books with practice exams) are available in almost all healthcare fields where licensure or certification requires an exam. Taking one or more practice exams well before the test date will help you see if you need to study certain areas more and will give you confidence for the actual exam.
- Keep the exam in mind throughout your school program. Hang on to materials that you think will help you study for the exam when the time comes.

Chapter Summary

- Help reduce test stress by taking care of your body by exercising, eating right, and getting enough rest.
- Meet stress head on with relaxation techniques, positive thinking, and by relying on your support network.
- Give yourself time to prepare and plan for tests. Talk with your instructor about what to expect, create a study plan, and take practice tests.
- With all kinds of tests, always read the directions and skim through the questions before you begin.
- When taking objective tests, work on the easier questions first to warm up your brain and jog your memory.
- For subjective tests, create an outline to help you get started on your essay.
- Review all graded tests to see where you can make improvements.
- Begin preparing well ahead for a licensure or certification exam, and take a practice test or two to ensure you've mastered the material and are confident for test day.

Review Questions

Objective Questions

1. Two best practices to employ on the day of a test include _____ and _____.
2. Question 1 is at the _____ level of Bloom's Taxonomy.
3. A student with a grade average of 80% at the end of a course will most earn the letter grade of _____.

Short-Answer Questions

1. Describe how to fight test anxiety.
2. Describe how to write an outline for an essay and why doing so is important.
3. Discuss two tips for doing well on multiple-choice questions, whether on a class test or licensure exam.

Applications

1. Form groups of two to four students. Each group member will come up with a five-question test for this course. The questions can be multiple choice, sentence completion, true/false, etc., or a mixture of question styles. Arrange a time to meet for 1 hour. Each of you will take a test you didn't write and complete it in 20 minutes. For the rest of the hour, go over the tests as a group, helping each other see where you made mistakes or did well. Discuss the strategies you used to answer the different types of test questions.
2. Find out whether you will be taking a licensure exam after finishing your education and visit the website of the licensing agency to learn about the exam.

Fundamental Writing Skills

The section in the writing skills chapter you should complete at the end of Chapter 9 is Section 11-9. You can find this section on page 232.

10

Writing, Presenting, and Researching for the Healthcare Professional

- Explain the importance of writing for classes.
- Explain the importance of the writing process.
- Describe the process or preparing and delivering presentations.
- Explain the importance of using appropriate research and citation tools.
- Describe strategies for researching.
- Explain the importance of good library skills.

Writing for Classes

Writing, like speaking, is an important communication skill. As a student, you'll most likely be required to write essays, reports, and research papers. The writing skills you develop in school will carry over into your professional career as well. As an allied health professional, you'll need solid writing skills for recording accurate and concise information in patient medical records.

Writing skills can be helpful for several other reasons, one of which is securing your first job. A well-written résumé and cover letter can help you get your foot in the door and get an interview, as discussed in Chapter 14. Even in email messages, being able to express yourself well shows that you are intelligent and competent. It also effectively gets your message across to the person with whom you are communicating. Good writing skills help you avoid misunderstandings that can result from poor communication.

Essay Structure

Whether you're writing a brief essay or a 15-page research paper, each writing assignment should be structured in roughly the same way. Formal academic writing includes an introduction, a body, and a conclusion. (For a discussion of paragraph structure, see Chapter 11.)

The Introduction

Always begin your written assignments with an introduction. The introduction should interest the reader in the topic you're about to discuss. Your introduction can be structured in a number of different ways. It can:

- center on a thesis statement (a thesis statement is a statement of the opinion or main idea to be discussed in your paper)
- present a problem or ask a question that you intend to answer
- describe a dramatic event or incident
- provide interesting statistics
- set a scene
- relate a short story

For example, in a persuasive essay, your introduction could begin by presenting a topic. Then, your thesis statement could include the main point you intend to argue about that topic.

Keep in mind that your introduction doesn't have to be the first thing you write. Even if you start with a basic outline and have a general idea of how you'd like to approach your topic, it's easy to get stuck on the introduction. If this happens, try working on other portions of the paper for a while and come back to it. Your introduction will be easier to write once you have a clear purpose in mind.

The introduction should be roughly 5% to 15% of the length of your entire paper. It needs to be informative but to the point. It should be interesting without giving away too much detail. For these reasons, it takes time and effort to write a good introduction. You may want to revise it again after you've completed your paper.

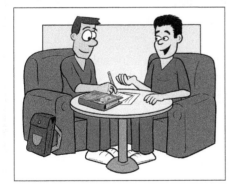

Sometimes It Is Easier to Write the Introduction Last—Michael

Michael frequently has to write essays for almost all of his courses, even for Anatomy and Physiology. At first, he found this very difficult because he always tried to write the introduction first. It seemed logical that you'd write the introduction first.

One day, when he was seeking some extra help on an essay in the college's writing center, one of the tutors suggested that Michael start with the body of the essay. "Just begin with the part you know best," the tutor told him, "and then go on from there. When you have all of the body written, you can go back and see what the essay is really about. Then you can write a paragraph introducing that. Of course, you will still have to revise the whole essay several times once you have a full draft."

This advice made starting his essays much easier for Michael. The revisions, though, are still difficult.

The Body

You do most of your writing in the body, which makes up about 70% to 90% of a paper's total length. The body of a paper presents details that support your thesis. The body may include:

- background information about your topic
- facts and supporting research
- explanations of key terms or phrases used throughout the paper
- quotes from other credible sources
- different arguments in opposition to your thesis and your responses to those arguments

The Conclusion

A strong conclusion ends the discussion presented in the paper and makes the reader think. To accomplish this, the conclusion needs to do more than blandly summarize main points. To write a strong conclusion, consider including:

- a quotation that relates to or sums up your thesis
- a question for the reader to consider
- encouragement for the reader to act in support of your idea
- one last example or story to reiterate your point

Works Cited List and References

The works cited list is a list of the sources you used to write your paper. It's important because it helps you back up the information included in your paper and gives credit to your sources of research. Whether you gathered information from a book, a website, a television program, or a magazine article, each source must be included in your works cited. A works cited list only shows the general sources, however. For quotations, specific statistics, and the theories and opinions of others, you'll need to include specific references in the text of the essay, usually as parenthetical citations. For more on this, see the "APA Style, an Explanation and an Overview" section.

Appendix

You probably won't need to include an appendix with each formal writing assignment you complete. An appendix is only necessary when you need to include other supportive materials that do not belong or cannot fit in the body of your paper. A few examples of such materials are:

- a list of key terms and definitions
- photos, illustrations, or figures
- tables, charts, maps, and other graphic elements

The Writing Process

You've decided on the type of paper you're going to write. You know it needs to have an introduction, a body, and a conclusion. What next? First, carefully reread the assignment to make sure you fully understand it. Is your topic appropriate? Are you expected to do research? How long should the final result be? When you are clear about all aspects of the assignment, you're ready to start the process.

Writing a paper involves multiple steps in a process. The writing process is a time-tested method to ensure you do your best on the paper. The process includes but is not limited to:

1. setting your schedule
2. selecting a topic

3. collecting information
4. organizing the information
5. evaluating the information
6. creating an outline
7. writing a first draft
8. revising the first draft
9. finalizing the paper

Scheduling

A good way to set up a schedule for writing a paper is to work backward from the due date listed in your syllabus. Then, mark the following on your calendar and weekly planner:

- Due date for the paper
- Amount of time you need to revise the paper
- Amount of time you need to write the first draft
- Date you should complete your research
- Date you need to begin research

When scheduling your time, be generous. Unexpected problems can arise, making some steps take longer than you anticipated. For example, you may go to the library to find that a book you need has already been checked out. Or you may find that you need extra time to evaluate and organize the materials you gathered. Whatever delays may occur, you can avoid stress by building in extra time for the full process.

Another aspect that may affect your writing schedule is the paper's length. Sometimes it's hard to predict how much work you'll need to do to complete the assignment. When considering how much time to allow yourself to write the paper, keep the following in mind:

- The required length of the paper
- The amount of time you have before the due date
- The amount of research you're expected to do
- The number of references your instructor requires you to have

Selecting a Topic

If your instructor assigns a specific topic, you won't have to worry about this stage of the writing process. If not, your instructor may give you a list of acceptable topics or guidelines for creating your own topic. When thinking about possible topics, select one that captures your interest. When you write about a subject that interests you, you'll be better motivated to work on the paper. Also, be sure to select a topic that you'll be able to research adequately. You'll have a hard time completing an assignment that requires a lot of research on an obscure topic.

Good places to search for topic ideas include:

- the table of contents in your textbook
- your lecture notes
- brainstorming sessions with your study group
- magazines, journals
- websites

Just remember to keep your topic fairly narrow. A more focused topic means a more focused writing process and a better paper. When looking for a topic, try to find a balance. Your topic should provide you with enough material to complete the assignment, but it should be focused enough that you can explain it fully in your paper.

One way to see if a topic is well defined or focused enough is to think about your thesis statement and the title of the paper. A good title is clear and appealing. The reader should know what the paper is about just by reading the title. However, if you come up with a title before writing the paper, keep in mind that the title isn't permanent and may need to change after the paper has been completed. Sometimes, it's simply a good exercise to think about the main point you'd like to communicate in your paper. Doing so may help you decide on a topic.

Giving Presentations

A formal presentation, another form of public speaking, involves preparation outside of class and sometimes significant research and planning. That part of the process is actually similar to writing a paper for a class or even studying for an exam. What's different is this preparation leads to a presentation given in class, in front of other students and the instructor—a situation that usually makes students nervous. But relax; with good planning and communication skills, you can develop the ability to give excellent presentations.

Begin by making sure you understand the exact requirements of the assignment. What's the topic and how long should it be? Then you can begin planning. Class presentations do not have to be difficult if you follow these six basic steps:

1. Analyze your audience and goals.
2. Plan, research, and organize your content.
3. Draft and revise the presentation.
4. Prepare visual aids.
5. Practice the presentation.
6. Deliver the presentation.

Who's Your Audience? What's Your Point?

In most class presentations, the answer to the first question seems obvious: other students and the instructor. Check the assignment, however—maybe you're supposed to address the class as if they were patients in a healthcare setting. Even if the audience is your class, you still need to think about what they already know and don't know about your topic. How much background information do they already have based on previous lectures and reading? Be careful not to give a boring recap of things they already know. However, it may be important to show how your specific topic fits in with subjects that have been discussed already in class.

Think also about your goal for the presentation. The assignment instructions from your instructor may provide the goal, but you may need to adjust it to what you can cover well in the time you're given for the presentation.

Plan, Plan, Plan

Start by brainstorming about your topic. You may also need do some more reading or research. Don't worry at first about how much material you're gathering. It's much better to know too much and then pick out the most important things to say in your allotted time than to rush ahead and then realize you don't have enough material.

Organizing a presentation or speech is similar to organizing topics in a paper for class (see "Essay Structure" in the "Writing for Classes" section). Introduce your topic and state your main idea, go into more detail about specific ideas in the body of the presentation, and conclude. Look for a logical order for the body of the presentation. Some topics might be covered in a chronological (time) order, whereas others are best developed through a compare-and-contrast organization.

If your goal is to persuade, sort out your separate arguments and build to the strongest or most important. Put similar ideas together and think about how you'll need to transition between very different ideas.

While researching your topic and outlining your main points, also start thinking about visual aids for the presentation.

Draft and Revise

You don't need to actually write out the presentation in full sentences and paragraphs because you shouldn't read it aloud—that makes for a dull presentation. Some students speak well from brief phrases written on note cards, whereas others prefer a more detailed outline.

You can't know for sure how long your presentation will last until you rehearse it, but try to estimate the time while drafting it. Figure that it takes 2 to 3 minutes to speak the amount of writing on a standard double-spaced page—but with visual aids, pauses, and audience interaction, it may take longer. This is only a rough guide, but you might start out thinking of a 10-minute presentation as the equivalent of a three- to four-page paper.

As you draft your speaking notes, consider questions like these:

- Am I going on too long about minor points?
- Do I have good explanations and reasons for my main points? Do I need more data or better examples? Where would visual aids be most effective?
- Am I using the best words for this topic and this audience? Should I be more or less informal in the way I talk about my topic?
- Does it all hold together and flow well from one point to the next? Do I need a transition when I shift from one idea to another?

Prepare Visual Aids

Most presentations gain from visuals, and with visual technology used in many classrooms, visual aids are often expected. Consider all possibilities when choosing appropriate visuals:

- PowerPoint, Google Slides, or Prezi slides, which may include:
  - charts
  - graphs
  - maps
  - photos, or other images
  - video clips
- A physical object
- Handouts (only when necessary—these can often be distracting)

Practice, Practice, Practice

Practice is the most important step in preparing. Practice also helps you get over stage fright and gain the confidence that you'll do a good job.

Practice first alone, either to a mirror or in an empty room where you imagine people sitting (so that you can move your eyes around the room to this "audience"). Do not read your notes aloud but speak in sentences natural for you. Glance down at your notes only briefly and then look up immediately to the mirror or around the room. Time yourself, but don't obsess about using precisely the exact number of minutes your instructor requested. If your presentation is way off, however, adjust your outlined notes.

Once you feel good about delivering your content from your notes, practice some more to work on your delivery. You might want to record your presentation on audio or video or ask a friend or roommate to watch your presentation.

Using Visual Aids

Use the available technology, whether a SMART Board or an ActivBoard, or even a flip chart or posters. Always check the assignment to confirm your instructor's expectations for your use of visual aids. You might also talk to your instructor about resources and applications for designing your visuals. Follow these guidelines:

- Design your visuals carefully. Use a simple, neutral background. Minimize the amount of text in visuals. Don't simply present word outlines of what you are saying.
- Don't use more than two pictures in a slide and use two only to make a direct comparison. Image montages are hard to focus on and can be distracting.
- Don't put a table of numbers in a visual aid. If you need to illustrate numerical data, use a graph. Don't use too many visuals or move through them so quickly that the audience gives all its attention to them rather than to you.
- Practice your presentation using your visual aids because they will affect your timing.
- Explain visuals when needed but not when they're obvious.
- Speak to the audience, not to the visual aid—glance at your visual aid only to make sure you are in synch with it.
- Practice a good opening to capture the audience's attention. Start with a striking fact or example (illustrating an issue, a problem), a brief interesting or humorous anecdote (historical, personal, current event), a question to the audience, or an interesting quotation. Then relate the opening to your topic and your main point and move into the body of the presentation.
- Try to speak in your natural voice, not a monotone as if you were just reading aloud.
- Practice making changes in your delivery speed and intensity to emphasize key points in your presentation.
- Don't keep looking at your notes. It's fine if you use words that are different from those you wrote down—the more you rehearse without looking at your notes, the more natural you will sound.
- Be sure you can pronounce all new words and technical terms correctly. Practice saying them slowly and clearly to yourself until you can say them naturally.
- Don't forget transitions. A reader notices it when a writer moves on to a new point (with a heading in the text, a paragraph break, or a transitional phrase), and listeners also need a cue that you're moving to a new idea. Practice phrases such as "Another important reason for this is . . . " or "Now let's move on to why this is so . . . "
- Watch out for all those little "filler" words people so often use in conversation, such as *like*, *you know*, *well*, and *uh*.
- Pay attention to your body language when practicing. Stand up straight and tall in every practice session so that you become used to it. Unless you have to use a fixed microphone in your presentation, practice moving around while you speak. Make natural gestures. Keep your eyes moving and making eye contact with the audience when you present. Practice smiling and occasionally pausing at key points.

Deliver the Presentation

On presentation day, get plenty of sleep and eat a healthy breakfast. Don't drink too many caffeinated drinks because that may make you hyper and nervous. Wear comfortable shoes and appropriate professional clothing that won't restrict you or make you self-conscious as you move around before the audience.

Remember: The audience is on your side. If you're still nervous before your presentation, take a few deep breaths. Rehearse your opening lines in your mind so that you don't have to look at your notes immediately when starting. Instead, look out and around your audience. Smile as you move to the front of the room. You'll see some friendly faces smiling back encouragingly.

Research

When researching for your paper, begin at your school's library. The librarian should be able to help you find specialized, health-related databases to which your school may subscribe as well as other sources that can provide you with preliminary information on your topic. Spend some time in the library familiarizing yourself with the information resources available to you. You'll surely need to return to them many times through the course of your studies. What's more, being information literate—that is, being able to effectively research topics using online and paper-based sources—is an important skill you will need to have as a student *and* as a healthcare professional (HCP).

Sources of Information

In addition to those you will find in the library, other excellent sources of information include the following:

- *Interviews with professors or experts in the field.* Conducting interviews will prepare you for future clinical work, when you may have to conduct information-gathering interviews with patients. In both cases, the process is similar:
  1. Be prepared. Make a list of the questions you'd like to ask. Make sure the most important questions are at the top of your list.
  2. During the interview, keep the conversation focused. If you only have a limited amount of time, try to avoid talking about things unrelated to your questions.
  3. Finally, when gathering information for a paper, you may wish to record the interview in addition to taking notes. This can help you remember quotes accurately. It also gives you a way to review any information you may have missed. *Just remember to ask permission first.* You can do this when scheduling the interview to avoid putting your interviewee on the spot when you meet; not everyone is comfortable being recorded.
- *Surveys and statistics.* The results of professional surveys may add to the information for your paper. You can conduct your own surveys as well using an online survey tool like SurveyMonkey. Statistics can be calculated after you receive responses to your survey. For example, suppose

Continued

you surveyed 50 subjects and 15 of those individuals answered *yes* to a question. The other 35 subjects answered *no*. Your statistics for that question would be 30% answering *yes* and 70% answering *no*. These results could then be used in your paper to support or argue against a particular point.

- *Unbiased observations.* Your own unbiased observations can be used as a source of information for your paper. However, the keyword here is *unbiased*. There are several methods you can use to avoid allowing your own opinions to cloud your observations. For example, you could create a checklist of things to look for as you observe a certain situation. During your observation, use the checklist to guide your note-taking. The checklist and thorough notes add reliability to your observations.
- *Personal experiences.* Some assignments called reflection essays allow you to use information gathered from your own experiences. Just be sure the experiences you draw from are directly related to the topic of your paper. For good measure, back up your experiences with more objective information from online or paper-based sources you trust.

Organizing Your Information

Index cards are still an excellent way to begin organizing your information. Fill out one index card per source, including main ideas and references to page numbers. (You'll need to know page numbers for the in-text references part of your paper.)

Start by creating cards for your general sources and then move to more specific sources. This is a good time to take notes on each source and look for quotes as well. Be sure to copy down quotes word for word and cite them accurately on your index cards. Also use individual cards for paraphrases or summaries, being sure to include the source information. In the sources themselves, use sticky notes to mark relevant chapters or sections if they are paper. For photocopied pages, you can use highlighters to mark important information. For online sources, save the links of your sources, either by bookmarking them or copying and pasting them into a savable document.

Next, sort your index cards according to topic. If you have several sources that provide the same information, discard the ones you won't need. Begin thinking about the basic layout of your paper at this point. Separate your cards into three stacks:

- The first stack is for information that belongs toward the beginning of your paper.
- The second stack is for material you plan to use toward the middle of your paper.
- The third stack holds the cards you'll need to consult when writing the end of your paper.

Evaluating Your Information

After you've organized your sources, you'll need to check each one for relevance to your topic:

- Check the publication date (for science-, technical-, and medical-related topics, try to avoid using sources published more than 5 years prior).
- Make sure each source contains supporting information.

If you find a source that argues against your thesis, it may still be relevant to your paper. You can write a stronger paper by including differing points of view and defending your thesis. Sources that contain countering material also help you determine how well your thesis holds up against arguments. If you find that your thesis is too weak, this is a good point in the writing process to rethink the focus of your paper. It would be much easier to rewrite your thesis than it would be to try to write an entire paper about an idea you're unable to support.

Once you've sorted relevant sources, make sure the information they contain is reliable. As you review each source, ask yourself:

- *Is the author biased?* Does the author merely present personal opinions without backing up statements with facts or research? Does the author criticize certain ideas without giving solid reasons why those ideas are faulty? Have statistics been presented in a misleading way to further the author's opinion?
- *Is the source primary or secondary?* A primary source contains firsthand information. A secondary source restates material from a primary source. Occasionally, secondary sources reproduce quotes made in primary sources. Out of context, those quotes may take on different meanings that affect their reliability. Whenever possible, use primary sources.

After evaluating your sources, keep only those that contain reliable information important to your topic. Then, set aside those index cards for sources you've decided not to use. Later, when you're sure you're not going to need those sources, you can discard them.

Creating an Outline

The next stage in the writing process is creating an outline. Your thesis statement can serve as the outline's introduction. This will help you stay focused on your main point as you write the rest of the outline. Another way to stay focused is to write a brief conclusion. You can expand this conclusion later when you write the first draft of your paper.

Next, refer to your index card notes as you map out the body of the outline. If you're required to submit a title page, table of contents, appendix, or works cited page with your final paper, use simple one-line entries to note these items on your outline as well.

When deciding how to organize the body of your outline, think about your three stacks of index cards for the beginning, middle, and end.

As you write your outline, and even as you write your paper, you're free to move sections around and reorganize information. The purpose of having an outline is to give yourself a guide, but it isn't set in stone. An outline allows you to see the organization of your paper at a glance and make necessary changes before you begin writing your first draft.

Anatomy of an Outline

Follow these guidelines when creating an outline for your paper:
I. Creating an outline
   A. Sections
      1. Introduction (use thesis statement)
      2. Body (consult index cards)
      3. Conclusion

Continued

      4. Other items (one-line entries)

        a. Title page

        b. Table of contents

        c. Appendix

        d. Works cited page

   B. Organization

      1. Use index cards to organize info in the body.

        a. Beginning of paper (first stack of cards)

        b. Middle of paper (second stack of cards)

        c. End of paper (third stack of cards)

      2. Move sections around as necessary.

Writing a First Draft

The first draft of your paper is just that—a draft. Don't worry about editing and polishing your writing at this point. There will be plenty of time for that later. The most important thing is to put your ideas into sentences and paragraphs.

While writing the first draft, you'll develop the introduction and body of your paper. You'll need to begin keeping track of references and works cited page sources. You'll also expand on the brief conclusion you wrote for your outline.

Another important part of writing a first draft involves developing the tone you'll use throughout your paper. To do this, think about your audience:

- Is this paper intended for your instructor?
- Will you be presenting it to the rest of the class?

To have a consistent tone in all sections of your paper, keep your audience in mind as you write.

Your outline should guide the process of writing the first draft. As you begin writing, however, feel free to make changes if the organization of your outline isn't working. Just be sure to save your work often.

The last step in writing your first draft is to put it away for a while. Depending on your schedule, this may mean 24 hours or several days. This gives your brain time to process what you've written. During the time you spend away from writing, you may think of ways to improve your paper. Whether you come up with the perfect introduction or a better way to state your conclusion, these ideas are valuable. Write them down so you can incorporate them later as you revise your first draft.

Revising the First Draft

After you've been away from your paper for some time, you can begin revising for the second draft. By this time, you should have a better idea of how the overall organization of your paper is working. If any big organizational changes need to be made, such as moving one whole section closer to the beginning or the end of the paper, now is the time to make them.

Be sure to save successive drafts as separate files (e.g., Draft 1, Draft 2, or Draft 3). That way, you can always refer to a previous version of your paper if you delete a section by mistake or if you decide to go back to your original organization.

With each draft, your paper should resemble more closely how it will look in its final stage. But how many drafts are needed? Reading your entire paper aloud is one way to help you notice parts that may need improvement. As you read, consider the following:

- *Organization.* Does the overall organization make sense? Does the paper move forward in a logical and clear way?
- *Paragraph structure.* Does each paragraph have a main idea and supporting details? Does the paper include transitions from one paragraph to the next?
- *Sentence flow.* Do the sentences flow smoothly from one to the next?

As you revise your paper, also keep the due date in mind. Be sure to allow yourself enough time for editing the final draft.

Once you're satisfied with the body of your paper, it's time to create the title page, table of contents (page numbers can be inserted after your final edit), references and works cited page, appendix, and any other items required by your instructor. Then, have someone else read the paper—it's always a good idea to have a fresh pair of eyes look for anything you may have missed. (Your school may also have a writing center staffed with people who can help. Remember, though, that their job is to indicate ways in which your paper can be improved—their job is not to correct your paper for you.) Your reviewer can look at things such as spelling, grammar, organization, logic, and any other elements your instructor may use to grade the paper. But keep in mind that any suggestions made by your reviewer are merely suggestions. In the end, you must decide yourself what changes to make.

Finalizing the Paper

The final stage in the writing process involves editing, formatting, and proofreading your paper.

1. During editing, it's helpful to consult other resources, such as a dictionary, thesaurus, and an English grammar and usage guide (see Chapter 11, for help with grammar and usage). As you edit your work, follow these guidelines:
   - Check the paper's tone to make sure it remains consistent.
   - Make sure terms are used consistently throughout the paper. For example, if you used *congestive heart failure* in one paragraph, avoid changing it to *heart failure* in another paragraph if it refers to the same condition.
   - Spell-check your paper with your own eyes. Check any words your spell-checker doesn't recognize (such as scientific terms). Remember that the spell-checker doesn't know the difference between "your" and "you're"—and can leave you with many confusing errors.
   - Check your grammar. For example, make sure all singular subjects have singular verbs and all plural subjects have plural verbs. ("He walks," not "He walk.")
   - Check your punctuation. All sentences should end with a period or other punctuation mark. All text in quotes should have both opening and closing quotation marks.
   - Check the spacing between lines of text. Most instructors require students to use double spacing to allow plenty of room for marks and comments.
   - Use Times New Roman or Arial for your font.
   - Make sure the font size is appropriate (12-point font is standard).
2. The next step in finalizing your paper is formatting. APA Style is the most commonly accepted format for health-related topics.

APA Style, an Explanation and an Overview

The most authoritative source for APA Style is the *Publication Manual of the American Psychological Association* (6th ed.). There exist, however, several excellent online resources that can help students with understanding and effectively using APA Style to complete their course writing assignments. This section provides a short explanation of the reasons for using citations and references, a brief overview of APA Style, and a list of online resources students can use while completing their writing assignments.

Why Should You Cite Other Sources? Where Can You Learn How to Do That?

When you write essays and research papers for your courses, you will frequently need to support your ideas and arguments by referring to the work of other HCPs and scholars. For example, as an allied health student, you could find yourself in a course similar to one we have taught called ENG206, Writing and Cultural Diversity. In this course, you may have decided to write an essay on the obstacles to therapeutic communication when providing care to the Hmong people of California's Central Valley. In any research on this topic, one of the sources you would absolutely need to consult is *The Spirit Catches You and You Fall Down*, Anne Fadiman's classic and disturbing account of one Hmong child's encounter with HCPs in a small county hospital. The book contains many striking examples of the ways in which the communication process can break down when an HCP is underprepared to work with patients and their families amid vast cultural differences. If you wanted to include some of Fadiman's examples in your essay, you would need to give credit to her research and writing in the book by citing her. Why and how do you do that?

Why Should You Cite Other Sources?

You should cite other sources that you use in your work for several reasons:

1. You should want to give credit to those people whose work you have used in support of your own work. When a reader encounters your work and comes across an interesting piece of information that you have included, the reader may want to know more about that. If that information comes from a source you have consulted in your research and properly cited in your essay, the reader can see the original source and follow up with it to learn more. This is one of the important ways in which learning and scholarship works.
2. You should want at all costs to avoid plagiarism. Plagiarism is the presentation of someone else's work as if it were your own. Plagiarism is a form of academic dishonesty and, as such, can be sufficient cause for failing an assignment or course or, in some cases, the expulsion from a school, college, or university. It is the student's responsibility to understand what plagiarism is and how it works. It is the student's responsibility to avoid committing plagiarism. Finally, it is the student's responsibility to accept the consequences when plagiarism has occurred.

Where Can You Learn How to Cite Other Sources?

The first place to start looking would be your school's library or the library's website. Several excellent online resources are included below:

Bunker Hill Community College Library's Citations Style Guides:
http://libguides.bhcc.mass.edu/c.php?g=396060&p=2690685

Bay State College Library's Research Fundamentals Guide:
https://libguides.baystate.edu/research101
Purdue's Online Writing Lab APA Style Guide:
https://owl.purdue.edu/owl/research_and_citation/apa_style/apa_style_introduction.html
American Psychological Association's APA Style Central:
http://www.apastyle.org/learn/index.aspx

Take a short break before you begin the last step—proofreading. Begin by printing a hard copy of your paper. Reviewing a hard copy is easier than looking at your paper on a computer screen, and you will more easily find errors in both the writing and formatting. Also, if you're too familiar with the text of your paper on a screen, your eyes might begin to skip over errors. By waiting a bit and then printing your paper out, you'll come back refreshed and ready to read your work closely. Here are some proofreading guidelines:

- Read your entire paper aloud (if possible).
- Remember your spellchecker will miss common errors and may actually create errors—you need to check every word yourself.
- Be on the lookout for any errors in punctuation or capitalization.
- When you come across an unfamiliar word, look it up in the dictionary to check its spelling and meaning.
- Read your paper from end to beginning, one sentence at a time. It sounds strange, but this will interrupt the rhythm you've developed from reading your paper many times and will help you see errors you might otherwise miss.

After completing this last step, you can hand in your final paper feeling confident about your work.

Researching for Writing or Presentations

As mentioned previously, you'll likely need to do some research for writing a paper or preparing a class presentation. The best place to start your research is in your school's library—and there are people in the library who can help you get started.

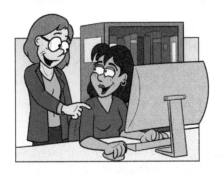

Asking an Expert for Help With Research—Amalia

Amalia was very excited when she received her first research paper assignment in college. The professor provided the students with a list of possible topics, and Amalia chose *How does sleep deprivation affect one's health?* She liked the topic, but she wasn't at first sure where to look for information. She typed the question into Google and came up with some good results, but she was concerned that she would need more and varied information for a short research paper.

Continued

She went to the college library's circulation desk, and the librarian there asked what kind of keyword searches Amalia had conducted and if Amalia had used the library's databases.

"I don't know how to do a keyword search or find a database," Amalia said.

"I can show you," the librarian offered. "Let's go over to one of the computers."

Amalia was amazed to learn how much great information was available once she learned how to look for it.

The Librarian Is There to Help

Librarians are highly trained experts on research techniques, as well as the information that can be found in the library. They will be happy to give you personal assistance, guiding you to relevant databases and other sources.

Databases

Your school's library likely subscribes to enormous stores of area-specific information called databases. Listed below are several of the most frequently used health-related databases, containing hundreds of thousands, and sometimes millions, of journal articles (* indicates that the database is accessible through subscription).

*CINAHL (Cumulative Index of Nursing and Allied Health Literature)
*HealthSource: Nursing/Academic
*ProQuest Health & Medicine
*Health Reference Center Academic
PubMed (https://www.ncbi.nlm.nih.gov/pubmed/)
PubMed Central (https://www.ncbi.nlm.nih.gov/pmc/)

Be sure to ask your school's librarian about the databases you can access through your school's library.

Websites

Because there are billions of websites on the Internet, it's helpful to have an idea of how to search for specific information and which websites to trust. By following some simple guidelines, your online research will go more smoothly.

Anatomy of a URL

Each webpage has an address, otherwise known as a URL (universal resource locator). If you know a site's URL, you'll have no trouble locating it among the many other sites on the Web.

Web addresses, especially lengthy ones, might look confusing, but each address is made up of the same basic components. Below is an explanation of each component, based on the fictional Web address http://www.acmehealthsupply.com.

- *http://* These letters stand for hypertext transfer protocol. Most Web addresses start out this way.
- *www.* This acronym for "World Wide Web" appears in many, but not all, URLs.

- *acmehealthsupply* This portion of the Web address indicates the name of the site. In this example, the site is named for the Acme Health Supply Company.
- *.com* This portion of the URL is called the suffix. The suffix provides additional information about the site.

URL Suffixes

Usually, you can gather certain information about a website just by looking at the suffix of its URL. Here's a list of common suffixes:

- *.com* This suffix usually indicates that a site is intended for commercial use. Most sites ending in .com are owned by businesses or individuals.
- *.edu* Web addresses ending in .edu indicate educational institutions (colleges and universities). If your school has a website, its URL probably ends in .edu.
- *.gov* This suffix indicates that a site is owned and operated by a government institution or agency.
- *.net* Web addresses ending in .net usually indicate Internet service providers (ISPs).
- *.org* This suffix indicates a nonprofit organization.

The Search Is On

What happens if you don't know the URL of the site you're looking for? Or what if you prefer to search for several different websites that deal with a specific topic? This is where search engines come in.

For example, suppose you needed to locate information on how to perform cardiopulmonary resuscitation (CPR). You use a search engine such as Google and enter keywords into the search box. For this search, *CPR* would be an appropriate keyword. The search engine then compiles a list of websites that may be relevant to your search. You view the results of your search and click on the links to websites that seemed applicable.

Most Web browsers now have one or more search engines, such as Google or Bing, built in on a toolbar for easy searching. Or you can go directly to a search engine's site, such as http://www.google.com or http://www.bing.com.

Improve Your Searching Skills

With so much information on the Web, it's sometimes tricky trying to locate the information you need. The following guidelines will help you perform better Internet searches.

Starting Your Search

- Begin by developing a list of keywords related to your research question. You can do this by looking at your research question and following these steps:
  1. Identify the main ideas in your research question.
  2. Think of *synonyms* (new words or phrases that have the same meaning as words or phrases in your research question).
  3. If appropriate, think of possible *antonyms* (words or phrases that have the opposite meaning of words or phrases in your research question).
  4. Use whole words only, that is, no abbreviations.

Continued

- For example, if your research question is "Do environmental issues impact human anatomy," main ideas and synonyms are the most likely to help. You could develop the following list of keywords:
  1. Main ideas—*environmental issues, human anatomy*
  2. Synonyms—*Environmental issues*: diet, living conditions, climate, air quality
     Human anatomy: body, skeleton, bones, tissue, muscles, vascular system, nervous system
- Avoid using words such as *a, an,* and *the* when entering keywords into a search bar. Most search engines ignore these words anyway.
- If you are looking for a specific phrase, enclose it in quotation marks. Most search engines recognize text contained within quotes as a single item. For example, if you needed to find information on heart disease in children, you would enter *"heart disease in children"* in the search bar.
- Be specific. Entering *diabetes education* in the search bar would give you more specific results to sort through than the more general search term *diabetes*.
- Avoid being overly specific. If your search returns few results, broaden your search terms.

Don't Give Up

- If your first search is unsuccessful, try rephrasing your keyword(s). You may find what you need by looking up a related word.
- For complicated searches, look for an "advanced search" button in the search engine. Advanced search features include the ability to exclude results with a certain key term and to search for synonyms in addition to an exact phrase.

  Again, don't forget the librarians. If you still have trouble with your searches after trying these techniques, a librarian may be able to help you find what you're looking for.

The Reliability Test

Remember: Just because information has been posted on the Internet doesn't make it trustworthy. When performing research online, be wary of unreliable websites. Use these guidelines when trying to spot the difference between reliable and unreliable sites:

- Compare sources to verify information. If a statement posted on a website seems too outrageous to be true, check it against a source you trust.
- Beware of sites that seem biased or push a specific agenda. These sites may skew facts or give blatant misinformation.
- Pay attention to URL suffixes. Usually, you can assume that sites ending in .gov or .edu contain reliable information. However, be wary of .edu sites that are owned by individual students at a university. These sites generally are not regulated for accuracy.
- As a general rule, the sites of well-known associations or agencies tend to post reliable information.
- Be especially critical of information posted on sites owned by individuals or small, unknown organizations. The owners of these sites often do not have the same accountability as reputable businesses or organizations.

Reliable Websites

Your instructor may be able to provide you with a more complete listing of reliable health professions websites related to your specific career area. Check the chart for a list to get you started.

Site Name	Address	Brief Summary
American Association of Medical Assistants	https://www.aama-ntl.org	Offers information for students and employers
American Dental Assistants Association	https://www.adaausa.org	Includes information on membership in the association, education, and employment
American Heart Association	https://www.heart.org	Includes information on continuing education and resources for professionals
American Red Cross	https://www.redcross.org	Offers health and safety information
American Society of Radiologic Technologists	https://www.asrt.org	Includes information on continuing education; provides links to online publications and an online learning center
Massage Therapy Foundation	http://www.massagetherapyfoundation.org	Provides resources for students, including a massage therapy research database
Mayo Clinic	http://www.mayoclinic.com	Provides health information from the scientists and doctors at the Mayo Clinic
National Institutes of Health (NIH)	https://www.nih.gov	Government-sponsored site; functions as the home page for all other NIH sites, such as the National Cancer Institute, National Institute on Aging, and others
PubMed	https://www.ncbi.nlm.nih.gov/pubmed	A medical information search engine from the National Library of Medicine, useful for professional medical material

Chapter Summary

- Develop good writing skills now for your future use in healthcare settings, such as writing accurate and concise reports in patient charts.
- Use the library, Internet, and other resources to research information for written assignments.
- Effectively outline and draft an APA-formatted paper.

Review Questions

Objective Questions

1. The three main sections of an academic essay are called the _____, the body, and the _____.
2. The most common format, or style, used for health-related writing is _____.
3. APA stands for _____.
4. To be information literate means to know all of the information on your course exam. (True or False)
5. A library online resource that holds hundreds of thousands of journal articles related to your general area of study, is called a _____.

Short-Answer Questions

1. List three ways to structure an introductory paragraph.
2. When gathering material for a paper, what are several sources where you can look to find information?
3. Why is it important to follow the full process for a writing assignment?
4. List three professional websites related to your area of study.

Applications

1. With a classmate, read the list of possible research questions below, and each choose a separate one to perform a keyword search on. Start by developing a list of keywords. Remember to break the research question down into *main ideas*, *synonyms*, and possible *antonyms*. Then, conduct your search online. Discuss the results. How did the results of your search differ with different keywords? Were some more helpful than others? Why?
   - Does diet affect the process of aging?
   - Is body posture related to cognitive performance?
   - Does forensic anatomy play a significant role in crime investigation?
   - How has the human body evolved through its history?
   - How does a person's emotional health impact his or her physical health?
   - Should children eat vegetarian food if their parents are vegetarians?
   - How does a child's relationship with his or her parents affect later eating/health habits?
   - How do behavioral factors influence the life expectancy?

11

Fundamental Writing Skills for the Healthcare Professional

OBJECTIVES

- Explain the functions and purposes of the parts of speech and punctuation.
- Illustrate correct sentence grammar.
- Identify common sentence errors and strategies for correcting them.
- Demonstrate effective paragraph basics.
- Describe the basics of electronic health records (EHRs).

Section 11-1 (To accompany Chapter 1, "Focusing on Success")

This chapter provides a basic guide to the essentials of grammar. Grammar is the foundation on which all good writing rests. Although we cannot promise that having an understanding of grammar alone will make you a better writer, we can say with confidence that without an understanding of grammar, you will have a much harder time becoming a good writer. Good writing skills are important in all healthcare professions. You will find that the further you advance in your healthcare career, the more you will have to write. The more you have to write, the stronger your writing skills need to be.

This chapter provides a thorough review of grammar, a basic overview of effective paragraph construction and a brief explanation of EHRs. You can use the chapter in one of three ways:

1. You can work through the chapter one section at a time, completing one of the nine sections along with each of the first nine chapters of the text. This step-by-step method will make completing the grammar section easier and less burdensome over the course of a semester. At the conclusion of each exercise, you can check your comprehension in the accompanying online answer key.
2. You can work through the nine sections of the chapter in sequence, completing the exercises and checking your answers in the online key.
3. You can work through the chapter exclusively online, completing the exercises independently.

Parts of Speech

- Nouns—words that are names of persons, places, things, or concepts
- Pronouns—words that substitute for nouns or refer to nouns
- Verbs—words that express or describe actions or states of being
- Adjectives—words that modify or describe nouns or pronouns
- Adverbs—words that modify or describe verbs, adjectives, or other adverbs
- Prepositions—words that show relationships of time or space
- Conjunctions—words that connect and show relationships between words, phrases, or clauses

Nouns

Nouns are words that are names of persons, places, things, or concepts. Examples of nouns are *stethoscope, patient, information, virus*, and *bed*.

Countable Nouns

Countable nouns name things that you can count: *two nurses, one scale, five desks, six books*.

Noncountable Nouns

Noncountable nouns name things that you cannot count, so they cannot take plural forms: *information, advice, patience, knowledge*.

Proper Nouns

Proper nouns name particular people, places, organizations, months, days of the week, and they are always capitalized: *Dr. Jones, Boston, Glendale Memorial Hospital, January, Tuesday*.

Common Nouns

Common nouns name general persons, places, organizations, things, or ideas: *doctor, city, hospital, month, day, treatment*.

Collective Nouns

Collective nouns name groups but are normally written in the singular form: *a committee, a healthcare team, a nursing pool, a faculty*.

Practice With: Nouns

Identify the types of nouns in bold print as proper nouns (PN), common nouns (CN), or collective nouns (CO). Underline all noncountable nouns.

1. **John** has been a **member** of the college **faculty** since he arrived in **Baltimore**.
2. Dr. **Martin** has some **experience** with elderly **patients**.
3. Mrs. Murphy's **daughter** will accompany her during the **examination**.
4. I think you can find the **thermometer** in the **cabinet** above the **sink**.
5. The **information** in the **chart** is not accurate, according to Dr. **Benson**.

Pronouns

Pronouns are words that replace or refer to nouns or other pronouns. The noun or pronoun it replaces or refers to is called its *antecedent*.

As examples, take the following sentences:

- Dr. Rodriguez brought his stethoscope to work this morning.
  - *Dr. Rodriguez* is the antecedent of *his*.
- Ms. Johnson brought her x-rays to the appointment with Dr. Rodriguez.
  - *Ms. Johnson* is the antecedent of *her*.
- Ms. Johnson told Dr. Rodriguez that she had chest pains.
  - *Ms. Johnson* is the antecedent of *she*.

Personal Pronouns

Personal pronouns refer to particular people, places, or things. Personal pronouns have several different categories.

Personal Pronouns

Subject Pronouns	Object Pronouns	Possessive Pronouns
I	me	my, mine
you	you	your, yours
he, she, it	him, her, it	his, her, hers, its
we	us	our, ours
they	them	their, theirs
who/whoever	whom/whomever	whose

Indefinite Pronouns

Indefinite pronouns do not refer to specific people, places, or things, and they do not need antecedents.

Indefinite Pronouns

Singular	Plural	Singular or Plural
someone, somebody, something	both	all
anyone, anybody, anything	few	any
everyone, everybody, everything	many	most
no one, nobody, nothing	several	none
every, each		some

Relative Pronouns

Relative pronouns introduce dependent clauses (see "Dependent Clauses" later in this chapter): *who, whom, whoever, whomever, whichever, that, which.*

- Ms. Jones is the patient *who* has a pulmonary function test this morning.
- Genuineness and empathy are two of the many important qualities *that* a healthcare professional must possess.
- Dr. Rodriguez is the cardiologist *whom* Ms. Jones wants to see.

Practice With: Pronouns

Identify the pronouns in bold print by marking them as personal pronouns (PP), indefinite pronouns (IP), or relative pronouns (RP).

1. Mr. Henin is the patient **who** insists on bringing **his** dog with **him** to all appointments.
2. Is there **anyone** here **who** can tell me where Dr. Jett left **his** stethoscope?
3. I understand what **you** just told **me**, but I still insist that the book is **mine**.
4. Mr. Pierre gave the nurse **his** medical history without having **his** daughter there to remember everything for **him**.
5. Martha said **she** knows **someone** in dining services **who** can come up and speak with **my** mother.

Verbs

Verbs are words that express actions or states of being. Examples of verbs are *examine, study, treat, wash,* and *sterilize.*

Auxiliary Verbs

Auxiliary verbs are forms of *to be, to do,* and *to have* that help the main verb.

- Dr. Pierre *was* examining Mr. North in Examination Room 3. (*to be: am, is, are, was, being, been*)
- Susan Chang *does* make sure to get a complete history with every patient. (*to do: do, does, did*)
- The x-rays *have* shown the scars on Mr. Frank's right lung. (*to have: have, has, had*)

Transitive Verbs

Transitive verbs show an action and transfer that action from the *subject* to a receiver, called a *direct object.*

- The radiology technician examined the medical record. (*Technician* is the subject, *examined* is the transitive verb, and *record* is the direct object.)
- The medical assistant took the patient's vital signs. (*Assistant* is the subject, *took* is the transitive verb, and *signs* is the direct object.)
- The doctor is prescribing a new medication. (*Doctor* is the subject, *prescribing* is the transitive verb, and *medication* is the direct object.)
- The nurse sees him. (*Nurse* is the subject, *sees* is the transitive verb, and *him* is the direct object.)

Intransitive Verbs

Intransitive verbs often show an action, but there is never a receiver of the action. Intransitive verbs can never take a direct object. Examples of intransitive verbs are sit, lie, sleep, die, breathe, and walk.

- The patient lies on the examination table. (The patient can lie *on* the examination table, but they cannot *lie* the examination table.)
- The medical assistant is sitting at the nursing station. (The medical assistant can sit *at* the nursing station, but they cannot *sit* the nursing station.)
- The nursing student slept through the night. (The nursing student can sleep *through* the night, but they cannot *sleep* the night.)

Linking Verbs

Linking verbs link a subject to a word after the verb. The word can be either an adjective or a noun that renames the subject. The most common linking verb is *to be* (am, is, are, was, were).

- Ms. Pontiac is asymptomatic. (*Asymptomatic* describes *Ms. Pontiac.*)
- Mr. Dodge was confused. (*Confused* describes Mr. Dodge.)
- Dr. Pound is a pulmonologist. (*Pulmonologist* renames *Dr. Pound.*)
- Jennifer is a radiology technologist. (*Radiology technologist* renames Jennifer.)

Other linking verbs can sometimes show a state of being. Examples of these are *feel, seem, look, taste, smell,* and *appear.*

- The medicine tastes bitter. (*Tastes* is the linking verb, and *bitter* describes the *medicine.*)
- The water looks clean. (*Looks* is the linking verb, and *clean* describes the *water.*)
- The child seems short of breath. (*Seems* is the linking verb, and *short of breath* describes the *child.*)
- The nursing staff appears busy. (*Appears* is the linking verb, and *busy* describes the *staff.*)

The verb *to feel* can sometimes be a linking verb and sometimes a transitive verb. When you use the verb *to feel* to describe a person's emotional state, you use it as a linking verb. When you describe an action of the subject, you use it as a transitive verb.

- The nurses felt bad after the patient died. (*Bad* describes the *nurses' emotional state.*)
- The doctor felt the patient's underarms for any sign of swelling. (*Underarms* is the direct object of *felt.*)

Practice With: Verbs

Identify the verbs in bold print in the sentences below as transitive verbs (TV), intransitive verbs (IV), or linking verbs (LV).

1. The nutritionist **gave** the patient a brochure on diabetic diets.
2. The nurse **looked** sad after hearing that her former patient **had died**.

Continued

3. Dr. Jameson **felt** the patient's neck for swollen lymph nodes.
4. The medical assistant **called** the pharmacist with the new prescription.
5. Mrs. Benitez **drove** her car to the oncologist's office for the first round of chemotherapy.
6. The basketball coach **felt** bad when one of his players was injured in the game.
7. The patient **slept** quietly after the surgery.
8. Martin **watched** the instructional video on the proper method of taking a patient's blood pressure.
9. This wound **looks** infected.
10. The doctor **wrote** the prescription, but the pharmacist could not **read** it.

Verb Tenses

Verb tenses show the time of an action.

Verb Tenses

To Examine (The Patient)	Present	Past	Future
Simple	She examines the patient.	She examined the patient.	She will examine the patient.
Progressive	She is examining the patient.	She was examining the patient.	She will be examining the patient.
Perfect	She has examined the patient.	She had examined the patient.	She will have examined the patient.

To Draw (The Patient's Blood)	Present	Past	Future
Simple	I draw the patient's blood.	I drew the patient's blood.	I will draw the patient's blood.
Progressive	I am drawing the patient's blood.	I was drawing the patient's blood.	I will be drawing the patient's blood.
Perfect	I have drawn the patient's blood.	I had drawn the patient's blood.	I will have drawn the patient's blood.

The progressive tense uses a form of *to be* and the *-ing* form of the verb to show actions that are continuing for a while.

- Ms. Johnson is coming in to the clinic three times this week to receive dialysis.
- Dr. Rodriguez was still examining Mr. Chen when the medical assistant arrived.

Practice With: Verbs and Verb Tenses

Underline the correct verb tense in each of the sentences.

1. Mr. Bernard **(came/will come)** in for his pulmonary function test yesterday.
2. As soon as I finish tomorrow's biology test, I **(will go/go)** to my internship site.
3. The patient **(has been waiting/was waiting)** for over an hour now.
4. The last time she was here, Miss Vega **(spoke/has spoken)** to the physical therapist.
5. Dr. Dickenson has not called me yet. I **(am still waiting/still wait)** by the phone.

Section 11-2 (To accompany Chapter 2, "Getting Organized and Managing Your Time as a Healthcare Professional")

Adjectives

Adjectives describe or modify nouns and pronouns. Adjectives can go before nouns or after linking verbs. Adjectives that go after linking verbs are called predicate adjectives because the predicate part of a sentence (or clause) includes the verb and objects or phrases connected to the verb. (See the section on "Subjects and Predicates" later in this chapter.)

- The infected wound needs to be treated. (*Infected* is describing the *wound*.)
- That wound looks infected and needs to be treated. (*Infected* is a predicate adjective that comes after the linking verb *looks* and describes the *wound*.)
- The sleeping patient shouldn't be disturbed. (*Sleeping* is describing the *patient*.)
- The patient is sleeping and shouldn't be disturbed. (*Sleeping* is a predicate adjective that comes after the linking verb *is* and describes the *patient*.)

Note: Writers should feel comfortable using adjectives in both of these ways. Both methods are equally effective.

Adverbs

Adverbs are words that describe or modify verbs, adjectives, other adverbs, or whole clauses and sentences. They usually end in *-ly*. They often explain the *how, when, where, why,* or *how much* of something that happens in a sentence.

- The phlebotomy nurse washed her hands thoroughly before leaving the patient's room. (The adverb *thoroughly* modifies the verb *washed*.)
- The patient's sprained ankle was very swollen. (The adverb *very* describes the adjective *swollen*.)
- The patient's blood pressure dropped extremely quickly during the surgery. (The adverb *extremely* modifies the adverb *quickly*, which is describing the verb *dropped*.)
- Unfortunately, the patient did not prepare for their positron emission tomography (PET) scan on Monday. (The adverb *unfortunately* modifies the entire sentence.)

Practice With: Adjectives and Adverbs

Identify the words in bold print below as adjectives (ADJ) or adverbs (ADV). Draw an arrow to the word each one modifies or describes.

1. The patient responded **quickly** to the **physical** therapy.
2. During his long convalescence from a **near-fatal** crash, Mr. Simpson made **good** use of his time by learning to speak Spanish **fluently**.
3. The ACE bandage was wrapped **tightly** around Mr. Pilgrim's **left** wrist.
4. The medicine tasted so **bad** that the patient **firmly** refused to take another swallow.
5. The doctor spoke **quietly** with the patient's family about the **upcoming** surgery.

Prepositions and Prepositional Phrases

Prepositions are words that often show relationships of time and space, that is, when or where something takes place.

- The patient interrupted the doctor during the visit. (The preposition *during* tells you *when* the patient interrupted the doctor.)
- The nurse is in the examination room. (The preposition *in* tells you *where* the nurse is.)

Examples of Prepositions

about	around	by	in front of	on	to
above	before	down	inside	onto	toward
across	behind	during	into	out of	until
after	below	except	like	outside	up
against	beneath	for	near	past	with
along	beside	from	next to	since	within
among	between	in	of	through	without

A *prepositional phrase* is a group of words made up of the preposition and the words that follow it. The noun or pronoun that follows the preposition is called the *object* of the preposition.

- Behind the desk (*Desk* is the object of *behind.*)
- In the hospital (*Hospital* is the object of *in.*)
- With the stethoscope (*Stethoscope* is the object of *with.*)

- Around the wound (*Wound* is the object of *around.*)
- Above the waist (*Waist* is the object of *above.*)
- Through a needle (*Needle* is the object of *through.*)

Prepositional phrases are important parts of sentences. It is usually helpful to remember that the subject of a sentence will not appear in a prepositional phrase.

- The radiology technologist placed the patient's elbow on the table. (*On the table* is a prepositional phrase in this sentence.)
- The nurse looked at the wound during the patient's visit. (This sentence has two prepositional phrases: *at the wound* and *during the patient's visit.*)
- The pharmacist spoke to the patient about the new medication after the doctor's appointment. (This sentence has three prepositional phrases: *to the patient, about the new medication,* and *after the doctor's appointment.*)

Practice With: Prepositions and Prepositional Phrases

Identify the prepositions below by circling them and then cross out any prepositional phrases.

1. The patient sat in the examination room waiting for the nurse.
2. Martha went to the library to find a book on gingivitis.
3. Both of the medical assistants enjoyed working with the phlebotomy nurse during blood gas draws.
4. After his MRI, Mr. Gilroy hoped to find out what the source of pain was in his right shoulder.
5. Drinking 2 L of contrast agent took John 30 minutes. When he was finished, he put the glass down on the bedside table and climbed out of bed.

Conjunctions

Conjunctions are words that join two or more parts of a sentence. They connect words, phrases, or clauses. The two kinds of conjunctions discussed here are coordinating conjunctions and subordinating conjunctions.

Coordinating Conjunctions

Coordinating conjunctions connect two or more words, phrases, or clauses. Coordinating conjunctions include *and, but, for, or, nor, so,* and *yet.*

- The nurse *and* the doctor included notes in the patient's chart. (The coordinating conjunction *and* connects the two words *nurse* and *doctor.*)
- The overworked medical assistant could not decide whether to prepare the examination room or to take the lab samples down to the pathology lab. (The coordinating conjunction *or* links the two phrases *to prepare the examination room* and *to take the lab samples.*)
- All members of the healthcare team went to the conference room for the weekly meeting, but the nurse manager had not arrived yet. (The coordinating conjunction

but connects the two clauses *all members of the healthcare team went to the conference room for the weekly meeting* and *the nurse manager had not arrived yet.*)
- Mary, the pharmacist, explained the medication's dosage, and she demonstrated how to load the syringe. (The coordinating conjunction *and* connects the two clauses *Mary, the pharmacist, explained the medication's dosage* and *she demonstrated how to load the syringe.*)

Subordinating Conjunctions

Subordinating conjunctions begin dependent clauses and connect them with independent clauses. (See "Dependent Clauses" and "Independent Clauses" later in this chapter.) The subordinating conjunction shows the relationship between the two clauses and generally explains *when, why,* or *under what circumstances.* Below is a list of the most common subordinating conjunctions.

Examples of Subordinating Conjunctions

after	as though	if	that	whenever
although	because	once	though	where
as	before	since	unless	whereas
as if	even if	so that	until	wherever
as long as	even though	than	when	while

- When the patient checked in for his appointment, the medical assistant escorted him to the examination room. (*When the patient checked in for his appointment* is a dependent clause. *When* is the subordinating conjunction. *The medical assistant escorted him to the examination room* is an independent clause.)
- Because the patient had not followed the directions to eat a carbohydrate-free/high-protein diet, she was not ready for the PET scan this morning. (*Because the patient had not followed the directions to eat a carbohydrate-free/high-protein diet* is a dependent clause. *Because* is the subordinating conjunction. *She was not ready for the PET scan this morning* is an independent clause.)

Practice With: Conjunctions and Prepositions

Identify the words in bold print as coordinating conjunctions (CC), subordinating conjunctions (SC), or prepositions (PREP).

1. **When** Mary arrived at the clinic, she turned **on** all the lights **and** unlocked the examination rooms.
2. Mr. Ford came **in** for his physical **after** work.

3. If Dr. Rodriguez calls **before** 6 PM, can you tell him that the patient is **at** the pharmacy waiting **for** the prescription?
4. I don't know the answer **to** that question **about** mitosis, **but** I know all the material **on** meiosis.
5. Can you explain the difference **between** white blood cells **and** red blood cells?
6. Mary has worked **as** a nurse **in** this clinic **since** she passed her licensure examination **in** 1997.
7. **Because** he was careful not to violate any of the hospital's patient privacy policies, Andrew told the newspaper reporters he could not confirm or deny **that** the star quarterback was currently undergoing knee surgery. He directed all calls **to** the hospital's public relations office **on** the fifth floor.
8. **During** the long surgery, the patient's family waited **in** the reception area eating cookies **and** drinking coffee.
9. **After** he finished answering the test's multiple-choice questions, Barry began answering the short-answer **and** matching questions.
10. David held the stethoscope **against** the mannequin's chest, **but** he could not hear a heartbeat.

Section 11-3 (To accompany Chapter 3, "Maintaining Your Health and Well-Being)

Punctuation

Punctuation helps you to be clear in your writing. Punctuation marks show relationships within a sentence and show the reader where the sentence ends.

Periods

Use periods at the ends of sentences, in abbreviations, and in decimals. These are examples of periods ending sentences:

- The doctor examined the patient.
- The medical assistant took the patient's vital signs.
- Sneezing is one symptom of allergies.

These are examples of periods used in abbreviations.

Examples of Periods in Abbreviations

Dr.	Mr.	Ms.	Mrs.	M.D.	R.N.	L.P.N.	N.A.	M.A.	M.S.
B.S.	B.A.	A.M.	P.M.	J.D.	Inc.	Co.	Corp.	Blvd.	Ave.

Remember that medical abbreviations can appear in upper or lower case letters and with or without a period. When you write measurements, be sure *not* to use periods.

Medical Abbreviations and Measurements

b.i.d.	a.c.	h.s.	MI	PFT	CBC	Hb	WBC	ETOH	
mm	cm	ml	L	cl	mcg	mg	kg	oz	ft

Use periods in decimals and to separate dollars and cents.

- My GPA is 3.49.
- He measured 0.56 cm.
- The per-visit copay is $10.50.

Question Marks and Exclamation Marks

Like periods, question marks and exclamation marks are used to end sentences. Each, however, is used to end a different kind of sentence.

Question Marks

Use a question mark at the end of a direct question.

- Do you feel any pain when I press your abdomen here?
- When did you first notice the ringing in your ears?
- Will the nurse draw any blood this evening?
- Does Mr. Jones have a living will?

Exclamation Marks

Use an exclamation mark to end a sentence showing urgency, emotion, or excitement.

- Call a code blue in Room C223!
- Take these bloods to the lab STAT!
- Do not let anyone except the doctor into that room!
- He survived a quadruple bypass!

Practice With: Periods, Question Marks, and Exclamation Marks

Proofread and correct the following passage, adding periods, question marks, and exclamation marks where necessary. You should find eight errors to correct.

David, a medical assistant, was working on Saturday at the nursing station in the Department of Hematology/Oncology Part of his job was to greet patients' friends and family members who came to the department on visits.

At about 10 AM, an elderly woman came up to the nursing station with a question She was a short woman who had to stand on her toes to see over the desk to speak to David. She seemed very confused.

Do you know where the Department of Cardiology is" she asked. "Is this the Department of Cardiology."

David knew that Cardiology was over in the next wing of the hospital and two floors up. He worried that if he gave the woman directions, she might get lost again He wanted to provide the best service possible to her.

"It's quite a way from here," he said. "I'd be happy to escort you there to make sure you find it."

The elderly woman smiled a bright smile to David "Thank you so much That's the nicest thing anyone's done for me today"

Commas

The comma, one of the most frequently used and misused pieces of punctuation, makes clear the relationships within a sentence.

Lists

Use commas between items in a list.

- The medical assistant noticed that the office first-aid kit lacked bandages, tape, gauze, and alcohol pads.
- The nursing student brought books, notepads, pens, and rulers.

   Note: In academic writing, be sure to use the final comma before the conjunction in a list (*and, but, yet, nor, or*).

Coordinate Adjectives

Use a comma between two adjectives that could be separated by *and*. Note that coordinate adjectives all modify the *same* noun.

- The basketball player came into the coach's office with a red, swollen knee. (The same sentence could be written with *and* between *red* and *swollen*.)
- James's asthma has shown a slow, steady improvement. (The same sentence could be written with *and* between *slow* and *steady*.)

Introductory Phrases or Clauses

Use a comma after an introductory phrase or a dependent clause.

- To help chemotherapy patients understand possible dietary restrictions, the American Cancer Society has produced this excellent pamphlet.
- Because the American Cancer Society has produced this excellent pamphlet, chemotherapy patients can have a better understanding of possible dietary restrictions.

   Note: If the independent clause comes before the dependent clause, do not use a comma.

- Chemotherapy patients can have a better understanding of possible dietary restrictions because the American Cancer Society produced this excellent pamphlet.

Coordinating Conjunctions

Use a comma before a coordinating conjunction (*and, but, or, for, nor, so, yet*) in a sentence with two independent clauses, called a *compound sentence*. (See "Independent Clauses" later in this chapter.)

- James's asthma is much improved, *but* it is still not completely controlled. (This sentence has two independent clauses: *James's asthma is much improved* and *it is still not completely controlled.*)

- James's asthma is not completely controlled, *yet* it is much improved. (This sentence has two independent clauses: *James's asthma is not completely controlled* and *it is much improved.*)
- James's asthma is much improved, *and* he will continue to see Dr. Rodriguez for more treatment. (This sentence has two independent clauses: *James's asthma is much improved* and *he will continue to see Dr. Rodriguez for more treatment.*)

Nonessential Clauses

Use commas around nonessential dependent clauses. Do not put commas around essential clauses. A clause is nonessential if you can take it out of the sentence without changing the sentence's meaning. The commas around the nonessential clause tell the reader that this clause contains extra, nonessential information.

- James, who is an avid video game player, is taking a new cortisone inhaler to control his asthma. (The clause *who is an avid video game player* is nonessential to the meaning of the sentence.)
- That cabinet, which the maintenance staff installed last week, contains all of the surgical prep kits we have left. (The clause *which the maintenance staff installed last week* is nonessential to the meaning of the sentence.)

You should not put commas around a clause that is essential to a sentence. The lack of commas tells the reader that the information in the clause is essential to the basic meaning of the sentence.

- The doctor who ordered this medication for James is not in the hospital today. (The clause *who ordered this medication for James* is essential to the meaning of the sentence. Without this information, the reader would not know which doctor the writer is referring to.)
- The medical records that contained the x-ray report were on the table in the conference room. (The clause *that contained the x-ray report* is essential to meaning of the sentence. Without this information, the reader would not know which medical records the writer is referring to.)

Note: Use the following guideline when deciding whether to use *which* or *that* to introduce a clause. Use *which* for a nonessential clause, and use *that* for an essential clause. Remember always to use *who* when referring to a person.

- The department of cardiology, **which is on the east end of the fourth floor**, is staffed by a team of dedicated healthcare professionals. (The clause *which is on the east end of the fourth floor* is nonessential to the meaning of the sentence. Note that the clause is set off by commas.)
- The only department **that has an open bed for the incoming patient** is cardiology. (The clause *that has an open bed for the incoming patient* is essential to the meaning of the sentence. Without this information, the sentence would read "The only department is cardiology," and the reader would not understand what the writer means.)

Appositive Phrases

Use commas around appositive phrases. (These are phrases that modify or describe nouns or pronouns with different words.)

- Jennifer Martinez, the nursing assistant who is on duty this evening, will check to see that all examination rooms are stocked with alcohol prep pads. (The phrase *the nursing assistant who is on duty this evening* identifies Jennifer Martinez by describing her.)

- Mr. Nguyen, a geriatric patient of Dr. Jones, is coming in with his daughter today. (The phrase *a geriatric patient of Dr. Jones* identifies Mr. Nguyen by describing him.)

Clarity

Use commas to make the meaning of your sentences clearer.

- Unclear: To Dr. Scott James was a pleasant patient because of his compliant and easy-going behavior.
- Clear: To Dr. Scott, James was a pleasant patient because of his compliant and easy-going behavior.

Other Uses for Commas

Also use commas in the following situations:

In addresses and geographic place names

- The clinic is at 1655 Highland Avenue, Glendale, California.
- Dr. Rodriguez did his residency in Glendale, Arizona, not Glendale, California.

In openings and closings of letters and emails

- Dear Ms. Johnson,
- Sincerely,

When you directly address another person

- Dr. Rodriguez, do you have the patient's medical record with you?
- Marcel, do you know where Dr. Rodriguez did his residency?

To separate a name from a title or degree and with Jr. and Sr.

- Be sure to address the letter to Michael Chen, M.D.
- Be sure to label the chart Carlos Ramirez, Jr. Carlos Ramirez, Sr. is his father.

In dates

- His date of birth is March 24, 1988.
- I was hired on International Nurses Day, which was May 12, 2010.

With numbers that have more than three digits

- She donated $5,000 to the hospital charity.
- The plane delivered 2,000,000 flu shot ampules last week.

Practice With: Commas

Proofread the following passage. Add commas where necessary. You should add at least 23 commas.

Michael a first-year nursing student has a medical terminology exam and a biology paper due tomorrow. He has been studying medical terminology all week and he has written much of the paper. In fact the biology paper is

Continued

almost finished. Michael figures that he has 4 maybe 5 more hours to work on it. He has just arrived in the library with his book bag. In the book bag he has his laptop computer his biology textbook his medical terminology textbook his note cards and his notebooks. If he finishes his biology paper he will not have enough time to study for his medical terminology exam. If he studies for medical terminology he will not have enough time to write his biology paper.

The library is crowded. After 15 minutes of looking around the library Michael cannot find an open seat at any of the tables or cubicles. The school has just over 7000 students and it seems to Michael that at least 6999 of them are already there in the library.

After another 10 minutes of looking Michael decides to go back to his room. His room is cramped cluttered and crowded. Still he figures that if he stays up all night he might have enough time to finish the biology paper and study for his medical terminology exam. It's going to be a long night.

Section 11-4 (To accompany Chapter 4, "Interacting With Others as a Healthcare Professional")

Semicolons

Use semicolons to connect parts of a sentence in the following ways.

Independent Clauses Without Conjunctions

Use a semicolon to connect two independent clauses that are not connected by a coordinating conjunction (*and, but, for, or, nor, so,* and *yet*) but are closely related.

- Ms. Augustin is calling for her test results; she had her bloods drawn last week. (The two ideas are closely related.)
- Dr. Clarke said she needed these blood cultures taken to the lab STAT; the patient is running a high fever. (The two ideas are closely related.)

Independent Clauses With Conjunctive Adverbs

Use a semicolon to connect independent clauses that are joined by a conjunctive adverb (*however, nevertheless, moreover, therefore*) or transitional phrases (*as a result, for example*).

- James's asthma is much improved; however, he still has trouble breathing in cold weather.
- The nursing supervisor has come up with many great ideas for improving patient care; for example, she suggested that the triage nurse speak to patients by phone before they arrive.

Items in a Long List

Use semicolons in a long list of items, especially if there are commas within some of the items.

- Please be sure that the first aid kit includes bandages, both adhesive and nonadhesive; tape; gauze; nonlatex gloves; alcohol wipes; and cotton swabs, especially that kind with wooden sticks.

Colons

Use a colon to present specific, important information.

Before a List, a Series, or a Quotation

- On the day of the exam, each nursing student should bring the following: one black pen, two blue books, a ruler, a stethoscope, and the exam study guide.
- Dr. Joe Shamir captured the spirit of our clinic's mission when he said on this day in 1976: "All of our patients deserve the very best care we can provide. That must be our number one priority. Nothing matters more than providing patients with the best care humanly and economically possible."

Other Uses for Colons

After the salutation in a formal letter or memorandum

- Dear Dr. Rodriguez:
- Dear Ms. Jones:
- To: Nursing Staff, 2CW

In the writing of time

- The doctor will arrive at 3:15 PM promptly.
- I've been waiting for the patient since 8:00 AM.

Practice With: Semicolons and Colons

Proofread the following passage from a letter, adding semicolons and colons where necessary. You should find at least eight places to correct errors.

Dear Mr. Pierre

At 915 last Wednesday morning, I called your office to ask about the status of my application for the open nursing assistant position that was advertised in *The Herald.* I left a message with Jane, the receptionist, who told me she would return my call later that day however, a week

Continued

has passed, and I have not heard back yet. I believe my credentials closely match those listed in the advertisement an associate's degree in a health-related major 2 years' experience working in a healthcare setting a desire to help patients, especially elderly patients and basic telephone and computer skills.

I would very much like to discuss with you the ways I may contribute to Longmeadow Medical Associates. I can be reached at my home phone 818-987-9876.

Sincerely,

Melanie Johnston

Apostrophes

Use apostrophes to show possessives and contractions.

Possessives

Use an apostrophe to show that a noun or indefinite pronoun is possessive.

Singular Nouns

Use -'s with singular nouns and pronouns.

- *Mrs. Nguyen's* medical record has been completely updated.
- *Everyone's* computer password will be reset next week.

Plural Nouns

Use -s' with plural nouns that form the plural by adding an *s*.

- All of the patients' records have been completely updated.
- Can you tell me where the nurses' report room is?

Two or More Nouns

Use -'s on the last noun to show joint ownership, and on each noun to show individual ownership.

- Susan and Barbara's car is parked behind the clinic. (Joint ownership)
- John's and Barbara's lab coats are still at the dry cleaners. (Individual ownership)

Important note: Possessive pronouns already show possession, so they never take apostrophes.

Possessive Pronouns

Followed by a noun	my	his	her	its	your	their
Not followed by a noun	mine	his	hers	its	yours	theirs

- This is my book. (The possessive pronoun *my* is followed by a noun, *book*.)
- This book is mine. (The possessive pronoun *mine* is not followed by a noun.)
- The patient's diet is his responsibility. (The possessive pronoun *his* is followed by a noun, *responsibility*.)
- The responsibility for the patient's diet is theirs. (The possessive pronoun *theirs* is not followed by a noun.)

Hyphens

Hyphens are important for clarity and should be used in the following ways.

Compound Modifiers

Use a hyphen to punctuate compound words that work together as adjectives to modify a noun.

- Mr. Wright needs to be scheduled for a *follow-up* appointment.
- I looked closely at the *grayish-black* area around the wound.
- The patient's father gave the doctor *second-hand* information.

   Do not use a hyphen if the compound modifier follows the noun.

- I looked closely at the surrounding tissue, which was grayish black.
- The doctor heard the information second hand.

   Note: When the first word in a compound modifier is an adverb (ending in *-ly*) or *very*, do not use a hyphen.

- Dr. Martin is an *internationally* known cardiologist.
- I looked closely at the *partially* removed tissue.
- Jennifer is a *very* sweet nurse.

Compound Words

Use a hyphen to form a compound word. A compound word has more than one word in it but works as a single word.

- John's *sister-in-law* is studying for her licensure examination.
- Dr. Rodriguez may seem like a *happy-go-lucky* guy, but he is really a very serious person.

Prefixes

Use a hyphen to connect many prefixes to words. Common hyphenated prefixes include *ex-*, *pro-*, and *self-*.

- The ex-president of the American Medical Association is going to speak at the seminar.
- The Surgeon General did not make a distinction between those who were pro-life and those who were pro-choice.

   Note: Always be sure to use a dictionary to see if you should use a hyphen with a prefix.

Other Uses for a Hyphen

- In written fractions: *one-fifth, two-thirds, one-fifteenth*
- In numbers from *twenty-one* to *ninety-nine*
- In numbers and dates that indicate a span of time: *1990-1998, 6:00-7:30*

Practice With: Apostrophes and Hyphens

Proofread the following sentences. Insert apostrophes and hyphens where needed.

1. Mrs. Smiths daughter in law is coming in to meet with Dr. Rodriguez to discuss Mrs. Smiths care plan.
2. Dr. Chen always sees the glass as half full. Dr. Johnson sees the glass as half empty. However, Dr. Chens nurse sees the glass as two thirds full.
3. Meghan came to visit Cara 23 times last week after Caras appendix was removed.
4. Dr. Martin wants to have a face to face meeting with Mr. Hernandez's future son in law.
5. One half of all babies born from 1960 1970 were inoculated.

Dashes

In some cases, you can use dashes instead of commas.

- For parenthetical information: *Mrs. Pontiac—the patient whose family always brings in a huge batch of chocolate chip cookies big enough for the entire nursing staff—has followed her sugar-free diet carefully.*
- For lists and explanations: *Mr. Lee asked for a complete list of what we do when we check vitals—blood pressure, respiratory rate, body temperature, and pulse rate.*

Parentheses

You can use parentheses in a few important ways.

- Around extra, additional information: *Mrs. Pontiac (the best baker in town) is on a strict sugar-free diet.*
- Around information that explains: *Mrs. Pontiac's third son (the one who started a bake shop on Fifth Avenue) has a monopoly on the market for chocolate chip cookies in Savannah.*
- Around numbers or letters in lists within sentences: *Remember to check Mr. Santiago's vitals: (1) pulse rate, (2) respiratory rate, (3) blood pressure, and (4) body temperature.*

Quotation Marks

Use quotation marks to enclose the exact words of a speaker or writer. You may need to use quotation marks to quote the exact words of a patient or family member.

- "Mark's behavior has become increasingly erratic over the past months," Mr. Smith said about his son.
- The patient said to his nurse, "I have a dull, heavy pain in my chest and a tingling in my neck and chin."
- "Never do harm" is part of the Hippocratic Oath.

Also use quotation marks to show part of a published work, such as a chapter, or to indicate that words or phrases are used in a particular way.

- The last chapter in this book is called "Fundamental Writing Skills."
- Write "Return to Sender" on the envelope.
- Put a sign on the door that says "Meeting in Progress."

Capital Letters

Use capital letters at the start of sentences, in proper nouns, in titles, and for adjectives derived from proper nouns.

Proper Nouns

Use capital letters to begin names of people, races, titles, geographical locations, months, seasons, and organizations. Do not use capital letters for general names of these things.

- The Mayo Clinic (a specific name) is the best clinic (a general name) in the state.
- President Simpson (a specific name) is the seventh president (a general name) this HMO has had in the last 5 years.
- Massachusetts has many great hospitals (a general name); the Brigham and Women's Hospital (a specific name) is just one of the best known.

Titles

Use capital letters to begin all words in titles except for articles (*the, a, an*), prepositions (e.g., *in, through, across, after*), and conjunctions (e.g., *and* or *but*). If an article, preposition, or conjunction is the first word of the title, you should capitalize it.

- *The Heirs of General Practice* is my favorite book by John McPhee.
- "The Use of Force" is one of *The Doctor Stories* by William Carlos Williams.

Other Uses for Capital Letters

Always use capital letters when writing the following:

- Nations and countries: United States of America, Mexico, Kenya, Haiti, Ukraine
- Planets: Earth, Mars, Jupiter
- Public place names: Copley Square, Ellis Island, Zuma Beach
- Names of streets: Broadway, Highland Avenue, Primrose Lane
- Days of week and names of months: Thursday, Sunday, March, September

- Holidays: Thanksgiving, Memorial Day, Martin Luther King, Jr. Day
- Religions: Catholicism, Buddhism, Judaism, Islam
- Languages: English, Spanish, German, Mandarin, Creole
- The first-person pronoun (always): I

Note: Always check a dictionary if you do not know whether a word or phrase should have capital letters.

Practice With: Quotation Marks and Capital Letters

Proofread the following sentences. Add quotation marks and capital letters where appropriate.

1. Suzanne has just published an article entitled meeting new patients' needs in the latest issue of *the journal of nursing*.
2. Mr. Keller's exact words were: just try to give me that flu shot. i'll show you.
3. Cheryl is going to madrid, spain, for thanksgiving.
4. The former president wanted to do more to restructure the hmo than president Cranston does.
5. Before he went in for his abdominal surgery, Mr. Martinez kept singing that old beatles song Don't let me down.

Numbers

Ordinal Numbers and Cardinal Numbers

Ordinal Numbers and Cardinal Numbers

Ordinal numbers show the order in which something happens.

Ordinal Numbers

Examples of ordinal numbers written as numerals are 1st, 2nd, 3rd, 5th, 10th, 15th, 21st, 22nd, 30th, 41st, 43rd, 52nd, 61st, 74th, 76th, 87th, 93rd, 99th, and 100th.

Examples of ordinal numbers written as words are first, second, third, fifth, twenty-first, twenty-eighth, thirtieth, forty-third, fifty-fourth, sixty-seventh, seventy-sixth, ninety-ninth, and one-hundredth.

Cardinal Numbers

Examples of cardinal numbers written as numerals are 1, 2, 3, 5, 10, 15, 21, 22, 30, 41, 43, 52, 61, 74, 76, 87, 93, 99, and 100.

Examples of cardinal numbers written as words are one, two, three, five, ten, twenty-one, twenty-two, thirty, forty-three, fifty-two, sixty-one, seventy-six, ninety-nine, and one hundred.

Arabic Numerals and Roman Numerals

Arabic Numerals and Roman Numerals

Arabic Numerals	Roman Numerals	Arabic Numerals	Roman Numerals
1	I	20	XX
2	II	30	XXX
3	III	40	XL
4	IV	50	L
5	V	60	LX
6	VI	70	LXX
7	VII	80	LXXX
8	VIII	90	XC
9	IX	100	C
10	X	200	CC
11	XI	300	CCC
12	XII	400	CD
13	XIII	500	D
14	XIV	600	DC
15	XV	700	DCC
16	XVI	800	DCCC
17	XVII	900	CM
18	XVIII	1,000	M
19	XIX		

Use the following guidelines when writing numbers as words or as numerals.

Guidelines for Writing Numbers as *Words* or as *Numerals*

Write numbers as words in these situations:

- When the number is ten or lower: one, two, four, seven, nine, ten.
- When the number is the first word in a sentence: Twenty-one blood cultures were run.
- When the number is an indefinite number: a couple hundred, a few million.
- When the number is a fraction alone in a sentence: He gave me one third of the pie.

Continued

- When the date is an ordinal number with no month: Tomorrow is my twenty-first birthday.
- When you use words for numbers everywhere else in the phrase, clause, or sentence: The doctor ordered two blood cultures and three urine samples in the next 24 hours.
- When you use a number under ten in a name: She lives on Fifth Avenue.

  Write numbers as numerals in these situations:

- When the number is over ten: 11, 15, 22, 27, 99.
- When you indicate a patient's age: The patient is 48 years old.
- When you use numerals everywhere else in the phrase, clause, or sentence: The patient in the emergency room received 157 stitches, 22 staples, and 3 small bandages on their back.
- When you use separate, unrelated numbers with a comma: On March 22, 112 people visited the emergency room.
- When you use numbers with symbols and abbreviations: 55%, #16 gauge needle, 10 cc, pH 7.5, 100 mg.
- When you write drug amounts: 1 mg of alprazolam, 50 mcg of fluticasone propionate.
- When the day precedes the month, write the date as an ordinal: the 5th of May.
- When you indicate amounts of money: $25, $9.95, 50 cents (Note: Always use the word cents for amounts under a dollar. Use the dollar sign for amounts over a dollar. Do not include .00 with even dollar amounts.)
- When you indicate a time with AM or PM: 10:15 AM, 7:30 PM (Note: Do not use :00 with exact hour times 6 AM, 9 PM. Do not use AM or PM with the word o'clock: 8 o'clock.)
- When you indicate numbers that have decimal fractions: 6.5 cm, 1.5 L. (Note: Always include a zero before a decimal that is not a whole number: 0.4 mg, 0.6%.)
- When you indicate dimensions, sizes, and temperatures as numerals: He wears a 10½ size shoe. It's 10 degrees below zero.

Practice With: Numbers

Proofread the following sentences. Make any corrections necessary with numbers.

1. 78 patients were sitting in the lobby for 30 minutes waiting for flu shots.
2. Marcia is very good at drawing blood. I'm sure she's drawn blood from a few 100 patients this year.
3. The article said that fifty-five % of newborns in that state had fewer than 2 siblings.
4. The new suture kits cost thirty-nine dollars each.
5. Dr. Rashad said he would be here at ten AM sharp.

Section 11-5 (To accompany Chapter 5, "Making the Most of Your Learning
Style as a Healthcare Professional")

Sentence Grammar

Effective communicators in any profession need to understand the parts of sentences and how they work together.

Subjects and Predicates

Subjects and predicates are the two parts of a sentence. The *simple* subject is the who or what the sentence is about, and the *simple* predicate shows the action (or, with linking verbs, what is called *the state of being*).

- The EMT arrived. (*EMT* is the subject; *arrived* is the predicate.)
- The patient is eating. (*Patient* is the subject; *is eating* is the predicate.)

A sentence can become more complicated when it includes other words, phrases, and clauses that modify the subject and the predicate, forming what is called a *complete* subject and *complete* predicate.

- The phlebotomy nurse went into Room 215C to take a blood gas on Mr. Jimenez. (*The phlebotomy nurse* is the complete subject, and the complete predicate is *went into Room 215C to take a blood gas on Mr. Jimenez.*)
- The patient in the examination room wants to talk to Dr. Chen before leaving. (*The patient in the examination room* is the complete subject, and the complete predicate is *wants to talk to Dr. Chen before leaving.*)
- The plastic syringes in that box don't have proper labeling. (*The plastic syringes in that box* is the complete subject, and the complete predicate is *don't have proper labeling.*)

Practice With: Subjects and Predicates

Underline the complete subjects (CS) and complete predicates (CP) in each sentence.

1. The patient survived.
2. These medications control James's asthma.
3. Mr. Adjani will call Dr. Williamson tomorrow morning about the test results.
4. The examination rooms are all clean.
5. Dr. Rodriguez is the only cardiologist who came out for the hospital charity's Valentine's Day party.

Phrases

A phrase is a group of words without a subject or a verb. A phrase never expresses a complete thought but always modifies a noun or a verb. Phrases are important parts of most sentences.

Prepositional Phrases

Prepositional phrases are the most common kind of phrases in English. A prepositional phrase contains a preposition and its object (the noun or pronoun in the phrase).

- The nurse looked at the patient's hands. (*At the patient's hands* is the prepositional phrase.)
- Dr. Schmidt will look at the patient's chart before he goes into the examination room. (*At the patient's chart* and *into the examination room* are prepositional phrases.)
- *Across the River and into the Trees* is one of my favorite books by Hemingway. (*Across the River* and *into the Trees* are both prepositional phrases.)

Verbal Phrases

Verbal phrases are formed by verbs but work as nouns or modifiers. The three types of verbal phrases include *infinitives*, *gerunds*, and *participles*.

Infinitive Phrases

Infinitives are formed by adding *to* in front of the verb (to examine, to write, to communicate). An infinitive phrase contains the infinitive and its modifiers.

- Jessica went to the library to study her nursing homework. (*To study her nursing homework* is the infinitive phrase.)
- Mrs. Ngogi came to the clinic to have her blood pressure taken. (*To have her blood pressure taken* is the infinitive phrase.)

Gerund Phrases

A gerund is formed by adding *-ing* to a verb. Gerunds work as nouns in sentences, frequently as the subject or direct object. A gerund phrase includes its modifiers.

- Understanding the principles of effective communication is important if you want to succeed professionally. (*Understanding the principles of effective communication* is a gerund phrase that works as the subject of the sentence.)
- Eating plenty of fruits and vegetables is a part of any healthy diet. (*Eating plenty of fruits and vegetables* is a gerund phrase working as the subject of the sentence.)
- Dr. Fritz likes examining patients who speak German. (*Examining patients* is a gerund phrase that works as a direct object of the verb *likes*.)

Participles

Participles are formed by adding *-ing* in present tense or *-ed* in past tense to verbs. They work as adjectives that modify nouns or pronouns. A participle phrase includes its modifiers.

- The patient, sitting on the examination table, told the nurse her medical history. (*Sitting on the examination table* is a present participle modifying the subject of the sentence, the noun *patient*.)
- Covering her eyes with her hands, she walked out of the conference room where her colleagues had gathered for a surprise birthday party. (*Covering her eyes with her hands* is a present participle modifying the subject of the sentence, the pronoun *she*.)
- Exhausted from studying all night for her biology exam, Barbara wanted to stop for another cup of coffee on her way to class. (*Exhausted from studying all night for her biology exam* is a past participle modifying the subject of the sentence, the noun *Barbara*.)

Practice With: Phrases

In the sentences below, identify the phrases in bold print as prepositional (P), infinitive (I), gerund (G), or participial (Part).

1. Mr. Vieira did not say a word to me **during the entire physical examination.**
2. **Skipping meals** is not a healthy way **to lose weight.**
3. Fists clenched, the little boy screamed **at the nurse** who had given him a shot **in his arm.**
4. **Helping patients better understand their treatment options** is the only responsible course to take.
5. Mrs. O'Donnell's daughter-in-law went out to the lobby to wait **during the 3-hour procedure.**

Clauses

A clause is a group of words that contains both a subject and a verb. Clauses can be independent clauses or dependent (also called subordinate) clauses.

Independent Clauses

An independent clause expresses a complete idea. An independent clause can stand alone as a complete sentence or as part of a longer sentence.

- Three staff members were late today. (This is an independent clause—a complete sentence.)
- Three staff members were late today because of a breakdown on the subway line. (*Three members were late today* is an independent clause in a longer sentence.)
- The patient seemed confused. (This is an independent clause—a complete sentence.)
- When the doctor asked her about taking her medication, the patient seemed confused. (*The patient seemed confused* is an independent clause in a longer sentence.)

Dependent Clauses

A dependent clause (also called a subordinate clause) cannot stand alone as a complete sentence. A dependent clause always has a subject and a verb, but it does not express a complete thought. A dependent clause has to be connected to an independent clause for its full meaning to be clear. A dependent clause always begins with a subordinating conjunction (*if, when, because, while,* and *although* are some examples) or a relative pronoun (*who, whom, that,* or *which*).

- Three staff members were late today because of a breakdown on the subway line. (*Because of a breakdown on the subway line* is a dependent clause that needs the independent clause *three staff members were late today* to form a complete sentence.)
- When the doctor asked her about taking her medication, Mrs. Jones seemed confused. (*When the doctor asked her about taking her medication* is a dependent clause that needs the independent clause *Mrs. Jones seemed confused* to form a complete sentence.)

- Josephine Martinique, who studied physical therapy with Dr. Johnson in Boston, is the strongest candidate for the new job opening. (*Who studied physical therapy with Dr. Johnson in Boston* is a dependent clause that needs the independent clause *Josephine Martinique is the strongest candidate for the new job opening* to form a complete sentence.)

Practice With: Independent and Dependent Clauses

Identify the clauses in bold print as either independent (I) or dependent (D).

1. **If Mrs. Robertson can come for her physical on Thursday morning at 11:00,** Dr. Rodriguez has an opening on his schedule.
2. **Mr. Solomon needs to go down to radiology for his chest CT.**
3. **The patient's prescription won't be ready for an hour** because the whole computer system went down and a backlog has formed.
4. Patients won't know about the women's health workshop **unless we tell them**.
5. **I don't know** where Dr. Marin put her stethoscope.

Section 11-6 (To accompany Chapter 6, "Listening, Taking Notes, and Reading as a Healthcare Professional")

Sentence Types

Use phrases and clauses to build clear and effective sentences. The three main kinds of sentences are simple, compound, and complex. All sentences use one of these three types.

Simple Sentences

A simple sentence has one independent clause. A simple sentence can be as short as two words, using just a subject and a verb. A simple sentence can also be longer, using many modifiers and phrases but never any other clauses.

- Alex studied. (This is a simple sentence—an independent clause—with a subject and a verb.)
- On Monday afternoon, Dr. Fredrickson consulted with radiology on Mrs. Lee's CT scan. (This is a simple sentence with three prepositional phrases: *Dr. Fredrickson consulted* are the subject and verb, and *on Monday afternoon, with radiology*, and *on Mrs. Lee's CT scan* are all prepositional phrases.)

Compound Sentences

A compound sentence has at least two independent clauses connected by a comma and then a coordinating conjunction (*and, but, for, or, nor, so,* or *yet*).

- Jermaine was downstairs at the pathology lab waiting, but the patient's unit of type O red blood wasn't ready. (*Jermaine was downstairs at the pathology lab waiting* and *the patient's unit of type O red blood wasn't ready* are both independent clauses, connected by a *comma* and then the coordinating conjunction *but*.)

- John read the doctor's orders, and then he called the pharmacy to make sure the patient's prescriptions were filled. (*John read the doctor's orders* and *then he called the pharmacy to make sure the patient's prescriptions were filled* are both independent clauses, connected by a *comma* and then the coordinating conjunction *and*.)

  A compound sentence can also have three independent clauses.

- Mr. Ortiz came in for his appointment, and then he began asking frantically for a drink of water, but he said he wasn't thirsty. (*Mr. Ortiz came in for his appointment, then he began asking frantically for a drink of water*, and *he said he wasn't thirsty* are all independent clauses, connected by *commas* and the coordinating conjunctions *and* and *but*.)

Complex Sentences

A complex sentence has one independent clause and at least one dependent clause. The dependent clause will always begin with a subordinating conjunction (*when, if, because, although*) or a relative pronoun (*who, which, that*).

- We will take Mr. Santos off the neutropenic diet when his white blood cell count rises to an acceptable level. (*We will take Mr. Santos off the neutropenic diet* is an independent clause, and *when his white blood cell count rises to an acceptable level* is a dependent clause started with the subordinating conjunction *when*.)
- Although Mrs. Kenney showed up on time for her colonoscopy, she hadn't prepared by fasting since the evening before. (*Although Mrs. Kenney showed up on time for her colonoscopy* is a dependent clause started with the subordinating conjunction *although*, and *she hadn't prepared by fasting since the evening before* is an independent clause.)

Sentence Errors

You should recognize early on what kinds of errors you might make when writing sentences. Learning how to identify these errors and correct them can help you become a much more effective writer. Here are a few important grammar points to remember, along with some of the most common sentence errors.

Subject-Verb Agreement Errors

A subject and a verb in a sentence must agree in number. If a subject is singular, the verb must be singular. If a subject is plural, the verb must be plural.

When a subject and verb in a sentence do not agree in number, the sentence contains a subject-verb agreement (S-V agreement) error.

- **With S-V agreement error**: Mr. Garbo have not completed his medical history forms. The subject and verb do not agree: The subject *Mr. Garbo* is singular; the verb *have* is plural.
- **Correct version**: Mr. Garbo has not completed his medical history forms. The subject and verb agree.
- **With S-V agreement error**: The faculty member do a good job helping students learn correct grammar. The subject and verb do not agree: the subject *faculty member* is singular; the verb *do* is plural.

- **Correct version**: The faculty member does a good job helping students learn correct grammar. The subject and verb agree.
- **With S-V agreement error**: Studying every day for many hours have made Mark a good medical assisting student but a boring friend. The subject and verb do not agree: The gerund phrase *studying for many hours* is the subject and is singular; the verb *have* is plural.
- **Correct version**: Studying every day for many hours has made Mark a good medical assisting student but a boring friend. The subject and verb agree.

The following indefinite pronouns often serve as subjects in sentences, and all of them are singular: *each, everyone, everybody, everything, either, neither, anyone, anything, anybody, nobody,* and *nothing.*

- **With S-V agreement error**: Neither of the doctors are on the cardiology unit. The subject and verb do not agree: The subject *neither* is singular and the verb *are* is plural.
- **Correct version**: Neither of the doctors is on the cardiology unit. The subject and verb agree.

Tip: Remember from the section on prepositions earlier in the chapter that the subject of a sentence will never be in a prepositional phrase—*of the doctors* and *on the cardiology unit* are both prepositional phrases.

Practice With: Subject-Verb Agreement

In the sentences below, choose the correct verb.

1. Both of the patients **(is/are)** in the examination rooms.
2. Bringing in family members to speak with the healthcare team members **(is/are)** what many elderly patients do to help them understand their treatment options.
3. Neither of the nurses **(has/have)** seen the patients' test results.
4. Many of the patients in this practice **(prefers/prefer)** the early morning schedule.
5. Each of the physicians in the department **(sees/see)** over 50 patients per week.

Run-Ons—Fused Sentences and Comma Splice Errors

A run-on occurs when two or more complete sentences are run together without adequate punctuation between them. There are two kinds of run-ons: *fused sentences* and *comma splice errors.*

A fused sentence has no punctuation between two complete sentences.

Fused sentence: David spent 30 minutes with Mrs. Briggs in her hospital room he came out and wrote three pages of notes on the encounter. (*Dave spent 30 minutes with Mrs. Briggs in her hospital room* and *He came out and wrote three pages of notes on the encounter* are both complete sentences.)

A comma splice error has a comma between two complete sentences. A comma is not adequate punctuation between two complete sentences without a conjunction.

Comma splice error: David spent 30 minutes with Mrs. Briggs in her hospital room, he came out and wrote three pages of notes on the encounter.

To correct the error, you must first identify the two complete sentences. Then you can choose one of four ways to complete the correct version.

1. Add a period between the two complete sentences and capitalize the first letter of the second sentence.
   David spent 30 minutes with Mrs. Briggs in her hospital room. He came out and wrote three pages of notes on the encounter.
2. Add a semicolon between the two complete sentences. (When you use a semicolon, you do not need to capitalize the first letter in the second sentence.)
   David spent 30 minutes with Mrs. Briggs in her hospital room; he came out and wrote three pages of notes on the encounter.
3. Add a comma and a coordinating conjunction between the two complete sentences.
   David spent 30 minutes with Mrs. Briggs in her hospital room, and he came out and wrote three pages of notes on the encounter.
4. Add a subordinating conjunction to one of the complete sentences.
   After David spent 30 minutes with Mrs. Briggs in her hospital room, he came out and wrote three pages of notes on the encounter. (Tip: If you begin the sentence with a dependent clause, you should place a comma after that dependent clause. You should not use a comma if you begin the sentence with an independent clause.)

Practice With: Correcting Run-Ons

Use any of the four methods described to correct these run-ons.

1. Not all elderly patients are good historians those who have trouble giving their medical histories should bring a family member to medical appointments.
2. Dr. Rodman wrote an order for a chest x-ray for Mr. Smith 2 hours ago, however, the medical assistant from radiology has not arrived yet to pick Mr. Smith up.
3. James Albertson called to renew his asthma prescription, Dr. Babson wants James to come in for an examination before renewing the prescription.
4. Maria studied all night for her medical ethics final, she's still not sure she understands the debate on stem cell research.
5. Mr. Matwick arrived 25 minutes late for his neurology appointment Dr. Lowe was still able to see Mr. Matwick promptly.

Section 11-7 (To accompany Chapter 7, "Study Skills")

Fragments

A sentence must have a subject and a verb, and it must be a complete thought. A *fragment* is missing either a subject or a verb, or it is not a complete thought (i.e., it cannot stand on its own as an independent clause). Sometimes, writers use fragments intentionally for emphasis.

- I want you to get out of bed and get dressed. Now! (*Now* is a fragment, having neither a subject nor a verb.)
- John studies day and night for his genetics class. Really, all the time. (*Really, all the time* is a fragment, having neither a subject nor a verb.)

It is important to be able to identify fragments and know how to correct them. Be on the lookout for the following three kinds of fragments.

Leaving Out the Verb

A fragment may occur by leaving out a verb.

- **Fragment**: The pharmacy filling hundreds prescriptions every day. (*Filling* is a participle, describing the pharmacy; the subject, *pharmacy*, has no real verb.)
- **Complete sentence**: The pharmacy fills hundreds of prescriptions every day. (*Fills* is the verb.)

Leaving Out the Subject

A fragment may occur also by leaving out the subject.

- **Fragment**: The pharmacy fills hundreds of prescriptions. *And delivers them every day.* (The verb *delivers* has no subject.)
- **Complete sentence**: The pharmacy fills and delivers hundreds of prescriptions every day. (*Pharmacy* is the subject; *fills* and *delivers* are the verbs describing what it does.)
- **Complete sentence**: The pharmacy fills hundreds of prescriptions every day. It also delivers those prescriptions. (*It*, a pronoun referring to the antecedent *pharmacy*, is the subject of the second sentence.)

Using Only a Dependent Clause

A dependent clause contains a subject and a verb, but it cannot stand alone. A dependent clause must be joined to an independent clause to form a complete sentence.

Tip: Dependent clauses always begin with a subordinating conjunction (*because, if, when, while*) or a relative pronoun (*who, which, that*).

- **Fragment**: Because the elderly patient appeared confused and frightened during the physical. (This group of words does have a subject *patient* and a verb *appeared*, but this is still a fragment. It is not a complete thought and cannot stand alone. The reader is left asking, "*What happened because the elderly patient appeared confused and frightened?*")

- **Complete sentence**: Because the elderly patient appeared confused and frightened during the physical, the doctor asked the patient's daughter to come into the examination room. (The dependent clause *Because the elderly patient appeared confused and frightened during the physical* is now connected to the independent clause *the doctor asked the patient's daughter to come into the examination room,* creating a complete sentence.)
- **Complete sentence**: The elderly patient appeared confused and frightened during the physical. (Dropping the subordinating conjunction *because* forms a complete sentence.)

Practice With: Correcting Fragments

Correct each of the fragments below. (Note: Not all of the groups of words are fragments.)

1. Marta is still not prepared for her anatomy test. Despite the fact that she began studying last week.
2. When the nurse gave the little boy his flu shot, he began to cry. Really loud.
3. Mr. Ortiz brought his daughter with him to his cardiology appointment. To help translate during the examination.
4. Dr. Simpson wants Mrs. Donaldson to come back for a follow-up appointment in 2 weeks. After she has been seen by neurology.
5. Because the nutritionist hasn't spoken to Mr. Barnes yet. Mr. Barnes is not ready to be discharged.

Verb Tense Errors

Try to remain consistent when using verb tense. Do not change verbs from one tense to another unless you indicate a change in time. Be sure that the tense you are using always matches the time you are describing.

- **Verb tense error**: When the doctor *came* into the examination room, the patient *asks* an important question.
- **Correct version**: When the doctor *came* into the examination room, the patient *asked* an important question.
- **Verb tense error**: The nurse *spoke* to the patient about taking medicine regularly because the patient *will not be following* the directions on the prescription.
- **Correct version**: The nurse *spoke* to the patient about taking the medicine regularly because the patient *had not followed* the directions on the prescription.
- **Verb tense error**: The patient states that when he closes his eyes he feels dizzy. He *closes* his eyes yesterday afternoon at work and *feels* so dizzy he has to sit down and take a break. (The second sentence is describing a specific time in the past, so the sentence should use the past tense.)
- **Correct version**: The patient states that when he closes his eyes he feels dizzy. He *closed* his eyes yesterday afternoon at work and *felt* so dizzy he had to sit down and take a break.

Practice With: Tenses

Underline the correct tense of each verb in parentheses.

1. Yesterday, Mr. Johnson (**calls/called**) to make an appointment for his physical examination.
2. Dr. Singh (**will be/has been**) out of the country until next Thursday. He has an opening at 3:30 PM on Friday.
3. When Dr. Gonzalez (**was/has been**) here last week, he renewed James's prescription for an asthma inhaler.
4. Janette (**works/has worked**) in this practice since 2002.
5. Before he finished school and passed his licensure exam, Jean (**works/had worked**) weekends as a unit clerk on the hematology ward.

Section 11-8 (To accompany Chapter 8, "Medical Math for the Healthcare Professional")

Paragraphing Basics

After the sentence, the most basic unit of writing is the paragraph. Writers use sentences to build paragraphs when describing or explaining ideas that are too complex to communicate with a single sentence. The length of paragraphs can vary, depending on the complexity of the idea the writer wants to communicate. Readers can often identify paragraphs easily because the first line of any paragraph may be indented. As readers, we are trained early in our education to recognize paragraphs as essential units of communicating important ideas.

Paragraph Structure

Paragraphs generally use a structure that contains three elements: (1) the topic sentence, (2) supporting sentences, and (3) the concluding sentence.

Topic Sentence

The topic sentence is often the first sentence in the paragraph, and it expresses the paragraph's main idea.

Supporting Sentences

The supporting sentences of a paragraph provide the reader with the details that make up the main idea of the paragraph. Each supporting sentence explains some aspect of the idea in the topic sentence.

Concluding Sentence

Usually the final sentence in the paragraph, the concluding sentence, summarizes the ideas of the paragraph and provides a closing. The closing can be any of the following: a solution to the problem discussed in the paragraph, a prediction based on the elements described in the paragraph, a recommendation based on the facts presented in the paragraph, or a restatement of the main idea of the paragraph.

Examples of Paragraph Elements

Example 1

Topic sentence: Effective communication skills are important in all of the health-care professions.

Supporting sentences: Good communication improves patient satisfaction, compliance, and healthcare outcomes. Professionals who can communicate effectively are better prepared to work with other members of the healthcare team.

Concluding sentence: Hospitals, practices, and other healthcare organizations rightly value good communication skills as one of the most important strengths employees can have.

Complete paragraph: Effective communication skills are important in all of the healthcare professions. Good communication improves patient satisfaction, compliance, and healthcare outcomes. Professionals who can communicate effectively are better prepared to work with other members of the healthcare team. Hospitals, practices, and other healthcare organizations rightly value good communication skills as one of the most important strengths employees can have.

Example 2

Topic sentence: Heart attacks can occur most often because of a condition called coronary artery disease or CAD.

Supporting sentences: This disease involves the buildup over many years of a fatty material, called plaque, on the inner walls of the coronary arteries. When such a buildup has occurred, a section of plaque can break open, causing a blood clot to form on the surface of the plaque.

Concluding sentence: A heart attack occurs if the clot becomes large enough to cut off most or all of the blood flow to the part of the heart muscle fed by the artery.

Complete paragraph: Heart attacks can occur most often because of a condition called coronary artery disease or CAD. This disease involves the buildup over many years of a fatty material, called plaque, on the inner walls of the coronary arteries. When such a buildup has occurred, a section of plaque can break open, causing a blood clot to form on the surface of the plaque. A heart attack occurs if the clot becomes large enough to cut off most or all of the blood flow to the part of the heart muscle fed by the artery.

Practice With: Paragraphs

For the paragraphs below, underline the topic sentence (TS), the supporting sentences (SS), and the concluding sentence (CS).

1. While the flu and the common cold are both respiratory illnesses that have similar symptoms and may be difficult to distinguish, these two illnesses are caused by different viruses. The flu generally is worse than the common cold, and symptoms such as fever, body aches, extreme tiredness, and dry cough are more common and intense. Colds are usually

Continued

milder than the flu. People with colds are more likely to have a runny or stuffy nose. Colds usually do not result in serious health problems, such as pneumonia, bacterial infections, or hospitalizations. Finally, the flu is caused by the influenza virus, which is a respiratory virus, whereas the common cold is caused by either the adenovirus or the corona virus, of which there are many different subsets.

2. A healthcare professional—any professional, for that matter—needs to have effective interpersonal skills. These are the skills one relies on most in order to have successful interaction with other people. These skills— which include tactfulness, courtesy, respect, empathy, genuineness, appropriate self-disclosure, and assertiveness—usually do not stand alone in isolation but rather exist in concert with each other. A healthcare professional who exhibits one of these skills as part of effective communication tends to exhibit others as well.

Section 11-9 (To accompany Chapter 9, "Test-Taking Skills")

Electronic Health Records

Healthcare organizations and networks in many countries across the world are making big changes in how they track and store patient information. These organizations moving away from using paper patient charts and toward EHR. An EHR is a digital version a patient's paper chart, a real-time record of the patient's history and care, and available to all authorized personnel within an organization or network.

According to HealthIT.gov, the official website of the Office of the National Coordinator for Health Information Technology (ONC), an EHR can:

1. Provide healthcare professionals with "a patient's medical history, diagnoses, medications, treatment plans, immunization dates, allergies, radiology images, and laboratory and test results"
2. Provide healthcare professionals with "access to evidence-based tools that providers can use to make decisions about a patient's care"
3. Allow healthcare organizations to "automate and streamline provider workflow"

An EHR is designed to be accessible to all healthcare professionals and healthcare entities involved in a patient's care, including, according to ONC, "laboratories, specialists, medical imaging facilities, emergency facilities, and school and workplace clinics—so they contain information from *all clinicians involved in a patient's care.*"

As a healthcare professional in the 21st century, you will have to use EHRs as part of your job every day. During your studies, you will likely take a course that introduces you to methods of contributing to and maintaining a patient's EHR. In the meantime, you can find more information online at https://www.healthit.gov/.

PART 3

ENTERING A HEALTHCARE PROFESSION

NOTES FOR PART 3

12

Preparing for Your Career Path as a Healthcare Professional

OBJECTIVES

- Understand the basic groups of different healthcare careers.
- Analyze detailed information about health careers in which you may be interested.
- Identify your personality traits and interests as they relate to health careers.
- Describe the personal characteristics needed for working successfully in various health professions.
- Recognize the importance of professional conduct.
- Distinguish between a job and a profession.

You may already be registered in a health career educational program and have already determined what courses you'll be taking as you prepare for a health profession. You may also have chosen your career—or at least an area of health care in which you're interested in working. Even so, students sometimes change their career choices as they learn more about what's involved in education and training and what they will do on the job. Other students are still in the process of choosing. However, all students should know what they will be getting themselves into in the future. This chapter helps you better understand different kinds of healthcare careers and the personal and professional traits needed to be successful in them.

The Health Professions

Who do you think of when you think about health care? Many people may say doctors and nurses. However, at this point in your education you should know about some of the many other health professionals also involved in health care. There are a multitude of different healthcare careers. This discussion will help you to find the career that best matches your interests and skills. The following strategies will get you started:

1. Learn about basic healthcare career groups.
2. Consider the education and training needed for possible careers.
3. Consider your personality and what you think you would like to do in your career. What personality traits and skills do you need to succeed in a given healthcare career? Take a self-assessment inventory to see how well you will fit in different professions.
4. Talk with an academic advisor about your choices.
5. Confirm your choice and commit to your educational path.

Health Career Groupings

The National Consortium for Health Science Education (NCHSE) has organized the 300 different health professions into five main groups. This is a good starting point for thinking about what different healthcare professionals (HCPs) do in their work. (See *Examples of Healthcare Professional Career Titles* for additional examples of careers in these groupings.)

- *Therapeutic services.* HCPs who work in therapeutic services deliver health care directly to patients. In addition to medicine, nursing, and dentistry, these careers include physician assistants, respiratory therapists, surgical technicians, dental assistants, home health aides, medical assistants, massage therapists, and pharmacy technicians. People who work in these careers usually enjoy working directly with patients and helping them maintain or regain their health.
- *Diagnostics services.* HCPs working in diagnostic services work closely with those in therapeutic services and often are also in direct contact with patients. Diagnostic health services, however, involve determining the nature of the patient's health problem, often using the latest technology. Examples of careers in diagnostic services are lab and radiography technology, ophthalmology, electrocardiography, and computed tomography technology. People who work in these careers usually enjoy working with scientific equipment and technology and knowing their work will help identify patients' health problems so that they can receive the appropriate therapy.
- *Health informatics.* Health informatics careers generally involve managing patient and other information—a crucial aspect of health care. Examples of these careers are health information management technicians, medical coders, medical transcriptionists, and patient account technicians. Because most medical information is now managed with computerized systems, people who work in these careers usually enjoy working on a computer, using written language, paying close attention to detail, and often working independently. Although these careers typically involve less direct patient contact, they are a very important part of the healthcare team.
- *Support services.* Many other health professionals contribute to the working of healthcare institutions and the full provision of health care. The general category of support services includes careers such as dietetic technicians, social workers, facilities managers, and food safety specialists. These careers may or may not involve direct patient contact and vary widely in terms of responsibilities and educational training.
- *Biotechnology research and development.* Because science and technology are continually developing new approaches within health care, many careers involve research. A few examples are laboratory technology, laboratory research, and quality control. Individuals in these careers, which often involve little patient contact, enjoy being part of a team focusing on science and the latest technology while they investigate new aspects of health care.

Examples of Healthcare Professional Career Titles

Therapeutic Services

- Anesthesiologist assistant
- Athletic trainer
- Audiologist
- Certified nurse assistant (CNA)

- Dental assistant
- Dental hygienist
- Dental lab technician
- Dentist
- Dietician
- Dosimetrist
- Emergency medical technician (EMT)
- Home health aide
- Licensed practical nurse (LPN)
- Massage therapist
- Medical assistant
- Occupational therapist
- Occupational therapy assistant
- Paramedic
- Pharmacy technician
- Physical therapist
- Physical therapy assistant
- Physician
- Physician assistant
- Recreation therapist
- Registered nurse
- Respiratory therapist
- Speech language pathologist
- Surgical technician
- Veterinarian technician

Diagnostic Services

- Cardiovascular technologist
- Clinical lab technician
- Computed tomography (CT) technologist
- Cytotechnologists
- Diagnostic medical sonographer
- Electrocardiographic (ECG) technician
- Electroencephalogram (EEG) technician
- Exercise physiologist
- Histotechnician
- Magnetic resonance imaging (MRI) technician
- Medical technologist
- Nuclear medicine technologist
- Pathology assistant
- Phlebotomist
- Positron emission tomography (PET) technician
- Radiologic technologist/radiographer
- Sonographer

Health Informatics

- Admitting clerk
- Community services specialists
- Data analyst

Continued

- Health educator
- Health information coder
- Health information services
- Medical biller
- Patient financial services
- Medical information technologist
- Medical librarian
- Reimbursement specialist, Healthcare Financial Management Association (HFMA)
- Transcriptionist
- Utilization manager

Support Services

- Biomedical/clinical technician
- Central services/sterile processing
- Environmental health and safety
- Environmental services
- Facilities manager
- Food service
- Hospital maintenance
- Industrial hygienist
- Materials management
- Transport technician

Biotechnology Research and Development

- Bioinformatics associate
- Biostatistician
- Clinical data management associate
- Clinical trials research associate
- Lab assistant
- Lab technician
- Manufacturing technician
- Product safety associate
- Processing technician
- Quality control technician
- Research assistant

ROLE PLAY

Healthcare Careers

With a partner, discuss which areas of career titles best fit your personality and career goals. Why? Which ones wouldn't be a good fit for you? Why?

Career Possibilities

With a general idea about one or more careers you may be interested in, it's easy to learn more about those specific professions. Your school likely has a student career office with directories and other books with detailed information about healthcare careers. Look for this information:

- Career titles
- Description of activities and roles performed

- Settings in which these professionals may work
- Education and training required
- Future job prospects and salary range

Online Resources

The U.S. Department of Labor, Employment and Training Administration maintains the "CareerOneStop" website with a wealth of information about many health careers. Start here: http://www.careeronestop.org. This takes you to the home page. Click on "Toolkit" and then "Occupation Profile" to reach a list of careers with detailed information. This site can also tell you about career facts in your own state. In addition, you can see videos of HCPs doing their work.

Exploring Majors for Healthcare Careers

Assuming you are already enrolled in an educational institution, the best way to learn more about preparing for a health career is to start with your school's catalog. You can find this on the school's website. In addition, individual departments and programs often post descriptions of the coursework for majors and certificate programs for working in different careers. Pay attention to information such as:

- prerequisites—courses or special background needed to enter the major or program
- the number of courses or semesters to fulfill degree or program requirements
- clinical experience required (usually through clinical labs or courses)
- options such as elective courses in other areas of your interest
- the associated costs of your education/training
- additional education needed later to advance your career options

Making Academic Choices

If you have questions or still aren't sure exactly what career path interests you the most, talk to your academic advisor or department representatives to learn more about the program or major. This is one of the most important decisions you'll make in your life, so consider your options carefully.

One of the first things many students notice about healthcare careers is the wide variation in educational preparation. Depending on the career and your state's requirements for education and training, the amount of time needed for this preparation can vary from 1 to 4 years of school or more. When making your choice, however, time should not be the key deciding factor. Instead, think about what you will actually be doing in your future career and how much you will enjoy it. Your choice may determine how you'll spend many years or even your whole life. Although you can always change careers at some later time, that might mean returning to school at additional cost.

It's also important to think about how your career might evolve over time. Will you be happy doing the same work for as long as 20 or 30 years? Does your chosen career allow you to move up a ladder within the same profession, taking on new responsibilities and challenges? This is called a "career path" because your education and your first job after school are only the first steps on a path that may take you onward and upward in your chosen profession. As you work within your profession, you continue to gain new skills and acquire new knowledge, allowing you to take on new responsibilities. You might become a supervisor and manage others who do what you once did. With experience or additional education, you may move up the ladder from an assisting role to a higher position or one with more independent functions.

If you're not sure where you can go in the future within a profession, talk to your advisor about this dimension of your choices as well.

Making Career Choices

People who are happiest in their work usually feel their career matches their personality and interests perfectly. They enjoy going to work because it's something they like to do and consider it a profession, not just a way to earn a living or a job.

How can you know what career is right for you? The process begins with understanding yourself.

Know Yourself

You already know a lot about yourself, even if you may not yet know everything about the health career in which you're interested. To get started, think about questions like these:

- Do you like working with people?
- Do you like helping people?
- Are you emotionally upset by the sight of blood, body fluids, or illness?
- Do you prefer being a team player or working independently?
- Are you more interested in the "human" side or the scientific side of health care?
- Can you work at a computer or lab bench for a long period without becoming restless?
- Do you enjoy communicating with others, whether by talking or writing?
- Do you like working with your hands?
- Do you prefer daily routines or frequently shifting activities?
- Do you like solving problems?
- Do you like learning new things frequently?

These are just a few of the ways people differ. There are no right or wrong answers to any of these questions; however, certain personality traits fit better with some careers than with others. Your goal is to find the perfect fit for you.

If you're still not sure, even after you have learned about specific careers and their educational requirements, an inventory of your personality and interests may help you decide. Recall the different learning styles from Chapter 5. In that chapter, you thought about how you best learn new information and skills. Do you learn more by seeing, hearing, or doing? Which kinds of learning activities are you most comfortable with? This can help you better understand your career style as well.

Choosing Your Healthcare Career

With a partner, discuss your answers to the questions above. If you have already selected a healthcare program, discuss how your answers led you to choose this field of study.

Personal and Professional Traits and Skills

As you prepare to enter a healthcare profession, think about what it means to be a professional. Having a career in a health profession is more than simply working a job. To be a professional involves demonstrating certain characteristics and behaving in certain ways. This begins with your personality traits, or who you are as a person.

Personal Characteristics

When you work in health care, your personality and conduct matter. Remember that patients need to believe that they can trust you to take care of them. Many patients will see you face to face, whether you're providing direct care or taking their insurance information. During this interaction, they will likely make decisions about whether you seem to care about them. Similarly, your coworkers need to be reassured that you can carry out your responsibilities.

Patients also give you information that is very private—sometimes information not even their families know. Therefore, you have to be the kind of person a patient can trust. The following are important characteristics you need to have to be a good HCP:

- *Caring.* Be someone who cares about the patients receiving health care.
- *Integrity.* Be recognized as someone who is honest and accountable and behaves ethically.
- *Dependability.* Be someone who always accepts your responsibilities and works hard to meet the expectations for a professional in your position.
- *Trustworthiness.* Be someone who consistently does the right thing and is always honest.
- *Teamwork.* Be a willing and effective member of the healthcare team.
- *Openness to change.* Be flexible and willing to keep learning.
- *Personal health.* Be a model of good health habits and behaviors.

Caring

Health care is all about caring for people's needs. Even if you're not in direct patient care—if you're working in a career behind the scenes—patients are still affected by the quality of your work. People who care about their work, who genuinely want to do their best, not only contribute more to the overall quality of health care but also are more successful in their career and experience more job satisfaction.

Caring begins now, as a student. A student who cares about learning, who sees the importance of learning for one's career, really wants to understand and be able to apply this knowledge or skill in the future.

Caring extends into all aspects of being a student. You should care enough to do your homework and assignments well and on time, to pay attention in class, and to show respect for your instructors and other students.

Caring also means caring for other people—making the effort to understand their feelings. This kind of caring, known as empathy, is essential for HCPs who work with patients. Empathy is to show that you understand—to the point of feeling—how another person feels. A caring person is also tactful, meaning that you consider the feelings of others before speaking in a way that might hurt another person.

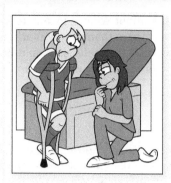

Empathy—Jenna

As a high school student, Jenna was a varsity soccer player. During a game in her senior year, she suffered a knee injury which required surgery and physical therapy. Jenna has since chosen a career as a physical therapist assistant. Because of her experience, she believes that she will be ideally suited to work with patients recovering from injuries. With a partner, discuss any experiences that you have had that will enable you to feel empathy for your patients.

Integrity

Integrity refers to the quality of your character. The character you develop as a student will influence the character you'll have as an HCP. That's why it's important to start thinking about your character now while you're in school.

People with integrity stand by their personal and professional codes of ethics. They're honest in everything they do and are accountable for their actions. This quality is especially important to have as an HCP. Someone with integrity will be sure to keep patient information private and will be honest about his or her actions—even after making a mistake.

Dependability

Dependability is crucial in health care. Medical facilities are busy places, making teamwork necessary for everyday office operations. Even one person not showing up to work or coming late can throw off the entire day. As a member of the health-care team, you need to be there—your colleagues are counting on you. Be someone who always makes it in to work on time.

Dependability also applies to the quality of your work. If you're asked to perform a task, you should always perform it when you are told to do so and to the exact specifications you are given. In the often hectic world of the healthcare facility, delays and mistakes add up to late hours and unhappy patients or potentially worse outcomes.

Being dependable means that you'll always follow through and do what you're asked. It means that your coworkers, supervisors, and patients can feel comfortable putting their trust in you and relying on you to get the job done.

Trustworthiness

Being trustworthy means people feel confident that you can be trusted in all situations and that you'll always do the right thing. You should never cut corners or do things that are not according to accepted procedure. Being trustworthy means you stand firm in your commitment to honesty, forthrightness, and doing things the right way. Not only will you feel good about yourself when you're trustworthy but you'll also earn and keep the respect of everyone around you.

Teamwork

Even while still a student, you're part of a team that includes instructors and other students. You will likely work on group projects with others, just as in your healthcare career you will be part of a team providing or supporting patient care.

To be an effective team player, you need to respect the other members of the team and what they have to offer. You need to make the effort to understand their point of view rather than thinking that you are always right. Commit yourself to working with others and doing your fair share, and avoid complaining if sometimes you believe you might be doing more than your share.

Working with others also requires patience. Be tolerant and understanding of others who may not be as quick to act. Being accepting helps you avoid feeling frustrated if things aren't going exactly as you'd prefer.

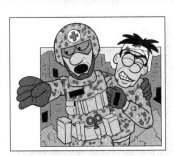

Teamwork—Michael

As a twice-deployed army veteran, Michael knows a lot about teamwork and how it is essential in health care. On more than one occasion he worked with others to save the life of an injured soldier. With a partner, discuss how teamwork is important in your current job. How do you expect it to be important in your chosen healthcare career?

Openness to Change

Health care is continually evolving as new technology and new diagnostic and therapeutic approaches develop and the healthcare system itself changes. Make an effort to stay open-minded and always willing to learn more. In fact, in health care more than in other professions, people are often required to take continuing education classes throughout their career so that they stay current in their field.

As a student, you are learning many new things. Most important is your attitude, so that you always stay open to continuing to learn. Don't view your education as something you *have to get through* and then be done with it. Accept the fact that you'll always be learning, that this is simply part of being an HCP, and learn to enjoy it! Once you relax and realize that education is an exciting benefit of having a healthcare career, not a *price to pay* or just a stage to go through to enter that career, you'll find you enjoy your daily life as a student more.

Openness to change also means being able to accept criticism from others. Your instructors, like supervisors in your career, will offer you feedback that is both positive and designed to help you improve in areas that need improvement. Try not to feel resentful; instead, accept criticism gracefully and continue to learn.

Personal Health

As an HCP, you will work to help others stay or become healthy, and health promotion is a key aspect of everything you will do. You will in fact be a model for others—family and friends as well as patients—and you should do your best to demonstrate good health habits yourself. That includes eating well and maintaining a healthy weight, exercising regularly, getting enough rest, and not using tobacco, drugs, or excessive alcohol. Not only is this important for your own health and well-being, but others will judge you in your career by your personal habits. Remember, people pay far more attention to what you *do* than what you say.

Professional Conduct

As you develop the personal characteristics just described, you're also learning how to act as a professional. Being a successful HCP isn't just about remembering the facts you learned in school. Doing your job well is not simply performing tasks exactly how you learned to do them. It's also about how you present yourself—with your conduct. The most knowledgeable person in the world will have trouble inspiring patients or coworkers with confidence if he or she seems rude, sarcastic, sloppy, or haphazard. Instead, we learn to behave like a professional.

Remember that as an HCP, every aspect of your conduct is scrutinized. Patients have to feel that they can trust you to take care of them. Your coworkers need to be reassured that you're capable of carrying out your responsibilities. You must present yourself as a responsible person who is focused on work.

For example, think back to doctors, nurses, and other healthcare providers you've encountered. How would you feel if they stood in the hall gossiping while you waited in the exam room? How would you feel if they seemed as though they were rushing, irritated, or impatient? Healthcare demands a high standard of professional conduct from its members. Here are some additional general behaviors that demonstrate professional conduct:

- *Act responsibly.* Follow the standards of practice in your work and take responsibility for your own actions. Admit failures and don't try to blame others if something goes wrong. Follow ethical standards in everything you do.
- *Accept diversity and embrace differences in others.* A professional knows people have different ideas, feelings, customs, and behaviors and does not judge them because of differences. Give the best possible care to all patients.
- *Communicate carefully and effectively.* Use the skills described in Chapter 4 when talking to patients, coworkers, and other health professionals. Avoid slang, sarcasm, and gossip—and never, ever violate the confidentiality of patients. You'll learn more about confidentiality in Chapter 13.
- *Show initiative.* If you see a problem, don't ignore it just because it may be outside your immediate work. Share your ideas if you see ways that things can be improved. Remember that in the healthcare team, everyone has an important role—and everyone can raise questions or offer ideas for the good of all.

Professional Conduct

With a partner, discuss how you apply the guidelines for professional conduct outlined above to your current job. How do you expect to apply them to your chosen healthcare career?

Characteristics of a Profession

How is a healthcare career more than just a job? What makes a career a profession rather than just a job to attend every day?

You've probably already worked in a job that does not require a specialized education or advanced training. Although there's certainly nothing wrong with working such a job, you might not have felt completely satisfied by your work. Maybe that's why you've chosen to enter a healthcare career instead.

A profession, on the other hand, is more fulfilling because you are more completely involved—your work becomes part of who you are. Healthcare professions, like other professions, have several characteristics that make them different from ordinary jobs. As you move into your chosen career, you will participate increasingly in the profession, so it's a good idea to be thinking ahead about these characteristics. This will also help prepare you for your clinical experiences in your education, the subject of Chapter 13. Even as a student, you will likely very soon be in *real* healthcare practice.

Education and Competence

No one enters any profession without education and training to gain specialized knowledge and skills. As a student, you already know about the education required. Along with this comes the expectation that in your healthcare career, you will have competence. That is, you have the knowledge and skills to do your work correctly and safely. It will not be necessary for a supervisor to stand over you at all times watching to make sure you're doing the right thing—you'll do your work well because you have learned how to do so and you care about it. That's one reason why it's important to care about your education now as a student. In the future you'll have the responsibility to act competently on your own when needed. It's a great feeling to know you can meet this challenge.

Self-Regulating Professions

Professions are generally said to be self-regulating. That means that even though the profession is in part governed by laws, the profession itself sets many of the standards by which people practice in it. For example, medical practice standards—such as the right way to perform medical procedures—are established by medical professionals. This makes good sense if you think about it: Who other than the professionals in a field would know best about how their work should be done?

Professions are also self-regulating in terms of proper behavior. Most professions have an ethical code that spells out how people in that profession should act toward each other, their clients, and the general public. Healthcare professions also have ethical codes for how people in those careers should behave toward patients, coworkers, and others. In Chapter 13, you'll learn about the ethical codes of health professions.

Professional Associations

As one entering a healthcare career, you may already know about one or more professional associations for practitioners in that career. A professional association is a nonprofit organization of people who work in a particular career, with many benefits for those who join. Most healthcare careers have professional associations, and many allow students to become members so that they can begin receiving the benefits right away. A few of these benefits are:

- subscriptions to professional publications
- access to online resources
- professional conferences, conventions, and workshops
- information on new technologies
- ethics guidelines
- patient educational materials
- networking opportunities
- grant and scholarship opportunities

Once you have decided which career you are preparing for, take a few minutes to learn about its professional associations. Ask your instructors or do an online search (search for "association + *name of career*"). Every association has a website that can provide you with benefits and help you to become more professional as you move into your career.

Networking

Another important aspect of most professions is networking among the people in the profession. Networking is a process of developing relationships with other people with whom you share common interests and who may be helpful to you in your career. Most networking is done in an informal way. You might have a conversation with an instructor after a course has ended. You might have expressed an interest in a particular type of work and maybe this instructor remembers this and later on tells you about a job opening he or she has learned about. That's networking in action. Or you might become friends with an older student who enters the profession ahead of you. If you stay in touch, you might one day learn of an available position where he or she works. That's also networking. In reality, more jobs are filled by people who have learned of an open position from someone they know than by people who respond to posted job openings.

Networking is not an attempt to use people, however. You shouldn't start networking motivated only by the thought of what you might get from them in the future. Rather, networking is more a matter of building relationships with people in your chosen field, whom you like and want to stay in touch with. You can start networking with other students right away. Forming a study group is a good way to spend time with other students in your career path. You get to know them as people, at the same time you increase your knowledge and skills in your courses. Many lifelong friendships—and networks—begin during one's education years.

Once you are practicing in your profession, your network continues to be valuable. You talk to people in your network about your work and learn new things about the field. You can problem-solve together, and you always have people to whom you can turn if you need advice for any work-related issues that may occur.

Chapter Summary

- Consider the five main groups of healthcare careers to determine or confirm which are most suitable for you.
- Research your chosen career through the Internet and resources available at your educational institution. Talk with your advisor if you have any questions.
- Use a self-assessment tool to explore your personality traits and personal interests to be sure your chosen career is a good match.
- Understand the personal characteristics that are important for working in a health profession. During your time as a student, work on developing your own characteristics and abilities so that you enter your career prepared to do your best.
- Accept what it means to be a professional. Conduct yourself in a way that inspires the trust and confidence of coworkers and patients.
- Begin participating in your profession right away through a professional association.
- Network with others in your profession to help you get started in your new healthcare career.

Review Questions

Objective Questions

1. Three essential characteristics of an HCP include _____, _____, and _____.
2. Concern for others that leads to a desire to help is referred to as _____.
3. Both your patients and your coworkers need to be assured that you are trustworthy. (True or False?)
4. In terms of personal health, HCP are models for their patients and should do their best to demonstrate good health habits. (True or False?)
5. Two distinguishing characteristics between a job and a profession include _____ and _____.

Short-Answer Questions

1. Which main group of healthcare careers interests you the most? Why?
2. What is the employment outlook for your chosen career?
3. Describe your personality traits and interests that match up with your chosen career.
4. List at least five personal characteristics that are important in all health professions.
5. Name three characteristics of a profession.

Applications

1. Online Exercise: Go to the U.S. Department of Labor website and look up a career in which you are interested in the Occupational Outlook Handbook. Type in a career title to search for it here: http://www.bls.gov/search/ooh.htm. Type in a career, for example, physical therapist assistants. Read the section "What Physical Therapist Assistants and Aides Do" to make sure people in this career do what you initially thought they do. Then read other information about that career you're interested in.
2. Group Discussion: With two or three other students, spend a few minutes talking about what you think are the most important personal characteristics for working in health care. Be sure each person has the opportunity to speak. Then compare your responses and talk about *why* each characteristic is important. As a group, try to come up with an example of a patient care problem that could occur if someone on the healthcare team did *not* manifest that characteristic in their work.
3. Role Playing and Discussion: In groups of two to four students, devise a role play for a patient care interaction. The healthcare provider(s) in this role play should demonstrate either professional or unprofessional behavior in the interaction with the patient. After each role play, other students should critique the behavior observed and provide rationales for how they evaluate this behavior.

13

Clinical Rotations

- Master new skills in a clinical environment.
- Exhibit the ability to effectively manage anxiety and stress.
- Demonstrate the standards of professionalism.
- Demonstrate the ability to maintain patient confidentiality and protect patient rights and safety.
- Succeed in a culturally diverse environment.
- Exhibit a high standard of personal conduct.
- Plan for your clinical rotation.

In this chapter, you will look ahead to your clinical rotation, which in many health-care educational programs is the first step toward a new career. This is an exciting time. You will learn about the professional standards of conduct you'll be expected to meet and about the importance of protecting patient rights and privacy. You will prepare for handling changes in your schedule, and you'll learn how your clinical instructor can help you before and after you begin your rotation. This chapter provides you with important information that will help you make your clinical rotation a positive experience.

Practical Experience in the Healthcare Setting

You have prepared for this next step by studying in the classroom and practicing in the clinical skills lab. You've probably imagined yourself in a healthcare setting, putting your knowledge into action. It's one thing to read about the tasks you will have to perform but quite another to carry out those tasks in the workplace. However, this is an exciting opportunity to use your skills and begin to experience what your future career will really be like. This chapter helps you to take full advantage of this important experience.

Embrace New Skills

You might think that in your clinical rotation you'll be taking on many new responsibilities. But the only thing that's really "new" about the tasks you'll perform is the fact that you'll be doing them for the first time in a clinical setting. After all, you've read about these tasks, practiced them in the classroom or laboratory, and you already know what to do. Of course, knowing what to do in your head is different from working with a patient or staff member.

The Clinical Skills Laboratory

Many programs require students to demonstrate certain skills in the laboratory before they perform these tasks during their clinical rotation. If you know there are tasks you'll be performing during your clinical experience and you'd like more practice, use the skills laboratory to brush up on them. Most schools schedule times when an instructor or student mentor works in the skills lab and provides assistance. Take advantage of those times to get extra help. If you're unsure how to get more practice, talk to your instructor.

The Healthcare Setting

Participating in skills labs will give you a good foundation for demonstrating skills during your clinical experience. Even so, it's natural to feel nervous the first time you have to do something in a real healthcare setting. You may feel like the only person in the room who hasn't performed a certain task a hundred times already. You might also feel as though coworkers or patients are judging you unfairly for your inexperience.

The best way to get started with hands-on experience is to jump in. You may feel awkward at first or reluctant to ask a question (especially in front of a patient or coworker), but with repetition you'll gain valuable practical experience very quickly.

Anxieties and Concerns

It's normal to be a little nervous about beginning a clinical experience, but remember that you *are* prepared. This is what you've been working toward every day. And you won't be alone—your clinical instructor or clinical mentor will be there to help you.

The Clinical Instructor

Although you're in a new environment and experiencing new things, you're not alone. Remember that the healthcare professionals (HCPs) you'll be working with were all novices at one time as well. You'll find camaraderie in sharing your experiences.

Your school may provide a clinical instructor to be with you during your clinical experience. Schools that do not send an instructor or coordinator to be with students usually arrange for someone on the job site to serve as a mentor. In either case, this person is there to help and answer questions.

Handling Anxiety

Whether you'll be assisting with patients in the examination room or hospital room, working in a lab, or handling medical coding and billing, you may feel some anxiety about doing the job. That's normal. If you ask people who are already working in health care, you'll probably find they felt the same way when they started.

It's important to address and deal with your anxiety. Mild anxiety probably won't affect your performance on the job, but a high level of anxiety would be a distraction. The following tips will help you minimize anxiety if necessary:

- Use the relaxation techniques described in Chapter 3 to help relieve your anxiety.
- Make an appointment to see your clinical mentor or instructor. He or she can reassure you that what you're feeling is normal and help you identify your anxieties and come up with a plan to reduce them.
- Take advantage of the resources offered by your school. Many schools also have counseling services that can help you cope with your stress.

Handling Stress

As you think about starting your clinical rotation, you may also be concerned about its additional demand on your time. You've already pushed your schedule to the limits with school and work. Your clinical experience will require even more schedule changes. But you can manage these changes by knowing what to expect and how to prepare for them.

For example, remember the support network you read about in earlier chapters. Family members, friends, classmates, and coworkers can all be sources of encouragement and support during your clinical experience. If you accept help from others during this busy time, you'll feel less stressed. (See *Your Safety Net: Family and Friends*.)

Your Safety Net: Family and Friends

Follow these steps to create a "safety net" of people you can rely on during your clinical experience:

1. Explain to your family that your schedule is going to change. Make sure they understand that this opportunity is important and that it's the next big step toward your new career.
2. Tell your family exactly what schedule changes are in store.
3. Offer concrete details about your new schedule.
   - If you have young children, talk with them about when or if they'll be in day care.
   - Talk with your family about which days or nights can be set aside for family time, such as family dinners.
   - Let your family know how much you appreciate their help.
4. Tell your friends about your new schedule, especially those you usually meet with for regularly scheduled events.
5. If you have roommates, make them aware of your schedule changes, especially if you do laundry together, share the cooking or cleaning, or have other commitments.
6. Most important, let your family and friends know that they are important to you and that this extra demand on your time isn't permanent. You may need their support to help get you through the busy days ahead.

Embrace Diversity

Chapter 4 describes the many benefits of experiencing diversity in school and society at large. You will also find a great diversity among both the HCPs and the patients you'll be working with in your clinical experience. This represents another great opportunity to meet a wide range of people and experience many kinds of differences. In this way, too, your clinical rotation is helping prepare you for your future career in health care.

You may want to review the section "What Is Cultural Diversity?" in Chapter 4 before your clinical experience. When working with others who are different from yourself in some way, respect them as individuals and remain open-minded. Do not expect everyone to look, dress, act, or think the same as you and your family or friends, but instead be accepting of differences. The more you interact with others, the more you will understand people with a different background—and the better you will become at serving a diverse patient population. Embrace the many differences that contribute so much to our multicultural world.

Personal and Professional Codes of Ethics

During much of your time at school, you've been focusing on acquiring information, whether that means memorizing key terms, reading about difficult concepts, or figuring out how to apply your new knowledge. There's so much to learn that everything else seems like an unimportant extra. But there's another area that's just as important to your future career in health care—your code of ethics. This becomes particularly important now in your clinical rotation.

In health care, you're often entrusted with personal information about people you don't know. You represent something to the patients you encounter—an ideal of a caring and educated HCP. You are expected to be trustworthy and to take your job seriously.

You should do everything in your power to live up to this ideal. Such an ideal may seem impossibly high, but it should be your goal. As you'll see, it's not about being perfect. It's about reminding yourself every day that what you do is not only special but also a privilege and a great responsibility as well.

A professional code of ethics addresses these areas:

- Professional and personal conduct
- Confidentiality
- Patient rights and safety

Professionalism

The first item in the professional code of ethics is professionalism itself. Professionalism means:

- maintaining professional conduct while in the clinical area
- working effectively with others on the healthcare team
- staying within the bounds of your knowledge and skills
- providing safe care through understanding and following policies and procedures

Professional and Personal Conduct

Chapter 12 describes what professional and personal conduct means. Remember that patients need to feel that they can trust you to take care of them. Many patients will see you face to face, whether you're providing direct care or taking their insurance information. During this interaction, they will likely decide whether you seem to care about them. Similarly, your coworkers need to be reassured that you're capable of carrying out your responsibilities. During your clinical rotation, strive to maintain the same conduct as the HCPs around you. You're not "just a student" any more.

The Healthcare Team

Your clinical rotation is a time for you to demonstrate how much you've learned and what you can do. However, it is also a time to show that you can be a successful member of a team.

Health care is all about teamwork. For example, an emergency medical technician takes critical vital signs and medical history before handing that information off to the doctor. The doctor makes evaluations based on this information and then orders lab work, x-rays, and medications—all of these are accomplished by other team members. Every link in the chain is important. Whether you are on the front line or in the front office, your work is critically important to the members of the team providing direct care. By sending the proper referrals and instructions to the lab, you enable lab personnel to perform necessary tests. In addition, you can protect a patient's safety by informing the pharmacy of any allergies the patient may have to certain drugs. By keeping patient records organized and up to date, you help ensure that the healthcare facility is providing the best care. Therefore, remember that you should not only excel in your own work; being a reliable team member is valuable as well.

Professional Limits

Just as professionalism involves being a team player, knowing the limits of your expertise and authority makes you a trustworthy and professional healthcare provider.

Verification

There probably will be times when you think you know how to perform a certain task, but you're not completely sure. You may feel reluctant to ask for verification—you might think it makes you look less knowledgeable. You may be tempted to go with a hunch.

Never ever proceed without being certain. If you have any questions about what you should do, ask someone who knows. Don't run the risk of making a mistake with a patient's records, medication, tests, or other procedures. Instead, get the help you need and then carry out the task.

Know Your Limits

What if your supervisor or another staff person asks you to do something you haven't yet been trained to do? You might be very reluctant to admit that you don't know how to do the task. However, this is a situation where you *must* say so. Remember, your clinical rotation is a learning experience. Everyone expects you to need guidance and training. No one expects you to know it all. It is critical that you stay within the bounds of your knowledge and skills.

In addition, letting your supervisor and coworkers know that you are aware of your capabilities and limitations is vital to keeping the team running properly. Your team will trust you more if they know that you never attempt to do anything unless you're sure you know how to do it.

Confidentiality

Maintaining patient confidentiality is both an ethical and legal obligation that is just as important for students on clinical rotation as for all HCPs. Only certain individuals can lawfully receive verbal, written, or electronic patient information. Those who need to know patient information include the patient's healthcare providers and those authorized by the patient to have access to that information. Private patient information is *any* information about a patient, including things, such as:

- health records
- data on billing and payment
- insurance information
- prescriptions

- symptoms and diagnoses
- test results
- personal information unrelated to health care

Keeping Patient Information Private

You might overhear coworkers sharing patient information with each other in a casual way, over lunch, or in the break room. If they encourage you to join in, remember that discussing private patient information is not only unprofessional but also it's illegal. Change the subject or just leave. If you never share information, others will not ask you. This may be difficult, but it's better than getting yourself and your workplace into legal trouble for breaching patient privacy.

The Health Insurance Portability and Accountability Act

The Health Insurance Portability and Accountability Act of 1996, or HIPAA, protects the privacy, confidentiality, and security of all medical records. During your program of study, you will learn about maintaining patient rights under HIPAA. During your clinical orientation, you will also receive information tailored to the healthcare facility where you're working as well as your own job tasks. Failure to comply with HIPAA regulations, whether intentional or unintentional, can result in civil penalties. (See *Patient Privacy Rights.*)

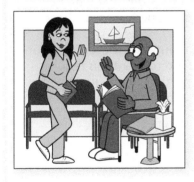

Patient Privacy—Thuy

Thuy was completing her clinical rotation at a major city hospital. Her preceptor and the other members of the healthcare team found her to be skilled and professional. Her next patient had complained of abdominal pain, and Thuy was to perform an ultrasound on his gallbladder. When she entered the waiting area to get the patient, she found that he was a professor in her program. She greeted him smiling warmly and brought him to the examination room. Thuy obtained the images she needed for the patient's diagnosis and he left. Later that day, she thought about how interested the other students would be about her patient, she but never forgot about HIPAA and how critical it was to maintain patient privacy.

Tips for Maintaining Patient Privacy

Follow these safeguards to help you maintain patient privacy:

- Protect your computer password and log off the computer when you're finished with it. Don't run the risk of an unauthorized person walking by and accessing patient information.
- Ensure faxes and computer printouts are not left unattended, especially in areas where curious patients are waiting, like the front desk.

- Dispose of unneeded patient information in designated receptacles before you leave the facility.
- Do not talk about patients in your casual conversations. This means no conversation about a patient even with the patient's visitors or your family and friends.
- Use a quiet voice when giving necessary information to others on the healthcare team, whether on the telephone or in person. A listening patient might spread details to other people.
- Remove patient identifying information before handing in written class work.

Patient Privacy Rights

The goal of HIPAA regulations is to provide safeguards against inappropriate use and release of personal medical information, including all medical records and identifiable health information in any form (electronic, paper, and verbal). HIPAA gives patients the right to:

- give consent before information is released for treatments, payment, or healthcare operations
- be educated about the provider's policy on privacy protection
- access their health records
- request that their health records be amended for accuracy
- access the history of nonroutine disclosures (disclosures that didn't occur in the course of treatment, payment, healthcare operations, or those not specifically authorized by the patient)
- request that the provider restrict the use and routine disclosure of information he or she has (Providers are not required to grant this request, especially if they think the information is important to the quality of patient care, such as disclosing HIV status to another medical treatment provider.)

Patient Rights and Safety

Concern for patients' rights and safety should be an important part of your professional ethics. You will not only protect your workplace from legal action but you'll also be providing the best care to patients. Patients have several rights about which you should be aware.

Collaboration Between the Patient and the Healthcare Professional in Determining Patient Care

Patients are more knowledgeable, assertive, and actively involved in their health care than ever before. They analyze their own symptoms and may question their doctors' diagnoses. Some patients even perform home testing before visiting a healthcare facility. Many patients also demand more information about the risks, alternatives, and benefits associated with the treatment recommended by their HCPs.

As a member of the healthcare team, you need to uphold all patient rights as you carry out your responsibilities. Become familiar with your employer's policy on patient rights. View your patients as partners in the healthcare process and help them get involved in their treatment and care.

Patient's Bill of Rights

The National League for Nursing (NLN) published a patient's bill of rights:

- People have the right to health care that is accessible and that meets professional standards, regardless of where they receive care.
- Patients have the right to courteous and individualized health care that is equitable, humane, and given without discrimination as to race, color, creed, sex, national origin, source of payment, or ethical or political beliefs.
- Patients have the right to information about their diagnosis, prognosis, and treatment, including alternatives to care and risks involved in care, in terms they and their families can easily understand, so they can give informed consent.
- Patients have the legal right to informed participation in all decisions concerning their health care.
- Patients have the right to information about the qualifications, names, and titles of personnel responsible for providing their health care.
- Patients have the right to refuse observation by those not directly involved in their care.
- Patients have the right to privacy during interview, exam, and treatment.
- Patients have the right to privacy in communicating and visiting with persons of their choice.
- Patients have the right to refuse treatments, medications, or participation in research and experimentation, without punitive action being taken against them.
- Patients have the right to coordination and continuity of health care.
- Patients have the right to appropriate instruction or education from healthcare personnel so they can achieve an optimal level of wellness and an understanding of their basic health needs.
- Patients have the right to confidentiality of all records (except as otherwise provided for by law or third-party payer contracts) and all communications, written or oral, between patients and healthcare providers.
- Patients have the right of access to all health records pertaining to them, the right to challenge and to have their records corrected for accuracy, and the right to transfer all such records in the case of continuing care.
- Patients have the right to information on the charges for services, including the right to challenge these.
- Above all, patients have the right to be fully informed as to all their rights in all healthcare settings.

Patient Safety

Patient safety is the responsibility of all members of the healthcare team, including you, whenever and wherever you are in the facility. Safety issues vary according to the type of facility and the capabilities and needs of individual patients. You can, however, take basic steps to reduce each patient's risk.

Trip and Fall Hazards

Falls can be caused by many factors: medication, debris on the floor, or out-of-place equipment. Be vigilant and protective of your patients. Even if you feel that your work area is well out of range for patient falls, remember that patients travel through most parts of a facility. As the unit clerk, for example, you would want to check the waiting area periodically to make sure there are no magazines on the floor, tables too close to chairs, or large potted plants too close to seats; all of these are potential trip-and-fall hazards. As a medical assistant walking down a hallway in a patient treatment area, for example, you would be alert for a wet spot that makes a floor slippery or an electrical cord over which a patient could trip; such conditions should be immediately reported or corrected.

Equipment Safety

You are responsible for making sure that the equipment you have been trained and authorized to use for patient care is free from defects. You're also responsible for using that equipment properly and following instructions in the procedure manual. If you have questions about equipment use, ask your supervisor or instructor.

Prevent Disease Transmission

To reduce the risk of transmitting disease, wash your hands frequently. Proper hand washing (with soap and water or waterless soap) is the single most effective thing you can do to prevent the spread of infection. Follow guidelines for washing or the use of hand sanitizer between patients, wearing gloves at appropriate times, and following other facility policies for preventing disease transmission.

Protect Yourself

While providing safe care for patients, you also must protect yourself. Prevention is the key to keeping yourself safe in the workplace.

Standard Precautions

To protect yourself from infection, you should handle the following as if they contain infectious organisms:

- All blood and other body fluids
- Human tissue
- Mucous membranes
- Broken skin

This means you should follow standard precautions at all times. For example, you must wear gloves for procedures that might expose you to a patient's blood or other body fluids. (See *Infection Control*.) Even if a patient appears healthy, the same precautions always apply.

Infection Control

The Centers for Disease Control and Prevention (CDC) publishes guidelines to provide the widest possible protection against the transmission of infection. CDC officials recommend that healthcare workers handle all blood and other body fluids, tissues, mucous membranes, and broken skin as if they contained infectious agents, regardless of the patient's diagnosis, and to take the following precautions:

- Wash your hands before and after patient care, after removing gloves, or immediately after contamination with blood, body fluids, excretions, secretions, or drainage.

- Wear gloves if you will or might come in contact with blood or other body fluids, specimens, tissues, secretions, excretions, mucous membranes, broken skin, or contaminated objects or surfaces.
- Change gloves and wash your hands between patients. When caring for the same patient, change gloves and wash your hands if you touch anything with a high concentration of microorganisms.
- Wear a fluid-resistant gown, eye protection, and a mask during procedures that are likely to generate droplets of blood or bodily fluids.
- Carefully handle used patient care equipment that's soiled with blood or body fluids; follow facility guidelines for cleaning and disinfecting equipment and environmental surfaces.
- Keep contaminated linens away from your body and place in properly labeled containers.
- Handle needles and sharps carefully, and immediately discard them in a designated disposal unit after use; use sharps with safety features whenever possible.
- Immediately notify your supervisor of a needlestick or sharp instrument injury, mucosal splash, or contamination of nonintact skin with blood or other body fluids to initiate appropriate investigation of the incident and care.
- Use mouthpieces, resuscitation bags, or ventilation devices in place of mouth-to-mouth resuscitation.
- If occupational exposure to blood is likely, you should be vaccinated against hepatitis B.
- Become familiar with your facility's infection control policies and procedures.

Hazardous Exposure

If you are injured by a sharp instrument, or if any of your mucous membranes are contacted by blood or other body fluids, notify your clinical instructor or supervisor immediately. This person will:

- help you with immediate first aid
- fill out an accident report
- ensure that you receive the proper follow-up care

Depending on your duties during your clinical rotation, you may be at risk of occupational exposure to hepatitis B. If so, your school might require you to get the hepatitis B vaccine series.

Preventing Back Injuries

Back injuries are common among healthcare employees. Many patient care facilities and laboratories require you to push, pull, lift, and carry heavy objects or equipment. By using proper body mechanics, you can avoid back injuries:

- Keep a low center of gravity by flexing your hips and knees instead of bending at the waist. This position distributes weight evenly between your upper and lower body and helps maintain balance.
- Create a wide base of support by spreading your feet apart. This tactic provides lateral stability and lowers your body's center of gravity.

- Maintain proper body alignment and keep your body's center of gravity directly over the base of support by moving your feet rather than twisting and bending at the waist.

Handle Chemicals With Care

Many potentially hazardous chemicals are used in healthcare facilities. Certain drugs, powerful cleaning solutions, and disinfectants are common hazards. A material safety data sheet (MSDS) provides you with information about the physical and chemical hazards that can occur from these substances. Each MSDS provides information about the chemicals found in a substance and how to treat exposure to that substance. Every healthcare facility has an MSDS manual. Make sure you know where the manual is located in your facility. Tell your clinical instructor immediately if you are exposed to any potentially hazardous chemical.

Prepare for the First Day of the Rotation

As you look forward to your upcoming clinical rotation, there are several things to become familiar with so you are prepared for your first day including the:

- dress code
- equipment
- mentor
- clinic

Dress Code

Professionalism starts with something that might seem trivial: clothes. You will need to dress appropriately for your clinical experience. You might be thinking that just wearing a uniform ensures you're dressing correctly. Yes, you probably will be wearing a uniform (e.g., scrubs). But there are other important points to keep in mind to make sure you're dressed appropriately:

- Keep your uniform clean. This can be hard to do in a clinical setting, but it's important. A stained or wrinkled uniform tells patients and staff members that you don't take your work seriously.
- Wear your identification badge pinned near your collarbone. Clipping it lower such as near your waist makes it less visible to people who need to see who you are.
- Choose shoes of a style worn by professionals in the facility's department. Don't wear sneakers or clogs unless you know for certain that they're allowed where you'll be working. Never wear sandals or open-toed shoes.

Aside from your uniform, there is another dress factor to keep in mind: Keep it simple. Many people are tempted to wear jewelry, perfume or cologne, or an unusual hairstyle. However, when you're at work, you shouldn't try to stand out with an original look. You should stand out because of your excellent skills and positive attitude. Professionals don't call attention to their looks on the job. They let their skills do the talking.

Some healthcare facilities have stricter guidelines about dress than others. Ask any questions you may have about dress code during your clinical orientation. Your clinical mentor or instructor will give you specific guidelines to follow. If you're ever unsure whether a particular item of clothing or accessory is appropriate, play it safe until you've checked with your instructor.

Equipment

You will be given a list of equipment you'll need for your clinical rotation. Make sure you have all the necessary supplies with you on your first day. You should also bring:

- a notebook
- a pen or pencil
- personal identification (such as a driver's license or student ID)

These additional items will come in handy in case you need to fill out any paperwork on your first day. You may need proof of identification to obtain a parking permit or an identification badge. If you drive to the facility, write down your car's license plate number in your notebook; you might need to register your car with the facility if you park in a garage.

Another helpful piece of equipment is a tablet. A tablet, like many cell phones, also may have functions that can simplify your life, such as a calculator, address book, calendar, to-do list, and memo pad.

As a rule, it's best to leave your cell phone turned off completely during work hours. Professionals do not allow themselves to be distracted by outside calls while on the job, and patients and other healthcare workers will be irritated if you take a call on the job or are even seen checking for messages while working. Use your cell phone only on your personal break time. If you must leave the phone on to receive a call in case of an emergency, such as from your child's school or day care provider, then set it to vibrate rather than ring and keep it in your pocket.

Your Mentor

Your clinical mentor (or preceptor) will coach you through your clinical experience. Do your best to start out on the right foot with your mentor—you just might learn something. Try to avoid making judgments about your mentor based on what you may have heard from other students. Remember that professionals interact with a wide range of other people without being influenced by personal opinions.

Addressing Your Mentor

Remember to be polite and respectful. Address your mentor as Mr., Ms., Dr., or by a first name, according to your mentor's stated preference. It's part of the mutual respect you want in your relationship.

Student–Mentor Relationship

You should have regular conversations with your mentor about what you are learning and doing. He or she will be happy to answer your questions and to see that you are eager to learn. If you believe that you are unable to develop a good relationship with your mentor, make an appointment to discuss your concerns. If you can't resolve the problems together, follow the procedures outlined in your student handbook for resolving problems.

The Facility

Because every healthcare facility is unique in some ways, you should enter your experience there with an open mind, ready to learn. Make an effort from the start to learn how the particular facility does things so you can fit in with the team as soon as possible. Important first steps include the following:

1. Attend your clinical orientation.
2. Work out the logistics before your first day.
3. Know the policies and rules.
4. Have a good attitude.

Clinical Orientation

Clinical orientation usually takes place at the facility where you'll be doing your rotation. It typically includes a welcome from a representative of the facility, followed by information about the facility. In addition to specifics about what you will be doing, you may learn:

- the facility's mission statement
- fire and safety procedures
- confidentiality rules

If you will be working with a computer, your orientation may also include computer training and password assignment.

Your mentor will explain the expectations for your rotation. You will receive a schedule along with any written assignments and due dates. Clinical objectives and evaluation procedures will also be reviewed at this time, so be sure to ask questions if you have them.

Logistics

You will need to consider many small but important details before you begin your clinical experience. Where should you park? Whom do you call if you're sick or will be late? Will your mentor need a way to contact you if you leave the facility for lunch?

Remember to ask these types of questions during orientation. The last thing you want at the end of your first day is to find that your car has been towed or to hear one day that your supervisor did not learn that you had called in sick until the day was half over. You certainly don't want to come back from lunch to find out that everyone has been looking for you.

Policies and Procedures

In health care, it's important to do things by the book. Facilities have policies and procedures for virtually every task, from filing to phlebotomy. These rules help ensure that everyone in the facility does things the same way, preventing errors or confusion about what was done or how it was done.

To prepare for your clinical experience, get a copy of the policy and procedures manual ahead of time so you can study it. When you are on the job, know where the manual is stored and refer to it before trying something new. You must always follow a facility's procedures, even if they are slightly different from what you learned in school.

Sometimes a policy or procedure may seem tedious, yet you must still follow it to the letter every time. One major reason for this is safety. Following procedures means you will be doing things correctly. If a patient develops a problem, you will know that you didn't contribute to it and you can confidently report to your supervisors that you performed your tasks accurately.

Attitude

This should be obvious but sometimes isn't: Just because you are in the facility for clinical rotation or an externship rather than working a "real job" there doesn't mean you shouldn't take it seriously. You are there working, but you're also there to learn. The facility doesn't *have* to invite you in and provide this valuable experience for you. In other words, be aware that as a student in a clinical rotation, you are a guest in the facility. Be sure you act like a good guest, behaving in a way that will lead to your being invited back. Furthermore, many students receive job offers from their rotation site. Consider your clinical rotation to be an extended interview where you want to excel and be valued.

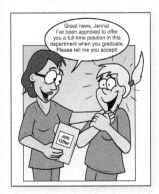

The Job Offer—Jenna

Jenna was completing her clinical rotation as a physical therapist assistant student. It was her last semester, and she was excited to graduate and get a job so that she and her daughter, Maddie, could get a place to live of their own. She had worked very hard at her studies as well as at her internship, always being professional and going the extra mile for her colleagues. One day in April, Jenna's preceptor called her into her office. Jenna's first thought was that she had done something wrong. However, when she went into the office, she found her preceptor with a big smile. "Jenna," her preceptor said, "you have been an outstanding student during this rotation and I have great news. I have been approved to offer you a full-time position in this department when you graduate. Please tell me you accept!"

Chapter Summary

- Because a clinical rotation or externship is a professional experience, practice good personal and professional conduct.
- Protect patients' rights by familiarizing yourself with the Patient's Bill of Rights.
- Guard patient privacy by following HIPAA rules.
- Work to ensure safety for all patients while also protecting yourself.
- Learn about your facility's safety rules by reading the policy and procedures manual.
- Plan for a successful clinical experience. Dress appropriately, bring the right books and supplies, and make sure you arrive on time.

Review Questions

Objective Questions

1. During a clinical rotation, a student must never perform a task that he or she has not yet been trained to do. (True or False?)
2. Private patient information includes _____, _____, and _____.
3. HIPAA protects patient _____.

4. The single most effective way to prevent the spread of infection is _____.
5. Infectious organisms may be found in _____ and _____.
6. MSDS provides information about the chemicals found in a substance and how to treat exposure to that substance. (True or False?)

Short-Answer Questions

1. How can you practice skills in a clinical setting before your rotation begins?
2. Why is it important to know your limits when you're working in health care?
3. Describe a mentor's role in your clinical experience.
4. List key steps to take in preparation for beginning your clinical experience.
5. Describe the importance of teamwork for the activities you will be engaged in during your clinical rotation.

Applications

1. Calm Your Fears: Make a list of any aspects of your upcoming clinical experience that you are concerned about. Then write down questions to ask your instructor that will help you better understand and prepare for these things.
2. Act It Out: Get together with three to five classmates. Each of you should write down the steps of a task or a clinical procedure you will perform during the clinical rotation. Then practice or act out each procedure or task until everyone in the group feels comfortable with the steps and ready for the clinical experience.

14

Succeeding in Your Future as a Healthcare Professional

OBJECTIVES

- Describe the elements of an effective résumé.
- Explain the importance and describe the elements of an effective cover letter.
- Understand the importance of interview preparation.
- Discuss the process of a successful interview.
- Explain the importance and describe the elements of an effective thank you letter.

Ultimately, your hard work in your academic program and training should lead to a satisfying and successful career as a healthcare professional (HCP). By the time you complete your program, you will have sat attentively through the lectures, diligently taking notes; you will have studied those notes and nearly memorized the texts; you will have performed the lab exercises and practicals; you will have taken and passed all of the tests; and you will have completed the required internships or clinical rotations. With all of that done, you will be ready to take that next exciting step to starting your career as an HCP.

The Résumé

There is an old saying: "You don't have a second chance to make a first impression."

This is especially true when considering your résumé. The first impression potential employers have of you will come from your résumé, and it should be the best impression you can possibly make. Simply, the importance of having an effective résumé cannot be overstated.

There are many styles, formats, and layouts that résumés can take. When the time comes, you should consult with the staff of your college's career services office to learn which style or format is most appropriate for your profession. Later in this chapter, you can find a listing of some of the online resources that can help you with résumé layout, in addition to two examples of résumé styles.

However, a good starting point is to list and discuss the main components of a résumé.

Résumé Components

- Your identifying and contact information
- Your résumé summary
- Your educational background
- Your work experience
- Your awards, certifications, and/or licenses

Your Identifying and Contact Information

This is the information at the top of the résumé. This should include your full name, your address, telephone numbers (your cell phone as well as your home phone if you have a land line), and email address.

Your Name

This should be your full legal name. For example, if your complete name is Joseph Albert Pierre, you may use your middle initial and list your name as Joseph A. Pierre. However, if you normally use your full middle name, you should list this as Joseph Albert Pierre. Do not use nicknames or abbreviated versions of your name if these are not part of your legal name. Your friends or family may call you "Joe" or "Al" or "Bert," but these would be inappropriate for identifying yourself at the top of your résumé. On the same line and immediately after your name, list any professional degrees, designations, or certifications you have completed. For example, if you have completed your associate's degree and are a surgical technologist, you would list your name as follows: Joseph A. Pierre, A.S., C.S.T.

Your Résumé Summary

Sometimes called a professional summary, or a career summary, this should be a two- to four-phrase statement that summarizes who you are, what you can offer professionally, and why an employer should want to hire you. In the past, the purpose of the résumé summary would have been fulfilled by the résumé objective. However, a résumé objective has become widely regarded as out-of-date and even obsolete. Your résumé summary is an opportunity for you to make your case in your own words in a concise and energetic manner. Below are two examples of résumé summaries—one effective and one ineffective.

An Effective Résumé Summary

Accomplished recent medical assisting graduate with strong, positive experiences in healthcare settings who is eager to provide quality, patient-centered care in a hospital, clinic, or private practice. An effective communicator who can work efficiently as a member of a healthcare team and who values the importance of collaboration between patients and their healthcare providers.

This summary succinctly states the applicant's strengths while emphasizing the motivations that make the applicant a strong candidate in a particular healthcare setting. Note that the description does not contain full sentences with subjects and agreeing verbs. Each of the groups of words, or "sentences," describes the applicant. The use of full sentences can often cause the summary to feel clunky, as we will see in the ineffective example.

An Ineffective Résumé Summary

I'm a recent graduate in medical assisting, and I want to work hard at providing good care to patients in your hospital. I've taken a course in communication skills for healthcare professionals. I know that communication skills are very important when working with coworkers and patients.

This second résumé summary, although clearly sincere in its intent, has a couple of problems. First, the writing, using three sentences that begin with the first person ("I"), feels repetitive and even wordy. Second, the writer has used contractions (e.g., "I'm," "I've"), which are informal constructions and inappropriate for a résumé.

ROLE PLAY	Using the example of an effective summary above, compose a short résumé summary of two to three sentences, describing yourself and what you have to offer as an HCP in your chosen field. Include those qualities that you believe would set you apart from other applicants for the same position. Then, exchange your summary with a partner in class. Read each other's summary and provide feedback that could help your class partner make their summary more effective. What was helpful about the feedback you received?
In-Class Summary Activity	

Your Educational Background

In this section of your résumé, you should provide a listing of your postsecondary experiences. You do not need to include high school information.

You should list these in reverse chronological order, that is, with the most recent at the top and then the next most recent below that, and so on. You should indicate the degree or certificate you earned and your program of study, the full name of the educational institution where you earned the credential, and the city and state in which the institution is located. You should not abbreviate the name of the school. For example, a school such as Bunker Hill Community College should not be identified by its abbreviation, BHCC, but by its full name. You should also include the year of graduation, or, if you are still enrolled as a student, the span of dates from your start to the present, for example, "2018 to present."

Your Work Experience

In this section of your résumé, you should provide your employment history, like your educational background, in reverse chronological order. You should include your job title, the name of the employer—that is, the organization or company—and the city and state. You should include the dates you worked there, including the months as numbers (e.g., "08/2016 to 06/2018"), or, if you still work there, the span of dates from your start to the present, for example, "10/2018 to present." You should not include the day you started or ended.

You should follow this information with a short list of concise bulleted descriptions of your responsibilities. You should write these using verbs in the past tense, but you do not need to include the first person pronoun "I." For example, in a résumé used to apply for a position as a dental assistant, a few of the items an applicant could list include the following:

- Prepared treatment room following prescribed procedures and protocols
- Prepared patients after escorting them to treatment room by seating and draping them
- Interviewed patients about current medications, diet, and recent dental history

Some pieces of information you should *not* include on your résumé include:

- your salary
- your supervisor's name
- your reason for leaving a position

Your Awards, Affiliations, Certifications, and/or Licenses

In this section, you should include any awards or honors you have received. Awards, scholarships, and other honors, such as being named to the Dean's List, are appropriate and reflect positively on your academic performance. You should also include any academic or extracurricular affiliations you have, such as membership in any of your school's clubs or societies that are relevant to your program of study. These, for instance, could include such organizations as the Medical Assistants Club, the Physical Therapist Assistants Society, or the Radiology Technologists Association.

You should also include any certifications or licenses you have already completed, such as certification in cardiopulmonary resuscitation (CPR) or phlebotomy. If you have completed a course and taken a certifying or licensing examination, but you have not yet learned the results of that examination, you should indicate that the results are pending.

Creating Your Résumé

Many colleges require students to create a résumé as part of their academic program's capstone or internship seminar. In such cases, students receive direct guidance from the instructor about résumé construction. Some schools have no such capstone or internship requirement, and do not require students to create a résumé before graduation.

In any case, your institution should have a career placement office where you can receive expert guidance and advice in putting together a strong résumé. Online resources also exist, although they frequently require a fee.

Among the best such websites are:

QuintCareers: https://www.quintcareers.com
My Perfect Resume: https://www.myperfectresume.com
CareerOneStop: http://www.careeronestop.org/JobSearch/Resumes/ResumeGuide
    /Introduction.aspx

Résumé Formats

Although there exist many different formats for résumés, two formats stand out as the most widely used: the functional résumé and the chronological résumé.

The functional résumé—this résumé emphasizes the skills and accomplishments of the applicant over the complete employment history. This format is most effective for jobseekers who have limited or little employment history—that is, those who are still students or recent graduates—or those who have professions in which the focus of the general skill set may not change very much over the course of a career (e.g., teaching or health care). This résumé includes only those periods of employment that are most relevant to the job sought. One possible drawback of this format is that prospective employers may believe that the emphasis on skills over employment history is an attempt by the applicant to conceal employment gaps or a history of job hopping. See an example of a functional résumé in Figure 14-1.

Amalia A. Torres

123 Main Street, Dorchester, MA 02121 • (508) 123-4567 • amalia.aa.torres@gmail.com

Professional Summary

Accomplished medical assisting student (anticipated 2020 graduate) with strong, positive experiences in laboratory and healthcare settings who is eager to provide quality, patient-centered care in a hospital, clinic, or private practice. An effective communicator who can work efficiently as a member of a healthcare team and who values the importance of collaboration between patients and their healthcare providers.

Skills

- Physical assessment
- Clinical judgment
- Interviewing skills
- Patient-centered care
- Electronic health record documentation
- Microsoft Word, Excel, PowerPoint

Work History

Medical Assistant Internship, 1/2020 to present
Dorchester Medical Associates – Dorchester, MA

- Updated patients' electronic health records, AthenaCare.
- Managed communications from patient messages to healthcare staff.
- Assisted medical assistants with escorting patients to examination rooms and logging vitals.
- Transported patient pathology samples to clinic laboratory.

Lab Assistant, 09/2018 to 12/2019
Bay City Community College – Boston, MA

- Cleaned and maintained lab equipment.
- Assisted faculty during lab practicals.
- Prepared lab kits and slides.
- Ordered supplies.

Education

Associate of Applied Science: Medical Assistant, anticipated 2020
Bay City Community College – Boston, MA

Honors, Affiliations, and Certifications

Dean's List, Fall 2018
Medical Assistants Society, 2018 to 2019
CPR Certification, June 2017

FIGURE 14-1 Example of a functional résumé.

The chronological résumé—this résumé emphasizes the entire employment history of the applicant. This format allows prospective employers to see the applicant's steady growth and development over the course of their employment history. See an example of a chronological résumé in Figure 14-2.

A Few Words to the Wise About Résumé Editing and Accuracy

Editing Your Résumé for Spelling, Grammar, and Punctuation

Simply put, your résumé must be letter-perfect. That is, there can be no misspelling, grammar, or punctuation errors. One misspelled name or one misplaced comma

Amalia A. Torres

123 Main Street, Dorchester, MA 02121 • (508) 123-4567 • amalia.aa.torres@gmail.com

Professional Summary

Accomplished medical assisting student (anticipated 2020 graduate) with strong, positive experiences in laboratory and healthcare settings who is eager to provide quality, patient-centered care in a hospital, clinic, or private practice. An effective communicator who can work efficiently as a member of a healthcare team and who values the importance of collaboration between patients and their healthcare providers.

Skills

- Physical assessment
- Clinical judgment
- Interviewing skills
- Patient-centered care
- Electronic health record documentation
- Microsoft Word, Excel, PowerPoint

Work History

Medical Assistant Internship, 1/2020 to present
Dorchester Medical Associates – Dorchester, MA

- Updated patients' electronic health records, AthenaCare.
- Managed communications from patient messages to healthcare staff.
- Assisted medical assistants with escorting patients to examination rooms and logging vitals.
- Transported patient pathology samples to clinic laboratory.

Lab Assistant, 09/2018 to 12/2019
Bay City Community College – Boston, MA

- Cleaned and maintained lab equipment.
- Assisted faculty during lab practicals.
- Prepared lab kits and slides.
- Ordered supplies.

Cashier, 09/2017 to 08/2018
Pathway Grocery – Dorchester, MA

- Checked customers out with their purchases.
- Maintained a clean storefront.
- Assisted shift manager with making change for cashiers.

Education

Associate of Applied Science: Medical Assistant, anticipated 2020
Bay City Community College – Boston, MA

Honors, Affiliations, and Certifications

Dean's List, Fall 2018
Medical Assistants Society, 2018 to 2019
CPR Certification, June 2017

FIGURE 14-2 Example of a chronological résumé.

can be enough for a hiring manager to reject a résumé. Employers want to hire people who are detail oriented and thorough, not people who are careless and sloppy. Remember the old saying from earlier in this chapter: "You don't get a second chance to make a first impression." If the first impression a recruiter or hiring manager has of you is that you really do not care about getting things right, down to the smallest detail, that's all that person needs to know about you—you are not the right person for the job.

Be sure to use a font and size that are easy to read and professional in appearance—the best choices are Times New Roman, Arial, and Cambria, size 12 font.

Proofread your résumé carefully and then ask a trusted friend to proofread your résumé. Once they have finished with it, proofread your résumé again!

Editing Your Résumé for Accuracy and Honesty

All dates and names in your résumé must be completely accurate.

You must also ensure that you are honest in your representation of your work history and skills. It would be wrong—and even potentially harmful to others and yourself—to embellish your skills or qualifications or the responsibilities you have undertaken in any part of your employment history. First, such dishonesty can lead to situations in which patients and others receive substandard care. Second, such unethical behavior can lead to immediate dismissal as well as possible legal liability.

Be honest. That is all that needs to be said.

Writing Your Cover Letter

The cover letter is the document you use to introduce yourself and your résumé. Your cover letter should get the attention of the hiring manager and make them want to learn more about you by reading your résumé. Your cover letter must be concise, interesting, and truthful. It should not simply be a letter version of the same information contained in your résumé. Also, you should never send just your résumé without a cover letter. Hiring managers in many industries consider an application that contains a résumé but no cover letter to be unprofessional. Finally, you should customize every cover letter for every specific job to which you apply.

In addition to your personal information at the top—which should be identical to that at the top of your résumé—a good cover letter should contain the following:

- **A personalized greeting**—you should do the necessary research to find the name and title of the hiring manager. A cover letter that begins "To Whom It May Concern" or "Dear Hiring Manager" will not be nearly as effective as one that begins with the hiring manager's name. The greeting should also be professional, using the appropriate title and last name, for example, "Dear Dr. Smith" or Dear Ms. Thomas." Do not try to be familiar or funny in the greeting. "Hey Danny" or "Hi Tina" are greetings likely to lead to an application's rejection.
- **A strong first paragraph**—this paragraph should include the exact title of the job for which you are applying, the name of the organization, and a couple of sentences about why you are interested in this *particular* job at this *particular* healthcare organization. Look again at the job listing, and be sure to use the exact same key words used in the listing. Show the hiring manager that you have researched the job and the organization and then indicate that your qualifications match those that the hiring manager wants in a new employee. A final word about the first sentence in this and all other business letters: *Do not begin by stating your name.* A first paragraph that begins "My name is Jeff Mason" can appear unprofessional. Remember, your name appears at the bottom of the letter—where it should appear—below the word "Sincerely."
- **A knockout second paragraph**—this paragraph should build on the indication in the first paragraph that your skills and qualifications are a great match for those required for this job. Read the job listing again, and use many of the exact words the employer used in the job description. For instance, if the listing indicates that the job requires familiarity with a certain electronic health record platform, say, athenahealth, and you have used and are familiar with this platform, say so explicitly in your cover letter. If the job listing indicates that the successful candidate will be a certified phlebotomist, and you are certified in phlebotomy, say so explicitly in your letter.

- This second paragraph is your opportunity to explain just what skills and qualifications you bring to this job. Take that opportunity. Again, though, just as with the résumé, do not embellish or exaggerate. Be honest.
- **A successful third and closing paragraph**—this paragraph should encourage the hiring manager to take the next step on your application, that is, invite you to an interview. This paragraph should be a bit shorter than the second paragraph. You should thank the hiring manager for taking the time read your materials. You should indicate your eagerness to meet with the hiring manager to further discuss your qualifications and how you can contribute in meaningful ways to the hiring healthcare organization. You should say that you look forward to hearing back from the hiring manager. See an example of a cover letter in Figure 14-3.

Amalia A. Torres

123 Main Street, Dorchester, MA 02121 • (508) 123-4567 • amalia.aa.torres@gmail.com

April 3, 2020

Nancy Johnson, RN
Nurse Manager
Women's Health Clinic
Danielson Medical Associates
567 Healthcare Way
Dorchester, MA 02121

Dear Ms. Johnson:

I am writing in response to your job listing on indeed.com for a medical assistant in Women's Health at Danielson Medical Associates. I am especially interested in the field of women's health, and I believe that I can use my experience and qualifications to contribute as a member of Danielson's patient-centered healthcare team.

My experience during my internship at Dorchester Medical Associates has allowed me to develop my skills in the taking of vitals, communicating with patients, and keeping electronic health records. I am very proficient with AthenaCare, the EHR system used by Danielson Medical Associates. Finally, Dorchester Medical Associates fosters collaborative relationships between patients and caregivers, much as Danielson Medical Associates does.

Thank you so much for considering my application materials. I look forward to an opportunity to meet with you so that we may discuss the new Medical Assistant position in Woman's Health at Danielson Medical Associates.

Sincerely,

Amalia A. Torres

Amalia A. Torres

FIGURE 14-3 Example of a cover letter.

Getting the Interview

Successful job interviews are the result of thorough preparation. Before arriving to the interview, you will want to ensure that you have completed the following tasks:

- Researching the job and the hiring organization
- Creating and completing a checklist of steps to prepare for the interview
- Practicing for the interview

Researching the Job and the Hiring Organization

You will want to be as familiar as possible with the responsibilities of the prospective job as well as the organization where you hope to work. Research the organization's website, reading each page carefully. Find the mission of the organization and try to understand how your role as an HCP in that organization supports the mission—that is, how someone in the job you are applying for contributes to making the organization better at serving patient's needs.

Try to learn about the history of the organization and any plans for expansion or change that are in the future. How does the department you are applying to fit into the larger organization? Finally, look to see what others in the healthcare community have to say about this organization. Can this information help you to achieve a "big picture" idea of how this organization functions in the larger community?

Your Interview Checklist

One week before the interview, you want to ensure that the following are prepared:

- **Your references**—you will want to make sure that you have three good references. Confirm with each that they will give you a positive reference. Have a printed copy of all three names with accurate titles and contact information.
- **Your résumé and other documents**—have several extra copies of your résumé printed on good quality paper. Have any necessary copies of official transcripts and/or certifications.

Three days before the interview, you want to ensure that the following are prepared:

- **The clothes you will wear to the interview**—does anything need to be ironed or dry cleaned? You want your appearance to be professional. Be prepared.
- **The folder or case in which you will carry your documents**—this should appear professional.
- **Paper on which to take notes**—you should have a clean tablet on which to write important information. Bring two pens: blue or black.

The day before the interview, you want to ensure that the following are prepared:

- **The exact location of the interview site**—do not assume you can figure this out the morning of the interview. Use Google Maps to find out where it is and how you will get there. Plan the route, whether you are taking public transportation or driving.
- **Parking and traffic**—if you are driving, do you know where available parking is? Have you accounted for rush hour traffic?

The day of the interview, you want to ensure that you do the following:

- **Eat at a time relative to the interview that will help you feel most comfortable**—you do not want to be hungry during the interview, but you also do not want to feel overfed. Eat at a time that you know will bring you to peak performance at the interview's start.
- **Have plenty of time to dress**—ensure that you look professional when you leave for the interview. This should not be something you rush.

Practicing for Your Interview

With a friend or family member, practice the interview at least 3 days before the actual date. Allow the practice interviewer to ask the questions in any order. Encourage them to try to think of follow-up questions to the answers you give and then answer those questions. Try to be completely familiar with the information you are providing during this important give-and-take. Ask the practice interviewer for feedback. Which answers could you improve on? Practice those again.

Possible Interview Questions

Although it is impossible to anticipate every possible interview question, you should come up with a list of those questions you believe you will likely be asked. Below is a list of possible questions an HCP could expect to receive during an interview. Are there any you can add?

Why do you believe you are qualified for this position?

- Your answer to this should be exclusively about your professional life. Your answer should be a brief but positive summary of your work or internship experience that is relevant to this position.
- Provide examples from past experience. Describe the importance these examples have for you and what you learned from them. How did you relate to them professionally?
- Try to emphasize how these experiences may be relevant to the job you are applying for.

Why did you leave your last job?

- Although this question is about your past, remember that you are in the interview to talk about your future. Do not let past experiences bog you down.
- Remain positive when describing your past employers or coworkers. Speaking negatively about them will only make you seem negative.

How well do you work under pressure?

- Be prepared for this question and have an answer ready. Provide an example of how you worked well under pressure in the past.
- Remember that the example you provide should demonstrate a positive attitude and that you are able to solve problems.

Why do you want to work here?

- You should learn as much as possible about the hiring organization before the interview.
- A hiring manager would want to hear how you see yourself contributing in positive ways in an environment you have taken the time to learn something about.

How would your coworkers describe you?

- This is an opportunity for you to describe your ability to work well as a member of a team.
- Explain how your communication skills have enhanced coworker relationships as well as the performance of the healthcare team.
- Remember, though, that hiring managers check references. They may ask this very same question to your former or current supervisor or coworker. You want the answers to be consistent. For this to happen, you must be honest.

What do you think are your strengths?

- When answering this question, be as specific as possible. Provide examples.
- As much as possible, try to ensure that the strengths you are describing are relevant to the job you are applying for.
- As with other answers you give, you will want this one to be consistent with those given by former supervisors and coworkers. Be honest.

What do you think are your weaknesses?

- Be prepared with an answer describing a weakness that is not essential to the job you are applying for.
- Be specific and provide an example.
- Since this answer is about your weaknesses, do not linger too long. After all, you are in the interview to discuss why you should be hired, not why you should not be hired. Again, be honest.

Where do you see yourself in 5 years?

- Hiring managers and recruiters expect and want you to have goals for the future, so describing these is good.
- Be sure, though, to explain how the job you are interviewing for plays a central role in those plans. This new job should not be simply a transition or stepping stone or something just to hold you over till a better opportunity comes along.
- Explain how the job you are interviewing for is part of your plans. Be as specific as possible.

Are you happy with your career choice?

- The first word in your answer to this should of course be "yes."
- Explain in some detail why you have decided to become an HCP.
- Have examples ready of those job aspects that you find most satisfying. Explain why you like them.

Tell me something about your internships/clinical rotations.

- Be prepared with specific details about where and when you completed your internships or clinical rotations.
- Explain what you learned at these sites. Be specific. The hiring manager will be interested in hearing not only about how well you worked with patients but also how well you worked as a member of a healthcare team. Be positive.

Tell me about a time when you had to work with someone culturally, racially, or ethnically different from you and any challenge that may have created. How did you deal with it?

- Be genuine when answering, and provide details of your experiences.
- Describe your commitment to serving an increasingly diverse patient population.
- Explain the importance of inclusiveness when working as a member of a team.

Tell me about the responsibilities in your last internship. Were there any you disliked?

- You should have a list of several specific job responsibilities that you performed.
- Explain what was satisfying about performing these responsibilities. Provide examples.
- When describing any responsibilities you did not like, be honest without sounding negative. Do not linger too long while describing what you did not like.

Tell me about a challenging patient with whom you worked.

- Be specific about the case, but remember that you cannot divulge any confidential patient information. Remember HIPAA. Do not use the patient's name or any identifying information.
- Be prepared for this question with an example ready. Use this as an opportunity to showcase your problem-solving skills. The patient was difficult, and you can explain why, but you should also be able to explain how you helped bring about a positive outcome. You do not want to describe a situation in which you failed. Be honest.

Do you have any questions for me?

- Your first word in response to this should be "yes."
- You should have prepared three or four specific questions before the interview. This will demonstrate professionalism and preparedness.
- These questions should make clear that you have researched the hiring organization before the interview. Answers to these questions should not be plainly available on the organization's website.
- These questions should demonstrate that you are interested in learning how the hiring manager sees you fitting in to the organization.

Your Thank You Letter (Email)

Do not wait to send this! Within a day of the interview—if not on the same day—you should send a note by email thanking the interviewer for taking the time to meet with you. The absence of a thank you letter can often be the reason a hiring manager decides against a particular candidate. A prompt letter shows courtesy and professionalism. After addressing the interviewer in the exact same manner as that used in the cover letter (e.g., Dear Dr. Smith, Dear Ms. Thomas), a thank you letter should contain the following:

- **The first paragraph**—this paragraph should have, at most, three sentences. The paragraph should begin with a sincere statement of thanks for the interview. You should follow this with a sentence expressing interest in the job. Conclude the paragraph by saying you believe the job will be exciting and interesting and include a reason why you think so.
- **The second paragraph**—this paragraph should emphasize again how your skills and qualifications make you a good fit for the job. You should provide at least one specific example of this. You should also use this paragraph to follow up on or clarify any questions from the interview.
- **The third paragraph**—this paragraph should explain that you are available to provide any additional information. Conclude the paragraph by saying you look forward to hearing from the hiring manager about the position. See an example of a thank you letter (email) in Figure 14-4.

To: Nancy Johnson

From: Amalia Torres

Re: Thanks for the interview

Dear Ms. Johnson:

Thank you so much for meeting me this morning to discuss the Medical Assistant opening in the Women's Health Clinic at Danielson Medical Associates. I am very interested in the position, and I believe working as a member of the Danielson team would be exciting, challenging, and fulfilling.

My clinical and administrative skills would serve me well in helping to bring the highest possible patient-centered care to the Danielson clients. I was especially pleased to learn that Danielson Medical Associates uses the AthenaCare electronic health record system. My experience using this system means I can quickly contribute to the clinic in meaningful ways.

If you have any questions or need any more information, please feel free to contact me. I look forward to hearing from you soon.

Sincerely,

Amalia A. Torres

FIGURE 14-4 Example of a thank you letter (email).

Review Questions

Objective Questions

1. There is only one format for a résumé that is appropriate for healthcare professionals. (True or False?)
2. A functional résumé is the kind of résumé an applicant should use when wanting to emphasize particular qualifications or skills. (True or False?)
3. A résumé summary is a short paragraph that a recruiter can read and save valuable time instead of reading the whole résumé. (True or False?)
4. A good cover letter is not just the applicant's résumé in letter form. (True or False?)
5. It is a good idea to be as informal as possible in a cover letter in order to put the hiring manager at ease. (True or False?)
6. If you have a strong résumé, you do not need to send a cover letter. (True or False?)
7. You should always assume that the interviewer will provide you with paper and pen to take notes during the interview. (True or False?)
8. The interview is a good place to first learn about the organization to which you are applying. (True or False?)
9. If you were fired from your last job, you should lie to the interviewer and say you quit. (True or False?)
10. Even if you say thank you and shake hands at the end of the interview, you should still send a thank you note. (True or False?)

Short-Answer Questions

1. What is the purpose of a cover letter?
2. List three possible questions an interviewer might ask you about your *specific* field of study?
3. Describe at least three elements of a résumé.
4. Explain what the purpose of a thank you letter is.

Applications

1. Write a cover letter that would be appropriate for a job in your area of study. Use the cover letter to sell yourself to a prospective employer. Then, with a classmate who has also written a cover letter, exchange the letters and provide feedback. Your feedback should address writing issues, such as grammar, punctuation, and spelling, as well as the effectiveness of the letter in selling the applicant.
2. Using the resources available through your college's career services office, find three employment opportunities that would be appropriate to a graduate in your field of study. What were the key words you used to conduct the search? Ask a representative from Career Services if there are other search terms you could have used? When you use these new terms, do you find other opportunities besides those you found the first time?

15

The Professionalism of the Healthcare Professional

OBJECTIVES

- Explain the importance of professionalism.
- Describe the characteristics of professional spoken and written communication.
- Describe the importance of professionalism in academic behaviors.
- Explain the importance of professionalism in interpersonal relationships.
- Describe the characteristics of professional dress.

You should know by now that as a future healthcare professional (HCP) you will be expected to demonstrate a high level of professionalism in every facet of your work. You should also know that as a health professions student you are already expected to exhibit those skills and behaviors that indicate your professionalism.

Those skills and behaviors—qualities that are essential to your success as a student now and as an HCP in the future—include aspects of communication, academic performance, interpersonal relationships, and appearance. These qualities usually do not stand alone but rather exist in concert with one another. What's more, they are often considered by many observers to be indicators of a person's character or personality. Most important of all, though, is that to become better at functioning at these higher levels of professionalism, one must often be prepared to grow personally as well as professionally. An allied health professional who exhibits any one of these skills tends to exhibit the others as well.

Spoken and Written Communication

Use Standard English and Not Slang

As a health professions student, you should always use standard English when speaking with a professor or, during clinical rotations, a patient. These people expect a high level of professionalism when interacting with you, and your use of standard English is one indication of your professionalism. Slang is not standard English and is used to communicate a common bond or commonality between members of a community or group, whose members may identify by age, gender, race, ethnicity, or other possible traits. Remember not to use slang when speaking with either a professor or a patient. This is also true for expletives, or, as they are more commonly called, curse words.

Grammar and Pronunciation

Be sure that you speak in grammatically correct sentences. Incorrect grammar can impede the clarity of the message you want to send and, just as important, can diminish the confidence the listener has that you know what you are talking about. The same holds true for pronunciation. Each setting in which human interaction takes place has agreed on pronunciations for commonly used words, and it is important that the speaker remain mindful of the setting and use appropriate pronunciation. In a healthcare setting, standard English language pronunciation is appropriate. Correct pronunciation enhances understanding and rapport between the speaker and listener. Incorrect pronunciation inhibits understanding and can cause mistrust.

Talk to Other People, Not at Them, and Be a Good Listener

Making sure that you talk *to* other people and not *at* them is a way of showing respect for them and their concerns. This involves providing some nonverbal cues as well, such as facing them directly and making appropriate eye contact, letting them know that when they speak you are listening carefully. Always try to let others finish speaking and never interrupt. Your attentiveness indicates that you value what the other person is saying to you, that you are trying to understand them, and that you have genuine concern for what they are telling you.

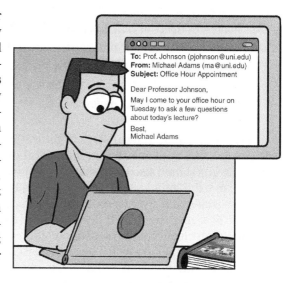

Email

Email is an almost instantaneous and essentially cost-free method of transmitting written information. It is faster and more spontaneous than a letter sent by the U.S. Postal Service; however, email is permanent like a posted letter. This may be of concern when there is a disagreement between the individuals involved.

Email messages are most effective when they are short and to the point. However, it is important to be mindful that these messages can seem very cold. When emailing a professor or school official, you should try to be as clear as possible, using correct grammar and vocabulary and avoiding slang. In emails to a patient, you must make an effort to compose a message that appears warm and caring.

Email may also be used to send longer documents as attachments. Be sure to open the document before sending the email to confirm that the correct document is attached.

Guidelines for the effective use of email in an educational or healthcare setting include the following:

- Check your school email account every day, and respond to messages within 24 hours.
- Use the subject line to inform the recipient about the content of the email—all too often students sending important email messages to professors forget this important part.

- Prepare an email with a message and a format that is appropriate for the intended recipient. Emails to professors, supervisors, or individuals with whom you are not acquainted may require a higher degree of formality than emails sent to friends or other students with whom you have a more casual relationship. Include a greeting such as Dear Dr. Roberts. Use complete sentences with correct capitalization. Check the spelling. Finally, sign the message and provide your contact information.
- Do not use all capital, or uppercase, letters. This may be interpreted as shouting.
- Avoid sending confidential messages via email without prior agreement by both the sender and the receiver.

Academic Professional Behaviors

While we have covered most of these areas earlier in the text, a few points deserve to be repeated in the context of professionalism.

Attendance

Attend every class. It's that simple. If you miss class, you miss the opportunity to understand the material covered firsthand, and you miss the opportunity to ask questions about something you might not understand. Furthermore, professors notice which students always attend and which students frequently do not attend class. If you miss class often and then show up at the professor's office hour asking for the material you've missed, the professor is likely to tell you that office hours are *not* intended to reteach the class to students who were absent but to help students who were in class with material for which they were present. Finally, different professors may have different policies on attendance. Some of your professors may have course policies stating that a certain number of absences may adversely affect a student's grade. The policy for any class will be stated on the syllabus. It's your job to know that policy.

Punctuality

Be on time for class—always. Frequent tardiness by a student is an indication that the student does not take the class material very seriously. Again, professors notice who comes on time and who comes late. Also, professors can have strict course policies about tardiness. For instance, it is not uncommon for some professors to have a policy stating that students who arrive late may not enter the class. A professor's tardiness policy will be on the syllabus.

Finally, never arrive late to a scheduled appointment during a professor's office hour, and never arrive late for a clinical rotation shift.

Preparedness

You should always come to class prepared, having completed the assigned reading or homework before the beginning of class. You want to get the most out of the lecture or discussion and having completed the reading will help you do that. Be sure that you have your textbook, your notebook, and pen or pencil.

Be prepared when you arrive for an appointment with your professor during office hour. If you're coming to ask for clarification on an assignment, be sure that you have read the assignment's instructions carefully before the appointment.

Deadlines

Meet all deadlines. Turn in every assignment on time. Again, different professors may have different policies regarding late assignments. Some may deduct points from the assignment's overall score, and some may not accept late assignments at all. It's your job to know each professor's policy. Of course, the best alternative for you is to turn in every assignment on time.

Presentation of Work

Your work should always be professional in appearance: in the correct format (see *APA Style, an Explanation and an Overview* in Chapter 10); typed; and free of grammar, punctuation, and spelling errors. If the professor has a specific policy around the submission of assignments by email or through the college's learning management system (LMS), you should know and follow that policy. Some professors want assignments to be turned in only electronically, and some professors require written assignments to be turned in *only* during class time and on paper. Make sure you know what the policy is for every one of your courses.

Cell Phones and Laptops

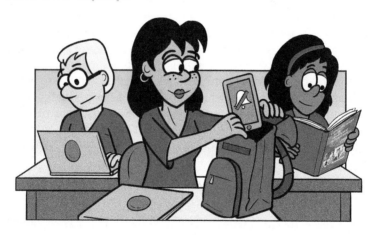

Cell Phones

It can seem that cell phones are everywhere and that everyone has one. According to the Pew Research Center in 2019, more than 5 billion people on earth have cell phones, and over half of those are smart phones. In the United States, 94% of people have cell phones, and 81% have smart phones. Despite their seeming ubiquity, one place cell phones frequently do not belong is in the classroom. It is your job to know the classroom policy on cell phones, as stated on the syllabus, for each of your courses. Generally speaking, though, unless your professor has asked you to bring your cell phone for a student-centered class activity—such as clicker voting with the use of an online program like ClassFlow—you should assume that your cell phone must remain out of sight and out of reach during class. You should not text during class, and you should make sure that your phone's ring setting is on silent.

Laptops

Again, different professors will have different policies regarding the use of laptops during class time. Courses may require students to use certain programs (e.g., Microsoft Excel) during class, and students may be allowed to use laptops for taking notes (see Chapter 6 on note-taking), but you should never use your laptop to do anything other than coursework during class time. You should not be on social media, and you should not be shopping online during class.

Interpersonal Relationships

Courtesy and Respect

In your interactions with others, you should show courtesy. In all situations, large and small, you should show consideration for other people's feelings and needs. You show courtesy when you do such things as making room at a table in the student lounge for another student who has come to join a study group. During a clinical rotation, you show courtesy when you ask a patient if he or she needs anything while waiting in the examination room for the doctor to arrive or by offering to get a blanket for the patient who looks cold while sitting in a wheelchair waiting to be taken down to radiology for x-rays. Showing courtesy is an important part of having good school and workplace manners.

When you show respect for another person, you show that you value that person. When a professor, another student, a patient, or coworker receives respect from you, that person feels that he or she is important to you. If that person is a professor, he or she will be eager to answer questions and provide feedback helpful to your learning the course material. If that person is a fellow student or a coworker, he or she will work more effectively with you. If that person is a patient and feels your respect, the patient will be more compliant and more able to help you provide the best care. You can show respect to others by using both nonverbal and verbal signals. Nonverbally, you can show respect to another person by shaking hands when first meeting, and especially by showing that you are paying attention to them: by maintaining a good posture toward that person when he or she speaks to you, by facing that person, and by making appropriate eye contact. Verbally, you can show respect to faculty and patients by using an appropriate title, such as Professor, Dr., Mr., Ms., or Mrs., and by using their name. You can show respect to another person by giving undivided attention.

Assertiveness Versus Aggressiveness

As a health professions student with professional communication skills, you will need to be assertive in your communication style; that is, you will need to be able to comfortably and confidently express your ideas, opinions, and feelings while still respecting the ideas, opinions, and feelings of others. To be an assertive communicator is to be able to stand up for what you believe is right without any undue anxiety about what others may think of you. It is important, however, not to confuse an assertive communication style with an aggressive communication style. When disagreeing with another student or a coworker, an assertive communicator will use clear and direct language while remaining relaxed and respectful, whereas an aggressive communicator tends to use confrontational and even sarcastic language, while maintaining a tense and often superior attitude. When you use an assertive style, you tell listeners that while you may disagree you remain honest and courteous with them. Their response, in turn, will be to feel respected and valued by you. They will trust you more easily.

Empathy

To show empathy is to show that you understand—to the point of feeling—how another person feels. When showing empathy to peers, coworkers, and patients, you demonstrate the use of some of the important skills discussed so far in this chapter—courtesy and respect—but you also show that you care. Your empathy tells the other person that you are there to fully acknowledge what they are feeling and that, within the appropriate limits, you will try to provide support and care. You show empathy to other students and coworkers by showing that you carefully listen to what they tell you and that you do your best to understand. You show empathy to patients during clinicals by showing them that you are paying attention to everything they attempt to communicate to you.

Genuineness

There is simply no substitute for showing genuineness or being genuine. To be genuine is to be completely open and honest in your words and actions when dealing with others. Friends and loved ones, family members, coworkers, and patients will all know when you are being genuine with them—and they will know when you are not. By being genuine, you let others know that they are getting the real you, that you are not putting on any sort of act or putting up any sort of front. When you are genuine in human interactions, you do not just go through the motions, but you engage fully. Other students and coworkers sense your genuineness when you show that you care about the quality of the work you do and their ability to do theirs. Patients in clinicals sense your genuineness when you show them courtesy, respect, and empathy and you show that you are doing your very best to serve them and their needs.

Respect for Diversity

An important part of being professional is showing respect for the worth and dignity of all individuals. As a future HCP, you should have a high regard for diverse cultures and the people who come from them. This regard is genuine in that it starts from within you and you do everything you can to foster it. From a genuine desire to do so, you actively pursue the development of your own cultural awareness and competence. As a future HCP, you advocate with, and on behalf of, populations who are traditionally underserved, and you recognize that you also have a role to play in eliminating disparities in healthcare availability and treatment to those who are underserved. (See Chapter 4.)

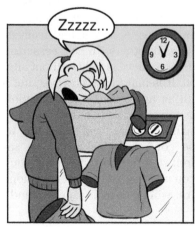 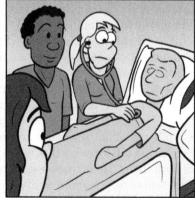

Professional Dress—Jenna

Jenna remembered late last night that the scrubs she needed to wear during today's lab section were dirty. She's happy now that she took the trouble to make sure the scrubs were clean and ready this morning.

Professional Dress

One more important way you can demonstrate your professionalism is by dressing appropriately in every situation. When making a presentation in front of a class filled with students or a meeting room filled with coworkers, you want to wear appropriate clothing. Dress professionally. When going to lab practicals, if scrubs are the required clothing, be sure you are wearing scrubs. Do not wear jewelry that may interfere with the performance of lab or patient care tasks. Dress professionally. If baseball caps are not a part of the expected professional dress code of your school or clinical rotation, do not wear a baseball cap. By dressing appropriately, you demonstrate your professionalism through the respect you show in each respective situation.

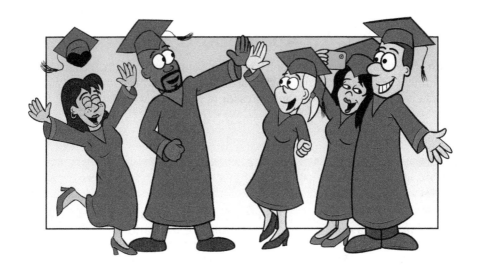

Chapter Summary

- You should recognize that demonstrating your professionalism in school and at work is important.
- You want to be sure your spoken and written communications are professional and appropriate.
- In all your academic endeavors, you want to comport yourself with the highest level of professionalism.
- All your interactions with others should illustrate your professionalism. This includes your interactions with faculty, staff, students, and coworkers.
- You recognize the importance of showing respect for the worth and dignity of everyone.
- You dress appropriately for each academic and professional situation.

Review Questions

Objective Questions

1. The quality you exhibit that tells others that it is the real you they perceive and that you don't just go through the motions but show you really care about what you're doing is called _____.
2. Checking your social media accounts during class lecture is okay as long as the professor doesn't find out. (True or False?)
3. Assertiveness is an important quality to have when dealing with friends only. (True or False?)
4. Checking your college email account regularly isn't really necessary because all of your real friends have your personal email address. (True or False?)

Short-Answer Questions

1. List three characteristics of a professional email.
2. List three characteristics of academic preparedness.

Applications

1. With a partner, evaluate yourself and then your partner with the Professional Readiness Score sheet below. What are some of the ways you could improve? What scores do you believe the professor of this class would give you?

PROFESSIONAL READINESS SCORE SHEET (A PRINTABLE VERSION IS AVAILABLE WITH THIS TEXT'S ONLINE RESOURCES)

Professional Behavior	Meets Expectations	Does Not Meet Expectations	Comments
Spoken and Written Communication			
Spoken communication with faculty, staff, and patients is clear and uses standard English	_____	_____	_____
Demonstrates good listening skills—appropriate eye contact and body language—with faculty, staff, peers, and patients	_____	_____	_____
Communicates professionally in email—messages to faculty, staff, peers, and patients are free of spelling, punctuation, and grammar errors. Word choice is appropriate (no slang).	_____	_____	_____
Responds promptly by email (within 24 hours)	_____	_____	_____

Professional Behavior	Meets Expectations	Does Not Meet Expectations	Comments
Academic Professional Behaviors			
Attends all classes	_____	_____	_____
Arrives on time to all classes	_____	_____	_____
Comes to class prepared	_____	_____	_____
Consistently turns in work on time	_____	_____	_____
Written work is correctly formatted and professional (proofread for errors in grammar, punctuation, and spelling).	_____	_____	_____
Does not allow cell phone to distract during class	_____	_____	_____
Uses a laptop appropriately—for note-taking or class exercises (not for social media, online shopping, etc.)	_____	_____	_____
Personal Interactions			
Demonstrates courtesy and respect in all interactions with faculty, staff, students, and patients	_____	_____	_____
Demonstrates empathy in interactions with others, including peers and patients	_____	_____	_____
Shows genuineness—others perceive that they are getting the "real" person in all interactions	_____	_____	_____
Shows a genuine respect for the worth and dignity of others	_____	_____	_____
Consciously works to develop own cultural competence and advocates for underserved populations	_____	_____	_____
Professional Dress			
Dresses appropriately in all school and work situations (including presentations and labs)	_____	_____	_____
Totals	_____	_____	_____

INDEX

Java™ Security

THE
JAVA™
SERIES

Exploring Java™

Java™ Threads

Java™ Network Programming

Java™ Virtual Machine

Java™ AWT Reference

Java™ Language Reference

Java™ Fundamental Classes Reference

Database Programming with JDBC™ and Java™

Developing Java Beans™

Java™ Distributed Computing

Also from O'Reilly

Java™ in a Nutshell

Java™ in a Nutshell, Deluxe Edition

Java™ Examples in a Nutshell

Netscape IFC in a Nutshell

Java™ Security

Scott Oaks

O'REILLY™

Cambridge · Köln · Paris · Sebastopol · Tokyo

Java™ Security

by Scott Oaks

Copyright © 1998 O'Reilly & Associates, Inc. All rights reserved.
Printed in the United States of America.

Published by O'Reilly & Associates, Inc., 101 Morris Street, Sebastopol, CA 95472.

Editor: Mike Loukides

Production Editor: Jane Ellin

Printing History:

May 1998:	First Edition

This book is printed on acid-free paper with 85% recycled content, 15% post-consumer waste. O'Reilly & Associates is committed to using paper with the highest recycled content available consistent with high quality.

ISBN: 1-56592-403-7

Table of Contents

Preface

When I first mentioned to a colleague of mine that I was writing a book on Java™ security, he immediately starting asking me questions about firewalls and Internet DMZs. Another colleague overheard us and started asking about electronic commerce, which piqued the interest of a third colleague who wanted to hear all about virtual private networks. All this was interesting, but what I really wanted to talk about was how a Java applet could be allowed to read a file.

Such is the danger of anything with the word "security" in its title: security is a broad topic, and everyone has his or her own notion of what security means. Complicating this issue is the fact that Java security and network security (including Internet security) are complementary and sometimes overlapping topics: you can send encrypted data over the network with Java, or you can set up a virtual private network that encrypts all your network traffic and remove the need for encryption within your Java programs.

This is a book about security from the perspective of a Java program. In this book, we discuss the basic platform features of Java that provide security—the class loader, the bytecode verifier, the security manager—and we discuss recent additions to Java that enhance this security model—digital signatures, security providers, and the access controller. The ideas in this book are meant to provide an understanding of the architecture of Java's security model and how that model can be used (both programmatically and administratively).

Who Should Read This Book?

This book is intended primarily for programmers who want to write secure Java applications. Much of the book is focused on various APIs within Java that provide security; we discuss both how those APIs are used by standard Java-enabled browsers and how they can be used in your own Java applications. From a programming perspective, this latter case is the most interesting: Java-enabled browsers have each adopted particular security models, but there's not much a programmer or administrator can do to alter those models. However, this is beginning to change, as technologies like Sun Microsystems' Activator bring Sun's basic security model to popular browsers.

For the end user or system administrator who is interested in Java security, this book will provide knowledge of the facilities provided by the basic Java platform and how those facilities are used by Java-enabled browsers and by Java applications. We do not delve into the specific security features of any Java-enabled browser, although we do point out along the way which security features of Java are subject to change by the companies that provide Java-enabled browsers. Hence, end users and system administrators can read this book (and skip over many of the programming examples) to gain an understanding of the fundamental security features of the Java platform, and they can understand from each of its parts how the security feature might be administrated (especially for Java applications). This is particularly true for end users and administrators who are interested in assessing the risk of using Java: we give full details of the implementation of Java's security model not only so that you can program within that model (and adjust it if necessary), but also so that you have a deep understanding of how it works and can assess for yourself whether or not Java meets your definition of security.

From a programming perspective, we assume that developers who read this book have a good knowledge of how to program in Java, and in particular how to write Java applications. When we discuss advanced security features and cryptographic algorithms, we do so assuming that the programmer is primarily interested in using the API to perform certain tasks. Hence, we explain at a rudimentary level what a digital signature is and how it is created and used, but we do not explain the cryptographic theory behind a digital signature or prove that a digital signature is secure. For developers who are sufficiently versed in these matters, we also show how the APIs may be extended to support new types of cryptographic algorithms, but again we leave the mathematics and rigorous definitions of cryptography for another book.

Versions Used in This Book

Writing a book on Java security has been a challenge for a number of reasons, not the least of which is that the security APIs have been radically changing over the past year. Java 1.1 introduced many of the APIs we'll be discussing in this book, including the notion of a security provider that supplies an implementation of the security package. Java 1.2 introduced significant changes to the security package as well as a new fundamental security object called the "access controller," which takes on much of the responsibility that has resided with the security manager since Java 1.0.

For the most part, we assume that developers using this book will be using Java 1.2, and our primary focus will be on the 1.2 release of the Java Development Kit (JDK) from Sun Microsystems. However, for developers using 1.1, we will provide full details of what's available in 1.1, and what has changed in 1.2; in some cases, this information has changed so radically that the information is relegated to an appendix. The information in this book is based on the 1.2 beta release; there may be slight differences in the 1.2 FCS release.

For the most part, we do not track changes between 1.0 and 1.1 in this book.

Most of the examples used in this book are available via ftp from the O'Reilly web site, *www.oreilly.com*. A few of the examples have been withheld from the online distribution because of U.S. restrictions on the export of cryptography.

Conventions Used in This Book

Constant width font is used for:

- Code examples
- Class, variable, and method names within the text

Italicized font is used for:

- Filenames
- Host and domain names
- URLs

When a new method or class is introduced, its definition will appear beginning with italicized text like this:

public void checkAccess(Thread t)
  Check whether the current thread is allowed to modify the state of the parameter thread.

In addition, one of the following symbols may appear next to a definition:

★   Indicates that the method/class is available only in 1.2.
☆   Indicates that the method/class has been deprecated in 1.2.

There are some examples of commands scattered through the book, especially in sections and appendices that deal with administration. By convention, all examples are shown as they would be executed on a Unix system, e.g.:

```
piccolo% keytool -export -alias sdo -file /tmp/sdo.cer
Enter keystore password:  ******
Certificate stored in file </tmp/sdo.cer>
```

In these examples, the text typed by the user or administrator is always shown in bold font; the remaining text is output from the command (the string `piccolo%` indicates a command prompt). On other systems, the names of the files would have to be changed to conform to that system (e.g., *C:\sdo.cer* for a Windows system). However, note that while Windows systems often use a forward-slash (/) for command-line options, Java tools (even on those systems) universally use a hyphen (-) to indicate command-line options. In these examples, then, only the filenames are different between platforms.

Organization of This Book

This book is organized in a bottom-up fashion: we begin with the very low-level aspects of Java security and then proceed to the more advanced features.

Chapter 1, *Java Application Security*

This chapter gives an overview of the security model (the Java sandbox) used in Java applications and sets the stage for the rest of the book.

Chapter 2, *Java Language Security*

This chapter discusses the memory protections built into the Java language, how those protections provide a measure of security, and how they are enforced by the bytecode verifier.

Chapter 3, *Java Class Loaders*

This chapter discusses the class loader, which is the class that reads in Java class files and turns them into classes. From a security perspective, the class loader is important in determining where classes originated and whether or not they were digitally signed (and if so, by whom), so the topic of class loaders appears throughout this book.

Chapter 4, *The Security Manager Class*

This chapter discusses the security manager, which is the primary interface to application-level security in Java. The security manager is responsible for arbitrating access to all local resources: files, the network, printers, etc.

Chapter 5, *The Access Controller*

The access controller is the basis for security manager implementations in Java 1.2. This chapter discusses how to use the access controller to achieve fine-grained levels of security in your application.

Chapter 6, *Implementing Security Policies*

This chapter ties together the information on the security manager and the access controller and shows how to implement one or both to achieve a desired security policy in your application.

Chapter 7, *Introduction to Cryptography*

This chapter provides an overview to the cryptographic algorithms of the Java security package. It provides a background for the remaining chapters in the book.

Chapter 8, *Security Providers*

This chapter discusses the architecture of the Java security package, and how that architecture may be used to extend or supplant the default cryptographic algorithms that come with the JDK.

Chapter 9, *Message Digests*

This chapter discusses message digests: how to create them, how to use them, and how to implement them.

Chapter 10, *Keys and Certificates*

This chapter discusses the APIs available to model cryptographic keys and certificates, and how those keys and certificates may be electronically transmitted.

Chapter 11, *Key Management*

This chapter discusses how keys can be managed within a Java program: how and where they may be stored and how they can be retrieved and validated.

Chapter 12, *Digital Signatures*

This chapter discusses how to create, use, and implement digital signatures. This chapter also contains a discussion of signed classes.

Chapter 13, *Encryption*

This chapter discusses the Java Cryptography Extension, which allows developers to encrypt and decrypt arbitrary streams of traffic.

Appendix A, *Security Tools*

This appendix discusses the administrative tools that come with Java that enable end users and administrators to work with the Java security model: `keytool`, `jarsigner`, and `policytool`.

Appendix B, *Identity-Based Key Management*

Key management in Java 1.1 was radically different than the systems we explored in the main text. This appendix discusses how key management was handled in Java 1.1; it uses classes that are still present (but not often used) in 1.2.

Appendix C, *Security Resources*

This appendix discusses how to keep up–to–date with information about Java's security implementation, including a discussion of Java security bugs and general resources for further information.

Appendix D, *Quick Reference*

This appendix is a simple reference guide to the classes that are discussed in this book.

Acknowledgments

I am grateful to the many people who have helped me with this book along the way; this book is as much a reflection of their support as anything else. I offer my heartfelt thanks to Mike Loukides for stewarding me through the editorial process.

Various drafts of this book were foisted upon my colleagues Mark Bordas, Charles Francois, David Plotkin, and Henry Wong; I am indebted to each of them for their feedback and support, and to Wendy Talmont for all her support. In addition, I was extremely fortunate to receive technical assistance from a highly talented group of individuals: to Jim Farley, Li Gong, Jon Meyer, Michael Norman, and especially to David Hopwood, I offer my deepest thanks for all your input. Finally, I must thank Roland Schemers for handling my last-minute barrage of questions with patience and insight.

The staff at O'Reilly & Associates was enormously helpful in producing this book, including Jane Ellin, the Production Editor; Robert Romano, who created the figures; Seth Maislin, who wrote the index; Hanna Dyer, the cover designer;

Nancy Priest, the interior designer; Mike Sierra for Tools support; and Claire Cloutier LeBlanc, Nancy Wolfe Kotary, and Sheryl Avruch for quality control.

Finally, I must offer my thanks to James for all his patience and support, and for putting up with my continual state of distraction during phases of this process.

Feedback for the Author

I welcome any comments on the text that you might have; despite the contributions of the people I've just listed, any errors or omissions in the text are my responsibility. Please send notice of these errors or any other feedback to *scott.oaks@sun.com.*

1

Java Application Security

When Java was first released by Sun Microsystems, it attracted the attention of programmers throughout the world. These developers were attracted to Java for different reasons: some were drawn to Java because of its cross-platform capabilities, some because of its ease of programming (especially compared to object-oriented languages like C++), some because of its robustness and memory management, some because of Java's security, and some for still other reasons.

Just as different developers came to Java with different expectations, so too did they bring different expectations as to what was meant by the ubiquitous phrase "Java is secure." Security means different things to different people, and many developers who had certain expectations about the word "security" were surprised to find that their expectations were not necessarily shared by the designers of Java.

This book discusses the features of Java that make it secure. In this book, we'll discuss why Java is said to be secure, what that security means (and doesn't mean), and—most importantly—how to use the security features of the Java platform within your own programs. This last point is actually the focus of this book: while some of Java's security features are automatically a part of all Java programs, many of them are not. In this book, we'll learn about all those features, and how to utilize them in our own Java applications.

What Is Security?

The first thing that we must do to facilitate our discussion of Java security is to discuss just what Java's security goals are. The term "security" is somewhat vague

1

unless it is discussed in some context; different expectations of the term "security" might lead us to expect that Java programs would be:

- *Safe from malevolent programs*: Programs should not be allowed to harm a user's computing environment. This includes Trojan horses as well as harmful programs that can replicate themselves—computer viruses.

- *Non-intrusive*: Programs should be prevented from discovering private information on the host computer or the host computer's network.

- *Authenticated*: The identity of parties involved in the program should be verified.

- *Encrypted*: Data that the program sends and receives should be encrypted.

- *Audited*: Potentially sensitive operations should always be logged.

- *Well-defined*: A well-defined security specification would be followed.

- *Verified*: Rules of operation should be set and verified.

- *Well-behaved*: Programs should be prevented from consuming too many system resources.

- *C2 or B1 certified*: Programs should have certification from the U.S. government that certain security procedures are included.

In fact, while all of these features could be part of a secure system, only the first two were within the province of Java's 1.0 default security model. Other items in the list have been introduced in later versions of Java: authentication was added in 1.1, encryption is available as an extension to 1.2, and auditing can be added to any Java program by providing an auditing security manager. Still others of these items will be added in the future. But the basic premise remains that Java security was originally and fundamentally designed to protect the information on a computer from being accessed or modified (including a modification that would introduce a virus) while still allowing the Java program to run on that computer.

The point driving this notion of security is the new distribution model for Java programs. One of the driving forces behind Java, of course, is its ability to download programs over a network and run those programs on another machine within the context of a Java-enabled browser (or within the context of other Java applications). Coupled with the widespread growth of Internet use—and the public-access nature of the Internet—Java's ability to bring programs to a user on an as-needed, just-in-time basis has been a strong reason for its rapid deployment and acceptance.

The nature of the Internet created a new and largely unprecedented requirement for programs to be free of viruses and Trojan horses. Computer users had always been used to purchasing shrink-wrapped software. Many soon began downloading software via ftp or other means and then running that software on their machines. But widespread downloading also led to a pervasive problem of malevolent attributes both in free and (ironically) in commercial software (a problem which continues unabated). The introduction of Java into this equation had the potential to multiply this problem by orders of magnitude, as computer users now download programs automatically and frequently.

For Java to succeed, it needed to circumvent the virus/trojan horse problems that plagued other models of software distribution. Hence, the early work on Java focused on just that issue: Java programs are considered safe because they cannot install, run, or propagate viruses, and because the program itself cannot perform any action that is harmful to the user's computing environment. And in this context, safety means security. This is not to say that the other issues in the above list are not important—each has its place and its importance (in fact, we'll spend a great deal of time in this book on the third and fourth topics in that list). But the issues of protecting information and preventing viruses were considered most important; hence, features to provide that level of security were the first to be adopted. Like all parts of Java, its security model is evolving (and has evolved through its various releases); many of the notions about security in our list will eventually make their way into Java.

One of the primary goals of this book, then, is to explain Java's security model and its evolution through releases. In the final analysis, whether or not Java is secure is a subjective judgment that individual users will have to make based on their own requirements. If all you want from Java is freedom from viruses, any release of Java should meet your needs. If you need to introduce authentication or encryption into your program, you'll need to use a 1.1 or later release of Java. If you have a requirement that all operations be audited, you'll need to build that auditing into your applications. If you really need conformance with a U.S. government-approved definition of security, Java is not the platform for you. We take a very pragmatic view of security in this book: the issue is not whether a system that lacks a particular feature qualifies as "secure" according to someone's definition of security. The issue is whether Java possesses the features that meet your needs.

When Java security is discussed, the discussion typically centers around Java's applet-based security model—the security model that is embodied by Java-enabled browsers. This model is designed for the Internet. For many users, this is not necessarily the most appropriate model: it is somewhat restrictive, and the security concerns on a private, corporate network are not the same as those on the Internet.

In this book, we take a different tack: the goal of this book is to show how to use the security model and how to write your own secure Java applications. While some of the information we present will be applicable to a browser environment, the security of any particular browser is ultimately up to the provider of the browser. Some browsers allow us to change the security policy the browser uses, but many do not. Hence, reading about the security manager in this book may help you understand how a particular browser works (and why it works that way), but that won't necessarily allow you to change the security model provided by that browser.

The Java Sandbox

Discussions of Java's security model often center around the idea of a sandbox model. The idea behind this model is that when you allow a program to be hosted on your computer, you want to provide an environment where the program can play (i.e., run), but you want to confine the program's play area within certain bounds. You may decide to give the program certain toys to play with (i.e., you may decide to let it have access to certain system resources), but in general, you want to make sure that the program is confined to its sandbox.

This analogy works better when you consider it from the view of a close relative rather than from the view of a parent. If you're a parent, you probably consider the purpose of a sandbox to be to provide a safe environment for your child to play in. When my niece Rachel visits me, however, I consider the purpose of a sandbox not (only) to be to protect her, but also to protect my grandmother's china *from* her. I love my niece, but I can't give her leave to run through my house; I enjoy running the latest cool applet on the Internet, but I can't give it leave to run through my filesystem.

The Java sandbox is responsible for protecting a number of resources, and it does so at a number of levels. Consider the resources of a typical machine as shown in Figure 1-1. The user's machine has access to many things:

- Internally, it has access to its local memory (the computer's RAM).
- Externally, it has access to its filesystem and to other machines on the local network.
- For running applets, it also has access to a web server, which may be on its local (private) net, or may be on the Internet.
- Data flows through this entire model, from the user's machine through the network and (possibly) to disk.

Each of these resources needs to be protected, and those protections form the basis of Java's security model.

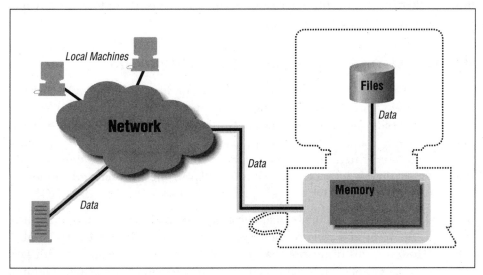

Figure 1-1. A machine has access to many resources

We can imagine a number of different-sized sandboxes in which a Java program might run:

- A sandbox in which the program has access to the CPU, the screen, keyboard, and mouse, and to its own memory. This is the minimal sandbox—it contains just enough resources for a program to run.

- A sandbox in which the program has access to the CPU and its own memory as well as access to the web server from which it was loaded. This is often thought of as the default state for the sandbox.

- A sandbox in which the program has access to the CPU, its memory, its web server, and to a set of program-specific resources (local files, local machines, etc.). A word-processing program, for example, might have access to the *docs* directory on the local filesystem, but not to any other files.

- An open sandbox, in which the program has access to whatever resources the host machine normally has access to.

The sandbox, then, is not a one-size-fits-all model. Expanding the boundaries of the sandbox is always based on the notion of trust: when my one-year-old niece comes to visit, there's very little in the sandbox for her to play with, but when my six-year-old godchild comes to visit, I trust that I might give her more things to play with. In the hands of some visitors, a toy with small removable parts would be dangerous, but when I trust the recipient, it's perfectly reasonable to include that item in the sandbox. And so it is with Java programs: in some cases, I might trust them to access my filesystem; in other cases, I might trust them to access only part of my filesystem; and in still other cases, I might not trust them to access my filesystem at all.

Applications, Applets, and Programs

It's no accident that this chapter has the word "application" in its title, because the Java security model is solely at the discretion of a Java application. When an applet runs inside the HotJava browser, HotJava is the Java application that has determined the security policy for that applet. And although other popular browsers are not written in Java, they play the role of a Java application: it is still the case that the choice of security model is up to the browser and cannot be changed by the applet.

This makes the distinction between applications and applets a crucial one: applications can establish and modify their security policies while applets (generally) cannot. However, this distinction has diminished over time. Beginning with Java 1.2, users of Java applications have the opportunity to run an application within a sandbox that the user or system administrator has constructed. In the next section, we'll see how the same functionality can be achieved with Java 1.1 as well. Under these scenarios, the Java security model for applications is solely at the discretion of the user or system administrator.

This is a major change of perception for many users and developers of Java, who are used to considering the security differences between applets and applications as a significant differentiator between the two types of programs. There will, of course, always be particular programming differences between applets and applications: an applet extends the `java.applet.Applet` class and is written as a series of callbacks, while an application can be any class that has a static method called `main()`. When this programming distinction is important, we'll use the terms "applet" and "application" as appropriate. But we'll typically use the term "program" to refer to the Java code that we're running.

Anatomy of a Java Application

The anatomy of a typical Java application is shown in Figure 1-2. Each of the features of the Java platform that appears in a rectangle plays a role in the development of the Java sandbox. In particular, the elements of the Java sandbox are comprised of:

The bytecode verifier

> The bytecode verifier ensures that Java class files follow the rules of the Java language. In terms of resources, the bytecode verifier helps enforce memory protections for all Java programs. As the figure implies, not all files are subject to bytecode verification.

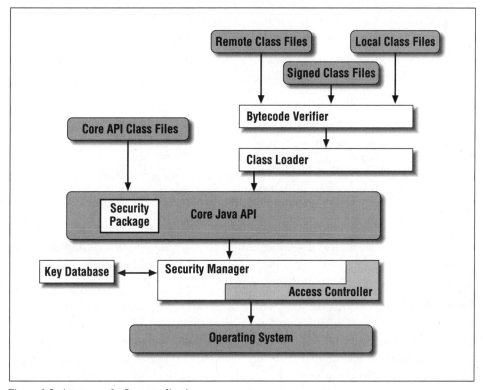

Figure 1-2. Anatomy of a Java application

The class loader

One or more class loaders load classes that are not found on the CLASSPATH. In 1.2, class loaders are responsible for loading classes that are found on the CLASSPATH as well.

The access controller

In Java 1.2, the access controller allows (or prevents) most access from the core API to the operating system.

The security manager

The security manager is the primary interface between the core API and the operating system; it has the ultimate responsibility for allowing or preventing access to all system resources. In 1.2, the security manager uses the access controller for most (but not all) of those decisions; in 1.0 and 1.1, the security manager is solely responsible for those decisions.

The security package

The security package (that is, classes that are in the java.security package) forms the basis for authenticating signed Java classes. Although it is only a small box in this diagram, the security package is a complex API, and discussion of it is broken into several chapters of this book. This includes discussions of:

- The security provider interface—the means by which different security implementations may be plugged into the security package
- Message digests
- Keys and certificates
- Digital signatures
- Encryption (an optional extension to the security package)

The security package was initially available in Java 1.1.

The key database

The key database is a set of keys used by the security manager and access controller to verify the digital signature that accompanies a signed class file. In the Java architecture, it is part of the security package, though it may be manifested as an external file or database.

The last two items in this list have broad applicability beyond expanding the Java sandbox. With respect to the sandbox, digital signatures play an important role, because they provide authentication of who actually provided the Java class. As we'll see, this provides the ability for end users and system administrators to grant very specific privileges to individual classes or signers. But a digital signature might be used for other applications. Let's say that you're deploying a payroll application throughout a large corporation. When an employee sends a request to view his payroll information, you really want to make sure that the request came from that employee rather than from someone else in the corporation. Often, this type of application is secured by a simple password, but a more secure system could require a digitially signed request before it sent out the payroll information.

We'll discuss security concerns in both these contexts in this book. In particular, two different examples will form the theme of the examples that are developed through this book:

- A browser-type program (called JavaRunner) that we'll use to explore the sandbox aspects of Java's security model
- The payroll application of a large company (XYZ Corporation) that we'll use to explore how the features of Java's security model can be used for purposes other than the sandbox (e.g., to sign a payroll request)

We'll develop a full implementation of the first of these examples; while we won't provide a complete payroll application, we will provide a number of examples of the security features required for such an application.

Running a Java Application

The parameters of the Java sandbox that we've outlined are possible elements of a Java application, but they are not required elements of an application. The remainder of this book will show us how and when those elements can be introduced into a Java application. First, however, we're going to discuss the techniques by which Java applications can be run.

There are two techniques that we'll introduce in this section: the JavaRunner technique and the Launcher technique. While both allow you to run an application securely, the examples in this chapter do not provide any security. We'll fill in the security pieces bit by bit, while we flesh out the security story. At that point, we'll show how to run Java applications securely.*

Typically, we're used to running Java applications simply by specifying on the command line the name of a class that contains a main() method. Consider this application that reads the file specified by a command-line argument:

```
public class Cat {
    public static void main(String args[]) {
        try {
            String s;
            FileReader fr = new FileReader(args[0]);
            BufferedReader br = new BufferedReader(fr);
            while ((s = br.readLine()) != null)
                System.out.println(s);
        } catch (Exception e) {
            System.out.println(e);
        }
    }
}
```

This is a regular Java application; if we wanted to run it and print out the contents of the password file on a Unix system, we could run the command:

```
piccolo% java Cat /etc/passwd
root:x:0:1:0000-Admin(0000):/:/usr/bin/csh
daemon:x:1:1:0000-Admin(0000):/:
bin:x:2:2:0000-Admin(0000):/usr/bin:
...
```

From a security point of view, this is a very rudimentary program. It contains none of the elements of the sandbox that we just listed; it has the default (wide-open) sandbox given by default to every Java application. This application can perform any operation it wants.

---

* See, for example, the end of Chapter 6.

Security and the Operating System

The security policy imposed by Java is augmented by the security features of the operating system on which Java is running. A Java application with a wide-open security policy may attempt to read the password file, but if the user running the application does not normally have permission to read the password file, the Java application will not succeed.

The actual security policy that is in effect for a Java application will be the intersection of the security policy built into the application and the security policy of the operating system when the application is run. For the purposes of this book, we ignore the security features that the operating system may provide.

There are two ways in which we can add security features to this application. One way is to add to the application a class loader, a security manager, use of the access controller, and so on. This additional programming would set the bounds of the sandbox for this particular application.

The other route we can take is to run this application under the auspices of another application that we'll call JavaRunner. This is completely analogous to the way in which we typically run applets: appletviewer is a Java application that runs applets, and JavaRunner is a Java application that runs other applications. JavaRunner is responsible for establishing the parameters of the Java sandbox (that is, it ensures that appropriate class loaders, a security manager, and the like are all in place) before it invokes the target application, just as appletviewer establishes the parameters of the Java sandbox before it invokes the target applet.

This technique removes the difference (in terms of security) between an applet and an application: both types of programs are now subject to the Java sandbox. There are a number of circumstances in which this is useful:

- If you download (or purchase) Java applications and want them to run in a sandbox.

- If you want to ensure that your internally developed applications all run in the desired sandbox (without having to include that code in every application).

- If you have a corporate or campus network and need to distribute Java applications under a new security model. Perhaps the new model will:

    — Give different security permissions to programs downloaded from within the corporate firewall than those from outside the corporate firewall (without requiring internal classes to be signed)

— Authenticate users on the corporate network before allowing sensitive payroll data to be sent (even over the corporate network)

— Encrypt that payroll data, so internal spies can't decipher it

— Allow the user greater discretion over the resources granted to a particular program

Although the JavaRunner program is designed to run other applications, there is no reason why it cannot be modified to run applets as well. Such a modification would require some extra code to parse the HTML containing the applet tag and set up an instance of the AppletStub and AppletContext classes for the applet itself. We're not showing the code to do that only because it's not really relevant to the discussion of Java security—but the JavaRunner could easily be extended to become an appletviewer (or, with an appropriate Java bean that interprets HTML, a full-fledged browser). The advantage, of course, is that as author of the browser you would have full control over the security model the browser employs.

Outline of the JavaRunner Application

Here's the basic implementation of the JavaRunner application:

```
public class JavaRunner implements Runnable {
    final static int numArgs = 1;
    private Object args[];
    private String className;

    JavaRunner(String className, Object args[]) {
        this.className = className;
        this.args = args;
    }

    void invokeMain(Class clazz) {
        Class argList[] = new Class[] { String[].class };
        Method mainMethod = null;
        try {
            mainMethod = clazz.getMethod("main", argList);
        } catch (NoSuchMethodException nsme) {
            System.out.println("No main method in " + clazz.getName());
            System.exit(-1);
        }

        try {
            mainMethod.invoke(null, args);
        } catch (Exception e) {
            Throwable t;
            if (e instanceof InvocationTargetException)
                t = ((InvocationTargetException) e)
                                .getTargetException();
```

```
            else t = e;
            System.out.println("Procedure exited with exception " + t);
            t.printStackTrace();
        }
    }

    public void run() {
        Class target = null;
        try {
            target = Class.forName(className);
            invokeMain(target);
        } catch (ClassNotFoundException cnfe) {
            System.out.println("Can't load " + className);
        }
    }

    static Object[] getArgs(String args[]) {
        String passArgs[] = new String[args.length - numArgs];
        for (int i = numArgs; i < args.length; i++)
            passArgs[i - numArgs] = args[i];

        Object wrapArgs[] = new Object[1];
        wrapArgs[0] = passArgs;
        return wrapArgs;
    }

    public static void main(String args[]) {
        if (args.length < 1) {
            System.err.println("usage:  JavaRunner classfile");
            System.exit(-1);
        }
        ThreadGroup tg = new ThreadGroup("JavaRunner Threadgroup");
        Thread t = new Thread(tg,
                new JavaRunner(args[0], getArgs(args)));
        t.start();
        try {
            t.join();
        } catch (InterruptedException ie) {
            System.out.println("Thread was interrupted");
        }
    }
}
```

This is a fully functional (if not full-featured) version of the JavaRunner program;
we can use it to run our Cat application like this:

```
piccolo% java JavaRunner Cat /etc/passwd
root:x:0:1:0000-Admin(0000):/:/usr/bin/csh
daemon:x:1:1:0000-Admin(0000):/:
bin:x:2:2:0000-Admin(0000):/usr/bin:
...
```

This will give us exactly the same results as when we ran the program by hand. The invokeMain() method will use the Java reflection API to find the static main() method of the Cat class and then construct an appropriate argument list to pass to that method. Note that the use of the reflection API introduces a dependency on Java 1.1 for this program. You can write a similar program under Java 1.0, but not without using the native (C) interface to Java.

Note also that we construct a new thread group and thread, and run the main() method under control of that thread. The primary reason we do that will become clear in Chapter 6 when we discuss thread security policies. But there's no reason why you couldn't expand this example to run multiple targets simultaneously, in which case each target should have its own thread and thread group anyway.

We've cheated a little bit here by using the forName() method of the Class class to find our target application class—we'll hear more about that in Chapter 3 when we discuss class loaders. For now, it will suffice to know that this will load our target class (assuming that the target class is found on the CLASSPATH). In addition, we still haven't done anything to set up a security manager or to enable the access controller. As a result, the sandbox for an application run under this program is non-existent: the bytecodes will not be verified, and there will be no restriction on any actions that the application may perform. But this is the example that we'll expand upon during the rest of this book as we add security features to it.

Don't think that the only function of a program like this is to run Java applications (or even Java applets). Consider the Java web server—it must dynamically invoke servlets for different web requests as those requests come in. An RMI server might operate similarly, perhaps even loading the code to perform its operations from a client machine. Although we stick with this example throughout the book, the need for security in server applications parallels the need for security in end-user applications.

Built-in Java Application Security

Beginning in Java 1.2, the Java platform itself comes with a security model built into applications it runs. This model is based upon information in the user's CLASSPATH. Setting the CLASSPATH is the same operation in Java 1.1 and Java 1.2, but in Java 1.2, classes that are found on the CLASSPATH may optionally be subject to a security model. This allows you to run the application code in a user- or administrator-defined sandbox: in particular, it uses the access controller of Java 1.2 to provide the same security environment for the target application as a Java-enabled browser provides for an applet.

The successful use of this facility depends upon the class loader that the built-in application runner will use, as well as depending upon the environment set up by the access controller and security manager. We'll examine how these facilities interact with this method of running applications in the next few chapters. For now, we'll just outline how this method operates.

As always, Java applications are run on the command line as follows:

```
piccolo% java Cat /etc/passwd
root:x:0:1:0000-Admin(0000):/:/usr/bin/csh
daemon:x:1:1:0000-Admin(0000):/:
bin:x:2:2:0000-Admin(0000):/usr/bin:
...
```

This example loads the *Cat.class* file from the user's CLASSPATH and runs the application with the single argument */etc/passwd*. As always, when an application is run in this manner, the sandbox in which the application runs is unlimited: the application can perform any activity it wants to.

There is a very important difference between running these examples in Java 1.1 and running them in 1.2: in 1.2, classes that are loaded from the CLASSPATH will be loaded by a class loader. The addition of the class loader to the CLASSPATH allows us to build a sandbox for the application. However, none of these examples actually builds a sandbox yet. In order to build a sandbox for these examples, we must specify the -usepolicy flag on the command line. This flag enables a security manager and access controller to be installed; we'll discuss the details of this option in Chapter 6.

The -usepolicy flag is only available in Java 1.2. Without it, Java applications in 1.2 behave exactly as they do in 1.1: they have a wide-open sandbox.

For historical reasons (and because it makes describing this facility easier), we'll refer to the ability to run applications with an optional argument to specify a sandbox as the Launcher. Given that the Launcher is a standard part of Java, you might ask why we're going to the trouble of implementing our own JavaRunner. One reason is simply to make our discussion clearer: it is easiest to understand the architecture of Java's security policy in the context of JavaRunner. Other reasons have to do with certain limitations that we'll discover about the Launcher:

• The Launcher comes only with Java 1.2 and later releases; if you're still using 1.1, you'll have to use the JavaRunner program.

• The Launcher can only run classes from the CLASSPATH—it cannot load classes from the network or from another location. However, simply because the program in question is an application does not mean we won't want to load its classes from a server—but we'll need JavaRunner to do that.

Secure Applications in 1.2 and 1.2 beta 2

In releases of 1.2 up through beta 2, running a secure application requires use of a special class: the Launcher class (sun.misc.Launcher). To run an application under control of the Launcher, you would execute this command:

```
piccolo% java sun.misc.Launcher Cat /etc/passwd
```

In 1.2 beta, classes that are loaded from the CLASSPATH are not subject to the sandbox. In order to load those classes through a class loader and subject them to the sandbox, you must specify an alternate classpath for the classes that make up the application:

```
piccolo% java -Djava.app.class.path=/classes sun.misc.Launcher \
Cat /etc/passwd
```

If the Cat class is found in */classes*, it will be subject to the sandbox. If it is found in the CLASSPATH, it will not.

Beginning in 1.2 beta 3, the Launcher class was incorporated into the virtual machine itself.

- The security manager used by the Launcher does not have all the features we might desire. While most of its features are configurable through the access controller (also a feature of Java 1.2), there are certain advanced policies that we cannot configure in that way. These features can only be achieved with some programming on our part.

Hence, both the Launcher and JavaRunner are useful mechanisms for running Java applications; which one you use depends on your particular requirements.

Summary

Security is a multifaceted feature of the Java platform. There are a number of facilities within Java that allow you to write a Java application that implements a particular security policy, and this book will focus on each of those facilities in turn. Java-enabled browsers (including those like HotJava™ that are written in Java) are the ultimate proof of these features: these browsers have used the features of the Java platform to allow users to download and run code on their local systems without fear of viruses or other corruption.

But the security features of Java need not be limited to the protections afforded to Java applets running in a browser: they can be applied as necessary to your own Java applications. This is done most easily by incorporating those features into a framework designed to run Java applications within a specified sandbox. The ability to define and modify that framework is one of the primary examples of this book. In addition, the security package allows us to create applications that use generic security features—such as digital signatures—for many purposes aside from expanding the Java sandbox. This other use of the security package will also be a constant theme throughout this book.

In the next chapter, we'll look into the security features of the Java language itself—the first set of security features that are available to any Java application.

2

Java Language Security

The first components of the Java sandbox that we will examine are those components that are built into the Java language itself. These components primarily protect memory resources on the user's machine, although they have some benefit to the Java API as well. Hence, they are primarily concerned with guaranteeing the integrity of the memory of the machine that is hosting a program: in a nutshell, the security features within the Java language want to ensure that a program will be unable to discern or modify sensitive information that may reside in the memory of a user's machine. In terms of applets, these protections also mean that applets will be unable to determine information about each other; each applet is given, in essence, its own memory space in which to operate.

In this chapter, we'll look at the features of the Java language that provide this type of security. We'll also look at how these features are enforced, including a look at Java's bytecode verifier. With a few exceptions, the information in this chapter is largely informational; because the features we are going to discuss are immutable within the Java language, there are fewer programming considerations than we'll find in later chapters. However, the information we'll present here is crucial in understanding the entire Java security story; it is very helpful in ensuring that your Java environment is secure and in assessing the security risks that Java deployment might pose. The security of the Java environment is dependent on the security of each of its pieces, and the Java language forms the first fundamental piece of that security.

As we discuss the language features in this chapter, keep in mind that we're only dealing with the Java language itself—as is the common thread of this book, all security features we're going to discuss do not apply when the language in question is not Java. If you use Java's native interface to run arbitrary C code, that C code will be able to do pretty much anything it wants to do, even when it violates the precepts we're outlining in this chapter.

Java Language Security Constructs

In this chapter, we're going to be concerned primarily with how Java operates on things that are in memory on a particular machine. Within a Java program, every entity—that is, every object reference and every primitive data element—has an access level associated with it. To review, this access level may be:

- `private`: The entity can only be accessed by code that is contained within the class that defines the entity.

- Default (or package): The entity can be accessed by code that is contained within the class that defines the entity, or by a class that is contained in the same package as the class that defines the entity.

- `protected`: The entity can only be accessed by code that is contained within the class that defines the entity, by classes within the same package as the defining class, or by a subclass of the defining class.

- `public`: The entity can be accessed by code in any class.

The notion of assigning data entities an access level is certainly not exclusive to Java; it's a hallmark of many object-oriented languages. Since the Java language borrows heavily from C++, it's not surprising that it would borrow the basic notion of these access levels from C++ as well (although there are slight differences between the meanings of these access modifiers in Java and in C++).

As a result of this borrowing, the use of these access modifiers is generally thought of in terms of the advantage such modifiers bring to program design: one of the hallmarks of object-oriented design is that it permits data hiding and data encapsulation. This encapsulation ensures that objects may only be operated upon through the interface the object provides to the world, instead of being operated upon by directly manipulating the object's data elements. These and other design-related advantages are indeed important in developing large, robust, object-oriented systems. But in Java, these advantages are only part of the story.

In a language like C++, if I create a `CreditCard` object that encapsulates my mother's maiden name and my account number, I would probably decide that those entities should be private to the object and provide the appropriate methods to operate on those entities. But nothing in C++ prevents me from cheating and accessing those entities through a variety of back-door operations. The C++ compiler is likely to complain if I write code that attempts to access a private variable of another class, but the C++ runtime isn't going to care if I convert a pointer to that class into an arbitrary memory pointer and start scanning through memory until I find a location that contains a string with 16 digits— a possible account number. In C++ systems, no one typically worried about such occurrences because all parts of the system were presumed to originate from the same place: it's my program, and if I want to work around my data model to get access to that data, so be it.*

Things change with Java. I might be surfing to play some cool game applet on *www.EvilSite.org,* and then I might go shopping at *www.Acme.com.* When my Java wallet applet runs, I'd hate for the applet that is still running from *www.EvilSite.org* to be able to access the private `CreditCard` object that's contained in my Java wallet—and while it's necessary for *www.Acme.com* to know that I have a valid `CreditCard` object, I don't necessarily feel comfortable telling them my mother's maiden name. Because I'm now in the midst of a dynamic system with active programs from multiple sites, I need to make sure that the data entities are accessed by only those objects that are supposed to have access to them. It's obvious that I want protection from *EvilSite.org,* whom I don't want to know about the `CreditCard` object contained in my Java wallet. But I also want to be protected from *Acme.com,* a site I feel relatively comfortable about, but who should not be granted access to all the data elements of an object that it must use.

This is only one example of why the Java platform must provide memory integrity—that is, it must ensure that entities in memory are accessed only when they are allowed to be, and that these entities cannot be somehow corrupted. To that end, Java always enforces the following rules:

Access methods are strictly adhered to.

In Java, you cannot be allowed to treat a `private` entity as anything but private: the intentions of the programmer must always be respected. Object serialization involves an exception to this rule; we'll give more details about that a little bit later.

Programs cannot access arbitrary memory locations.

This is easy to ensure, as Java does not have the notion of a pointer. For example, casting between an `int` and an `Object` is strictly illegal in Java.

Entities that are declared as `final` *must not be changed.*

Final variables in Java are considered constants; they are immutable once they are initialized. Consider the havoc that could ensue if the `final` modifier were not respected:

- A `public` `final` variable could be changed, drastically altering the behavior of a program. If a rogue applet swapped the values of the variables `EAST` and `WEST` in the `GridBagConstraints` class, for example, any new applets would be laid out incorrectly (and probably incomprehensibly). That's a rather benign example of what could potentially be a dramatic security flaw.

---

* In a large project with multiple programmers, there's a strong argument that such an attitude on the part of an individual programmer is not to be dismissed so lightly, but we'll let that pass.

- A subclass could override a `final` method, altering the behavior of a class. One of the features of the Java API is that threads are not allowed to raise their priority above a certain maximum priority (typically, the priority of the thread group to which the thread belongs). This feature is enforced by the `setPriority()` method of the `Thread` class, which is a `final` method; allowing that method to be overridden would defeat the security mechanisms.

  This feature is used for virtually all of Java's security checks: performing an operation requires calling a `final` method in a Java class; only that `final` method can trap into the operating system to execute the operation. That `final` method is responsible for making sure the operation does not proceed if it would violate the security policy in place.

- A subclass could be created from a `final` class, with similar results. In Java, strings are considered as constants—their value may not be changed once the string has been created. If the `String` class could be subclassed, this rule could not be enforced.

Variables may not be used before they are initialized.

If a program were able to read the value of an uninitialized variable, the effect would be the same as if it were able to read random memory locations. A Java class wishing to exploit this defect might then declare a huge uninitialized section of variables in an attempt to snoop the memory contents of the user's machine. To prevent this type of attack, all local variables in Java must be initialized before they are used, and all instance variables in Java are automatically initialized to a default value.

Array bounds must be checked on all array accesses.

Like the access modifiers that started this discussion, bounds checking is generally thought of in terms other than security: the prime benefit to bounds checking is that it leads to fewer bugs and more robust programs. But it has security benefits as well: if an array of integers happens to reside in memory next to a string (which, in memory, is an array of characters), writing past the end of the array of integers would change the value of the string. The effect of this is generally a bug, but it could be exploited as a security hole as well: if the string held the destination account number for an electronic funds transfer, we could change the destination account number by willfully writing past the end of the array of integers.*

---

* This type of attack is not as far-fetched as it might seem; an early version of Netscape Navigator suffered from just this type of security hole. When long URLs were typed into the Goto field, the Netscape C code that read the string overwrote the bounds of the array where the characters were to be stored and clobbered a key location in memory, which allowed a security breach.

Objects cannot be arbitrarily cast into other objects.

Given the class fragment:

```
public class CreditCard {
    private String acctNo;
}
```

and the rogue class:

```
public class CreditCardSnoop {
    public String acctNo;
}
```

then the following code cannot be allowed to execute:

```
CreditCard cc = Wallet.getCreditCard();
CreditCardSnoop snoop = (CreditCardSnoop) cc;
System.out.println("Ha!  Your account number is " + snoop.acctNo);
```

Hence, Java does not allow arbitrary casting between objects; an object can only be cast to one of its superclasses or its subclasses (if, in the latter case, the object actually is an instance of that subclass). Note that the Java virtual machine is much stricter about this rule than the Java compiler is. In the example above, the compiler would complain about an illegal cast. We could satisfy the compiler by changing the code as follows:

```
Object cc = Wallet.getCreditCard();
CreditCardSnoop snoop = (CreditCardSnoop) cc;
```

Only the virtual machine will know if the returned object actually is of type CreditCard or not. In this case, then, the virtual machine is responsible for throwing a ClassCastException when the snoop variable is assigned to thwart the attack.

These are the techniques by which the Java language ensures that memory locations are read and written only when such access should normally be allowed. This restriction protects the user's machine from the outside: if I download an applet onto my machine, I don't want that applet accessing the private variables of my CreditCard class. However, if that applet has a private variable within it, nothing prevents me (depending on my operating system) from using a program outside of the browser to scan the memory on my system and figure out somehow what value that particular variable has. Similarly, nothing prevents me from having another program outside the browser change the value of a particular variable that is held in memory on my machine.

If you're an applet developer and are worried about this type of problem, you're pretty much on your own to come up with a solution to it. This might be particularly troublesome if you had, say, a variable somewhere in your applet that held a Boolean value indicating whether or not the user was licensed for a particular operation; a very clever user can go outside the browser and manipulate the machine's memory so that the integrity of your licensing scheme is violated. This problem is not new to Java, but it's not solved by Java either.

Object Serialization and Memory Integrity

There is one general exception to the rules about public, private, and protected access in Java. Object serialization is a feature of Java that allows an object to be written as a series of bytes; when those bytes are read someplace else, a new object is created that has the same state as the original object. Object serialization has two main purposes: it's used extensively in the RMI API to allow clients and servers to exchange objects, and it's used whenever you need to save a particular object to disk and want to recreate the object at some later point in time.

The murky issue here is just what constitutes an object's state. In the case of our CreditCard object, the account number is pretty basic to creating that object, but it's a variable that needs to be private for the reasons we've been discussing. In order for object serialization to work, it must have access to those private variables so it can correctly save and restore the object's state. That's why the object serialization API can access and save all private variables of an object (as well as its default, protected, and public variables). Similarly, the object serialization API is able to store those values back into the private data members when the object is actually reconstituted.

Depending on your perspective, this is a good thing or a bad thing. From a security perspective, it can be a bad thing: if the CreditCard object is saved to disk, something else can come along and read all that information from the disk file. Worse yet, the file could be edited in such a way that the object will be recreated in a completely different state than it originally had, with potentially damaging results.

In theory, this is the same problem we just discussed about influences outside the browser being able to read and write the private data of objects that are held in memory (which may help to explain why object serialization works this way by default). In practice, however, it's much easier to change the data in a binary file than to figure out how to access and change the value of an object in memory. Hence, object serialization has two additional mechanisms associated with it that make it more secure.

The first of these is that object serialization can only occur on objects that implement the java.io.Serializable interface (or its subclass, the java.io.Externalizable interface). The Serializable interface requires no methods, so it can be thought of simply as a flag to the virtual machine that says: "Hey, virtual machine—I've thought about the security aspects of this class, and it's okay if you serialize it by writing out all its data." By default, an object is not serializable, lest its internal private state be violated.

The second of these mechanisms is that object serialization respects the transient keyword associated with a variable: if our account number in the

CreditCard class were declared as private transient, then object serialization would not be allowed to read or write that particular variable. This lets us design classes that can be stored and reconstituted without showing their private data to the world.

Of course, a CreditCard object without an account number is worthless; what we really need is something that can save and reconstitute the transient data in such a way that the data cannot be compromised. This can be achieved by having our class implement the writeObject() and readObject() methods. The write-Object() method is responsible for writing out the transient data to the given output stream, while the readObject() method is responsible for reading the data corresponding to the transient data and storing that data into the field. It's your decision how to save and reconstitute the data so that its integrity is preserved, but typically this will mean that you'll want to use one of the encryption APIs we'll discuss in Chapter 13.

Storing and reconstituting the transient data can also be achieved by implementing the Externalizable interface and implementing the writeExternal() and the readExternal() methods of that interface. The difference in this case is that these two methods are now responsible for saving and reconstituting the entire state of the object—no data is stored or reconstituted for you.

Using either of these techniques, you have the ability to protect any sensitive data contained in your objects, even if you choose to share those objects over the network or save those objects to some sort of persistent storage.

Enforcement of the Java Language Rules

The list of rules we outlined above are fine in theory, but they must be enforced somehow. We've always been taught that overwriting the end of an array in C code is a bad thing, but I somehow still manage to do it accidentally all the time. There are also those who willfully attempt to overwrite the ends of arrays in an attempt to breach the security of a system. Without mechanisms to enforce these memory rules, they become simply guidelines and provide no sort of security at all.

This necessary enforcement happens at three different times in the development and deployment of a Java program: at compile time, at link time (that is, when a class is loaded into the virtual machine), and at runtime. Not all rules can be checked at each of these points, but certain checks are necessary at each point in order to ensure the memory security that we're after. As we'll see, enforcement of these rules (which is really the construction of this part of the Java sandbox) varies depending on the origin of the class in question.

Compiler Enforcement

The Java compiler is the first thing that is tasked with the job of enforcing Java's language rules. In particular, the compiler is responsible for enforcing all of the rules we outlined above except for the last two: the compiler cannot enforce array bound checking nor can it enforce all cases of illegal object casts.

The compiler does enforce certain cases of illegal object casts—namely, casts between objects that are known to be unrelated, such as the following code:

```
Vector v = new Vector();
String s = (String) v;
```

But the validity of a cast between an object of type X to type Y where Y is a subclass of X cannot be known at compile time, so the compiler must let such a construct pass.

The Bytecode Verifier

Okay, the compiler has produced a Java program for us, and we're about to run the Java bytecode of that program. But if the program came from an unknown source, how do we know that the bytecodes we've received are actually legal?

Bytecode Verification of Other Languages

Throughout this section, we're discussing the bytecode verifier as if it were tied to the Java language. This is somewhat imprecise: the bytecode verifier is actually independent of the original source language of the program. If we had a C++ compiler that generated Java bytecodes from C++ source, the bytecode verifier would still be able to verify (or not) the bytecodes.

However, the verification of the bytecodes would still depend upon the semantics of the Java language, and not the semantics of C++; just because the bytecodes in question originated from C++ code is no reason that they should suddenly be allowed to cast an arbitrary memory location into an object.

For this reason, I prefer to think of the bytecodes in terms of the Java language itself. There are tools to produce Java bytecodes from other languages (like Scheme), but in general, producing Java bytecodes from another language severely limits the constructs that can be written in that other language.

This brings us to the need for the bytecode verifier—the second link in the chain of responsibility of enforcing the rules of the Java language. Normally when the need for the bytecode verifier is discussed, it's in terms of an evil compiler—that is, a compiler that someone has written in such a way that the code produced by the compiler is not legal Java code. The theory is that code from such a compiler could be constructed in order to create and exploit a security hole by ignoring a rule in the Java language. Such an attack might seem to be difficult to achieve, in that it would require some detailed knowledge of the Java compiler.

It turns out that the evil compiler issue is a red herring—it doesn't really matter whether such an attack is likely or not, because it's trivial to create non-conforming Java code with any standard Java compiler. Assume that we have these classes:

```java
public class CreditCard {
    public String acctNo = "0001 0002 0003 0004";
}

public class Test {
    public static void main(String args[]) {
        CreditCard cc = new CreditCard();
        System.out.println("Your account number is " + cc.acctNo);
    }
}
```

If we run this code, we'll create a CreditCard object and print out its account number. Now say that we realize the account number should really have been private, so we go back and change the definition of acctNo to be private and recompile only the CreditCard class. We then have two class files, and the Test class file contains Java code that illegally accesses the private instance variable acctNo of the CreditCard class.

The above example shows an innocent mistake, but a malicious programmer could use just this technique to produce illegal Java bytecodes. In order to modify the contents of a string, for example, all we need to do is:

1. Copy the java.lang.String source file into our CLASSPATH.

2. In the copy of the file, modify the definition of value—the private array that holds the actual characters of the string—to be public.

3. Compile this modified class, and replace the *String.class* file in the JDK.

4. Compile some new code against this modified version of the String class. The new code could include something like this:

```java
public class CorruptString {
    public static void modifyString(String src, String dst) {
        for (int i = 0; i < src.length; i++) {
```

```
        if (i == dst.length)
                return;
        src.value[i] = dst.value[i];
    }
  }
}
```

Now any time you want to modify a string in place, simply call this modi-fyString() method with the string you want to corrupt (src) and the new string you want it to have (dst).

5. Remove the modified version of the String class.

Now the CorruptString class can be referenced by a Java program, which can use it to attempt to corrupt any string that it has a reference to. Even though the program will run with the original version of the String class, the CorruptString class will be able to access the private value array within the String class—unless the bytecode verifier rejects the CorruptString class.

Inside the bytecode verifier

The bytecode verifier is an internal part of the Java virtual machine and has no interface: programmers cannot access it and users cannot interact with it. The verifier automatically examines most bytecodes as they are built into class objects by the class loader of the virtual machine (see Figure 2-1). We'll give just a brief overview of how the bytecode verifier actually works.

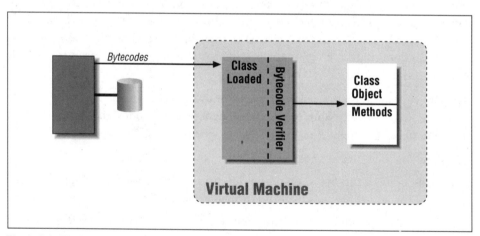

Figure 2-1. The bytecode verifier

The verifier is often referred to as a mini-theorem prover (a term first used in several documents from Sun). This sounds somewhat more impressive than it is; it's not a generic, all-purpose theorem prover by any means. Instead, it's a piece of code that can prove one (and only one) thing—that a given series of (Java) bytecodes represents a legal set of (Java) instructions.

Specifically, the bytecode verifier can prove the following:

- The class file has the correct format. The full definition of the class file format may be found in the Java virtual machine specification; the bytecode verifier is responsible for making sure that the class file has the right length, the correct magic numbers in the correct places, and so on.

- Final classes are not subclassed, and final methods are not overridden.

- Every class (except for java.lang.Object) has a single superclass.

- There is no illegal data conversion of primitive data types (e.g., int to Object).

- No illegal data conversion of objects occurs. Because the casting of a superclass to its subclass may be a valid operation (depending on the actual type of the object being cast), the verifier cannot ensure that such casting is not attempted—it can only ensure that before each such attempt is made, the legality of the cast is tested.

- There are no operand stack overflows or underflows.

  In Java, there are two stacks for each thread. One stack holds a series of method frames, where each method frame holds the local variables and other storage for a particular method invocation. This stack is known as the data stack and is what we normally think of as the stack within a traditional program. The bytecode verifier cannot prevent overflow of this stack—an infinitely recursive method call will cause this stack to overflow. However, each method invocation requires a second stack (which itself is allocated on the data stack) that is referred to as the operand stack; the operand stack holds the values that the Java bytecodes operate on. This secondary stack is the stack that the bytecode verifier can ensure will not overflow or underflow.

Hence, when the bytecode verifier has completed its task, we know that the code in question follows many of the constraints of the Java language—including most of the rules that the compiler was also responsible for ensuring. The remaining rules are verified during the actual running of the program.

Delayed bytecode verification

When we began this section, we said that the bytecode verifier is responsible for *examining* all the bytecodes of the class—we explicitly did not say that the verifier is responsible for *verifying* all the bytecodes. This is because the bytecode verifier may delay some of the checks it is responsible for, as long as those checks are performed before the code is actually executed. In typical verifier implementations, the bytecode verifier does not immediately test to see if all field and method accesses are legal according to the access modifiers associated with that field or method.

This is driven by a desire to be efficient—our Test class may reference the acctNo field of our CreditCard class, but it may do so only if a particular branch in the code is taken. In the following code, there's no need to verify that the access to acctNo is legal unless an IllegalArgumentException has been generated:

```
CreditCard cc = getCreditCard();
try {
    Wallet.makePurchase(cc);
} catch (IllegalArgumentException iae) {
    System.out.println("Can't process for account " + cc.acctNo);
}
```

Hence, the bytecode verifier delays all tests for field and method access until the code is actually executed. The process by which this happens is implementation independent; one technique that is often used is to ensure during verification that all accesses test the validity of the field access. If the access is valid, the standard bytecodes are then replaced during execution with a special bytecode indicating that the test has been performed and access to the field in question no longer needs to be tested. On the other hand, if the validity test fails, the virtual machine throws an IllegalAccessException.

This gives us the best of both worlds—verification of the access is performed during the actual running of the program (after traditional bytecode verification has occurred), but the verification is still only performed once (unlike the runtime verification we'll examine later).

Controlling bytecode verification

Bytecode verification seems like a great thing: not only can it help to prevent malicious attacks from violating rules of the Java language, it can also help detect simple programmer errors—such as when we changed the access modifier of acctNo in our CreditCard class, but forgot to recompile our Test class.

Nonetheless, bytecode verification is not used on all classes. Like many security-related features of Java, bytecode verification only applies to certain classes. In Java 1.1 and earlier, classes that are loaded from the CLASSPATH are deemed to be trusted and are not subject to bytecode verification, whereas classes that are loaded from another location (e.g., a file- or HTTP-based URL) are not deemed to be trusted and must be verified. In Java 1.2, this policy has changed and all classes except those in the core Java API are verified. This difference really reflects the class loader that is used to load the class, as we'll see in the next chapter.

In typical usage, this is a workable policy. Browsers always ensure that the code imported to run an applet is verified, and Java applications are typically not verified. Of course, this may or may not be the perfect solution:

- If a remote site can talk an end user into installing a local class into the browser's CLASSPATH, the local class will not be verified and may violate the rules we've discussed here. In 1.2, this is much harder, since the class must be added to the zip file containing the core API classes.

- You may implicitly rely upon the verifier to help you keep files in sync so that when one is changed, other files are verified against it.

As a user, you (theoretically) have limited control over the verifier—though such control depends on the browser you are using. If you are running a Java application, you can run java with the -verify option, which will verify all classes. Similarly, if you are using a browser written in Java—including the appletviewer—you can arrange for the java command to run with the -noverify option, which turns verification off for all classes. Occasionally, a browser not written in Java will allow the user to disable bytecode verification as well—e.g., Internet Explorer 3.0 for the Mac had this capability, although it was present only because the bytecode verifier could not run in certain limited memory configurations.

However, although these options to the virtual machine are well-documented, they are not implemented on all platforms. One way to ensure that application code is run through the bytecode verifier is to use the final version of the JavaRunner program (once we add a class loader to it in the next chapter) or the Launcher in Java 1.2.

Runtime Enforcement

Like the compiler, the bytecode verifier cannot completely guarantee that the bytecodes follow all of the rules we outlined earlier in this chapter: it can only ensure that the first four of them are followed. The virtual machine must still take responsibility for ultimately determining that the Java bytecodes provide the security we expect them to.

The remaining security protections of the Java language must be enforced at runtime by the virtual machine:

Array bounds checking

In theory, the bytecode verifier can detect certain cases of array bounds checking, but in general, this check must take place at runtime. Consider the following code:

```
void initArray(int a[], int nItems) {
    for (int i = 0; i < nItems; i++) {
```

```
        a[i] = 0;
    }
}
```

Since nItems and a are parameters, the bytecode verifier has no way of determining whether this code is legal. Hence, array bounds checking is always
done   at   runtime.   Failure   to   meet   this   rule   results   in   an
ArrayIndexOutOfBoundsException.

Object casting

The verifier can and will detect the legality of certain types of casts, specifically, whenever unrelated classes are cast to each other. The virtual machine
must monitor when a superclass is cast into a subclass and test that cast's
validity; failure to execute a legal cast results in a ClassCastException. This
holds for casts involving interfaces as well, since objects that are defined as an
interface type (rather than a class type) are considered by the verifier to be of
type Object.

Summary

Because the notion of security in Java is pervasive, its implementation is equally
pervasive. In this chapter, we've explored the security mechanisms that are built
into the Java language itself. Essentially, at this level the security mechanisms are
concerned with establishing a set of rules for the Java language that creates an
environment where an object's view of memory is well-known and well-defined, so
that a developer can ensure that items in memory cannot be accidentally or intentionally read, corrupted, or otherwise misused. We also took a brief look at Java's
bytecode verifier, including why it is necessary, and why you should turn it on,
even for Java applications.

It's important to keep in mind that the purpose of these security constraints is to
protect the user's machine from a malicious piece of code and not to protect a
piece of code from a malicious user. Java does not (and could not) prevent a user
from acting on memory from outside the browser (with possibly harmful results).

3

Java Class Loaders

In this chapter, we're going to explore Java's class loading mechanism—the mechanism by which files containing Java bytecodes are read into the Java virtual machine and converted into class definitions. The operation of Java programs depends on the class loader; given Java's desire to ensure security throughout its architecture, it should come as no surprise that class loaders are also a very important piece of the Java security story. The class loader normally works in conjunction with the security manager and access controller to provide the bulk of the protections associated with the Java sandbox.

The class loader is important in Java's security model because initially, only the class loader knows certain information about classes that have been loaded into the virtual machine. Only the class loader knows where a particular class originated, and only the class loader knows whether or not a particular class was signed (although the class loader arranges for the Class object itself to carry its signature with it). Hence, one of the keys to writing a secure Java application is to understand the role of the class loader and to write (or at least use) a secure class loader.

We'll address both those points in this chapter. We begin with an overview of how the class loader functions, and the features that its basic functions add to the overall security of the Java platform. We'll then look into writing our own class loader, the motivation for which will vary depending on the release of Java you're using and the type of application you are running.

As with the other elements of the Java sandbox, the ability to create and use a class loader is limited to Java applications. Java applets use the class loader provided for them by the browser in which they are running, and they are generally prohibited from creating their own class loader.

Security and the Class Loader

There are two instances where the class loader plays an important role in the Java security model: it must coordinate with Java's security manager or access controller, and it must enforce certain rules about the namespace used by Java classes.

Class Loaders and Security Enforcement

The class loader must coordinate with the security manager and access controller of the virtual machine in order to determine the security policy for a Java program. We'll explore this in more detail in the next few chapters when we discuss these various security mechanisms; for now, we'll just consider the motivation for the following connection.

As we know, a Java applet cannot (normally) read a file when the applet is being run in a browser such as HotJava.* The HotJava browser itself, however, can read files, even while it is also running applets. Both the browser and the applets are using the same classes to (attempt to) read a file, so clearly there must be something that allows the `java.io` classes to determine that one case should fail while the other case should succeed. That differentiation is the by-product of the class loader: the class loader allows the security manager to find out particular information about the class, which allows the security manager to apply the correct security policy depending on the context of the request. When we discuss the security manager, we'll discuss the specific mechanics by which this can be achieved. For now, it is only important to keep in mind that the class loader is the piece of the Java architecture that is able to make this distinction. Since it loaded the class, it knows if the class came from the network (i.e., the class is part of the applet and should not be trusted) or if the class came from the local filesystem (i.e., the class is part of the browser and should be trusted). It also knows if the class was delivered with a digital signature, and the exact location from which the class was loaded. All these pieces of information may be used by the security manager and access controller to establish a security policy.

Class Loaders and Namespaces

The second place where the class loader provides security in Java is more subtle and has to do with Java's namespace rules. Recall that the full name of a Java class is qualified by the name of the package to which the class belongs; there is no standard class called `String` in the Java API, but there is the class

---

* This is true of all Java-enabled browsers, of course, but the point is clearer when we consider the HotJava browser since that browser is written in Java.

java.lang.String. On the other hand, a class does not need to belong to a package, in which case its full name is just the name of the class. It's often said that these classes are in the default package, but that's slightly misleading: as it turns out, there is a different default package for each class loader in use by the virtual machine.

Consider what happens if you surf to a page at *www.sun.com* and load an applet that uses a class called Car (with no package name); after that, you surf to a page at *www.ora.com* and load a different applet that uses a class called Car (also with no package name). Clearly, these are two different classes, but they have the same fully qualified name—how can the virtual machine distinguish between these two classes?

The answer to that question lies in the internal workings of the class loader. When a class is loaded by a class loader, it is stored in a reference internal to that class loader. A class loader in Java is simply an object whose type is some class that extends the ClassLoader class. When the virtual machine needs access to a particular class, it asks the appropriate class loader. For example, when the virtual machine is executing the code from *sun.com* and needs access to the Car class, it asks the class loader that loaded the applet (r1 in Figure 3-1) to provide that class.

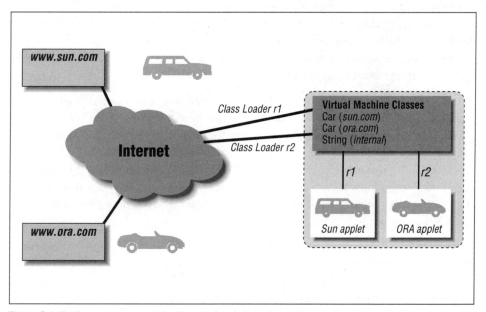

Figure 3-1. Different instances of the class loaders help to disambiguate class names

In order for this scheme to work, the Car class from *www.ora.com* must be loaded using a different class loader than that which loaded the Car class from *www.sun.com*. That way, when the virtual machine asks the class loader r2 for the definition of the Car class, it will get back (correctly) the definition from *ora.com*. The class loader does not need to be a different class; as this example implies, it must merely be a different *instance* of the class. Hence, applets that have a different CODEBASE (even if they originate on the same host) are always loaded by different instances of the browser's class loader. Applets on the same page with the same CODEBASE, however, may use the same class loader so that they may share class files (as well as sharing other information). Some browsers also allow applets on different pages to be loaded by the same class loader as long as those applets have the same CODEBASE, which is generally a more efficient and useful implementation.

This differentiation between class files loaded from different class loaders occurs no matter what packages are involved. Don't be confused by the fact that there were no explicit package names given in our example. A large computer company might define a class named com.sun.Car, a large oil company might also define a class called com.sun.Car, and the two classes need to be considered as distinct classes—which they will be if (and only if) they are loaded by different instances of the class loader.

So far we've given a logical reason why the class loader is involved in the namespace resolution of Java classes. You might think that if everyone were to follow the convention that the beginning of their package name must be their Internet domain in reverse order—e.g., com.sun for Sun Microsystems—this idea of different class loaders wouldn't be necessary. But there are security reasons for this namespace separation as well.

In Java, classes that are members of the same package have certain privileges that other classes do not have—they can access all the classes of the package that have the default protection (that is, the classes that are neither public, private, nor protected). Additionally, they can access any instance variable of classes in the package if the instance variable also has the default protection. As we discussed in Chapter 2, the ability to reference only those items to which a class has access is a key part of the security restrictions Java places on a program to ensure memory and API integrity.

So let's assume that no class loader based package separation exists, and that we rely on Sun Microsystems to name its classes com.sun.Car and so on. Everything would proceed reasonably, until we surf to *www.EvilSite.org*, where someone has placed a class called com.sun.DoSomethingEvil. Without the namespace separation introduced by the class loader, this class would suddenly have access to all the default protected classes and default protected variables of every class that had been downloaded from Sun. Worse, that site could supply a class called com.sun.Car with a much different implementation than Sun's—such that when the user (metaphorically, of course) applied the car's brakes, the new implementation sped up instead. Clearly, this is not a desirable situation.

Note too that with a badly written class loader, the hackers at *EvilSite.org* have the potential to supply new classes to override the core classes of the Java API. When the class loader that loaded the applet from *EvilSite* is asked to provide the java.lang.String class, it must provide the expected version of that class and not some version from *EvilSite.org*. In practice, this is not a problem, because the class loader is written to find and return the core class first.

Without enforcement of the namespace separation that we've just outlined, there is no way to ensure that the hackers at *EvilSite.org* have not forged a class into the com.sun package. The only way to prevent such forgeries would be to require that every class be a signed class which authenticated that it did in fact come from sun.com (or wherever its package name indicates that it should have come from). Authenticated classes certainly have their place in Java's security model, but it would be unmanageable to require that every site sign and authenticate every class on its site.

Hence, the separation of classes based on the class loader that loaded them—and the convention that applets on different pages are loaded by different class loaders—has its benefits for Java security as well as solving a messy logistical problem. We'll now look into the details of how the class loader actually works.

Anatomy of a Class Loader

When the Java virtual machine needs access to a particular class, it is up to a class loader to provide the class. The class loader goes through the following steps to load and define a class:

1. If the class loader has already loaded this class, it should find the previously defined class object and return that object immediately.

2. The security manager is consulted to see if this program is allowed to access the class in question. If it is not, a security exception is thrown. This step may be considered optional.

3. Otherwise, an internal class loader is consulted to attempt to load the class from the CLASSPATH. If that succeeds, the class loader returns. This ensures that classes within the Java API will not be superseded by classes loaded from the network (or other location).

   The way this is done varies between 1.1 and 1.2. In 1.1, there is a single method (the findSystemClass() method) that handles this step. In 1.2, a class loader must delegate to another class loader to find classes that are on the CLASSPATH and call the findSystemClass() method to find classes that are in the core API.

4. The security manager is consulted to see if this program is allowed to create the class in question. If it is not, a security exception is thrown. This step may be considered optional.

5. The class file is read into an array of bytes. The mechanism by which the class loader reads the file and creates the byte array will vary depending on the class loader (which, after all, is one of the points of having different class loaders).

6. The byte codes are run through the bytecode verifier.

7. A Class object is constructed from the bytecodes. In the process, the methods defining the class are created. In Java 1.1 and later, this process also ensures that the name in the class file matches the name that the class loader thought it was asked to load.

8. Before the class can be used, it must be resolved—which is to say that any classes that it immediately references must also be found by this class loader. The set of classes that are immediately referenced contains any classes that the class extends as well as any classes used by the static initializers of the class. Note that classes that are used only as instance variables, method parameters, or local variables are not normally loaded in this phase: they are loaded when the class actually references them (although certain compiler optimizations may require that these classes be loaded when the class is resolved).

Step 5 of this process varies depending on the policy of the particular class loader—the data for the class may be read from the network or the filesystem (or from any other location, such as a database). The other steps of this process will remain fixed for a well-defined class loader.

There are a number of class loaders that are used in Java programs, described in the following sections.

The Internal Class Loader

All Java programs must have the capability of loading certain classes—the Java API classes and any otherslocated in the user's CLASSPATH. Some of these classes are bootstrapped into the virtual machine. The first thing the virtual machine typically does is load the Java API class files (the *classes.zip* file) for future use.

The internal class loader uses the native operating system's file access methods to open and read the class files into byte arrays. When one of these classes contains a reference to another class, the internal class loader is again consulted to load the referenced class.

Unlike other class loaders we'll explore, the internal class loader cannot be overridden. Most of the internal class loader, in fact, is written in native code so that it can be accessed directly by the virtual machine (a requirement for the virtual machine to be able to bootstrap the API classes).

The internal class loader is often referred to as the default class loader or the primordial class loader. Due to some details of the Class class, we often speak of classes that are loaded by the internal class loader as having no class loader at all (and as a result, the internal class loader is sometimes called the null class loader).

There is a significant change in the use of the primordial class loader between Java 1.1 and 1.2. In 1.1, the primordial class loader was used to load all classes on the CLASSPATH. In 1.2, the primordial class loader is used only to load the Java API class files; the virtual machine constructs an instance of the URLClassLoader class to load the classes from the CLASSPATH.

The Applet Class Loader

An applet needs the ability to load classes via HTTP from the network. Hence, applet class loaders typically use the URL class to read in the data for a class file from the applet's CODEBASE host.

There is no standard applet class loader in the Java API—each Java browser is responsible for implementing its own class loader. In practice, the class loaders of various browsers are indistinguishable (and are usually based on the reference class loader implemented in Sun's appletviewer), but a Java programmer cannot simply instantiate an applet class loader in a platform-independent way.[*]

The RMI Class Loader

Beginning with JDK 1.1, the Java API includes an RMI class loader that can be used by any application. Despite its name, the RMI class loader needn't be used in an RMI application, and it is not truly a class loader—that is, it does not extend the ClassLoader class. In function, the RMIClassLoader class (java.rmi.server.RMIClassLoader) is very similar to the applet class loader—it uses the HTTP protocol to load the desired class file from a remote machine and then defines the class from the data in that file.

The RMI class loader cannot be instantiated directly; you must use one of its static methods to load a class. Once an initial class is loaded by the RMI class loader, any classes it references will also be loaded by the RMI class loader. In addition, the RMI class loader can only load classes from the URL specified by the

---

[*] If you want, you can figure out which class in the JDK on your system is the applet class loader, instantiate an instance of that class, and use it, but all virtual machines will not necessarily have that class available.

`java.rmi.server.codebase` property, so it is not a generic solution to all applications where a class loader might be used.

If you are loading individual, unsigned classes (i.e., classes that are not in a JAR file) from a single URL (i.e., a single directory, whether a file-based or an HTTP-based URL), using the RMI class loader is the simplest option for Java 1.1 applications. For Java 1.2 applications, you can use the RMI class loader for this purpose, or you can use the URL class loader; the URL class loader will offer you more flexibility.

The Secure Class Loader

Beginning with Java 1.2, the Java API includes a class loader in the `java.security` package called `SecureClassLoader`. This class has a protected constructor, so its real use is to provide the basis for the development of other class loaders. The distinguishing feature of the secure class loader is that it associates a protection domain with each class that it loads. Protection domains form the basis of the operation of the access controller; we'll see more about them in Chapter 5. For now, just accept the fact that if you want to use the access controller to establish your security policy, you'll need to use a class loader that extends the `Secure-ClassLoader` class.

The URL Class Loader

Also beginning with Java 1.2, the Java API includes a general-purpose class loader that can load classes from a set of URLs: the `URLClassLoader` class (`java.net.URLClassLoader`). This class is public and fully implemented, so for 1.2-based applications, it provides a truly useful, general purpose class loader:

public class URLClassLoader extends SecureClassLoader ★
> Load classes from a set of URLs. A URL in this set may be a directory-based URL, in which case the class loader will attempt to locate individual class files under that directory. A URL in this set may also be a JAR file, in which case the JAR file will be loaded, and the class loader will attempt to find a class in the JAR file.

An instance of the `URLClassLoader` class is created via one of these constructors:

public URLClassLoader(URL urls[]) ★
public URLClassLoader(URL urls[], ClassLoader parent) ★
> Construct a class loader based on the given array of URLs. This class loader attempts to find a class by searching each URL in the order in which it appears in the array.

> The second of these constructors constructs a URL class loader that uses the 1.2-based delegation model for loading classes (which we discuss at the end of

this chapter). In that case, the parent class loader will be asked to load the class first; if it fails, this URL class loader proceeds to load the class. This is the preferred constructor to use.

We can construct a URL class loader like this:

```
URL urls[] = new URL[2];
urls[0] = new URL("http://piccolo.East/~sdo/");
urls[1] = new URL("file:/home/classes/LocalClasses.jar");
URLClassLoader ucl = new URLClassLoader(urls, parent);
```

When we use this class loader to load the class com.sdo.Car, the class loader first attempts to load it via the URL *http://piccolo.East/~sdo/com/sdo/Car.class*; if that fails, it looks for the class in the *LocalClasses.jar* file.

It should come as no surprise that this class is the basis for running the Launcher. In that case, the array of URLs is created based on the list of URLs that make up the CLASSPATH (but not including the core Java API classes).

Choosing the Right Class Loader

With all these class loaders to choose from, which is the better choice: an existing class loader or your own custom class loader? The answer depends upon your needs. It is better not to write your own class loader if an existing one can fit your needs, but that's not always possible. Here are some guidelines:

1. Start by trying to use an instance of the URLClassLoader class. This class can load classes from multiple sites, using file-based and HTTP-based URLs. It can process individual class files and JAR files (including signed JAR files, which will become important later in our discussion). This class is the basis of the Launcher, although with the Launcher itself, you're limited to file-based URLs.

   When would you not use the URL class loader? Here are some possible cases:

   — When you want to load classes other than via HTTP or the file system. You may have classes that are held in a database, or you may want to define the bytecodes for a class programmatically.

   — When you want to load classes from different hosts and you have *a priori* knowledge of which class is on which host. The URL class loader will search for classes in its list of URLs sequentially; prior knowledge may allow you to load classes more efficiently.[*]

---

[*] In the beta release of 1.2, URLClassLoader fails to handle multiple HTTP-based URLs correctly. It is hoped that this will be fixed for FCS; if it is not and you need to load classes from multiple web servers, you will need to use your own class loader—see the information about the MultiLoader class in the section "Loading from Multiple Sites" later in this chapter .

2. If you're on a 1.1-based system and only need to load classes from a single site, use the RMI class loader. Remember that you will have to define as a property the location where those classes are found.

3. Otherwise, you'll need to provide a custom class loader.

Loading Classes

We'll now explore the details of how a class loader actually loads classes. There is a single method of the ClassLoader class (and all its subclasses) that accomplishes this:

public Class loadClass(String name)

   Load and resolve the named class. A ClassNotFoundException is thrown if the class cannot be found.

This is the simplest way to use a class loader directly: it simply requires that the class loader be instantiated and then be used via the loadClass() method. Once the Class object has been constructed, there are four ways in which a method in the class can be executed:

- A static method of the class can be executed using the native method interface of the Java virtual machine. This is the technique the Java virtual machine uses to execute the main() method of a Java application once the initial class has been loaded, but this is not generally a technique used by Java applications.

- An object of the class can be constructed using the newInstance() method of the Class class, but only if the class has an accessible constructor that requires no arguments. Once the object has been constructed, methods with well-known signatures can be executed on the object. This is the technique that a program like appletviewer uses: it loads the initial class of the applet, constructs an instance of the applet (which calls the applet's no-argument constructor), and then calls the applet's init() method (among other methods).

- Starting with JDK 1.1, the reflection API can be used to call a static method on the class, or to construct instances of the object and execute methods on that object. The reflection API allows more flexibility than the second choice, since it allows arguments to be passed to the constructor of the object. This is the technique that is used by our JavaRunner program.

- In the URLClassLoader class, the invokeClass() method may be called to call the static main() method of the class (assuming that one exists), passing it an array of strings. This is the technique the Launcher uses.

The second case is more commonly implemented, if only because it's simpler (and it is applicable in all versions of Java). But consider the following modifications to our JavaRunner program:

```java
public class JavaRunner implements Runnable {
    final static int numArgs = 2;
    ClassLoader cl;
    String className;
    Object args[];

    JavaRunner(ClassLoader cl, String className, Object args[]) {
        this.cl = cl;
        this.className = className;
        this.args = args;
    }

    void invokeMain(Class clazz) {
        .. unchanged ..
    }

    public void run() {
        Class target = null;
        try {
            target = cl.loadClass(className);
            invokeMain(target);
        } catch (ClassNotFoundException cnfe) {
            System.out.println("Can't load " + className);
        }
    }

    static Object[] getArgs(String args[]) {
        .. unchanged ..
    }

    public static void main(String args[])
                                    throws ClassNotFoundException {
        Class self = Class.forName("JavaRunner");
        JavaRunnerLoader jrl = new
                    JavaRunnerLoader(args[0], self.getClassLoader());
        JavaRunnerLoader jrl = new JavaRunnerLoader(args[0], parent);
        ThreadGroup tg = new ThreadGroup("JavaRunner Threadgroup");
        Thread t = new Thread(tg,
                new JavaRunner(jrl, args[1], getArgs(args)));
        t.start();
        try {
            t.join();
```

```
      } catch (InterruptedException ie) {
         System.out.println("Thread was interrupted");
      }
   }
}
```

We've replaced the forName() method that we used in our example in Chapter 1 with the highlighted code here: now we construct a class loader (an instance of the JavaRunnerLoader class, the definition of which we'll see in just a bit) and are now using the loadClass() method to find our target class.

In Java 1.2, constructing the class loader requires that we find the class loader that loaded our class and pass that to the constructor of the JavaRunnerLoader class. In 1.1, we would not use the self instance variable.

We've also changed the arguments required to run this program, which is why we've changed the definition of numArgs. Previously, we required the name of the class and any arguments the class requires. Now we require an additional argument: the name of the URL from which to load all the classes. Hence, if our Cat class was on the web server named *piccolo*, we could run our JavaRunner example like this:

```
piccolo% java JavaRunner http://piccolo/ Cat /etc/passwd
root:x:0:1:0000-Admin(0000):/:/usr/bin/csh
daemon:x:1:1:0000-Admin(0000):/:
bin:x:2:2:0000-Admin(0000):/usr/bin:
...
```

Note the difference between this implementation and the one we showed in Chapter 1. In this case, the Cat class is loaded from the JavaRunner class loader, and any classes the Cat class needs are dynamically loaded from that class loader. In Chapter 1, what happened was a product of the release of Java. In 1.1, the Cat class was loaded from the primordial class loader; any classes it required were loaded from the primordial class loader as well. In 1.2, the Cat class was loaded from an instance of the URLClassLoader class, and any classes it required were loaded from that class loader as well.

The practical result is that the security manager and access controller will give different permissions to the Cat class depending on which class loader loaded it: the permissions that are assigned to a class may be different depending upon whether the class was loaded from the URL class loader, the JavaRunner class loader, or the primordial class loader. Exactly how those permissions differ depends upon the internal implementation of the class loader as well as the security manager and access controller that are in effect. In a nutshell, these differences will be based upon where the class loader found the class, and whether or not that class was signed.

Implementing a Class Loader

Part of the security implications of a class loader depend upon its internal implementation. When you implement a class loader, you have two basic choices: you can extend the ClassLoader class, or you can extend the SecureClassLoader class. The second choice is preferred, but it is not an option for Java 1.1. If you're programming in 1.2, you may choose to use the URL class loader rather than implementing your own, but the information in this section will help you understand the security features of the URL class loader. In this section, then, we'll look at how to implement both default and secure class loaders.

Implementing the ClassLoader Class

Aside from the primordial class loader, all Java class loaders must extend the ClassLoader class (java.lang.ClassLoader). Since the ClassLoader class is abstract, it is necessary to subclass it to create a class loader.

Protected methods in the ClassLoader class

In order to implement a class loader, we start with this method:

protected abstract Class loadClass(String name, boolean resolve) ☆
protected Class loadClass(String name, boolean resolve) ★
> Using the rules of the class loader, find the class with the given name and, if indicated by the resolve variable, ensure that the class is resolved. If the class is not found, this method should throw a ClassNotFoundException. This method is abstract in 1.1, but not in 1.2. In 1.2, you typically do not override this method.

The loadClass() method is passed a fully qualified class name (e.g., java.lang.String or com.xyz.XYZPayrollApplet), and it is expected to return a class object that represents the target class. If the class is not a system class, the loadClass() method is responsible for loading the bytes that define the class (e.g., from the network).

There are four final methods in the ClassLoader class that a class loader can use to help it achieve its task:

protected final Class defineClass(String name, byte data[], int offset, int length)
> Create a Class object from an array of bytecodes. The defineClass() method runs the data through the bytecode verifier and then creates the Class object. This method also ensures that the name in the class file is the same as the name of the argument—that is, that the bytes actually define the desired class.

protected final Class findSystemClass(String name)

Attempt to find the named class by using the internal class loader to search the user's CLASSPATH. If the system class is not found, a ClassNotFoundException is generated. In 1.2, this method searches only the classes in the Java API.

protected final Class findLoadedClass(String name)

Find the class object for a class previously loaded by this class loader. If the class is not found, a null reference is returned.

Finding Previously Loaded Classes

According to the Java specification, a class loader is required to cache the classes that it has previously loaded, so that when it is asked to load a particular class, it is not supposed to re-read the class file. Not only is this more efficient, it allows a simpler internal implementation of many methods, including the resolveClass() method.

The Java specification hedges this somewhat by stating that this requirement may change in the future, when the classes will be cached by the virtual machine itself. Hence, the ClassLoader class in JDK 1.0 did not do any caching, and it was up to concrete implementations of class loaders to perform this caching.

Beginning with JDK 1.1, however, caching within the class loader was considered important enough that the base ClassLoader class now performs this caching automatically: a class is put into the cache of the class loader in the defineClass() method and may be retrieved from the cache with the findLoadedClass() method. Since these methods are final, and since the cache itself is a private instance variable of the ClassLoader class, this permits a class loader to be written without any knowledge of whether the class loader or the virtual machine is doing the caching.

---

protected final void resolveClass(Class c)

For a given class, resolve all the immediately needed class references for the class; this will result in recursively calling the class loader to ask it to load the referenced class.

The loadClass() method is responsible for implementing the eight steps of the class definition list given above. Typically, implementation of this method looks like this:

```
protected Class loadClass(String name, boolean resolve) {
    Class c;
    SecurityManager sm = System.getSecurityManager();

    // Step 1 -- Check for a previously loaded class
```

```
    c = findLoadedClass(name);
    if (c != null)
        return c;

    // Step 2 -- Check to make sure that we can access this class
    if (sm != null) {
        int i = name.lastIndexOf('.');
        if (i >= 0)
            sm.checkPackageAccess(name.substring(0, i));
    }

    // Step 3 -- Check for system class first
    try {
        // In 1.2 only, defer to another class loader if available
        if (parent != null)
            c = parent.loadClass(name, resolve);
        else

        // Call this method in both 1.1 and 1.2
            c = findSystemClass(name);

        if (c != null)
            return c;
    } catch (ClassNotFoundException cnfe) {
        // Not a system class, simply continue
    }

    // Step 4 -- Check to make sure that we can define this class
    if (sm != null) {
        int i = name.lastIndexOf('.');
        if (i >= 0)
            sm.checkPackageDefinition(name.substring(0, i));
    }

    // Step 5 -- Read in the class file
    byte data[] = lookupData(name);

    // Step 6 and 7 -- Define the class from the data; this also
    //       passes the data through the bytecode verifier
    c = defineClass(name, data, 0, data.length);

    // Step 8 -- Resolve the internal references of the class
    if (resolve)
        resolveClass(c);

    return c;
}
```

For most of the class loaders we're interested in, this skeleton of a class loader is sufficient, and all we need to change is the definition of the `lookupData()` method (as well as the constructor of the class, which might need various initialization parameters).

This method might be used to implement a 1.1-based class loader, where the `loadClass()` method is abstract. In 1.2, however, it is easier to use the existing `loadClass()` method and override only the existing `findLocalClass()` method:

protected Class findLocalClass(String name) ★

>   Load the given class according to the internal rules of the class loader. This method should assume that it is responsible for implementing only steps 5, 6, and 7 in our list: that is, it should read the data and call the `defineClass()` method, but it needn't look for an existing implementation of the class or check to see if it is a system class. If the class cannot be found, this method should return null (which is what the default implementation of this method returns in all cases).

We'll use this method in our example of a secure class loader. If you must implement a 1.1-based class loader, you can use the code from that example to implement a `lookupData()` method that could be used by the above implementation of the `loadClass()` method.

From a security point of view, the `loadClass()` method is important because it codifies several aspects of how Java handles security. One example of this is that the order in which the `loadClass()` method looks for classes is significant. Much of the security within Java itself depends on classes in the Java API doing the correct thing—e.g., the `java.lang.String` class is `final` and holds the array of characters representing the string in a private instance variable; this allows strings to be considered constants, which is important to several aspects of Java security. When a class loader is asked to find the `java.lang.String` class, it is very important that it return the class from the Java API rather than returning a class (possibly having different and insecure semantics) it loaded from a different location.

Hence, it is important that the class loader call the `findSystemClass()` method immediately after it attempts (and fails) to find the class in its internal cache (via the `findLoadedClass()` method). By codifying this behavior in the `loadClass()` method, the `ClassLoader` class ensures that the class loader will have the correct behavior to enforce the overall security of the virtual machine. This is why the `loadClass()` method is no longer abstract in 1.2. This method really should be made `final` now, but that would break compatibility with previously written class loaders.

Violating security by returning the incorrect class would have required the cooperation of the class loader. This might have happened accidentally, if the author of the class loader did not provide a correct implementation. It might also have

---

Secure Class Loaders and the defineClass() Method

When a class is defined by a secure class loader, one of the parameters that it must specify is a CodeSource object or a ProtectionDomain object. A CodeSource object encapsulates certain information about the class—where it was loaded from and whether or not it was signed (and if so, by whom); a ProtectionDomain object encapsulates information about the specific permissions that have been granted to the class.

We're deferring discussion of these classes until Chapter 5, when we can discuss them in their proper context. For now, we'll just use the getCodeSource() method whenever a code source is necessary and trust it to provide us with the correct object.

---

happened maliciously, if the author of the class loader intentionally wrote an incorrect implementation. The new implementation solves the first problem, but not the second: the author of the class loader can still override the loadClass() method directly to do whatever he wants. In general, you have to trust the author of your class loader anyway, so the new implementation enhances security mostly by assisting developers in writing more robust programs.

Implementing the SecureClassLoader Class

Starting with JDK 1.2, there is an extension of the ClassLoader class that any Java developer can use as the superclass of her own class loader: the SecureClassLoader class (java.security.SecureClassLoader).

In terms of security, the benefit of the SecureClassLoader class comes because it is fully integrated with the notion of protection domains that was introduced in 1.2. We'll discuss this integration more fully in Chapter 5, when we have an understanding of what a protection domain is.

Protected methods of the SecureClassLoader class

The SecureClassLoader class provides these two new methods:

protected final Class defineClass(String name, byte buf[], int offset, int length,
    CodeSource cs, Object signers[])
protected final Class defineClass(String name, byte buf[], int offset, int length,
    ProtectionDomain pd, Object signers[])
    Define a class that is associated with the given code source or protection domain and the given array of signers. Either of these last two parameters

may be null; if both are null, this method is the equivalent of the define-Class() method in the base ClassLoader class.

protected CodeSource getCodeSource(URL url, Object signers[])

Construct a code source based on the given URL and signers; this is the code source that would then be passed to the defineClass() method. It is preferable to construct a code source via this method rather than directly instantiating a code source object, since this method will keep a cache of code source objects, which may be reused.

As our first example of a class loader, we'll use the same paradigm for loading classes that a Java-enabled browser uses, namely an HTTP connection to a web server:

```java
public class JavaRunnerLoader extends SecureClassLoader {
    protected URL urlBase;
    public boolean printLoadMessages = true;

    public JavaRunnerLoader(String base, ClassLoader parent) {
        super(parent);
        try {
            if (!(base.endsWith("/")))
                base = base + "/";
            urlBase = new URL(base);
        } catch (Exception e) {
            throw new IllegalArgumentException(base);
        }
    }

    byte[] getClassBytes(InputStream is) {
        ByteArrayOutputStream baos = new ByteArrayOutputStream();
        BufferedInputStream bis = new BufferedInputStream(is);
        boolean eof = false;
        while (!eof) {
            try {
                int i = bis.read();
                if (i == -1)
                    eof = true;
                else baos.write(i);
            } catch (IOException e) {
                return null;
            }
        }
        return baos.toByteArray();
    }

    protected Class findLocalClass(String name) {
        String urlName = name.replace('.', '/');
        byte buf[];
```

```
        Class cl;

        SecurityManager sm = System.getSecurityManager();
        if (sm != null) {
            int i = name.lastIndexOf('.');
            if (i >= 0)
                sm.checkPackageDefinition(name.substring(0, i));
        }
        try {
            URL url = new URL(urlBase, urlName + ".class");
            if (printLoadMessages)
                System.out.println("Loading " + url);
            InputStream is = url.openConnection().getInputStream();
            buf = getClassBytes(is);
            CodeSource cs = getCodeSource(urlBase, null);
            cl = defineClass(name, buf, 0, buf.length, cs, null);
            return cl;
        } catch (Exception e) {
            System.out.println("Can't load " + name + ": " + e);
            return null;
        }
    }

    public void checkPackageAccess(String name) {
        SecurityManager sm = System.getSecurityManager();
        if (sm != null)
            sm.checkPackageAccess(name);
    }
}
```

The key decision in using this class loader is where the classes are located—that is, the URL that needs to be passed to the constructor. If we were using this class loader in a browser, that URL would be the applet's CODEBASE; for an application, this location is up to the application to decide, using whatever means it deems appropriate (in the JavaRunner application, we used a command-line argument for that purpose). Note that the URL that is passed to the constructor must be a directory; in order to compose that directory into a URL later in the findLocal-Class() method, the name must end with a slash.

The logic of the findLocalClass() method itself is simple: we need to convert the class name (e.g., com.XYZ.HRApplet) to a URL, which we can do by replacing the package-separating periods with slashes. Once the URL has been created, we simply obtain an input stream to the URL, read the bytes from that stream, and pass the bytes to the defineClass() method.

Note that the findLocalClass() method encompasses most of the logic that is necessary for the lookupData() method we'd need if we were writing a 1.1-based class loader. The only difference for a 1.1-based class loader is that we would not need to call the defineClass() method, as that is called in our 1.1-based implementation of the loadClass() method.

The implementation we've just shown is the basis for the implementation of the URLClassLoader class. The basic difference between the two is that our implementation operates on a single URL, while the URLClassLoader class operates on an array of URLs. The URLClassLoader class can also read JAR files while our present implementation can only read individual class files; we'll remedy both those situations in the next section.

Implementing Security Policies in the Class Loader

When we discussed the algorithm used to load classes, we mentioned that you could test to see if the class loader was allowed to access or define the package that the class belonged to. You might, for example, want to test whether the program should be allowed to access classes in the sun package, or define classes in the java package.

It is up to the author of the class loader to put these checks into the class loader—even in 1.2. In 1.2, the loadClass() method does not call the checkPackageAccess() method of the security manager directly (as we did in our skeleton of the loadClass() method): instead, it calls the checkPackageAccess() method of the ClassLoader class. In the ClassLoader class, the checkPackageAccess() method simply returns. Hence, if you want to make the check for package access that we showed earlier, you must override the checkPackageAccess() method in your class loader and insert the appropriate call to the security manager. In 1.1, of course, you have to write the loadClass() method from scratch, so you can call the security manager or not as you deem appropriate.

In the case of defining a class in a package, the necessary code in a 1.2-based class loader must be inserted into the findLocalClass() method as we did in our example class loader. Note that the URL class loader—the only concrete implementation of a class loader in the core API—does not make such a call; it allows you to define a class in any package whatsoever.

For the Launcher (and any applications built on the URLClassLoader class), then, the default security model does not perform either of these checks. This is unfortunate: if a program is allowed to define a class in the java package, then that class will have access to all the package-protected classes and variables within that package, which carries with it some risk. The reason this model is the default has to do with the way in which the access controller defines permissions; we'll explore it more in depth when we write our own security manager in Chapter 6.

Extensions to the Class Loader

When we implemented a class loader above, we had a fully operational class loader that paralleled the first class loaders that were used by Java's `appletviewer` or by a Java-enabled browser. However, there are other extensions to the class loader that are often useful.

Class Loaders and Other Protocols

Long before HTTP and the Web became popular, IP networks like the Internet had dozens of other protocols upon which a class loader could be based—FTP, NFS, RCP, and others. It's possible to write a class loader based on any of these protocols, although it's not as easy as using HTTP. The standard Java URL class will handle all the low-level details of the HTTP protocol for us, whereas we'd have to write the low-level details of the ftp (or whichever) protocol ourselves. We won't show an example of any of these protocols, since the concepts are all the same.

One advantage these protocols have is that they typically offer some level of user authentication: FTP requires a password, NFS requires appropriate credentials to be sent, etc. Hence, some of these protocols might seem well-suited to an implementation where security is a concern—except that this level of authentication is often no stronger than simply putting the classes to be downloaded on a web server that requires a password to get into a particular directory.

Loading from Multiple Sites

We started with a complete class loader suitable for use in `appletviewer`-type programs where the classes are to be loaded from the network. This is good as far as it goes, but let's delve a little more into the security issues that surround that class loader.

In the world of Java-enabled browsers, an applet can retrieve classes from only one site—the CODEBASE specified in the applet's HTML tag. There are other reasons why an applet can only make a network connection to its CODEBASE (which we'll discuss in Chapter 4), but one of the reasons is contained in the discussion we outlined above: because classes loaded by the same class loader are considered to be in the same package, and an applet that loaded classes from multiple sites could run the risk of classes from different sites interfering with each other.

In an ideal world, however, a Java program may want to load classes from several locations on the network. Consider the deployment outlined in Figure 3-2 for XYZ Corporation: XYZ Corporation employs a network support group to manage its departmental servers, and within each department, there are programmers who are responsible for deploying the department's applications on those servers.

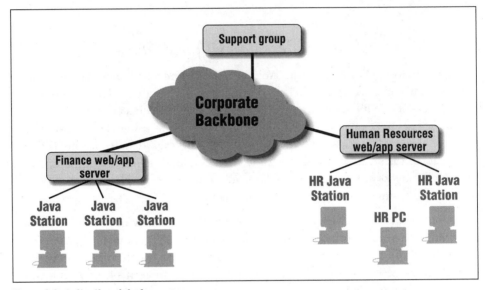

Figure 3-2. A distributed deployment

When the corporate network support group develops some useful JavaBeans™ components, everyone in the corporation is encouraged to use them in their departmentally developed applications. This gives the applications a certain consistency between departments as well as promoting reuse of the efforts of the network support group. But as it stands now, the support group must distribute the Java Bean class files to each department so that these beans can be used by programs that are hosted on each departmental server.

Of course, there are technologies outside of Java that can manage distribution, but this is just a variation of the same application distribution problem that Java was originally hailed for solving. Unfortunately, the single-host-based class loader employed by standard Java-enabled browsers doesn't address this situation.

One improvement that we might make is to allow our class loader to load classes from multiple hosts on the network. There's some overhead involved here: when a program running on a machine on the HR network needs to load a class, does it check for the class on the HR server first or on the support group server first? Either way, there will be a number of lookups that check the wrong server first, which is somewhat inefficient. Judicious use of package names could help: if the support group beans were all placed in a single package, the class loader could be smart enough to contact the support group server only when asked to load classes from that package.

Remember that this intelligence about package names solves a logistical problem as well. Say that the support group writes a Java bean called Check that provides a nice graphical representation of a checkbox; this graphical representation is part of the look-and-feel on which XYZ Corporation wants to standardize. Now the HR group wants to create a payroll application, so they create a Check class representing the financial instrument that is used to pay their employees. Now when an HR applet wants to instantiate a Check object, what is it referring to—a GUI class or a financial instrument?

Solving this problem in the intranet world is straightforward—it's easy for the support and HR groups to coordinate their namespace so that the class loader won't see these collisions (e.g., by having the support group use names in a particular package, which again could make the class loader more efficient). In the case of the freewheeling Internet, this type of coordination is not possible: there can be no guarantee that two unrelated sites won't use classes that are in the same package. So the multiple-site class loader is really only appropriate for intranet use.

There are various ways in which the multiple-site class loader could be implemented—for this example, we'll assume that any classes that are in the com.XYZ.support package should be loaded from the network support group's server (which we'll hardcode into the class loader, though we would normally configure this to be a property). Any other classes should come from the server that initialized the class loader. So our new class loader looks like this:

```
public class MultiLoader extends JavaRunnerLoader {
    private static final String server = "support.xyz.com/";

    public MultiLoader(String url, ClassLoader parent) {
        super(url, parent);
    }

    protected Class findLocalClass(String name) {
        URL codeURL;

        SecurityManager sm = System.getSecurityManager();
        if (sm != null) {
            int i = name.lastIndexOf('.');
            if (i >= 0)
                sm.checkPackageDefinition(name.substring(0, i));
        }

        try {
```

```
            String codeName = name.replace('.', '/') + ".class";
            if (name.startsWith("com.xyz.support"))
                codeURL = new URL("http://" + server + codeName);
            else codeURL = new URL(urlBase, codeName);
            if (printLoadMessages)
                System.out.println("Loading " + name);
            InputStream is = codeURL.openConnection().getInputStream();
            byte buf[] = getClassBytes(is);
            return defineClass(name, buf, 0, buf.length, cs, null);
        } catch (Exception e) {
            return null;
        }
    }
}
```

If you're thinking clearly about the security ramifications of this code, then you've already spotted a potential error: just because we're asked to load a class named com.xyz.support.Car doesn't necessarily mean that we should contact our internal server to do so—we should only contact that internal server if the other classes that we are loading are also from our internal network. That is, if we use this class loader in a browser that is loading an applet from *www.EvilSite.org* that requests the class com.xyz.support.Car, we should attempt to load that class from *EvilSite* and not from our support group's server; we should only load com.xyz.support classes from *support.xyz.com* when the other classes in the program come from another machine in the *xyz.com* domain.

We could have put the logic to deal with that possibility into the class loader itself; however, it's equally possible to put that logic elsewhere into our application. The JavaRunner program, for example, must instantiate a new class loader for each program it loads, and it's simpler to instantiate a MultiLoader class loader when the program is being loaded from a machine within the *xyz.com* domain, and to instantiate a regular JavaRunnerLoader when the program is being loaded from a machine outside the *xyz.com* domain.

Note the different approach taken here and in the URLClassLoader class: in this case, we contact a second machine only when we have classes in a particular package that we expect to find on that machine. If we had constructed a URLClassLoader as follows:

```
URL urls[] = new URL[2];
url[0] = new URL("http://hr.xyz.com/");
url[1] = new URL("http://support.xyz.com/");
URLClassLoader ucl = new URLClassLoader(urls);
```

then we would have functionally achieved something similar. However, with the URL class loader, when we search for a class named com.xyz.support.Check, we'll always contact the HR server first, which is slightly less efficient. On the other hand, the technique used by the URL class loader is clearly more flexible than the approach we've outlined above.

A JAR File Class Loader

There is one important feature present in many class loaders that we haven't yet mentioned, and that is the ability to load a single file that contains many classes. JAR files have a significant advantage over individual class files: loading several classes in a single file can be orders of magnitude faster than loading those same classes through individual HTTP connections. The reason for this comes from a property of the HTTP protocol: it takes a relatively long time to set up an HTTP connection. In fact, the time it takes to transfer the data in a Java class file over a network is usually much shorter than the time required to set up the HTTP connection. Hence, JAR files are often preferred because they can greatly speed up the time it takes to download an applet.

In browsers based on 1.0.2, support for JAR files is browser-dependent; those browsers that support them refer to the JAR file as an archive. In browsers based on 1.1, support for JAR files is present within the JDK itself using classes in the java.util.zip package, because a JAR file is really just a zip file with some additional information. In Java 1.2, there is an additional set of classes in the java.util.jar package that can help to process these files as well (including the additional information in the JAR file).

Of course, there's a flip side to using JAR files. If you use a large word-processing program in Java, you'll probably want to avoid loading a lot of the classes when you download the program: there's no need to spend the time downloading all the class files that implement the spellchecker until it is actually time to check the document's spelling. With JAR files, you don't have that luxury; you must load all the classes in a single shot. Even in those browsers in which you can specify multiple JAR files, the class loader has no way of knowing which particular JAR file contains which particular classes, so it still has to load all of them at once.*

Nevertheless, JAR files are very popular, and they certainly have their place for programs where all (or at least most) of the classes are likely to be used every time the program is run. So we'll look into the additions that must be made to our class loader in order for it to support loading a JAR file. This may seem to be taking us somewhat far afield of our discussion about application security, but there is another reason JAR files are important: they provide the necessary support for digitally signed classes. We typically speak of a signed class as an entity

---

* A Java application could be more clever about this: it could know to load the archive containing the classes to perform the spellcheck when it was time to run the spellchecker. But an applet cannot do that, because an applet has no mechanism that it can use to tell the browser to load a new archive.

unto itself; in fact, a signed class can only be delivered as part of a JAR file. Hence, a class loader that can process JAR files is very important.

So, to complete our understanding of the class loader and to prepare us for those future examples, we'll show how to add JAR support to our custom class loader. In order to support a JAR file, we'll create a new class. Although the logic is similar to our JavaRunnerLoader class, we get no benefit from extending that class, so we'll show the full implementation here. Changes to the JavaRunnerLoader class are shown in bold.

```
public class JarLoader extends SecureClassLoader {
    private URL urlBase;
    public boolean printLoadMessages = true;
    Hashtable classArrays;
    CodeSource cs;

    public JarLoader(String base, ClassLoader parent) {
        super(parent);
        try {
            if (!(base.endsWith("/")))
                base = base + "/";
            urlBase = new URL(base);
            classArrays = new Hashtable();
            cs = getCodeSource(urlBase, null);
        } catch (Exception e) {
            throw new IllegalArgumentException(base);
        }
    }

    private byte[] getClassBytes(InputStream is) {
        ByteArrayOutputStream baos = new ByteArrayOutputStream();
        BufferedInputStream bis = new BufferedInputStream(is);
        boolean eof = false;
        while (!eof) {
            try {
                int i = bis.read();
                if (i == -1)
                    eof = true;
                else baos.write(i);
            } catch (IOException e) {
                return null;
            }
        }
        return baos.toByteArray();
    }

    protected Class findLocalClass(String name) {
        String urlName = name.replace('.', '/');
        byte buf[];
        Class cl;
```

```
    SecurityManager sm = System.getSecurityManager();
    if (sm != null) {
        int i = name.lastIndexOf('.');
        if (i >= 0)
            sm.checkPackageDefinition(name.substring(0, i));
    }

    buf = (byte[]) classArrays.get(urlName);
    if (buf != null) {
        cl = defineClass(name, buf, 0, buf.length, cs, null);
        return cl;
    }

    try {
        URL url = new URL(urlBase, urlName + ".class");
        if (printLoadMessages)
            System.out.println("Loading " + url);
        InputStream is = url.openConnection().getInputStream();
        buf = getClassBytes(is);
        cl = defineClass(name, buf, 0, buf.length, cs, null);
        return cl;
    } catch (Exception e) {
        System.out.println("Can't load " + name + ": " + e);
        return null;
    }
}

public void readJarFile(String name) {
    URL jarUrl = null;
    JarInputStream jis;
    JarEntry je;

    try {
        jarUrl = new URL(urlBase, name);
    } catch (MalformedURLException mue) {
        System.out.println("Unknown jar file " + name);
        return;
    }
    if (printLoadMessages)
        System.out.println("Loading jar file " + jarUrl);

    try {
        jis = new JarInputStream(
                    jarUrl.openConnection().getInputStream());
    } catch (IOException ioe) {
        System.out.println("Can't open jar file " + jarUrl);
        return;
    }
```

```
        try {
            while ((je = jis.getNextJarEntry()) != null) {
                String jarName = je.getName();
                if (jarName.endsWith(".class"))
                    loadClassBytes(jis, jarName);
                // else ignore it; it could be an image or audio file
                jis.closeEntry();
            }
        } catch (IOException ioe) {
            System.out.println("Badly formatted jar file");
        }
    }


    private void loadClassBytes(JarInputStream jis, String jarName) {
        if (printLoadMessages)
            System.out.println("\t" + jarName);
        BufferedInputStream jarBuf = new BufferedInputStream(jis);
        ByteArrayOutputStream jarOut = new ByteArrayOutputStream();
        int b;
        try {
            while ((b = jarBuf.read()) != -1)
                jarOut.write(b);
            classArrays.put(jarName.substring(0, jarName.length() - 6),
                            jarOut.toByteArray());
        } catch (IOException ioe) {
            System.out.println("Error reading entry " + jarName);
        }
    }


    public void checkPackageAccess(String name) {
        SecurityManager sm = System.getSecurityManager();
        if (sm != null)
            sm.checkPackageAccess(name);
    }
}
```

The bulk of the change in this example is the addition of two new methods (the readJarFile() and loadClassBytes() methods). These two new methods are used to process the JAR file.

The classes in the java.util.jar package handle all the details about the JAR file for us, and we're left with a simple implementation: we use the getNext-JarEntry() method to obtain each file in the archive and process each one sequentially. For maximum efficiency, we don't actually need to create the class from the bytes until necessary: the loadClassBytes() method just creates an array of bytes for each class in the JAR file.

This necessitates a slight change to the logic in our findLocalClass() method: now when we need to provide a class that is not a system class, we check first to see if that class is in the `classArrays` hashtable. If it is, we obtain the bytes for the class from that hashtable (where they were stored in the `readJarFile()` method) rather than opening a URL to obtain the bytes for the class over the network.

If you need to produce a similar class loader under 1.1, you can use the `java.util.zip` package instead of the `java.util.jar` package. In this example, the two are functionally equivalent, and you may simply substitute `Zip` every time you see `Jar` (and `zip` for `jar`) with one exception: replace the `getNextJarEntry()` method with the `getNextEntry()` method. Later, when we deal with signed JAR files, that substitution will not work: the difference between the two packages is that the `jar` package understands the signature format and manifest of the JAR file.

This implementation is similar to the procedure followed by the `URLClassLoader` class; in that case, the JAR files occur as elements in the array of URLs passed to the class.

Miscellaneous Class Loading Topics

There are a few details that we haven't yet covered. These details are not directly related to the security aspects of the class loader, which is why we've saved them until now. If you're interested in the complete details of the class loader, we'll fill in the last few topics here.

Delegation

Beginning with Java 1.2, class loading follows a delegation model. This new model permits a class loader to be instantiated with this constructor:

protected ClassLoader(ClassLoader delegate) ★

Create a class loader that is associated with the given class loader. This class loader delegates all operations to the delegate first: if the delegate is able to fulfill the operation, this class loader takes no action. For example, when the class loader is asked to load a class via the `loadClass()` method, it first calls the `loadClass()` method of the delegate. If that succeeds, the class returned by the delegate will ultimately be returned by this class. If that fails, the class loader then uses its original logic to complete its task:

```
public Class loadClass(String name) {
    Class cl;
    cl = delegate.loadClass(name);
    if (cl != null)
        return cl;
    // else continue with the loadClass() logic
}
```

You may retrieve the delegate associated with a class loader with this method:

public ClassLoader getParent() ★

> Return the class loader to which operations are being delegated. If there is no
> such class loader, return null.

You'll notice that we used delegation in all of our examples. This is pretty much a
requirement: when the virtual machine starts, it creates a URL class loader that is
based on the directories and JAR files present in your CLASSPATH. That class
loader is the class loader that will be used to load the first class in your application
(i.e., the JavaRunner class in our example).

That URL class loader is the only class loader that knows about the CLASSPATH. If
the application will reference any other classes that are part of the CLASSPATH,
you will be unable to find them unless you use the delegation model of class
loading: the JavaRunner loader will first ask the URL class loader to load the
class. If the class is on the CLASSPATH, the URL class loader will succeed; otherwise, the JavaRunner loader will end up loading the class itself. This logic is built
into the loadClass() method; you do not need to concern yourself with it at a
programming level, but it is the reason why you must use delegation.

Loading Resources

A class loader can load not only classes, but any arbitrary resource: an audio file,
an image file, or anything else. Instead of calling the loadClass() method, a
resource is obtained by invoking one of these methods:

public URL getResource(String name)
public InputStream getResourceAsStream(String name)
public URL getLocalResource(String name) ★

> Find the named resource and return either a URL reference to it or an input
> stream from which it can be read. Implementations of class loaders should
> look for resources according to their internal rules, which are typically (but
> need not be) the same rules as are used to find classes. In our first JavaRun-
> nerLoader class, that would mean simply constructing a URL based on the
> urlBase concatenated with the name parameter.

> In 1.1, the default behavior for these methods is to return null.

> In 1.2, the getResource() method calls the getSystemResource() method;
> if it does not find a system resource, it returns the object retrieved by a call to
> the getLocalResource() method (which by default will still be null). The
> getResourceAsStream() method simply calls the getResource() method
> and, if a resource is found, open the stream associated with the URL.

public static URL getSystemResource(String name)
public static InputStream getSystemResourceAsStream(String name)

> Find the named resource and return either a URL reference to it or an input stream from which it can be read. By default, these methods look for the resource on the CLASSPATH and return that resource (if found).

public final Enumeration getResources(String name) ★
public Enumeration getLocalResources(String name) ★

> Return an enumeration of resources with the given name. In the first method, an enumeration of the local resources of all delegated class loaders (including the present class loader) is returned; in the second method, only the local resources of the present class loader are returned.

Summary

The class loading mechanism is integral to Java's security features. Typically this integration is considered in light of the relationship between the class loader and the security manager. However, the class loader is important in its own right. The class loader must enforce the namespace separation between classes that are loaded from different sites (especially when these different sites are untrusted). Newer versions of the class loader (in Java 1.2) provide an easier route for developers of class loaders, and they provide more hooks into the access controller.

For sites that need a more flexible security policy, a different class loader may be desirable. For example, a class loader that allows programs within a protected, internal network to load class files from several machines on that internal network is particularly useful for extending the advantages that the Java model brings to program distribution. Other variations on this theme are possible—as long as the implementor remembers to keep the security requirements of Java's namespace model in mind when such variations are designed.

In the next chapters, we'll look in depth at Java's security manager and Java's protection domains, and see how the class loader and these features together further enforce Java's security policies.

4

In this chapter:
- *Overview of the Security Manager*
- *Trusted and Untrusted Classes*
- *Using the Security Manager*

The Security Manager Class

When most people think of Java security, they think of the protections afforded to a Java program—and, more particularly, only by default to a Java applet—by Java's security manager. As we've seen, there are other important facets of Java's security story, but the role played by the security manager is of paramount importance in the degree to which your machine will be safe from malicious Java programs.

On one level, the Java security manager is simple to understand, and it's often summarized by saying that it prevents Java applets from accessing your local disk or local network. The real story is more complicated than that, however, with the result that Java's security manager is often misunderstood. In this chapter, we'll look into how the security manager actually works, what it can and can't do, and when it does—and doesn't—protect you. In this chapter, we're only going to look at the security manager in terms of its capabilities, with an emphasis on how those capabilities are used by popular browsers; we'll look into writing our own security manager in the next few chapters.

Overview of the Security Manager

On a simple level, the security manager is responsible for determining most of the parameters of the Java sandbox—that is, it is ultimately up to the security manager to determine whether many particular operations should be permitted or rejected. If a Java program attempts to open a file, the security manager decides whether or not that operation should be permitted. If a Java program wants to connect to a particular machine on the network, it must first ask permission of the security manager. If a Java program wants to alter the state of certain threads, the security manager will intervene if such an operation is considered dangerous.

The security manager is of particular concern to authors and users of Java applets. In general, Java applications do not have security managers—unless the author of the application has provided one. Historically, that's been a somewhat unusual occurrence, even though there are many times when you might want a security manager in your Java application; this stems from the fact that before Java 1.2, writing a security manager was more difficult than it is now. Beginning in 1.2, there is a default, user-configurable security manager that is suitable for most applications, one which can even be installed via a command-line argument when starting an application. This brings the benefits of a security manager to an application without requiring any programming. And we'll show how to write your own (non-default) security manager for the JavaRunner program in Chapter 6.

But this point cannot be overemphasized: Java applications (at least by default) have no security manager, while Java applets (again, by default) have a very strict security manager. This leads to a common misconception that exists in the arena of Java security: it's common to think that because Java is said to be secure, it is always secure, and that running Java applications that have been installed locally is just as secure as running Java applets inside a Java-enabled browser. Nothing is further from the truth.

To illustrate this point, consider the following malicious code:

```
public class MaliciousApplet extends Applet {
    public void init() {
        try {
            Runtime.getRuntime().exec("/bin/rm -rf .");
        } catch (Exception e) {}
    }
    public static void main(String args[]) {
        MaliciousApplet a = new MaliciousApplet();
        a.init();
    }
}
```

If you compile this code, place it on your web server, and load it as an applet, you'll get an error reflecting a security violation. However, if you compile this code, place it in a directory, and run it as an application, you'll end up deleting all the files in your current directory.* As a user, then, it's crucial that you understand which security manager is in place when you run a Java program so that you understand just what types of operations you are protected against.

---

* The example will only delete the files in your current directory if you run it on a Unix system, but we could have included similar code for any other operating system.

Security Managers and the Java API

The security manager can be considered a partnership between the Java API and the implementor of a specific Java application or of a specific Java-enabled browser. There is a class in the Java API called SecurityManager (java.lang.SecurityManager) which is the linchpin of this partnership—it provides the interface that the rest of the Java API uses to check whether particular operations are to be permitted. The essential algorithm the Java API uses to perform a potentially dangerous operation is always the same:

1. The programmer makes a request of the Java API to perform an operation.

2. The Java API asks the security manager if such an operation is allowable.

3. If the security manager does not want to permit the operation, it throws an exception back to the Java API, which in turn throws it back to the user.

4. Otherwise, the Java API completes the operation and returns normally.

Let's trace this idea with the example that we first saw in Chapter 1:

```
public class Cat {
    public static void main(String args[]) {
        try {
            String s;
            FileReader fr = new FileReader(args[0]);
            BufferedReader br = new BufferedReader(fr);
            while ((s = br.readLine()) != null)
                System.out.println(s);
        } catch (Exception e) {
            System.out.println(e);
        }
    }
}
```

The FileReader object will in turn create a FileInputStream object, and constructing the input stream is the first step of the algorithm. When the input stream is constructed, the Java API performs code similar to this:

```
public FileInputStream(String name) throws FileNotFoundException {
    SecurityManager security = System.getSecurityManager();
    if (security != null) {
        security.checkRead(name);
    }
    try {
        open(name); // open() is a private method of this class
    } catch (IOException e) {
        throw new FileNotFoundException(name);
    }
}
```

This is step two of our algorithm and is the essence of the idea behind the security manager: when the Java API wants to perform an operation, it first checks with the security manager and then calls a private method (the open() method in this case) that actually performs the operation.

Meanwhile, the security manager code is responsible for deciding whether or not the file in question should be allowed to be read and, if not, for throwing a security exception:

```
public class SecurityManagerImpl extends SecurityManager {
    public void checkRead(String s) {
        if (theFileIsNotAllowedToBeRead)
            throw new SecurityException("checkRead");
    }
}
```

The SecurityException class is a subclass of the RuntimeException class. Remember that runtime exceptions are somewhat different than other exceptions in Java in that they do not have to be caught in the code—which is why the check-Read() method does not have to declare that it throws that exception, and the FileInputStream constructor does not have to catch it. So if the security exception is thrown by the checkRead() method, the FileInputStream constructor will return before it calls the open() method—which is simply to say that the input file will never be opened, because the security manager prevented that code from being executed.

Typically, the security exception propagates up through all the methods in the thread that made the call; eventually, the top-most method receives the exception, which causes that thread to exit. When the thread exits in this way, it prints out the exception and the stack trace of methods that led it to receive the exception. This leads to the messages that you've probably seen in your Java console:

```
sun.applet.AppletSecurityException: checkread
        at sun.applet.AppletSecurity.checkRead(AppletSecurity.java:427)
        at java.io.FileOutputStream.<init>(FileOutputStream.java)
        at Cat.init(Cat.java:7)
        at sun.applet.AppletPanel.run(AppletPanel.java:273)
        at java.lang.Thread.run(Thread.java)
```

If the security exception is not thrown—that is, if the security manager decides that the particular operation should be allowed—then the method in the security manager simply returns, and everything proceeds as expected.

Several methods in the SecurityManager class are similar to the checkRead() method. It is up to the Java API to call those methods at the appropriate time. You may want to call those methods from your own Java code (using the technique shown above), but that's never required. Since the Java API provides the interface to the virtual operating system for the Java program, it's possible to isolate all the necessary security checks within the Java API itself.

You Don't Know About All Security Violations

Since a violation of the rules of the security manager manifests itself as a security exception, it's possible to hide the attempted violation from the user running the program by catching that exception.

To portray this feature in a positive light, it allows the author of a Java program to provide a more intelligent program that might be delivered to an end user in different ways. If the program is delivered as an application, the author may want to save some state from the program in a file on the user's disk; if the program is delivered as an applet, the author will need to save that state by sending it to the web server. So the program might have code that looks like this:

```
OutputStream os;
try {
    os = new FileOutputStream("statefile");
} catch (SecurityException e) {
    os = new Socket(webhost, webport).getOutputStream();
}
```

Now the Java program has an appropriate output stream where it can save its data.

On the other hand, this technique can be used by the author of an applet to probe your browser's security manager without your knowledge—because the applet is catching the security exceptions, you'll never see them. This is one reason why it's important to understand the ramifications of adjusting your browser's security policy.

One exception to this guideline occurs when you extend the virtual operating system of the Java API, and it is important to ensure that your extensions are well-integrated into Java's security scheme. Certain parts of the Java API—the `Toolkit` class, the `Provider` class, the `Socket` class, and others—are written in such a way that they allow you to provide your own implementation of those classes. If you're providing your own implementation of any of these classes, you have to make sure that it calls the security manager at appropriate times.

It's important to note that there is (by design) no attempt in the Java API to keep any sort of state. Whenever the Java API needs to perform an operation, it checks with the security manager to see if the operation is to be allowed—even if that same operation has been permitted by the security manager before. This is because the context of the operation is often significant—the security manager might allow a `FileOutputStream` object to be opened in some cases (e.g., by certain classes) while it might deny it in other cases. The Java API cannot keep track of this contextual information, so it asks the security manager for permission to perform every operation.

Trusted and Untrusted Classes

In the discussion that follows, we make the distinction between trusted and untrusted classes. Generally, an implementation of a security manager allows more operations for trusted classes than for untrusted classes. Whether or not a class is trusted is a complex decision based upon many factors—not the least of which is the release of Java under which the program is running. The default notion of what constitutes a trusted class has changed significantly between releases of Java:

- In Java 1.0, a class that is loaded from the CLASSPATH is considered trusted, and a class that is loaded from a class loader is considered untrusted.

- In Java 1.1, that same rule applies, but a class that is loaded from a JAR file may carry with it a digital signature that allows it to be given extra privileges.

- In Java 1.2, a class that is loaded from the core API is considered trusted and may perform any operation it wants to. Otherwise, classes are (by default) given privileges based upon where they were loaded from, including if they were loaded from the CLASSPATH. However, this applies only when certain command-line arguments are present; in the default method of loading applications, items from the CLASSPATH are generally considered trusted.

Nothing inherent in the design of the security manager requires security to be enforced as an all-or-nothing proposition for each class. It's possible to write a security manager that gives access to certain parts of the filesystem only to certain classes (even classes that came from the network), or to write a security manager that prohibits classes loaded from the CLASSPATH from performing operations that are normally permitted to classes loaded from the filesystem. A security manager can be as simple or as sophisticated as its author desires, with the result that the security manager can enforce a simple binary yes-or-no policy for operations, or it can enforce a very specialized, very detailed policy. This is true of all security managers in all versions of Java, though as we'll see in Chapter 5, one of the prime benefits of Java 1.2 is that it makes it much easier to achieve fine-grained security policies.

However, even though a sophisticated security manager can enforce a very detailed security policy, most implementations of the security manager (especially implementations that occur within popular Java-enabled browsers) assume that a trusted class is one that has been loaded from the CLASSPATH, while an untrusted class is one that has been loaded from a class loader. Furthermore, trusted classes are normally permitted to perform any operation, while an untrusted class is normally subjected to the full extent of the provisions of the security manager.

This dichotomy is essentially the same as the one we normally make between applications and applets: since an application is loaded entirely through the CLASSPATH, all of its classes are considered trusted, and the application can perform any operation that it wants to. On the other hand, the classes that comprise an applet are generally loaded from the network; hence they are considered untrusted and denied any operation that has the potential to violate the browser's security policy.

Beginning with Java 1.1, this distinction became less clear (and Java 1.2 made it even fuzzier): classes now have the ability to be signed, and classes that are signed can be treated as trusted or untrusted. We discuss the rationale behind that idea in Chapter 7 and we fully explore signed classes in the last part of this book; for now, we'll just keep in mind that some classes are trusted and some are not.

Using the Security Manager

We're now going to examine the public methods of the security manager so that we may understand how the security manager is used by applications and by the Java API.

Setting a Security Manager

There are two methods in the System class that are used to work with the security manager itself:

public static SecurityManager getSecurityManager()
> Return a reference to the currently installed security manager object (or null if no security manager is in place). Once obtained, this object can be used to test against various security policies.

public static void setSecurityManager(SecurityManager sm)
> Set the system's security manager to the given object. This method can only be called once, and once installed, the security manager cannot be removed. Attempting to call this method after a security manger has already been installed will result in a SecurityException.

These methods operate with the understanding that there is a single security manager in the virtual machine; the only operations that are possible on the security manager are setting it (that is, creating an instance of the security manager class and telling the virtual machine that the newly created object should be the security manager), and getting it (that is, asking the virtual machine to return the object that is the security manager so that a method might be invoked upon it).

We've already seen how you might use the getSecurityManager() method to retrieve the security manager and invoke an operation on it. Setting the security manager is a predictably simple operation:

```
public class TestSecurityManager {
    public static void main(String args[]) {
        System.setSecurityManager(new SecurityManagerImpl());
        ... do the work of the application ...
    }
}
```

However, there's an important detail here: the setSecurityManager() method is written in such a way that it can only be called once. Once a particular security manager has been installed, that security manager will be used by every other class that runs in this virtual machine. Once the policy is established, it cannot be changed (although the policy itself might be very fluid).

This fact has two important ramifications. First, as the author, it's up to you to write a security manager that embodies all the security policies you want your Java application to have. Second, in a Java-enabled browser, the security manager is always set as the browser initializes itself. This makes it impossible for an applet to set the security manager—it must live with the policy established by the author of the browser. This, of course, is a crucial feature of the security manager: since the security manager is responsible for fencing in the applet, it would be a catastrophe if the applet could change the security manager and hence the security policies of the browser.

The real significance of this last point, however, is that it is up to the developer of a browser to set the security policy. There is no absolute security policy that is common to every Java-enabled browser; each company that supports one is free to develop its own security manager and, accordingly, the security policies of that browser.

Now that we have an understanding of how the security manager works, we'll look into what protection the security manager actually provides. We'll discuss the public methods of the security manager that perform security checks and when those methods are called, along with the rationale behind each of the methods. Since these methods are all public, they can be called anywhere, including in your own code, although as we've mentioned, that's a rare thing.

When we discuss the rationale for each of the methods in the SecurityManager class, we'll discuss them from the point of view of untrusted classes. For now, consider an untrusted class as one loaded from the network (i.e., as part of an applet), while a trusted class is one that has been loaded from the filesystem through the user's CLASSPATH (including the classes that are part of the Java-enabled browser itself).

Methods Relating to File Access

The most well-known methods of the security manager class handle access to files on the local network. This includes any files that are on the local disk as well as files that might be physically located on another machine but appear (through the use of NFS, NetWare, Samba, or a similar network-based filesystem) to be part of the local filesystem.

These are the methods the security manager uses to track file access:

public void checkRead(FileDescriptor fd)
public void checkRead(String file)
public void checkRead(String file, Object context)

    Check whether the program is allowed to read the given file. The last method in this list is not used by the Java API itself.

public void checkWrite(FileDescriptor fd)
public void checkWrite(String file)

    Check whether the program is allowed to write the given file.

public void checkDelete(String file)

    Check whether the program is allowed to delete the given file.

Interestingly, although as developers we tend to think of other file operations—such as creating a file or seeing when the file was last modified—as being distinct operations, as far as security is concerned, the Java API considers all operations to be either reading, writing, or deleting.

Table 4-1 lists the Java API interaction with the checkRead(), checkWrite(), and checkDelete() methods, listing when and why each check is invoked. In all the tables in this chapter, the syntax may imply that the calling methods are all static, but that of course is not the case: the entry File.canRead() means the canRead() method invoked on an instance of the File class.

This table lists only those classes that directly call the security manager method in question. There may be many routes through the Java API that lead to one of these checks; for example, when a FileReader object is constructed, it will construct a FileInputStream object, which will result in a call to checkRead().

Table 4-1. Check Methods

Method	Calling Methods	Rationale
checkRead()	File.canRead()	Test if the current thread can read the file
	FileInputStream() RandomAccessFile()	Constructing a file object requires that you must be able to read the file
	File.isDirectory() File.isFile()	Determining whether a file object is an actual file or a directory requires that you must be able to read the file
	File.lastModified()	Determining the modification date requires that you read the file's attributes
	File.length()	Determining the length requires that you read the files attributes
	File.list()	Determining the files in a directory requires that you read the directory
checkWrite()	File.canWrite()	Test if the current thread can write the file
	FileOutputStream() RandomAccessFile()	To construct a file object, you must be able to write the file
	File.mkdir()	To create a directory, you must be able to write to the filesystem
	File.renameTo()	To rename a file, you must be able to write to the directory containing the file
	File.createTemp-File() ★	To create a temporary file, you must be able to write the file
checkDelete()	File.delete()	Test if the current thread can delete a file
	File.deleteOnExit() ★	Test if the current thread can delete the file when the virtual machine exits

By default, in most Java-enabled browsers, untrusted classes are not allowed any sort of file access, for these reasons:

- If an untrusted class is allowed to read an arbitrary file, it might read your password file, or the data file from your tax preparation program, or the temporary file containing an edit log of the sensitive document you're working on.

- If an untrusted class is allowed to write an arbitrary file, it might overwrite data on your machine, essentially erasing the file. Worse, it might insert a virus into an existing file (or create a new file with a virus), with catastrophic results. Less damaging, but still a problem, would be the ability for the applet to completely fill the available disk space.

- If an untrusted class is allowed to delete files, it could destroy any data in your local filesystem.

The Real Reason Applets Cannot Access Files

If you're a Java developer chafing at the restriction that an applet cannot access the user's local files, you're missing one of the points of developing in Java. The real reason your applet can't access local files is that there may not be any: what if your applet is being run on a network computer or a Java-enabled TV webtop? If your applet requires a local disk, it will be unable to run on the next generation of computing devices. Java is leading-edge technology; if you're riding the next wave, you may as well take full advantage of it—there is a wealth of middleware Java tools that will allow you to easily read and write files from and to a remote web server or file server.

Some Java developers consider this strict restriction on file access unnecessarily draconian—they'd seek a compromise where at least some access to some local files is possible. The types of suggested compromises are things like:

- Untrusted classes should be allowed access to the system's temporary directory.

  The problem with this is that other programs might have left sensitive data in that directory. If I'm editing salary data on my machine, I wouldn't want some untrusted class to come along and see the edit log that exists in the system's temporary directory.

- A single directory could be set up for the exclusive use of untrusted classes.

  This does not prevent a bad untrusted class from accessing, erasing, or corrupting the data files of other untrusted programs.

- An individual directory could be set up for each applet (or for each package of untrusted classes).

  This would work in theory, but such a scheme would be unwieldy. It also leaves potential attack routes for an applet. On the Internet, one site can pretend to be another site by engaging in IP spoofing (see the discussion in "The Need for Authentication" in Chapter 7); applets from such sites could read data from the original applet. In addition, an applet could still fill the available disk space.

- The user could be prompted before an untrusted class accessed a file.

  This issue is less black-and-white. On the one hand, there's a persuasive argument that computer users are pretty intelligent, and they'll know whether or not a program should be allowed to access the file in question. In the real world, however, there are users who will not pay enough attention to such prompts and always grant access, to the detriment of their system's security. You may not have much sympathy for users on home computers who grant an applet access to the data file of their financial package, but the user on a corporate or campus network who allows an applet access to his or her password file harms other users of the network as well.

Nonetheless, as with all policies enforced by the security manager, it is up to the author of a particular program (or web browser) to establish the policy the security manager will enforce. Hence, while Netscape Navigator, Internet Explorer, and HotJava all have a default policy that prevents untrusted classes from all file access, some of them allow the user to configure a different policy. HotJava and the JDK's `appletviewer`, for example, allow the user to create a set of directories in which applets can read and write files, and some versions of Internet Explorer allow the user to grant file access to all untrusted classes.

There is one exception to the rule about file access: applets that are loaded from a CODEBASE that specifies `file` as its protocol (e.g., *file:/myapplets*) are allowed to read (but not create or delete) files in the CODEBASE directory (and any of its subdirectories). This is required to allow the applet to load other resources—audio files, images, as well as other classes—in the same manner in which it would load those resources through an HTTP-based URL.

If you carefully considered the list of methods in the tables above, you were probably surprised not to see an obvious method to check: the actual `read()` or `write()` methods of any of the `File` classes. The assumption here is that a trusted class is responsible for determining the security policy associated with any particular `File` object; if the trusted class decides that it is okay for an untrusted class to perform I/O on a particular `File*Stream` object, then it is free to deliver that object to the untrusted class, and the untrusted class is free to read or write to that object. This implementation also allows for much greater efficiency: if the program had to check with the security manager every time it called the `read()` or `write()` methods, I/O performance would drastically suffer.

Methods Relating to Network Access

Network access in Java is always accomplished by opening a network socket, whether directly through the `Socket` class or indirectly through another class like the `URL` class. An untrusted class can only (by default) open a socket to the machine from which it was actually downloaded; typically, this is the location given by the CODEBASE tag in the HTML for the browser page containing the applet or—in the absence of such a tag—the web server for the page. In either case, the machine in question is a web server, so we'll use that terminology in this discussion.

This restriction on untrusted classes is designed to prevent two types of attack. The first attack concerns a rogue applet using your machine for malicious purposes by connecting to a third machine over the network. The canonical description of this attack is an applet that connects to the mail server on someone else's machine and sends people on that machine offensive email from your address. There are more severe attacks possible with this technique, however—such an applet could use a connection from your machine to break into a third computer; auditors on that third computer will think the break-in attempts are coming from you, which can cause you all sorts of legal problems.

The second sort of attack concerns network information on your local network that you might not want to be broadcast to the world at large. Typically, computers at corporations or campuses sit behind a firewall so that users on the Internet cannot access those computers (see Figure 4-1). The firewall allows only certain types of traffic through (e.g., HTTP traffic), so that users on the local network can access the Internet, but users on the Internet cannot glean any information about the local network.

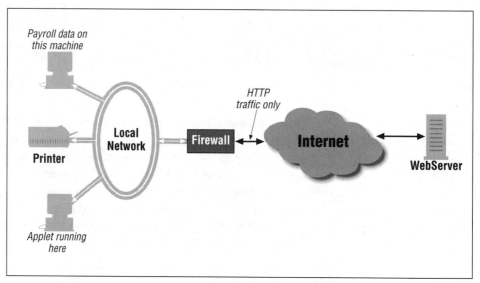

Figure 4-1. A typical firewall configuration

Now consider what happens if an applet downloaded onto a machine on the local network can connect to other machines on the local network. This allows the applet to gather all sorts of information about the local network topology and network services and to send that information (via HTTP, so that it will pass through the firewall) back out onto the Internet. Such an opportunity for corporate spying would be very tempting to would-be hackers. Worse, if the applet had access to arbitrary network services, it could break into the local HR database and steal employee data, or it could break into a network file server and steal corporate documents. Hence, applets (and untrusted classes in general) are prevented from arbitrary network access.

The Real Reason Why Network Access Is Limited

Just when you realized that your applet couldn't access files in the new network computing model and thus had to send all its data over the network comes this restriction of limited network access.

But even if this restriction didn't exist in Java, the configuration of many sites dictates a harsher restriction for network access anyway—the corporate or campus firewall. The firewall often restricts all traffic between the applet's web server and the user's browser to a set of protocols and, possibly, a set of hosts. If you're going to write really effective network applets with Java, you have to take this into account anyway—which means that all your network access really needs to use something called HTTP-tunneling to work.

HTTP-tunneling means that all requests between the applet and the network service running on the web server are encapsulated to look like normal HTTP (web browsing) traffic. This allows the data to go through firewalls that filter out traffic based on protocol. And by only connecting back to the web server, the data will pass through firewalls that filter out traffic based on the destination. There are a variety of well-known techniques for accomplishing HTTP-tunneling via the URL class, and RMI gives you such tunneling transparently.

So, once again, if you're going to write applets that take advantage of the full power of Java, Java's network security restrictions won't get in your way—you'll have worked around them anyway.

Network sockets can be logically divided into two classes: client sockets and server sockets. A client socket is responsible for initiating a conversation with an existing server socket; server sockets sit idle waiting for these requests to come from client sockets. Untrusted classes are often restricted from creating server sockets. Normally, this is not a problem: since an applet can only talk to its web server, it could only answer requests from that machine—and the applet can already open a connection to that machine at will; there's no algorithmic or logistic reason why an operation between the applet and the web server cannot always start with the applet as the client. In situations where the applet is allowed to open client sockets to other machines, however, this reasoning doesn't apply, and the ability to create a server socket is often granted in such situations (and, sometimes, in all situations).

The security manager uses the following methods to check network access:

public void checkConnect(String host, int port)
public void checkConnect(String host, int port, Object context)

    Check if the program can open a client socket to the given port on the given host. The second form of this method is never called directly from the Java API.

public void checkListen(int port)

> Check if the program can create a server socket that is listening on the given port.

public void checkAccept(String host, int port)

> Check if the program can accept (on an existing server socket) a client connection that originated from the given host and port.

public void checkMulticast(InetAddress addr)
public void checkMulticast(InetAddress addr, byte ttl)

> Check if the program can create a multicast socket at the given multicast address (optionally with the given time-to-live value).

public void checkSetFactory()

> Check if the program can change the default socket implementation. When the Socket class is used to create a socket, it gets a new socket from the socket factory, which typically supplies a standard TCP-based socket. However, a socket factory could be used to supply SSL-based sockets, or any other socket variant.

The instances where these methods are used and the rationale for such uses are shown in Table 4-2.

Table 4-2. Security Manager Methods to Protect Network Access

Method	Called by	Rationale
checkConnect()	DatagramSocket.send() DatagramSocket.receive() ☆ MulticastSocket.send() Socket()	Test if the untrusted class can create a client-side connection
checkConnect()	DatagramSocket.getLocalAddress() InetAddress.getHostName() InetAddress.getLocalHost() InetAddress.getAllByName()	Test if the untrusted class can see any hosts on the local network
checkListen()	DatagramSocket() MulticastSocket() ServerSocket()	Test if the untrusted class can create a server-side socket
checkMulticast()	DatagramSocket.send() DatagramSocket.receive() MulticastSocket.send() MulticastSocket.receive() MulticastSocket.joinGroup() MulticastSocket.leaveGroup()	Test if the untrusted class can operate on a multicast socket
checkAccept()	ServerSocket.accept() DatagramSocket.receive() ★	Test if the untrusted class can accept a server connection

Table 4-2. Security Manager Methods to Protect Network Access (continued)

Method	Called by	Rationale
checkSetFactory()	ServerSocket.setSocketFactory() Socket.setSocketFactory() URL.setURLStreamHandlerFactory() URLConnection.setContentHandler- Factory() RMI.setSocketFactory()	Test if the untrusted class can alter the manner in which all sockets are created
checkSetFactory()	HttpURLConnection.setFollowRedi- rects()	Test if the untrusted class can change redirection behavior

Some notes are in order. As in the case with file access, these methods sometimes check operations that are logically different from a programming view, but are essentially the same thing at a system view. Hence, the checkConnect() method not only checks the opening of a socket but also the retrieval of hostname or address information (on the theory that to know the name of a host, you need to be able to open a socket to that host). This last test may seem somewhat odd— under what circumstances, you might wonder, should an untrusted class not be able to know the name or address of the machine on which it is running? Recall that we want to prevent the outside world from knowing our network topology; this includes the name and address of the user's machine as well.*

There was a change in the default security policy supplied in 1.0 and in 1.1 with respect to untrusted classes and server sockets (either instances of class Server-Socket or datagram sockets that received data from any source). In 1.0, untrusted classes were typically not allowed to create a server socket at all, which meant that the checkListen() and checkAccept() methods always threw a security exception when an applet attempted such an operation. In 1.1 and later, untrusted classes are allowed to create a server socket so long as the port number of that socket is greater than the privileged port number on the machine (typically 1024). Note too that the receive() method of the DatagramSocket class in 1.2 now calls the checkAccept() rather than the checkConnect() method.

Some applet publishers consider it to be very inconvenient to have to put both the applet and any network services that the applet requires on the same machine (the applet's web server). When you're configuring a network of machines, it certainly is more natural to have a database server that is separate from the web server; the scaling and flexibility that such separation gives is the cornerstone of network computing. Hence, an applet that is running on the browser shown in

---

* On the other hand, there's a good chance that the outside web server already knows that information, since our browser sent along a hostname and other information when it retrieved the file to begin with. If our request passed through a firewall or proxy server, there's a chance that some of this information was prevented from passing to the outside web server, but that's not necessarily the case either.

Figure 4-2 would consider it more convenient to access the database server directly. Sites with this configuration may therefore attempt to convince you to adjust your browser's network connection policy so their applet will work in this multitiered environment.

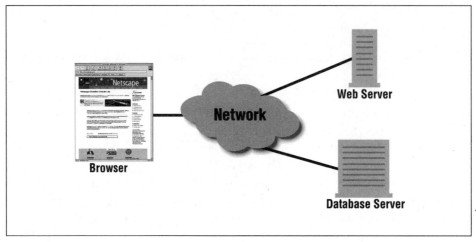

Figure 4-2. An untrusted class cannot directly connect to the database server

However, it's relatively trivial for applet publishers to set up a proxy service on their web server that forwards requests to the third machine, so that the applet only connects to the web server while the proxy service can connect to the third machine (e.g., the database server). Such a configuration may not be ideal—there's still a lot of traffic on the web server going through the proxy—but it's an effective compromise.

The requirement to use a proxy should not prove onerous to developers, either; it's common for network software providers to deliver such proxies with their Java code. Many JDBC-driver vendors, for example, provide such a proxy HTTP server that their JDBC drivers can access. Writing a simple proxy from scratch for other services is well within the grasp of good Java programmers.

Nonetheless, if in your view the reward of reduced network traffic outweighs the security considerations behind preventing arbitrary network access by untrusted classes, the Sun browsers (HotJava and `appletviewer`) and some versions of Internet Explorer allow you to configure them so that untrusted classes can connect to any host on the network.

The `checkSetFactory()` method of the security manager class is responsible for arbitrating the use of several low-level aspects of Java's network classes. Most of the tests made by this method have to do with whether or not the untrusted class is allowed to create some variety of socket factory. Socket factories are classes that are responsible for creating sockets that implement a particular interface while having a nonstandard feature: for example, a Java server might want to encrypt all of its traffic, so it would create and install a socket factory that creates only SSL-enabled sockets. Predictably, untrusted classes cannot change the socket factory in use.

This method is also used to determine whether the Java program will automatically follow redirect messages when opening a URL. When a Java program opens a URL, the server to which it is connected may send back a redirect response (an HTTP response code of 3xx). Often, browsers follow these redirects transparently to the user; in Java, the programmer has the ability to determine if the redirection should automatically be followed or not. An untrusted class is not able to change whether redirection is on or off. The HttpURLConnection class that uses this method is abstract, so the actual behavior of this class may be overridden in a particular implementation.

Methods Protecting the Java Virtual Machine

There are a number of methods in the SecurityManager class that protect the integrity of the Java virtual machine and the security manager. These methods fence in untrusted classes so that they cannot circumvent the protections of the security manager and the Java API itself. These methods are summarized in Table 4-3.

Table 4-3. Security Manager Methods Protecting the Virtual Machine

Method	Called by	Rationale
checkCreateClass-Loader()	ClassLoader()	Class loaders are protected since they provide information to the security manager
checkExec()	Runtime.exec()	Other processes might damage the user's machine
checkExec()	System.setIn() ☆ System.setOut() ☆ System.setErr() ☆	Don't let important messages be redirected away from the user
checkLink()	Runtime.load() Runtime.loadLibrary()	Don't let untrusted code import native code
checkExit()	Runtime.exit()	Don't let untrusted code halt the virtual machine
checkExit()	Runtime.runFinalizers-OnExit()	Don't let untrusted code change if finalizers are run
checkPermission() ★	many	See if the current thread has been granted a particular permission

public void checkCreateClassLoader()

The distinction we keep mentioning between trusted and untrusted classes is often based on the location from which the class was loaded (i.e., if the class came from the filesystem or from the network). As a result, the class loader we examined in Chapter 3 takes on an important role, since the security manager must ask the class loader where a particular class came from. The class loader is also responsible for marking certain classes as signed classes. Hence, an untrusted class is typically not allowed to create a class loader. This method is only called by the constructor of the `ClassLoader` class: if you can create a class loader (or if you obtain a reference to a previously created class loader), you can use it.

public void checkExec(String cmd)

This method is used to prevent execution of arbitrary system commands by untrusted classes—an untrusted class cannot, for example, execute a separate process that removes all the files on your disk.* In addition, this method is used to test whether a Java program is able to redirect the standard input, output, or error streams to another source—with the predictable result that untrusted classes are not allowed to perform such redirection.

In Java 1.2, this method is no longer used to determine whether the standard streams may be redirected. Redirection of those streams in 1.2 is determined instead by the `checkPermission()` method.

public void checkLink(String lib)

System commands aren't the only code that is out of reach of the security manager—any native (C language) code that is executed by the virtual machine cannot be protected by the security manager (or, in fact, by any aspect of the Java sandbox). Native code is executed by linking a shared library into the virtual machine; this method prevents an untrusted class from linking in such libraries.

It may seem as if this check is very important. It is, but only to a point: the programmatic binding from Java to C is such that Java code cannot just call an arbitrary C function—the C function must have a very specialized name that will not exist in an arbitrary library. So any C function that the untrusted class would like to call must reside in a library that you've downloaded and placed on your machine—and if the program's author can convince you to do that, then you don't really have a secure system anyway, and the author could find a different line of attack against you.

---

* The separate process would not need to be written in Java, of course, so there would be no security manager around to enforce the prohibition about deleting files.

public void checkExit(int status)

Next, there is the continuing processing of the virtual machine itself. This method prevents an untrusted class from shutting down the virtual machine. This method also prevents an untrusted class from changing whether or not all finalizers are run when the virtual machine does exit. This means that an untrusted class—and in particular, an applet—cannot guarantee that all the finalize methods of all the objects will be called before the system exits (which cannot be guaranteed in any case, since the browser can be terminated from the operating system without an opportunity to run the finalizers anyway).

public void checkPermission(Permission p) ★
public void checkPermission(Permission p, Object context) ★

Check to see if the current thread has the given permission. This method is at the heart of the access controller, which we'll explain in Chapter 5, where we'll also list when it is called. The second form of this method is never used by the Java API. The default for untrusted classes is to be given only a few explicit permissions, which we'll also list in Chapter 5.

Methods Protecting Program Threads

Java depends heavily on threads for its execution; in a simple Java program that uses images and audio, there may be a dozen or more threads that are created automatically for the user (depending on the particular implementation of the VM). These are system-level threads responsible for garbage collection, the various input and output needs of the graphical interface, threads to fetch images, etc. An untrusted class cannot manipulate any of these threads, because doing so would prevent the Java virtual machine from running properly, affecting other applets and possible even the browser itself.

The security manager protects threads with these methods:

public void checkAccess(Thread g)

Check if the program is allowed to change the state of the given thread.

public void checkAccess(ThreadGroup g)

Check if the program is allowed to change the state of the given thread group (and the threads that it holds).

public ThreadGroup getThreadGroup()

Supply a default thread group for newly created threads to belong to.

Table 4-4 shows the methods of the Java API that are affected by the policy set in the checkAccess() methods.

Table 4-4. Security Manager Methods Protecting Thread Access

Method	Called by	Rationale
CheckAccess(Thread g)	Thread.stop() Thread.interrupt() Thread.suspend() Thread.resume() Thread.setPriority() Thread.setName() Thread.setDaemon() Thread.setClassLoader() ★ Thread()	Untrusted classes may only manipulate threads that they have created
checkAccess(Thread-Group g)	ThreadGroup() ThreadGroup.setDaemon() ThreadGroup.setMaxPriority() ThreadGroup.stop() ThreadGroup.suspend() ThreadGroup.resume() ThreadGroup.destroy() ThreadGroup.interrupt() ★	Untrusted classes can only affect thread groups that they have created
getThreadGroup()	Thread()	Threads of untrusted classes must belong to specified groups

Most of the rationale behind these methods is straightforward: an untrusted class can manipulate its own threads, and it can manipulate threads that are in its thread group. This prevents an untrusted class from suspending the threads responsible for loading images; for example, those threads were not created by the untrusted class, and so the untrusted class cannot affect them.

Threads in a Java program are organized into a hierarchy (see Figure 4-3). In theory, the policy of the security manager should also apply to this hierarchy such that threads may only manipulate threads that are below them in the hierarchy. Hence, the calculating thread really should not be able to manipulate the state of the I/O reading thread—regardless of whether the calculating thread is executing trusted code or untrusted code. Similarly, the processing thread ought to be able to manipulate the state of the I/O reading thread even if the code to do so is in an untrusted class, since that implies that the untrusted class created the processing thread and the I/O thread anyway.

In practice, however, it does not work that way in Java 1.1: in that release, by default each applet is given an individual thread group, and the threads within that group can manipulate other threads within that group without respect to any hierarchy. In Java 1.2, the default is for the thread hierarchy to operate as expected.

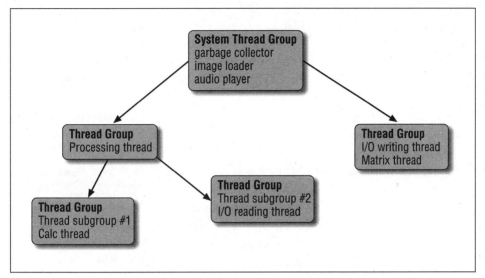

Figure 4-3. A Java thread hierarchy

Unlike the other public methods of the security manager, the getThreadGroup() method is not responsible for deciding whether access to a particular resource should be granted or not, and it does not throw a security exception under any circumstances. The point of this method is to determine the default thread group that a particular thread should belong to. When a thread is constructed and does not ask to be placed into a particular thread group, the getThreadGroup() method of the security manager is used to find a thread group to which the thread should be assigned. By default, this is the thread group of the calling thread, but a security manager can implement different logic so that the thread hierarchy we've described above becomes possible.

The getThreadGroup() method is only present in Java 1.1 and subsequent releases. In Java 1.0 (and browsers built on that release), thread security was generally non-existent: any thread could manipulate the state of any other thread, and applets weren't able to create their own thread groups. This additional method provided the infrastructure by which security managers built in Java 1.1 and later releases can implement the security policy that we've described here.

Methods Protecting System Resources

The Java-enabled browser has access to certain system-level resources to which untrusted classes should not be granted access. The next set of methods (outlined in Table 4-5) in the SecurityManager class handles those system-level resources.

Table 4-5. Security Manager Protections of System Resources

Method	Called by	Rationale
`checkPrintJobAccess()`	`Toolkit.getPrintJob()`[a]	Untrusted classes can't initiate print jobs
`checkSystemClip-boardAccess()`	`Toolkit.getSystem-Clipboard()`	Untrusted classes can't read the system clipboard
`checkAwtEventQueue-Access()`	`Event-Queue.getEvent-Queue()`	Untrusted classes can't manipulate window events
`checkPropertiesAc-cess()`	`System.getProper-ties()` `System.setProper-ties()`	Untrusted classes can't see or set system properties
`checkPropertyAc-cess()`	`System.getProp-erty()`	Untrusted classes can't get a particular system property
`checkPropertyAc-cess()`	`Locale.setDefault()`	Can't change the locale unless the `user.language` property can be read
`checkPropertyAccess()`	`Font.getFont()`	Can't get a font unless its property can be read
`checkTopLevelWindow()`	`Window()`	Windows created by untrusted classes should have an indentifying banner

[a] The `Toolkit` class is abstract and hence may vary by implementation; it's assumed that the implementation on a particular platform will call the correct method of the security manager.

public void checkPrintJobAccess()

Untrusted classes are not allowed access to the user's printer. This is another example of a nuisance protection; you wouldn't want a rogue applet sending reams of nonsense data to your printer. This method is never actually called by the standard Java API—it's up to the platform-specific implementation of the AWT toolkit to call it.

Note that this doesn't prevent the user from initiating a print action from the browser—it only prevents an applet from initiating the print action. The utility of such a check is subtle: the user always has to confirm the print dialog box before anything is actually printed (at least with the popular implementations of the AWT toolkit). The only sort of scenario that this check prevents is this: the user could surf to *www.EvilSite.org* and then to *www.sun.com*; although the applets from *EvilSite* are no longer on the current page, they're still active, and one of them could pop up the print dialog. The user will associate the dialog with the *www.sun.com* page and presumably allow it to print—and when the *EvilSite* applet then prints out offensive material, the user will blame the Sun page.

public void checkSystemClipboardAccess()

The Java virtual machine contains a system clipboard that can be used as a holder for copy-and-paste operations. Granting access to the clipboard to an untrusted class runs the risk that a class will come along, examine the clipboard, and find contents a previous program left there. Such contents might be sensitive data that the new class should not be allowed to read; hence, untrusted classes are prevented from accessing the system clipboard. This restriction applies only to the system clipboard: an untrusted class can still create its own clipboard and perform its own copy-and-paste operations to that clipboard. Untrusted classes can also share non-system clipboards between them.

This method is also never actually called by the Java API; it's up to the platform-specific implementation of the AWT toolkit to call it.

public void checkAwtEventQueueAccess()

Similarly, the Java virtual machine contains a system event queue that holds all pending AWT events for the system. An untrusted class that had access to such a queue would be able to delete events from the queue or insert events into the queue. This protects against the same sort of scenario we saw for printing—an applet on a previously visited page could insert events into the queue which would then be fed to an applet on the existing page.

Since this means that an untrusted class cannot get the system event queue, it is unable to call any of the methods of the EventQueue class—specifically the postEvent() and peekEvent() methods. Note, however, that an applet may still post events to itself using the dispatchEvent() method of the Component class.

public void checkPropertiesAccess()
public void checkPropertyAccess(String key)

The Java virtual machine has a set of global (system) properties that contains information about the user and the user's machine: login name, home directory, etc. Untrusted classes are generally denied access to some of this information in an attempt to limit the amount of spying that an applet can do. As usual, these methods only prevent access to the system properties; an untrusted class is free to set up its own properties and to share those properties with other classes if it desires.

Note that security managers are typically written to allow access to some system properties based on the name of the property.

public boolean checkTopLevelWindow(Object window)

Java classes, regardless of whether they are trusted or untrusted, are normally allowed to create top-level windows on the user's desktop. However, there is a concern that an untrusted class might bring up a window that looks exactly like another application on the user's desktop and thus confuse the user into doing something that ought not be done. For example, an applet could bring up a window that looks just like a telnet session and grab the user's password when the user responds to the password prompt. For that reason, top-level windows that are created by untrusted classes have some sort of identifying banner on them.

Note that unlike other methods in the security manager, this method has three outcomes: if it returns true, the window will be created normally; if it returns false, the window will be created with the identifying banner. However, this method could also throw a security exception (just like all the other methods of the security manager class) to indicate that the window should not be created at all. However, all the popular security manager implementations allow an untrusted class to bring up a window, subject to the identifying banner.

Methods Protecting Security Aspects

There are a number of methods in the security manager that protect Java's idea of security itself. These methods are summarized in Table 4-6.

Table 4-6. Security Manager Methods Protecting Java Security

Method	Called by	Rationale
checkMemberAccess()	Class.getFields() Class.getMethods() Class.getConstructors() Class.getField() Class.getMethod() Class.getConstructor() Class.getDeclaredClasses() Class.getDeclaredFields() Class.getDeclaredMethods() Class.getDeclaredConstructors() Class.getDeclaredField() Class.getDeclaredMethod() Class.getDeclardConstructor()	Untrusted classes can only inspect public information about other classes
checkPackageAccess()	not called	Check if the untrusted class can access classes in a particular package

Table 4-6. Security Manager Methods Protecting Java Security (continued)

Method	Called by	Rationale
checkPackageDefinition()	not called	Check if the untrusted class can load classes in a particular package
checkSecurityAccess()	Identity.setPublicKey() Identity.setInfo() Identity.addCertificate() Identity.removeCertificate() IdentityScope.setSystemScope() Provider.clear()[a] Provider.put() Provider.remove() Security.insertProviderAt() Security.removeProvider() Security.setProperty() Signer.getPrivateKey() Signer.setKeyPair() Identity.toString()[b] Security.getProviders() Security.getProvider() Security.getProperty()	Untrusted classes cannot manipulate security features

[a] The provider methods only call the security manager in 1.2.
[b] The last four methods in this list no longer call the security manager in 1.2.

public void checkMemberAccess(Class clazz, int which)

In Chapter 2, we examined the importance of the access modifiers to the integrity of Java's security model. Java's reflection API allows programs to inspect classes to determine the class's methods, variables, and constructors. The ability to access these entities can impact the memory integrity that Java provides.

The reflection API is powerful enough that, by inspection, a program can determine the private instance variables and methods of a class (although it can't actually access those variables or call those methods). Untrusted classes are allowed to inspect a class and find out only about its public variables and methods.

public void checkSecurityAccess(String action)

In the last half of this book, we'll be examining the details of the Java security package. This package implements a higher-order notion of security, including digital signatures, message digests, public and private keys, etc. The security package depends on this method in the security manager to arbitrate which classes can perform certain security-related operations. As an example, before a class is allowed to read a private key, this method is called with a string indicating that a private key is being read.

Predictably, an untrusted class is not allowed to perform any of these security-related operations, while a trusted class is.* Although the string argument gives the ability to distinguish what operation is being attempted, that argument is typically ignored in present implementations. As we discuss the features of the security package itself, we'll examine more in depth how the security package uses this method.

public void checkPackageAccess(String pkg)
public void checkPackageDefinition(String pkg)

These methods are used in conjunction with a class loader. When a class loader is asked to load a class with a particular package name, it will first ask the security manager if it is allowed to do so by calling the checkPackageAccess() method. This allows the security manager to make sure that the untrusted class is not trying to use application-specific classes that it shouldn't know about.

Similarly, when a class loader actually creates a class in a particular package, it asks the security manager if it is allowed to do so by calling the checkPackageDefinition() method. This allows the security manager to prevent an untrusted class from loading a class from the network and placing it into, for example, the java.lang package.

Note the distinction between these two methods: in the case of the checkPackageAccess() method, the question is whether the class loader can reference the class at all—e.g., whether we can call a class in the sun package. In the checkPackageDefinition() method, the class bytes have been loaded, and the security manager is being asked if they can belong to a particular package.

By default, these methods are never called. If you write a class loader, you should make sure that you call these methods as we indicated in Chapter 3.

That's all the methods of the security manager class that are used by the Java API to perform checks on certain operations. There are two more public methods of the SecurityManager class that we have not examined in this section; even though those methods are public, they are generally only used when you implement your own security manager, so we will defer their discussion. Remember that the discussion we followed in this chapter about the behavior of the system is

---

* This is not quite true: most browsers (including Netscape Communicator 4.0 and Internet Explorer 4.0) do not implement the Java security package at all. For classes loaded over the network, the effect is the same: you cannot use the methods of the security package. In these browsers, a trusted class in the browser's CLASSPATH, however, is also unable to use the security package.

based on a default set of behaviors exhibited by popular Java-enabled browsers—but since each browser is free to implement its own security policies, your particular browser may have a variation of the features we've just discussed.

Summary

In this chapter, we've had an overview of the most commonly known feature of Java's security story: the security manager. The security manager is responsible for arbitrating access to what we normally consider operating system features—files, network sockets, printers, etc. The goal of the security manager is to grant access to each class according to the amount of trust the user has in the class. Often, that means granting full access to trusted classes (that is, classes that have been loaded from the filesystem) while limiting access when the access is requested from an untrusted class (that is, a class that has been loaded from the network).

Although the security manager is the most commonly known feature of Java's security story, it's often misunderstood: there is no standard security manager among Java implementations, and Java applications, by default, have no security manager at all. Even with the popular Java-enabled browsers, the user often has latitude in what protections the security manager will be asked to enforce.

We examined in this chapter all the times when the security manager is asked to make a decision regarding access; such decisions range from the expected file and network access to more esoteric decisions, such as whether a frame needs a warning banner or what thread group a particular thread should belong to. This gave us a basic understanding of how the security manager can be used to enforce a specific policy, and the issues involved when defining such a policy. This knowledge will be used as a basis in the next few chapters, when we'll look at how to implement our own security manager.

5

The Access Controller

In this chapter, we're going to examine Java's access controller. While the security manager is the key to the security model of the Java sandbox, the access controller is the mechanism that the security manager actually uses to enforce its protections. The security manager may be king, but the access controller is really the power behind the throne.

The access controller is actually somewhat redundant. The purpose of the security manager is to determine whether or not particular operations should be permitted or denied. The purpose of the access controller is really the same: it decides whether access to a critical system resource should be permitted or denied. Hence, the access controller can do everything the security manager can do.

The reason there is both an access controller and a security manager is mainly historical: the access controller is only available in Java 1.2 and subsequent releases. Before the access controller existed, the security manager had to rely on its internal logic to determine the security policy that should be in effect, and changing the security policy required changing the security manager itself. Starting with 1.2, the security manager is able to defer these decisions to the access controller. Since the security policy enforced by the access controller can be specified in a file, this allows a much more flexible mechanism for determining policies. The access controller also gives us a much simpler method of granting fine-grained, specific permissions to specific classes. That process was theoretically possibly with the security manager alone, but it was simply too hard to implement.

But the large body of pre-1.2 Java programs dictates that the primary interface to system security—that is, the security manager—cannot change; otherwise, existing code that implements or depends on the security manager would become obsolete. Hence, the introduction of the access controller did not replace the security manager—it supplemented the security manager. This relationship is illustrated in Figure 5-1. Typically, an operation proceeds through the program code into the Java API, through the security manager to the access controller, and finally into the operating system. In certain cases, however, the security manager may bypass the access controller. And native libraries are still outside the domain of either the security manager or the access controller (although the ability to load those libraries may be restricted, as we've seen).

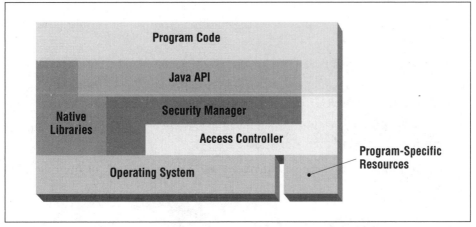

Figure 5-1. Coordination of the security manager and the access controller

The access controller plays another role in this picture as well: it allows a program to determine that access to any arbitrary resource must require explicit permission. A program that accesses employee payroll information from a corporate database may want to assign permission to each employee to access only his or her own data in the database. While global access to the database may be controlled by the security manager (e.g., because it's necessary to open a file or socket to get to the database), access to the particular record can be controlled by the access controller alone. Because the access controller (unlike the security manager) is easily extensible, it is simple for a program to use the same security framework to access both the general resources of the operating system and any specific resources of the program.

Keep in mind, however, that the core Java API never calls the access controller unless a security manager is in place, and that the access controller will not be initialized until it is called. If you call it directly for a program-specific resource, it will initialize itself automatically. But by default, Java applications run without a security manager will not use the access controller. We'll discuss later in this chapter and in Chapter 6 the use of the -usepolicy flag to install a security manager into the application, which will initialize the access controller for us.

In this chapter, then, we'll look into the access controller, including its implementation and its use. This will give us the necessary knowledge of how the access controller works, how it can be used to change the security of a Java program without requiring code changes, and how it is used to implement the security manager. This last point will also give us the necessary information to write our own security manager. In Java 1.2, there are only rare cases where such a task is necessary.

The access controller is built upon four concepts:

- *Code sources*: An encapsulation of the location from which certain Java classes were obtained

- *Permissions*: An encapsulation of a request to perform a particular operation

- *Policies*: An encapsulation of all the specific permissions that should be granted to specific code sources

- *Protection domains*: An encapsulation of a particular code source and the permissions granted to that code source

Before we examine the access controller itself, we'll look each of these building blocks.

The CodeSource Class

When we examined class loaders, we introduced the notion of a code source. A code source is a simple object that merely reflects the URL from which a class was loaded and the keys (if any) that were used to sign that class. The SecureClass-Loader class (and its subclasses) are responsible for creating and manipulating these code source objects.

The CodeSource class (java.security.CodeSource) has a few interesting methods:

public CodeSource(URL url, PublicKey key[]) ★

Create a code source object for code that has been loaded from the specified URL. The optional array of keys is the array of public keys that have signed the code that was loaded from this URL. These keys are typically obtained from reading a signed JAR file, which we'll show in Chapter 12; if the code was not signed, this argument should be null.

public boolean equals(Object o) ★

Two code source objects are considered equal if they were loaded from the same URL (that is, the equals() method for the URL of the objects returns true) and the array of keys is equal (that is, a comparison of each key in the array of keys will return true).

public final URL getLocation() ★

Return the URL that was passed to the constructor of this object.

public final PublicKey[] getKeys() ★

Return a copy of the array of keys that was passed to the constructor of this object. The original keys are not returned so that they cannot be modified accidentally (or maliciously).

That's the extent of the CodeSource class. When we discussed the SecureClass-Loader class in Chapter 3, we showed that the defineClass() method expected a CodeSource object as a parameter. It's up to the implementor of the Secure-ClassLoader to provide this object. In the URLClassLoader class, this happens automatically, based on the URL where the class was actually located. By default, each URL in the URLClassLoader class will have its own distinct code source object, so all classes that are loaded from that URL are considered to have the same code source. This does not have to be the case (though it's much simpler); you could have a different code source for each class, or even different code sources for sets of classes from the same URL (although we question the wisdom of doing that).

In Chapter 3, we obtained code source objects from the getCodeSource() method of the class loader source. The relationship between that method (which requires a URL and an array of objects as parameters) and the constructor of the code source should be fairly obvious. The advantage of the getCodeSource() method is that it allows each class loader to maintain a cache of code source objects, which is more efficient than constructing a new code source object each time one is needed. Hence, in our examples we will not construct code source object directly.

Permissions

The basic entity that the access controller operates on is a permission object—an instance of the Permission class (java.security.Permission). The Permission class itself is an abstract class that represents a particular operation. The nomenclature here is a little misleading, because a permission object can reflect two things. When it is associated with a class (through a code source and a protection domain), a permission object represents an actual permission that has been granted to that class. Otherwise, a permission object allows us to ask if we have a specific permission.

For example, if we construct a permission object that represents access to a file, possession of that object does not mean that we have permission to access the file. Rather, possession of the object allows us to ask if we have permission to access the file.

An instance of the `Permission` class represents one specific permission. A set of permissions—e.g., all the permissions that are given to classes signed by a particular individual—is represented by an instance of the `Permissions` class (`java.security.Permissions`). As developers and administrators, we'll make extensive use of these classes, so we'll need to investigate them in depth.

The Permission Class

Permissions have three properties:

A type

>All permissions carry a basic type that identifies what the permission pertains to. A permission object to access a file will have a type of `FilePermission`; an object to create a window will have a type of `AWTPermission`; permission to use the XYZ company payroll application would have a type of `XYZPayrollPermission`.

A name

>All permissions have a name that identifies the specific object that a permission relates to. A `FilePermission` has a name that is the name of the file to be accessed; an `AWTPermission` to create a window has a name of `topLevel-Window`; permission to access a particular employee's payroll record would have the name of that employee. Names are often based on wildcards, so that a single file permission object may represent permission to access several files, and so on.

>The name of a permission is fairly arbitrary. In the case of file permissions, the name is obviously the file. But the name of the `topLevelWindow` permission (among many others) is chosen by convention, and it is up to all Java programs to adhere to that convention. This is only a concern to programmers when dealing with your own permission classes; as a developer you rarely need to create permission objects for the types of permissions defined in the Java API.

>On the other hand, this naming convention is of concern to end users and administrators, who must know the name of the permission they want to grant to the programs they are going to run. These names must go into the policy file (which we'll discuss in just a bit).

Actions

>Some permissions carry with them one or more actions. The presence of these actions is dependent upon the semantics of the specific type of permission. A file permission object has a list of actions that could include read, write, and delete; an XYZ payroll permission object could have a list of actions that includes view and update. On the other hand, a window permission does

not have an action: you either have permission to create the window, or you don't. Actions can also be specified by wildcards. The terms used to specify a list of actions are also arbitrary and handled by convention.

Permissions can serve two roles. They allow the Java API to negotiate access to several resources (files, sockets, and so on). Those permissions are defined by convention within the Java API, and their naming conventions are wholly within the domain of the Java API itself. Hence, you can create an object that represents permission to read a particular file, but you cannot create an object that represents permission to copy a particular file, since the copy action is not known within the file permission class.

On the other hand, you can create arbitrary permissions for use within your own programs and completely define both the names of those permissions as well as the actions (if any) that should apply. If you are writing a payroll program, for example, you could create your own permission class that uses the convention that the name of the permission is the employee upon whose payroll information you want to act; you could use the convention that the permissible actions on the payroll permission are view and update. Then you can use that permission in conjunction with the access controller to allow employees to view their own payroll data and to allow managers to change the payroll data for their employees.

We'll look at both of these cases, starting with the classes that are provided within the Java API itself. These classes are used by the Java API (and in particular, by the security manager) to protect access to certain resources in ways that are fairly intuitive, given our knowledge of the security manager (but we'll examine that interaction in detail later).

Permissions of the Java API

There are 11 standard permissions in the Java API, each of which is implemented as a class:

1. The FilePermission class (java.io.FilePermission)

   This class represents permissions for files. This class implements two wildcard patterns for filenames: an asterisk matches all files in a given directory, and a hyphen matches all files that reside in an entire directory hierarchy. Valid actions for file permissions are read, write, delete, and execute.

   File permissions must be constructed with their platform-specific name. Hence, */myclasses/xyz* is a valid name for a file permission on a Unix system, but not on a Macintosh (where an equivalent name might be *System Disk:myclasses:xyz*). When these strings are specified programmatically, they are not too difficult to construct (using the file separator property);

when these strings need to be specified in an external file, an appropriate syntax must be used.

Keep in mind the difference between an asterisk and a hyphen: an asterisk only traverses a single directory, while a hyphen traverses an entire filesystem. Hence */myclasses/** will not include */myclasses/xyz/HRApplet.class*, but */myclasses/-* will. A single asterisk will access all files in the current directory, and a single hyphen will access all files in the current directory and its subdirectories.

If you want to access all files on a particular machine, you specify the special token <<ALL FILES>>.

A `FilePermission` object is constructed by providing the name of the file and a list of actions on that file:

```
FilePermission p1 = new FilePermission("-", "execute");
FilePermission p2 = new FilePermission("/myclasses/*", "read, write");
FilePermission p3 = new FilePermission("<<ALL FILES>>", "read");
```

Here, p1 represents permission to execute all files that are in the filesystem hierarchy under the current directory, p2 represents permission to read and write all files that exist in the directory */myclasses*, and p3 represents permission to read all the files on the machine.

2. The `SocketPermission` class (`java.net.SocketPermission`)

   This class represents permissions to interact with network sockets. The name of a socket permission is *hostname:port*, where each component of the name may be specified by a wildcard. In particular, the hostname may be given as a hostname (possibly DNS qualified) or an IP address. The leftmost position of the hostname may be specified as an asterisk, such that the host *piccolo.East.Sun.COM* would be matched by each of these strings:

   ```
   piccolo
   piccolo.East.Sun.COM
   *.Sun.COM
   *
   129.151.119.8
   ```

   The port component of the name can be specified as a single port number or as a range of port numbers (e.g., 1–1024). When a range is specified, either side of the range may be excluded:

   ```
   1024 (port 1024)
   1024- (all ports greater than or equal to 1024)
   -1024 (all ports less than or equal to 1024)
   1-1024 (all ports between 1 and 1024, inclusive)
   ```

   Valid actions for a socket permission are accept, connect, listen, and resolve. These map into the socket API: accept is used by the `ServerSocket` class to see if it can accept an incoming connection from a particular host; connect is used by the Socket class to see if it can make a connection to a particular host, listen is used by the ServerSocket class to see if a server socket can be created at all, and resolve is used by the Socket class to see if the IP address for a particular host can be obtained.

Constructing a socket permission, then, is simply a matter of putting together the desired strings in the correct format:

```
SocketPermission s1 = new SocketPermission("piccolo:6000", "connect");
SocketPermission s2 = new SocketPermission("piccolo:1024-",
                                           "accept, listen");
```

Here s1 represents permission to connect to the X server (port 6000) on machine *piccolo*, and s2 represents permission for *piccolo* to start a server on any nonprivileged port.

3. The PropertyPermission class (java.util.PropertyPermission)

This class represents permissions for Java properties. Property permission names are specified as dot-separated names (just as they are in a Java property file); in addition, the last element can be a wildcard asterisk: *, a.*, a.b.*, and so on.

The valid actions for this class are read and write. Hence, to construct a property permission, you would do something like:

```
PropertyPermission p1 = new PropertyPermission("java.version", "read");
PropertyPermission p2 = new PropertyPermission("xyz.*", "read,write");
```

Here, p1 represents permission to read the version of the virtual machine that's in use, and p2 represents permission to read or write all properties that begin with the token xyz.

4. The RuntimePermission class (java.lang.RuntimePermission)

This class represents permissions for the Java runtime—essentially, permissions to perform any of the operations encapsulated by the Runtime class, including most thread operations. The names recognized by this class are dot-separated names and are subject to the same wildcard asterisk matching as the property permission class.

Runtime permissions have no associated actions—you either have permission to perform those operations, or you don't. Hence, a runtime permission is constructed as:

```
RuntimePermission r1 = new RuntimePermission("exit");
RuntimePermission r2 = new RuntimePermission("package.access.*");
```

Here, r1 represents permission to exit the virtual machine, and r2 represents permission to access any package.

5. The AWTPermission class (java.awt.AWTPermission)

This class represents permissions to access certain windowing resources. In particular, as we might assume from the corresponding methods in the security manager, there are three conventional names in this class: topLevelWindow, systemClipboard, and eventQueue.

There are no actions associated with this class. In addition, this class technically supports wildcard matching, but since none of the conventional names are in dot-separated format, that facility is unused. Hence, an AWT permission is constructed like this:

```
AWTPermission a = new AWTPermission("topLevelWindow");
```

6. The NetPermission class (java.net.NetPermission)

This class represents permissions to interact with three different classes. The first is the Authenticator class: there are no concrete implementations of the Authenticator class within the JDK, but implementations of that class provide HTTP authentication for password-protected web pages. The valid names associated with this class are Authenticator.setDefault and Authenticator.requestPasswordAuthentication. Wildcard asterisk matching applies to these names.

In addition, the ability to create multicast sockets is encapsulated in the NetPermission class, with a name of multicast.

Finally, the ability to create a listener for the URLClassLoader class is encapsulated in the NetPermission class with a name of URLClassLoader.setListener.

There are no associated actions with a net permission, so they are constructed as follows:

```
NetPermission n1 = new NetPermission("multicast");
NetPermission n2 = new NetPermission("Authenticator.*");
```

7. The SecurityPermission class (java.security.SecurityPermission)

This class represents permission to use the security package. Names passed to this class are subject to wildcard asterisk matching, and there are no actions associated with this class. The valid names to this class include all the valid strings that can be passed to the checkSecurityAccess() method of the security manager; as we discuss the security API in the last half of this book, we'll list these names for each class.

8. The SerializablePermission class (java.io.SerializablePer-mission)

This class represents various permissions relating to the serialization and deserialization of an object. No wildcards or actions are accepted by this class. This permission has one valid name: enableSubstitution. If granted, this permission allows the `enableResolveObject()` method of the `ObjectInputStream` and the `enableReplaceObject()` method of the `ObjectOutputStream` classes to function.

9. The `ReflectPermission` class (`java.lang.reflect.ReflectPermis-sion`)

   This permission represents the ability to set the accessible flag on objects that are to be used with the reflection API. This class has a single name (access) and no actions.

10. The `UnresolvedPermission` class (`java.security.UnresolvedPermis-sion`)

   This class is used internally in the Java API to represent external permissions (i.e., permissions that are implemented by third-party APIs) before the class that defines that permission is found. This permission is only needed if you are writing an implementation of the `Policy` class.

11. The `AllPermission` class (`java.security.AllPermission`)

   This class represents permission to perform any operation—including file, socket, and other operations that have their own permission classes. Granting this type of permission is obviously somewhat dangerous; this permission is usually given only to classes within the Java API and to classes in Java extensions. This class has no name or actions; it is constructed as follows:

   ```
   AllPermission ap = new AllPermission();
   ```

Using the Permission Class

We'll now look into the classes upon which all these permissions are based: the `Permission` class. This class abstracts the notion of a permission and a name. From a programmatic standpoint, the `Permission` class is really used only to create your own types of permissions. It has some interesting methods, but the operations that are implemented on a permission object are not generally used in code that we write—they are used instead by the access controller. Hence, we'll examine this class primarily with an eye towards understanding how it can be used to implement our own permissions.

`Permission` is an abstract class that contains these public methods:

public Permission(String name) ★
   Construct a permission object that represents the desired permission.

public abstract boolean equals(Object o) ★
   Subclasses of the `Permission` class are required to implement their own test for equality. Often this is simply done by comparing the name (and actions, if applicable) of the permission.

public abstract int hashCode() ★

Subclasses of the `Permission` class are required to implement their own hash code. In order for the access controller to function correctly, the hash code for a given permission object must never change during execution of the virtual machine. In addition, permissions that compare as equal must return the same hash code from this method.

public abstract String getName() ★

Return the name that was used to construct this permission.

public abstract String getActions() ★

Return the canonical form of the actions (if any) that were used to construct this permission.

public String toString() ★

The convention for printing a permission is to print in parentheses the class name, the name of the permission, and the actions. For example, a file permission might return:

```
("java.io.FilePermission","/myclasses/xyz/HRApplet.class","read")
```

public abstract boolean implies(Permission p) ★

This method is one of the keys of the `Permission` class: it is responsible for determining whether or not a class that is granted one permission is granted another. This method is normally responsible for performing wildcard matching, so that, for example, the file permission */myclasses/-* implies the file permission */myclasses/xyz/HRApplet.class.* But this method need not rely on wildcards; permission to write a particular object in a database would probably imply permission to read that object as well.

public PermissionCollection newPermissionCollection() ★

Return a permission collection suitable for holding instances of this type of permission. We'll discuss the topic of permission collections in the next section. This method returns `null` by default.

public void checkGuard(Object o) ★

Call the security manager to see if the permission (i.e., the `this` variable) has been granted, generating a `SecurityException` if the permission has not been granted. The object parameter of this method is unused. We'll give more details about this method later in this chapter.

Implementing your own permission means providing a class with concrete implementations of these abstract methods. Note that the notions of wildcard matching and actions are not generally present in this class—if you want your class to support either of these features, you're responsible for implementing all of the necessary logic to do so (although the `BasicPermission` class that we'll look at next can help us with that).

Say that you are implementing a program to administer payroll information. You'll want to create permissions to allow users to view their payment history. You'll also want to allow the HR department to update the pay rate for employees. So we'll need to implement a permission class to encapsulate all of that:

```java
public class XYZPayrollPermission extends Permission {

    protected int mask;
    static private int VIEW = 0x01;
    static private int UPDATE = 0x02;

    public XYZPayrollPermission(String name) {
        this(name, "view");
    }

    public XYZPayrollPermission(String name, String action) {
        super(name);
        parse(action);
    }

    private void parse(String action) {
        StringTokenizer st = new StringTokenizer(action, ",\t ");

        mask = 0;
        while (st.hasMoreTokens()) {
            String tok = st.nextToken();
            if (tok.equals("view"))
                mask |= VIEW;
            else if (tok.equals("update"))
                mask |= UPDATE;
            else throw new IllegalArgumentException(
                                "Unknown action " + tok);
        }
    }

    public boolean implies(Permission permission) {
        if (!(permission instanceof XYZPayrollPermission))
            return false;

        XYZPayrollPermission p = (XYZPayrollPermission) permission;
        String name = getName();
        if (!name.equals("*") && !name.equals(p.getName()))
            return false;
        if ((mask & p.mask) != p.mask)
            return false;
        return true;
    }

    public boolean equals(Object o) {
```

```
        if (!(o instanceof XYZPayrollPermission))
            return false;

        XYZPayrollPermission p = (XYZPayrollPermission) o;
        return ((p.getName().equals(getName())) && (p.mask == mask));
    }

    public int hashCode() {
        return getName().hashCode() ^ mask;
    }

    public String getActions() {
        if (mask == 0)
            return "";
        else if (mask == VIEW)
            return "view";
        else if (mask == UPDATE)
            return "update";
        else if (mask == (VIEW | UPDATE))
            return "view, update";
        else throw new IllegalArgumentException("Unknown mask");
    }

    public PermissionCollection newPermissionsCollection() {
        return new XYZPayrollPermissionCollection();
    }
}
```

The instance variables in this class are required to hold the information about the actions—even though our superclass makes references to actions, it doesn't provide a manner in which to store them or process them, so we have to provide that logic. That logic is provided in the parse() method; we've chosen the common convention of having the action string treated as a list of actions that are separated by commas and whitespace. Note also that we've stored the actual actions as bits in a single integer—this simplifies some of the later logic.

As required, we've implemented the equals() and hashCode() methods—and we've done so rather simply. We consider objects equal if their names are equal and their masks (that is, their actions) are equal, and construct a hash code accordingly.

Our implementation of the getActions() method is typical: we're required to return the same action string for a permission object that was constructed with an action list of "view, update" as for one that was constructed with an action list of "update, view". This requirement is one of the prime reasons why the actions are stored as a mask—because it allows us to construct this action string in the proper format.

Finally, the `implies()` method is responsible for determining how wildcard and other implied permissions are handled. If the name passed to construct our object is an asterisk, then we match any other name; hence, an object to represent the permissions of the HR department might be constructed as:

```
new XYZPayrollPermission("*", "view, update")
```

When the `implies()` method is called on this wildcard object, the name will always match, and because the action mask has the complete list of actions, the mask comparison will always yield the mask that we're testing against. If the `implies()` method is called with a different object, however, it will only return true if the names are equal and the object's mask is a subset of the target mask.

Note that we also might have implemented the logic in such a way that permission to perform an update implies permission to perform a view simply by changing the logic of testing the mask—you're not limited only to wildcard matching in the `implies()` method.

The BasicPermission Class

If you need to implement your own permission class, the `BasicPermission` class (`java.security.BasicPermission`) provides some useful semantics. This class implements a basic permission—that is, a permission that doesn't have actions. Basic permissions can be thought of as binary permission—you either have them, or you don't. However, this restriction does not prevent you from implementing actions in your subclasses of the `BasicPermission` class (as the `PropertyPermission` class does).

The prime benefit of this class is the manner in which it implements wildcards. Names in basic permissions are considered to be hierarchical, following a dot-separated convention. For example, if the XYZ corporation wanted to create a set of basic permissions, they might use the convention that the first word of the permission always be `xyz`: `xyz.readDatabase`, `xyz.writeDatabase`, `xyz.runPayrollProgram`, `xyz.HRDepartment.accessCheck`, and so on. These permissions can then be specified by their full name, or they can be specified with an asterisk wildcard: `xyz.*` would match each of these (no matter what depth), and `*` would match every possible basic permission.

The wildcard matching of this class does not match partial names: `xyz.read*` would not match any of the permissions we just listed. Further, the wildcard must be in the rightmost position: `*.readDatabase` would not match any basic permission.

The `BasicPermission` class is abstract, although it does not contain any abstract methods, and it completely implements all the abstract methods of the `Permission` class. Hence, a concrete implementation of the `BasicPermission` need only contain a constructor to call the correct constructor of the superclass (since there is no default constructor in the BasicPermission class). Subclasses must call one of these constructors:

public BasicPermission(String name) ★

Construct a permission with the given name. This is the usual constructor for this class, as basic permissions do not normally have actions.

public BasicPermission(String name, String action) ★

Construct a permission with the given name and action. Even though basic permissions do not usually have actions associated with them, you must provide a constructor with this signature in all implementations of the BasicPermission class due to the mechanism that is used to construct permission objects from the policy file (which we will see later in this chapter).

Permission Collections

The access controller depends upon the ability to aggregate permissions so that it can easily call the implies() method on all of them. For example, a particular user might be given permission to read several directories: perhaps the user's home directory (*/home/sdo/-*) and the system's temporary directory (*/tmp/-*). When the access controller needs to see if the user can access a particular file, it must test both of these permissions to see if either one matches. This can be done easily by aggregating all the file permissions into a single permission collection.

Every permission class is required to implement a permission collection, then, which is a mechanism where objects of the same permission class may be grouped together and operated upon as a single unit. This requirement is enforced by the newPermissionCollection() method of the Permission class.

The PermissionCollection class (java.security.PermissionCollection) is defined as follows:

public abstract class PermissionCollection

Implement an aggregate set of permissions. While permission collections can handle heterogeneous sets of permissions, a permission collection typically should be used to group together a homogeneous group of permissions (e.g., all file permissions or all socket permissions, etc.).

There are three basic operations that you can perform on a permission collection:

public abstract void add(Permission p) ★

Add the given permission to the permission collection.

public abstract boolean implies(Permission p) ★

Check to see if any permission in the collection implies the given permission. This can be done by enumerating all the permission objects that have been added to the collection and calling the `implies()` method on each of those objects in turn, but it is typically implemented in a more efficient manner.

public abstract Enumeration elements() ★

Return an enumeration of all the permissions in the collection.

The *javadoc* documentation of this class claims that a permission collection is a collection of heterogeneous permission objects. Forget that idea; introducing that notion into permission collections vastly complicates matters, and the issue of a heterogeneous collection of permission objects is better handled elsewhere (we'll see how a little bit later). As far as we're concerned, the purpose of a permission collection is to aggregate only permission objects of a particular type.

Permission collections are typically implemented as inner classes, or at least as classes that are private to the package in which they are defined. There is, for example, a corresponding permission collection class for the `FilePermission` class, one for the `SocketPermission` class, and so on.

None of these collections is available as a public class that we can use in our own program. Hence, in order to support the `newPermissionCollection()` method in our `XYZPayrollPermission` class, we'd need to do something like this:

```
public class XYZPayrollPermissionCollection extends
                                PermissionCollection {
    private Hashtable permissions;
    private boolean addedAdmin;
    private int adminMask;

    XYZPayrollPermissionCollection() {
        permissions = new Hashtable();
        addedAdmin = false;
    }

    public void add(Permission p) {
        if (!(p instanceof XYZPayrollPermission))
            throw new IllegalArgumentException(
                                "Wrong permission type");
        XYZPayrollPermission xyz = (XYZPayrollPermission) p;
        String name = xyz.getName();
        XYZPayrollPermission other =
                    (XYZPayrollPermission) permissions.get(name);
        if (other != null)
            xyz = merge(xyz, other);
        if (name.equals("*")) {
            addedAdmin = true;
            adminMask = xyz.mask;
```

```
        }
        permissions.put(name, xyz);
    }

    public Enumeration elements() {
        return permissions.elements();
    }

    public boolean implies(Permission p) {
        if (!(p instanceof XYZPayrollPermission))
            return false;
        XYZPayrollPermission xyz = (XYZPayrollPermission) p;
        if (addedAdmin && (adminMask & xyz.mask) != 0)
            return true;
        Permission inTable = (Permission)
                            permissions.get(xyz.getName());
        if (inTable == null)
            return false;
        return inTable.implies(xyz);
    }

    private XYZPayrollPermission
            merge(XYZPayrollPermission a, XYZPayrollPermission b) {
        String aAction = a.getActions();
        if (aAction.equals(""))
            return b;
        String bAction = b.getActions();
        if (bAction.equals(""))
            return a;
        return new XYZPayrollPermission(a.getName(),
                            aAction + "," + bAction);
    }
}
```

Note the logic within the implies() method—it's the important part of this example. The implies() method must test each permission in the hashtable (or whatever other container you've used to store the added permissions), but it should do so efficiently. We could always call the implies() method of each entry in the hashtable, but that would clearly not be efficient—it's better to call only the implies() method on a permission in the table that has a matching name.

The only trick is that we won't find a matching name if we're doing wildcard pattern matching—if we've added the name "*" to the table, we'll always want to return true, even though looking up the name "John Smith" in the table will not return the administrative entry. Implementing this wildcard pattern matching efficiently is the key to writing a good permission collection.

When you use (or subclass) one of the concrete permission classes that we listed earlier, there is no need to provide a permission collection class—all concrete implementations provide their own collection. In addition, there are two other cases when you do not need to implement a permission collection:

- When you extend the Permission class, but do not do wildcard pattern matching.

  Hidden internally within the Java API is a PermissionsHash class, which is the default permission collection class for permission objects. The PermissionsHash class stores the aggregated permissions in a hashtable, so the implementations of its add() and elements() methods are straightforward. The implementation of its implies() method is based on looking up the name of the permission parameter in the hashtable collection: if an entry is found, then the implies() method is called on that entry.

- When you extend the BasicPermission class and do not provide support for actions.

  The newPermissionClass() method of the BasicPermission class will provide a permission collection that handles wildcard pattern matching correctly (and efficiently).

The Permissions Class

So far, we've spoken about permission collections as homogeneous collections: all permissions in the XYZPayrollPermissionCollection class are instances of the XYZPayrollPermission class; a similar property holds for other permission collections. This idea simplifies the implies() method that we showed above. But to be truly useful, a permission collection needs to be heterogeneous, so it can represent all the permissions a program should have. A permission collection really needs to be able to contain file permissions, socket permissions, and other types of permissions.

This idea is present within the PermissionCollection class; conceptually, however, it is best to think of heterogeneous collections of permissions as encapsulated by the Permissions class (java.security.Permissions):

public final class Permissions extends PermissionCollection

Implement the PermissionCollection class. This class allows you to create a heterogeneous collection of permissions: the permission objects that are added to this collection need not have the same type.

This class contains a concrete implementation of a permission collection that organizes the aggregated permissions in terms of their individual, homogenous permission collections. You can think of a permissions object as containing an aggregation of permission collections, each of which contains an aggregation of individual permissions.

For example, let's consider an empty permissions object. When a file permission is added to this object, the permissions object will call the `newPermissionCollec-tion()` method on the file permission to get a homogeneous file permission collection object. The file permission is then stored within this file permission collection. When another file permission is added to the permissions object, the permissions object will place that file permission into the already existing file permission collection object. When a payroll permission object is added to the permissions object, a new payroll permission collection will be obtained, the payroll permission added to it, and the collection added to the permissions object. This process will continue, and the permissions object will build up a set of permission collections.

When the `implies()` method of the permissions object is called, it will search its set of permission collections for a collection that can hold the given permission. It can then call the `implies()` method on that (homogenous) collection to obtain the correct answer.

The `Permissions` class thus supports any arbitrary grouping of permissions. There is no need to develop your own permission collection to handle heterogeneous groups.

In addition to the methods that are inherited from the `PermissionCollection` class, the `Permissions` class has these public methods:

public void setReadOnly() ★

> Mark the permissions object as read-only. Once a permissions object is marked as read-only, attempts to add a permission to it (via the `add()` method) will throw a `SecurityException`.

public boolean isReadOnly() ★

> Return whether or not this permissions object has been marked as read-only.

The Policy Class

The third building block for the access controller is the facility to specify which permissions should apply to which code sources. We call this global set of permissions the security policy; it is encapsulated by the `Policy` class (`java.security.Policy`):

public abstract class Policy ★

> Establish the security policy for a Java program. The policy encapsulates a mapping between code sources and permission objects in such a way that

classes loaded from particular locations or signed by specific individuals have the set of specified permissions.

A policy class is constructed as follows:

public Policy() ★

Create a policy class. The constructor should initialize the policy object according to its internal rules (e.g., by reading the *java.policy* file, as we'll describe later).

Like the security manager, only a single instance of the policy class can be installed in the virtual machine at any time. However, unlike the security manager, the actual instance of the policy class can be replaced. These two methods install and retrieve the policy:

public static Policy getPolicy() ★

Return the currently installed policy object.

public static void setPolicy(Policy p) ★

Install the given policy object, replacing whatever policy object was previously installed.

Getting and setting the policy object requires going through the `checkProperty()` method of the security manager. By default, this succeeds only if you already have been granted a security permission with the name of `Policy.getPolicy` or `Policy.setPolicy` (as appropriate). There's a bootstrapping issue involved when setting the policy, since granting permissions requires the policy to have been set. Hence, the initial policy is typically set by a class in the core API, as those classes always have permission to perform any operation.

There are two other methods in the `Policy` class:

public abstract Permissions evaluate(CodeSource cs) ★

Create a permissions object that contains the set of permissions that should be granted to classes that came from the given code source (i.e., loaded from the code source's URL and signed by the keys in the code source).

public abstract void refresh() ★

Refresh the policy object. For example, if the initial policy came from a file, re-read the file and install a new policy object based on the (presumably changed) information from the file.

In programmatic terms, writing a policy class is a matter of implementing these methods. The default policy class is provided by the `PolicyFile` class (`java.security.PolicyFile`), which constructs the set of permissions based on the information found in a file on the user's local disk (a process we're just about to examine).

Unfortunately, the `PolicyFile` class that parses that file and builds up the set of permissions is a package-protected class; it is not accessible to us as programmers. Hence, while it's possible to write your own policy class, it is a fairly involved process. You might want to write your own `Policy` class if you want to define a set of permissions through some other mechanism than a URL (e.g., loading the permissions via a policy server database). That implementation is fairly straightforward: you need only provide a mechanism to map code sources to a set of permissions. Then, for each code source, construct each of the individual permission objects and aggregate them into a permissions object to be returned by the `evaluate()` method.

Property Expansion and the Policy Class

You'll notice an unusual syntax in the list of policy properties in the *java.security* file: `${foo.bar}`. This syntax uses property substitution to fill in the given target; for example, the string `${user.home}` might expand to */home/sdo* on my Unix desktop machine and to *C:* on my Windows desktop machine. As you might have guessed, the string `${/}` expands to the file separator character on the platform that is reading the file.

This property substitution allows us to use one set of configuration files no matter what the underlying platform, since we can use standard Java properties to hide those platform-specific details. This is particularly important when specifying filenames for file permissions in a policy file.

If the `policy.expandProperties` property in the *java.security* file is set to `false`, however, substitution will not occur and these strings should not be used. If they are used, they will be treated as literal strings and fail.

The Default Policy

The `Policy` and `PolicyFile` classes give system administrators or end users the ability to define in a file a security policy for any Java program; this allows changes to the security model for the program without modifying the program's code. The policy that you can specify in this file is extremely flexible, since it's based on the permission model we examined earlier. If you want a Java program to be able to read a single directory, you can specify the appropriate file permission in the policy file. If you want a Java program to be able to connect to particular hosts on the network, you can specify the appropriate socket permissions in the policy file. And if you want a Java program to be able to administer payroll records, you can specify the appropriate payroll permissions in the policy file.

By default, the policy for a Java program is read from two locations, but this is controlled by the system security file. This file is a set of properties that apply to the security package in general; it is named *$JAVAHOME/lib/security/java.security.*

In terms of the `Policy` class, here are the relevant entries in the *java.security* file:

```
policy.provider=java.security.PolicyFile
policy.expandProperties=true
policy.allowSystemProperty=true
policy.url.1=file:${java.home}/lib/security/java.policy
policy.url.2=file:${user.home}/.java.policy
```

The first of these properties defines the class that should be instantiated to provide the initial instance of the `Policy` class: in this case, the `PolicyFile` class (which implements the behavior we're now describing). Here's the algorithm that the `PolicyFile` class uses to read in policy files. The entire set of entries in the resulting policy is composed of all the specific entries read from all of the following files:

1. If the `policy.allowSystemProperty` property in the *java.security* file is set to `true` (which it is by default), then the first file to be read is a file specified on the command line with the `-usepolicy` argument. For example, the following command would first load the policy file from */globalfiles/java.policy*:

   ```
   piccolo% java -usepolicy:/globafiles/java.policy Cat /etc/passwd
   ```

   If the `policy.allowSystemProperty` property is set to `false`, then   the -usepolicy file will be ignored. On the other hand, if this property is set to `true` and the filename given as the `-usepolicy` argument begins with an equals sign:

   ```
   piccolo% java -usepolicy:=/globalfiles/java.policy Cat /etc/passwd
   ```

   then the given file is the *only* policy file that will be read (and hence the only file that will define permissions).

   Note that you may also specify the `-usepolicy` flag with no argument, in which case the policy files from the *java.security* file (see the next step) are used and no additional files are consulted:

   ```
   piccolo% java -usepolicy Cat /etc/passwd
   ```

   This last example is the typical usage. Any of these examples set up the default sandbox for us in Java 1.2—the parameters of this sandbox are defined by the entries in the policy file.

2. Next, the `PolicyFile` class looks for properties of the form `policy.url.n` where n is an integer starting with 1. As it finds each property, it reads in the policy from the given URL; in the default set of properties we listed above, this means that the first URL to be read is the *java.policy* file in the *$JAVA-HOME/lib/security* directory and the second URL to be read is the *.java.policy*

file in the user's home directory. You may specify as many or as few of these URLs as desired, but they must be numbered consecutively starting with 1.

3. If no files have been loaded (because there was no -usepolicy argument and there were no policy.url properties), then an internal static set of permissions is loaded (which is the same set of permissions defined by the default *java.policy* file we list below).

The policy files are designed to map code sources to sets of permissions. For example, this entry:

```
grant codeBase http://www.xyz.com/ {
    permission java.io.FilePermssion "${user.home}${/}docs${/}-",
                                        "read, write, delete";
};
```

means that any code loaded from the top-level directory of *www.xyz.com* is granted permission to use any files under the user's *docs* directory. The code base in this case is used to construct a code source with no public keys.

The above example is one case of a policy entry, also called a grant entry, and a policy file is a collection of policy entries. Each entry is specific to one code source and should list all the permissions for that code source—but a single policy file can have several entries and thus work effectively for code that originated from multiple sources. The syntax of a policy entry is as follows:

```
grant [signedBy <signer>] [, codeBase <code source>] {
        permission <class> [<name> [, <action list>]];
        ...
        permission <class> [<name> [, <action list>]];
};
```

As indicated by the bracket syntax, the signedBy and codeBase entries are optional. If both are missing, the list of permissions applies to a class with any code source. The signer entry should be a name that matches an entry in the system's key management system—a concept we'll explore in Chapter 11. The codeBase should be the URL that applies to the location from which the classes were loaded—including a file-based or HTTP-based URL.

Note that omitting the signedBy and codeBase fields in the policy file means that the given permissions should apply to all code sources. It does not mean that the listed permissions should apply only to classes that had a code source with no URL and no public key. This point about the code source is important: permissions given within the policy file apply only to classes that have a code source. Classes that are loaded by the primordial class loader do not have a code source— these classes are given permission to perform any operation. Hence, the Java API itself has no restrictions placed upon what operations it may perform.

The permissions themselves should have the fully package-qualified class name for the permission—including any permission classes (like the XYZPayrollPermission class) that you may have defined for your own application. The name will be used to construct the permission, along with the action list (if present). An internal (private) method of the PolicyFile class is used to construct the permission object; this method expects to find a constructor that takes both a name and an action. If the action is not present, then null will be passed to the constructor. This requirement forces you to include a constructor with both arguments in all your permission classes, including those that are extensions of the BasicPermission class.

Here's the default policy file that comes with the Java 1.2. This is the system security file (i.e., the one loaded from *$JAVAHOME/lib/security/java.policy*); there is no default file for each user. This is also the set that will be loaded when no policy files are found:

```
// Standard extensions get all permissions by default
grant codeBase "file:${java.home}/lib/ext/" {
    permission java.security.AllPermission;
};


// default permissions granted to all domains
grant {
    // allows anyone to listen on un-privileged ports
    permission java.net.SocketPermission "localhost:1024-", "listen";

    // "standard" properies that can be read by anyone
    permission java.util.PropertyPermission "java.version", "read";
    permission java.util.PropertyPermission "java.vendor", "read";
    permission java.util.PropertyPermission "java.vendor.url", "read";
    permission java.util.PropertyPermission
                            "java.class.version", "read";
    permission java.util.PropertyPermission "os.name", "read";
    permission java.util.PropertyPermission "os.version", "read";
    permission java.util.PropertyPermission "os.arch", "read";
    permission java.util.PropertyPermission "file.separator", "read";
    permission java.util.PropertyPermission "path.separator", "read";
    permission java.util.PropertyPermission "line.separator", "read";

    permission java.util.PropertyPermission
                            "java.specification.version", "read";
    permission java.util.PropertyPermission
                            "java.specification.vendor", "read";
    permission java.util.PropertyPermission
                            "java.specification.name", "read";

    permission java.util.PropertyPermission
                            "java.vm.specification.version", "read";
```

```
        permission java.util.PropertyPermission
                        "java.vm.specification.vendor", "read";
        permission java.util.PropertyPermission
                        "java.vm.specification.name", "read";
        permission java.util.PropertyPermission "java.vm.version", "read";
        permission java.util.PropertyPermission "java.vm.vendor", "read";
        permission java.util.PropertyPermission "java.vm.name", "read";
    };
```

When you use this policy file, then, all classes that are loaded from the Java extensions directory will be granted all permissions. All other non-system classes will have read access to the system properties listed as well as being able to listen on a socket with a port number of 1024 or greater (which means that the class will be able to create a server socket on an unprivileged port).

A policy file may contain an additional entry:

```
    keystore ".keystore";
```

This entry specifies the name of the URL that will be used to process the keystore in which public keys for the signers listed in the policy file should be found. This entry is missing from the default policy file, as it does not contain any entries that are signed. The name of this file is relative to the URL that was used to load the file; if the `policy.url` property was *file:/${user.home}/.java.policy*, the URL to load the keystore will be *file:/${user.home}/.keystore*. The keystore entry may be an absolute URL if desired.

Policy files may be constructed by hand, or you may use the `policytool` application that comes with the JDK to administer those files (see Appendix A).

Protection Domains

A protection domain is a grouping of a code source and permissions—that is, a protection domain represents all the permissions that are granted to a particular code source. In the default implementation of the `Policy` class, a protection domain is one grant entry in the file. A protection domain is an instance of the `ProtectionDomain` class (`java.security.ProtectionDomain`) and is constructed as follows:

public ProtectionDomain(CodeSource cs, Permissions p) ★

    Construct a protection domain based on the given code source and set of permissions.

When associated with a class, a protection domain means that the given class was loaded from the site specified in the code source, was signed by the public keys specified in the code source, and should have permission to perform the set of operations represented in the permissions object. Each class in the virtual machine may belong to one and only one protection domain, which is set by the class loader when the class is defined.

However, not all class loaders have a specific protection domain associated with them: classes that are loaded by the primordial class loader have no protection domain. In particular, this means that classes that exist as part of the system class path (that is, the Java API classes) have no explicit protection domain. We can think of these classes as belonging to the system protection domain.

A protection domain is set for a class inside the `defineClass()` method. A protection domain is assigned to a class depending upon one of the following cases:

- The `defineClass()` method accepts a protection domain as a parameter. In this case, the given protection domain is assigned to the class. This technique is typically used when you want to define some permissions for a particular class in addition to (or perhaps instead of) the set of permissions that were found by the `Policy` class. We'll show how to do this in Chapter 6, since this is a useful technique for defining an enhanced security model for checking thread access.

- The `defineClass()` method accepts a code source as a parameter. In this case, a protection domain is defined based on the given code source and a set of permissions that have been defined by the system's security policy. This set of permissions is returned from the `evaluate()` method of the `Policy` class.

- The `defineClass()` method accepts neither of these parameters. In this case, a protection domain is defined based on a code source with `null` parameters and a set of permissions that have been defined by the system's security policy (retrieved with the `evaluate()` method). This case will include the default grant entry we listed earlier.

There are three utility methods of the `ProtectionDomain` class:

public CodeSource getCodeSource() ★
Return the code source that was used to construct this protection domain.

public Permissions getPermissions() ★
Return the permissions object that was used to construct this protection domain.

public boolean implies(Permission p) ★
Indicate whether the given permission is implied by the permissions object contained in this protection domain.

The AccessController Class

Now we have all the pieces in place to discuss the mechanics of the access controller. The access controller is represented by a single class called, conveniently, `AccessController`. There are no instances of the `AccessController` class (`java.security.AccessController`)—its constructor is private, so that it cannot be instantiated. Instead, this class has a number of static methods that can be called in order to determine if a particular operation should succeed. The key method of this class takes a particular permission and determines, based on the policy specified by the policy file, whether or not the permission should be granted:

public static void checkPermission(Permission p) ★

> Check the given permission against the policy in place for the program. If the permission is granted, this method returns normally; otherwise, it throws an `AccessControlException`.

We can use this method to determine whether or not a specified operation should be permitted:

```
public class AccessTest extends Applet {
    public void init() {
        SocketPermission sp = new SocketPermission(
                        getParameter("host") + ":6000", "connect");
        try {
            AccessController.checkPermission(sp);
            System.out.println("Ok to open socket");
        } catch (AccessControlException ace) {
            System.out.println(ace);
        }
    }
}
```

Whether the access controller allows or rejects a given permission depends upon the set of protection domains that are on the stack when the access controller is called. Figure 5-2 shows the stack that might be in place when the `init()` method of the `AccessTest` applet is called. In the *appletviewer*, an applet is run in a separate thread—so the bottom method on the stack is the `run()` method of the `Thread` class.* That `run()` method has called the `run()` method of the `Applet-Panel` class. This second `run()` method has done several things prior to calling the `init()` method: it first created an HTTP-based class loader (from an internal class that is a subclass of the `URLClassLoader` class) and has used that class loader to load the `AccessTest` class. It then instantiated an instance of the `AccessTest`

---

* In fact, the `run()` method is always the bottom method on a stack, since stacks apply on a per-thread basis.

class and called the init() method on that object. This left us with the stack shown in the figure—the run() method of the Thread class has called the run() method of the AppletPanel class, which has called the init() method of the Test class, which has called the checkPermission() method of the AccessController class.

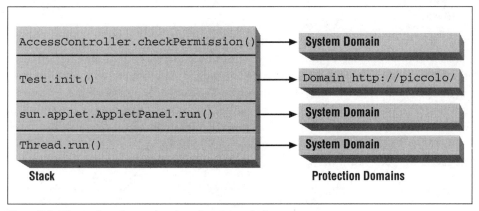

Figure 5-2. The stack and protection domains of a method

The reason we need to know the stack trace of the current thread is to examine the protection domains that are on the stack. In this example, only the AccessTest class has been loaded by a class loader: the AppletPanel class and the Thread class were loaded from the core API with the primordial class loader. Hence, only the AccessTest class has a nonsystem protection domain (associated with the URL from which we loaded it, *http://piccolo/* in this case).

The permissions for any particular operation can be considered to be the intersection of all permissions of each protection domain on the stack when the checkPermission() method is called. When the checkPermission() method is called, it checks the permissions associated with the protection domain for each method on the stack. It does this starting at the top of the stack, and proceeding through each class on the stack.

If this entry appeared in the policy file:

```
grant codeBase http://piccolo/ {
    permission java.net.SocketPermission "*:1024-", "connect";
}
```

the protection domain that applies to the AccessTest class will have permission to open the socket. Remember that the system domain implicitly has permission to perform any operation; as there are no other nonsystem protection domains associated with any class on the stack, the checkPermission() method will permit this operation—which is to say that it will silently return.

For most implementations of Java browsers, and many Java applications, there will only be a single nonsystem protection domain on the stack: all the classes for the applet will have come from a single CODEBASE (and hence a single protection domain). But the checkPermission() method is more general than that, and if you use a class loader that performs delegation, there will be multiple protection domains on the stack. This is a common occurrence if you're using a Java extension.

Let's say that you've written a payroll application that uses a class loader that loads classes from two sources: the server in the XYZ HR department and the server in the XYZ network services department.* This might lead to a call to the checkPermission() method with the stack shown in Figure 5-3. Note that this stack trace is a little more complicated than the one we've just shown—in this case, we're relying on the fact that the constructor of the Socket class will (indirectly) call the access controller. That is what actually happens, and we'll explore that process in our next chapter. For now, we'll just accept the fact that this is the correct stack trace.

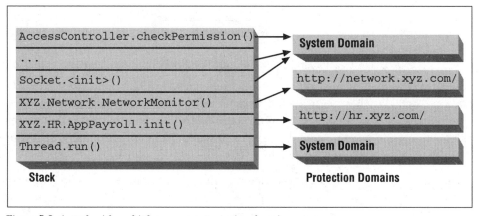

Figure 5-3. A stack with multiple nonsystem protection domains

In this example, the access controller first checks the protection domain for the Network class to see if a class loaded from *http://network.xyz.com/* is allowed to connect to the socket. If that succeeds, it then checks the protection domain of the PayrollApp class to see if a class loaded from *http://hr.xyz.com/* is allowed to connect to a the socket. Only if both code sources are granted permission in the policy file (either individually or via an entry that does not specify a code base at all) does the checkPermission() method succeed.

Whether or not this is the appropriate behavior depends upon your intent. Let's say that the policy file for the payroll application specifies that classes with a code

---

* We showed this example and class loaders to implement it in Chapter 3.

base of *http://network.xyz.com/* are allowed to create sockets, but that no other protection domains (other than the system protection domain, of course) are granted that permission. That leads to the situation where a class from the network services department might not be able to open a socket (even though it has that permission in the file): if there is any class in the HR protection domain on the stack, the operation will fail. All classes on the stack must have permission for an operation to succeed.

Often, however, you want a class to be temporarily given the ability to perform an action on behalf of a class that might not normally have that ability. In this case, we might want to establish a policy where the classes from the HR department cannot create a socket directly, but where they can call classes from the network services department that can create a socket.* In this case, you want to tell the access controller to grant (temporarily) the permissions of the network services department to any methods that it might call within the current thread.

That facility is possible with these two methods of the access controller class:

public static void beginPrivileged() ★

> Extend the permissions of the calling class within the calling thread to any subsequent method calls.

public static void endPrivileged() ★

> Retract the permissions of the calling class.

The `beginPrivileged()` and `endPrivileged()` methods form a block of code; all code within this block will be executed as if it had the privileges of the class that called the `beginPrivileged()` method. Hence, we might write our network class like this:

```
public class NetworkMonitor {
    public NetworkMonitor() {
        try {
            AccessController.beginPrivileged();
            Socket s = new Socket("net.xyz.com", 4000);
        } catch (Exception e) {
            // Do exception processing here for
            // a possible AccessControlException
            // and for exceptions from creating the socket
        } finally {
            AccessController.endPrivileged();
        }
    }
}
```

---

* Consider this in terms of writing a file: an applet might not be able to write a file, but it can call a method of the JDK to play audio data—which means that the JDK class must write to the audio device file.

Note the use of the `finally` clause here; this is typical for the `endPrivileged()` method. The rationale behind this is that if the socket constructor were to throw an uncaught exception—for example, a runtime exception or a thread death—it is still important for the `endPrivileged()` method to be called to make sure that the privileges are not in effect when the network monitor constructor returns. Using the `finally` clause ensures that this happens.

As it turns out, however, the access controller is smart enough to realize when a method that has called `beginPrivileged()` has returned, so if that method somehow forgets to call the `endPrivileged()` method, security will not be compromised. No errors are thrown to the user; the access controller simply (and silently) adjusts its internal state to reflect that the `beginPrivileged()` call should no longer be in effect.

Let's examine the effect these calls have on the access controller. The access controller begins the same way, by examining the protection domains associated with each method on the stack. But this time, rather than searching every class on the stack, the access controller stops searching the stack when it reaches the class that has called the `beginPrivileged()` method. In the case of Figure 5-3, this means that the access controller does not continue searching the stack after the `NetworkMonitor` class, so as long as the policy file has a valid entry for the *http://network.xyz.com/* code base, the monitor will be able to create its socket.

There's an important (but subtle) distinction to be made here: the `beginPrivileged()` method does not suddenly establish a global permission based on the protection domain of the class that called it. Rather, it specifies a stopping point as the access controller searches the list of protection domains on the stack. In the previous example, we assumed that *http://network.xyz.com/* had permission to open the socket. When the access controller searched the protection domains on the stack, it first reached the protection domain associated with *http://network.xyz.com/*. Since that domain had been marked as the privileged domain, the access controller returned at that point: it never got to the point on the stack where it would have checked (and rejected) the protection domain associated with *http://hr.xyz.com/*.

Now consider what would happen if the permissions given to these protection domains were reversed; that is, if the *http://network.xyz.com/* protection domain is not given permission to open the socket, but the *http://hr.xyz.com/* protection domain is. We might be tempted to write the `PayrollApp` class (knowing that it will have permission to open the socket) like this:

```
public class PayrollApp {
    NetworkMonitor nm;
```

```
    public void init() {
        try {
            AccessController.beginPrivileged();
            nm = new NetworkMonitor();
        } finally {
            AccessController.endPrivileged();
        }
    }
}
```

When the code within the Socket constructor calls the checkPermission()
method, the access controller searches the same stack shown in Figure 5-3. When
the access controller reaches the protection domain associated with
http://network.xyz.com, it immediately throws an AccessControlException,
because that protection domain does not have permission to open sockets. Even
though a protection domain lower in the stack does have such a permission, and
even though that protection domain has called the beginPrivileged() method
of the access controller, the operation is rejected when the access controller finds
a protection domain that does not have the correct permission assigned to it.

This means that a protection domain can grant privileges to code that has called
it, but it cannot grant privileges to code that it calls. This rule permits key operations of the Java virtual machine; if, for example, your nonprivileged class calls the
Java API to play an audio clip, the Java API will grant permission to the calling
code to write data to the audio device on the machine. When you write your own
applications, however, it's important to realize that the permission granting goes
only one way.

Guarded Objects

The notion of permissions and the access controller can be encapsulated into a
single object: a guarded object, which is implemented by the GuardedObject class
(java.security.GuardedObject). This class allows you to embed another object
within it in such a way that all access to the object will first have to go through a
guard (which, typically, is the access controller).

There are two methods in the GuardedObject class:

public GuardedObject(Object o, Guard g) ★
> Create a guarded object. The given object is embedded within the guarded
> object; access to the embedded object will not be granted unless the guard
> allows it.

public Object getObject() ★

> Return the embedded object. The `checkGuard()` method of the guard is first
> called; if the guard prohibits access to the embedded object, an `AccessCon-`
> `trolException` will be thrown. Otherwise, the embedded object is returned.

The guard can be any class that implements the `Guard` interface (`java.secu-`
`rity.Guard`). This interface has a single method:

public void checkGuard(Object o) ★

> See if access to the given object should be granted. If access is not granted,
> this method should throw an `AccessControlException`; otherwise it should
> silently return.

Although you can write your own guards, the `Permission` class already implements the guard interface. Hence, any permission can be used to guard an object
as follows:

```
public class GuardTest {
    public static void main(String args[]) {
        GuardedObject go = new GuardedObject(new XYZPayrollRequest(),
                       new XYZPayrollPermission("sdo", "view"));
        try {
            Object o = go.getObject();
            System.out.println("Got access to object");
        } catch (AccessControlException ace) {
            System.out.println("Can't access object");
        }
    }
}
```

When the `getObject()` method is called, it in turn calls the `checkGuard()`
method of the `XYZPayrollPermission` class, which (as it inherits from the
`Permission` class) will call the `checkPermission()` method of the access
controller, passing the XYZ payroll request object as an argument.

Summary

In this chapter, we've looked at Java's access control mechanism. The access
controller is the most powerful security feature of the Java platform: it protects
most of the vital resources on a user's machine, and it allows users (or system
administrators) to customize the security policy of a particular application simply
by modifying entries in the *java.policy* (and/or other similar) files.

The access controller is able to control access to a well-established set of system
resources (files, sockets, etc.), but it is extensible as well: you can create your own

permission classes that the access controller can use in order to grant or to deny access to any resource that you like.

In the next chapter, we'll look into more details of implementing a security policy, including the important relationship between the access controller and the security manager. And, because the access controller is only available with Java 1.2, we'll look at how the security manager can be used to implement a security policy in earlier releases of Java as well.

6

In this chapter:
- *Protected Methods of the Security Manager*
- *Security Managers and the Class Loader*
- *Implementation Techniques*
- *Running Secure Applications*

Implementing Security Policies

In Chapter 4, we examined the security manager in the context of existing implementations of the security manager for use in Java-enabled browsers; we followed that with a discussion of the access control mechanism and Java's ability to define access policies.

In this chapter, we'll put that information together and look at how the security manager is actually implemented, and how you can implement your own security manager. There are three times when it's important to write your own security manager:

In an RMI server

RMI wants you to provide a security manager for all RMI servers; for RMI servers that load client classes, a security manager is required. There is a default RMI security manager that you may use for this purpose, or you may write your own.

In a customized browser

If you're writing your own Java-enabled browser, you'll want to provide a security manager. In addition, if you're using an existing browser, you may want to use a different security manager in that browser. Some browsers already allow the user to specify a different security manager via a property; other browsers can be licensed for this type of customization.

In a Java application

If you download, install, and run Java applications on your machine, you may want to provide a security manager to protect your system against those applications the same way that it is protected against Java applets. In Java 1.1 and earlier releases, this requires you to write a security manager. In Java 1.2, you can use the access control mechanism instead of writing a complete security manager. However, even in Java 1.2 you may need to write your own security manager in certain circumstances. There are methods (like the getThread-Group() method) of the security manager that are outside the scope of the access controller, and there are certain types of permissions (like those typically given to the checkConnect() method) that cannot be specified in a *java.policy* file.

Access Control and the Security Manager

When the access controller was introduced into Java 1.2, it made a big difference to the role of the security manager. Previously, the security manager was paramount in allowing or rejecting operations on files and sockets and other system resources. In Java 1.2, the security manager began to defer permission checking to the access controller.

However, the security manager remains an important interface to system security. The Java API still calls the methods of the security manager to enforce system security—and now most of these methods call the access controller. This allows for upward compatibility—if you wrote a 1.1-based security manager that implements your desired security policy, you can still use that security manager with Java 1.2; your program will run exactly the same as it used to. In this case, you needn't worry about policy files and code sources and secure class loaders—the security model that you've already encapsulated into your security manager will be respected.

Protected Methods of the Security Manager

We've often said that the distinction between trusted and untrusted code has its roots in information that the security manager must obtain from the class loader. There are two ways in which this happens: through a set of generic methods of the SecurityManager class that inform the security manager about the state of the class loader, and through an agreed-upon interface between the security manager and the class loader. We'll look at the first of these mechanisms in this section, and we'll discuss the second mechanism later when we actually develop a security manager.

The use of these protected methods is vital in Java 1.1 and previous releases. In Java 1.2, they are much less important—some of them have even been deprecated. This is not surprising, since the access controller now gives us much of the information that initially could only be obtained from the class loader. We'll give a complete overview of these methods here, although it is information that you'll only need to complete a 1.1-based security manager.

The methods of the security manager that provide us with generic information about the class loader are all protected methods of the security manager class; they are summarized in Table 6-1.

Table 6-1. Protected Methods of the Security Manager Class

Method	Purpose
getClassContext()	Return all the classes on the stack to see who has called us
currentClassLoader()	Return the most recent class loader
currentLoadedClass()	Return the class that was most recently loaded with a class loader
classLoaderDepth()	Return the depth in the call stack where the most recent class loader was found
classDepth()	Return the depth in the call stack of the given class
inClass()	Return true if the given class is on the stack
inClassLoader()	Return true if any class on the stack came from a class loader

protected native Class[] getClassContext()
　　Return an array of all classes on the stack of the currently executing thread.

The first such method we'll discuss lets us retrieve all the classes involved in making the current call to the security manager. This method itself is rarely used in a security manager, but it is the basis for many of the methods we'll discuss in this section.

The getClassContext() method returns an array of Class objects in the order of the call stack for the current method. The first element of the array is always the Class object for the security manager class, the second element is the Class object for the method that called the security manager, and so on.

Accessing all the classes in this array is one way to determine whether the call originally came from code that is in the Java API or whether it came from other code. For example, we could put the following method into our custom security manager:

```
public class MySecurityManager extends SecurityManager {
    public void checkRead(String s) {
        Class c[] = getClassContext();
        for (int i = 0; i < c.length; i++) {
            String name = c.getName();
            System.out.println(name);
        }
    }
}
```

If we then try to create a `FileReader` object:

```
public class Test {
    public static void main(String args[]) {
        System.setSecurityManager(new MySecurityManager());
        FileReader f = new FileReader("/etc/passwd");
    }
}
```

we see the following output from the `checkRead()` method:

```
MySecurityManager
java.io.FileInputStream
java.io.FileReader
Test
```

In other words, a method in the `Test` class invoked a method in the `FileReader` class, which invoked a method in the `File InputStream` class, which invoked a method (the `checkRead()` method, in fact) in the `MySecurityManager` class.

The policies you want to enforce determine how you use the information about these classes—just keep in mind that the first class you see is always your security manager class and the second class you see is normally some class of the Java API. This last case is not an absolute—it's perfectly legal, though rare, for any arbitrary class to call the security manager. And as we saw in Chapter 4, some methods are called by platform-specific classes that implement particular interfaces of the Java API (such as methods that implement the `Toolkit` class).

Also keep in mind that there may be several classes from the Java API returned in the class array—for example, when you construct a new thread, the `Thread` class calls the `checkAccess()` method; the classes returned from the `getClassContext()` method in that case are:

```
MySecurityManager
java.lang.Thread
java.lang.Thread
java.lang.Thread
java.lang.Thread
Test
Test
```

We get this output because the `Thread` class constructor calls three other internal methods before it calls the security manager. Our `Test` class has created a thread in an internal method as well, so the `Test` class also appears twice in the class array.

protected native ClassLoader currentClassLoader()
  Search the array of classes returned from the `getClassContext()` method for the most recently called class that was loaded via a program-defined class loader, and return that class loader.

The objects in the class array returned from the getClassContext() method are generally used to inspect the class loader for each class—that's how the security manager can make a policy decision about classes that were loaded from disk versus classes that were loaded from the network (or elsewhere). The simplest test that we can make is to see if any of the classes involved in the current method invocation are loaded from the network, in which case we can deny the attempted operation. This is the method we use to do that.

To understand currentClassLoader(), we need to recall how the class loader works. The class loader first calls the findSystemClass() method, which attempts to find the class in the user's CLASSPATH (or system classpath in 1.2). If that call is unsuccessful, the class loader loads the class in a different manner (e.g., by loading the class over the network). As far as the Java virtual machine is concerned, the class loader associated with a class that was loaded via the find-SystemClass() method is null. If an instance of the ClassLoader class defined the class (by calling the defineClass() method), then (and only then) does Java make an association between the class and the class loader. This association is made by storing a reference to the class loader within the class object itself; the getClassLoader() method of the Class object can be used to retrieve that reference.

Hence, the currentClassLoader() method is equivalent to:*

```
protected ClassLoader currentClassLoader() {
    Class c[] = getClassContext();
    for (int i = 1; i < c.length; i++)
        if (c[i].getClassLoader() != null)
            return c[i].getClassLoader();
    return null;
}
```

We can use this method to disallow writing to a file by any class that was loaded via a class loader:

```
public void checkWrite(String s) {
    if (currentClassLoader() != null)
        throw new SecurityException("checkWrite");
    }
}
```

With this version of checkWrite(), only the Java virtual machine can open a file for writing. When the Java virtual machine initializes, for example, it may create a thread for playing audio files. This thread will attempt to open the audio device

---

* The truth is that the currentClassLoader() method is written in native code, so we don't know how it actually is implemented, but it is functionally equivalent to the code shown. This is true about most of the methods of this section, which for efficiency reasons are written in native code.

on the machine by instantiating one of the standard Java API file classes. When the instance of this class is created, it (as expected) calls the checkWrite() method, but there is no class loader on the stack. The only methods that are involved in the thread opening the audio device are methods that were loaded by the Java virtual machine itself and hence have no class loader. Later, however, if an applet class tries to open up a file on the user's machine, the checkWrite() method is called again, and this time there is a class loader on the stack: the class loader that was used to load in the applet making the call to open the file. This second case will generate the security exception.

A number of convenience methods of the security manager class also relate to the current class loader:

protected boolean inClassLoader() ☆

Test to see if there is a class loader on the stack:

```
protected boolean inClassLoader() {
    return currentClassLoader() != null;
}
```

protected Class currentLoadedClass() ☆

Return the class on the stack that is associated with the current class loader:

```
protected Class currentLoadedClass() {
    Class c[] = getClassContext();
    for (int i = 0; i < c.length; i++)
        if (c[i].getClassLoader() != null)
            return c[i];
    return null;
}
```

protected native int classDepth(String name) ☆

Return the index of the class array from the getClassContext() method where the named class is found:

```
protected int classDepth(String name) {
    Class c[] = getClassContext();
    for (int i = 0; i < c.length; i++)
        if (c[i].getName().equals(name))
            return i;
    return -1;
}
```

protected boolean inClass(String name) ☆

Indicate whether the named class is anywhere on the stack:

```
protected boolean inClass(String name) {
    return classDepth(name) >= 0;
}
```

Many of these convenience methods revolve around the idea that an untrusted class may have called a method of a trusted class and that the trusted class should not be allowed to perform an operation that the untrusted class could not have performed directly. These methods allow you to write a Java application made up of trusted classes that itself downloads and runs untrusted classes. The HotJava browser is the best-known example of this sort of program. For example, the security manager of the HotJava browser does not allow an arbitrary applet to initiate a print job, but HotJava itself can.

HotJava initiates a print job when the user selects the "Print" item from one of the standard menus. Since the request comes from a class belonging to the HotJava application itself (that is, the callback method of the menu item), the browser is initiating the request (at least as far as the security manager is concerned). An applet initiates the request when it tries to create a print job.

In both cases, the getPrintJob() method of the Toolkit class calls the check-PrintJobAccess() method of the security manager. The security manager must then look at the classes on the stack and determine if the operation should succeed. If there is an untrusted (applet) class anywhere on the stack, the print request started with that class and should be rejected; otherwise, the print request originated from the HotJava classes and is allowed to proceed.

Note the similarity between this technique and the manner in which the access controller works. In Java 1.2, the HotJava classes belong to the system domain, so they are allowed to do anything; the classes that make up the applet, however, are prohibited from initiating the print job (unless, of course, an entry that enables printing for that applet's code source is in the policy file). This is why these methods have been deprecated in 1.2, where the access controller is the desired mechanism to provide this functionality.

The Class Loader Depth

The example that we just gave is typical of the majority of security checks the security manager makes. You can often make a decision on whether or not an operation should be allowed simply by knowing whether or not there is a class loader on the stack, since the presence of a class loader means that an untrusted class has initiated the operation in question.

There's a group of tricky exceptions to this rule, however, and those exceptions mean that you sometimes have to know the exact depth at which the class loader was found. Before we dive into those exceptions, we must emphasize: the use of the class loader depth is not pretty. Fortunately, beginning with Java 1.2, this method has been deprecated, and we need no longer concern ourselves with it. If you need to write a 1.1-compatible security manager, however, you need to use the information in this section.

The depth at which the class loader was found in the class context array can be determined by this method:

protected native int classLoaderDepth() ☆

Return the index of the class array from the getClassContext() method where the current class loader is found:

```
protected int classLoaderDepth() {
    Class c[] = getClassContext();
        for (int i = 0; i < c.length; i++) {
            if (c[i].getClassLoader() != null)
                return i;
        }
    return -1;
}
```

Let's look at this method in the context of the following applet:

```
public class DepthTest extends Applet {
    native void evilInterface();

    public void init() {
        doMath();
        infiltrate();
    }

    public void infiltrate() {
        try {
            System.loadLibrary("evilLibrary");
            evilInterface();
        } catch (Exception e) {}
    }

    public void doMath() {
        BigInteger bi = new BigInteger("100");
        bi = bi.add(new BigInteger("100"));
        System.out.println("answer is " + bi);
    }
}
```

Under normal circumstances, we would expect the doMath() method to inform us (rather inefficiently) that 100 plus 100 is 200. We would further expect the call to the infiltrate() method to generate a security exception, since an untrusted class is not normally allowed to link in a native library.

The security exception in this case is generated by the checkLink() method of the security manager. When the infiltrate() method calls the System.loadLibrary() method, the loadLibrary() method in turn calls the checkLink() method. If we were to retrieve the array of classes (via the getClassContext()

method) that led to the call to the checkLink() method, we'd see the following classes on the stack:

```
MySecurityManager (the checkLink() method)
java.lang.Runtime (the loadLibrary() method)
java.lang.System  (the loadLibrary() method)
DepthTest         (the infiltrate() method)
DepthTest         (the init() method)
... other classes from the browser ...
```

Because the untrusted class DepthTest appears on the stack, we are tempted to reject the operation and throw a security exception.

Life is not quite that simple in this case. As it turns out, the BigInteger class contains its own native methods and hence depends on a platform-specific library to perform many of its operations. When the BigInteger class is loaded, its static initializer attempts to load the math library (by calling the System.loadLibrary() method), which is the library that contains the code to perform these native methods.

Because of the way in which Java loads classes, the BigInteger class is not loaded until it is actually needed—that is, until the doMath() method of the DepthTest class is called. If you recall our discussion from Chapter 3 regarding how the class loader works, you'll remember that when the doMath() method is called and needs access to the BigInteger class, the class loader that created the DepthTest class is asked to find that class (even though the BigInteger class is part of the Java API itself). Hence, the applet class loader (that is, the class loader that loaded the DepthTest class) is used to find the BigInteger class, which it does by calling the findSystemClass() method. When the findSystemClass() method loads the BigInteger class from disk, it runs the static initializers for that class, which call the System.loadLibrary() method to load in the math library.

The upshot of all this is that the System.loadLibrary() method calls the security manager to see if the program in question is allowed to link in the math library. This time, when the checkLink() method is called, the class array from the getClassContext() method looks like this:

```
MySecurityManager        (the checkLink() method)
java.lang.Runtime        (the loadLibrary() method)
java.lang.System         (the loadLibrary() method)
java.math.BigInteger     (the static intializer)
java.lang.ClassLoader    (the findSystemClass() method)
AppletLoader             (the loadClass() method)
java.lang.ClassLoader    (the loadClassInternal() method)
DepthTest                (the doMath() method)
DepthTest                (the init() method)
... various browser classes ...
```

As we would expect, the first three elements of this list are the same as the first three elements of the previous list—but after that, we see a radical difference in the list of classes on the stack. In both cases, the untrusted class (DepthTest) is on the stack, but in this second case, it is much further down the stack than it was in the first case. In this second case, the untrusted class indirectly caused the native library to be loaded; in the first case the untrusted class directly requested the native library to be loaded. That distinction is what drives the use of the class-LoaderDepth() method.

So in this example, we need the checkLink() method to obtain the depth of the class loader (that is, the depth of the first untrusted class on the stack) and behave appropriately. If that depth is 3, the checkLink() method should throw an exception, but if that depth is 7, the checkLink() method should not throw an exception. There is nothing magical about a class depth of 7, however—that just happens to be the depth returned by the classLoaderDepth() method in our second example. A different example might well have produced a different number, depending on the classes involved.

Testing the Security Manager

If you want to know whether or not the security manager will permit a certain operation, you might be tempted to ask the security manager directly. If you want to know, for example, if you can change the state of a particular thread, you might be tempted to write this code:

```
SecurityManager sm = System.getSecurityManager();
boolean canModify = true;
if (sm != null) {
    try {
        sm.checkAccess(myThread);
    } catch (SecurityException se) {
        canModify = false;
    }
}
```

Sometimes this procedure works, and sometimes it doesn't. The methods of the security manager that depend on the depth of the class loader usually test for a specific value. In the code fragment above, the depth of the class loader is 1—which is a depth that most security managers will not complain about, so the canModify variable is set to true. When an actual operation on the thread is attempted, however, the depth of the class loader will be different, and the security manager will reacts differently.

Hence, the only certain way to know if the security manager will prohibit an operation is to attempt that operation and see if a security exception is thrown.

There is, however, something special about a class depth of 3 in this example: a class depth of 3 always means that the untrusted class called the `System.loadLibrary()` method, which called the `Runtime.loadLibrary()` method, which called the security manager's `checkLink()` method.* Hence, when there is a class depth of 3, it means that the untrusted class has directly attempted to load the library. When the class depth is greater than 3, the untrusted class has indirectly caused the library to be loaded. When the class depth is 2, the untrusted class has directly called the `Runtime.loadLibrary()` method—which is to say again that the untrusted class has directly attempted to load the library. When there is a class depth of 1, the untrusted class has directly called the `checkLink()` method— which is possible, but that is a meaningless operation. So in this case, a class depth that is 3 or less (but greater than -1, which means that no untrusted class is on the stack) indicates that the call came directly from an untrusted class and should be handled appropriately (usually meaning that a security exception should be thrown).

But while 3 is a magic number for the `checkLink()` method, it is not necessarily a magic number for all other methods. In general, for most methods the magic number that indicates that an untrusted class directly attempted an operation is 2: the untrusted class calls the Java API, which calls the security manager. Other classes have other constraints on them that change what their target number should be.

The class depth is therefore a tricky thing: there is no general rule about the allowable class depth for an untrusted class. Worse, there's no assurance that the allowable class depth may not change between releases of the JDK—the JDK could conceivably change its internal algorithm for a particular operation to add another method call, which would increase the allowable class depth by 1. This is one reason why the class depth is such a bad idea: it requires an intimate knowledge of all the trusted classes in the API in order to pick an appropriate class depth. Worse, a developer may introduce a new method into a call stack and completely change the class depth for a sensitive operation without realizing the effect this will have on the security manager.

Nonetheless, in order for certain classes of the Java API to work correctly, you need to put the correct information into your 1.1-based security manager (such as in the `checkLink()` method that we just examined). The methods that need such treatment are summarized in Table 6-2.

---

* Theoretically, it could also mean that an untrusted class has called a trusted class that has called the `Runtime.loadLibrary()` method directly. However, the Java API never bypasses the `System.loadLibrary()` method, so that will not happen in practice. If you expect trusted classes in your Java application to work under the scenario we're discussing here, you must also follow that rule.

Table 6-2. Methods of the SecurityManager Class Affected by the Depth of the Class Loader

Method	Depth to Avoid	Remarks
checkCreateClass-Loader()	2	Java beans create a SystemClassLoader
checkPropertiesAccess()	2	Java API calls System.getProperties()
checkPropertyAccess()	2	Java API gets many properties
checkAccess(Thread t)	3	Java API manipulates its own threads
checkAccess(Thread-Group tg)	3 (sometimes 4)	Java API manipulates its own thread groups
checkLink()	2 or 3	Java API loads many libraries
checkMemberAccess()	3	Java API uses method reflection
checkExec()	2	Toolkit implementations of getPrintJob() may execute a print command
checkExit()	2	The application may call exit
checkWrite()	2	Toolkit implementations may create temporary files; the Java API needs to write to audio and other device files
checkDelete()	2	Toolkit implementations may need to delete temporary files
checkRead()	2	Java API needs to read property files
checkTopLevelWindow()	3	Trusted classes may need pop-up windows

In all cases in Table 6-2, the Java API depends on being allowed to perform an operation that would normally be rejected if an untrusted class performed it directly. The JavaBeans classes, for example, create a class loader (an instance of SystemClassLoader) in order to abstract the primordial class loader. So if an untrusted class creates a Java bean, that Java bean must in turn be allowed to create a class loader, or the bean itself won't work.

Note that not every target depth in this table is 2. In the case of the Thread and ThreadGroup classes, operations that affect the state of the thread call the check-Access() method of the Thread or ThreadGroup class itself, which in turn calls the checkAccess() method of the SecurityManager class. This extra method call results in an extra method on the stack and effectively increases the target depth by 1. Similarly, the checkTopLevelWindow() method is called from the constructor of the Window class, which in turn is called from the constructor of the Frame class, resulting in a target depth of 3.

Remember that this table only summarizes the methods of the security manager where the actual depth of the class loader matters to the core Java API. If you're writing your own application, you need to consider whether or not your application classes want to perform certain operations. If you want classes in your application to be able to initiate a print job, for example, and you don't want untrusted classes that your application loads to initiate a print job, you'll want to put a depth check of 2 into the checkPrintJobAccess() method. In general, for methods that aren't listed in the above table, a depth of 2 is appropriate if you want your application classes (i.e., classes from the CLASSPATH) to be able to perform those operations.

There is once again a nice similarity between these ideas and the access controller. When you call the beginPrivileged() method of the access controller, you're achieving the same thing a security manager achieves by testing the class depth. The point to remember about the class depth is that it allows the security manager to grant more permissions to a class than it would normally have—just like the beginPrivileged() method grants its permissions to all protection domains that have previously been pushed onto the stack. Of course, the access controller is a much smarter way to go about this, since it doesn't depend upon someone getting the class depth right; it only depends upon the actual characteristics of the stack during execution of the program.

Protected Instance Variables in the Security Manager

There is a single protected instance variable in the security manager class, and that is the inCheck instance variable:

protected boolean inCheck ☆

Indicate whether a check by the security manager is in progress.

The value of this variable can be obtained from the following method:

public boolean getInCheck() ☆

Return the value of the inCheck instance variable.

Since there is no corresponding public method to set this variable, it is up to the security manager itself to set in check appropriately.*

This variable has a single use: it must be set by the security manager before the security manager calls most methods of the InetAddress class. The reason for this is to prevent an infinite recursion between the security manager and the InetAddress class. This recursion is possible under the following circumstances:

---

* Don't get all excited and think that your untrusted class can use this method to see when the security manager is working. As we'll see, it's only set by the security manager in a rare case, and even if it were set consistently, there's no practical way for your untrusted class to examine the variable during the short period of time it is set.

1. An untrusted class attempts to open a socket to a particular host (e.g., *sun.com*). The expectation is that if the untrusted class was loaded from *sun.com* that the operation will succeed; otherwise, the operation will fail.

2. Opening the socket results in a call to the checkConnect() method, which must determine if the two hosts in question are the same. In the case of a class loaded from *sun.com* that is attempting to connect to *sun.com*, a simple string comparison is sufficient. If the names are the same, the checkConnect() method can simply return immediately. In fact, this is the only logic performed by some browsers—if the names do not literally match, the operation is denied immediately.

3. A complication arises if the two names do not match directly, but may still be the same host. My machine has a fully qualified name of *piccolo.East.Sun.COM*; browsers on my local area network can access my machine's web server as *piccolo, piccolo.East,* or *piccolo.East.Sun.COM*. If the untrusted class is loaded from a URL that contained only the string *piccolo,* and the class attempts to open a socket to *piccolo.East,* we may want that operation to succeed even though the names of the hosts are not equal.

   Hence, the checkConnect() method must retrieve the IP address for both names, and compare those IP addresses.

4. To retrieve the IP address for a particular host, the checkConnect() method must call the InetAddress.getByName() method, which converts a string to an IP address.

5. The getByName() method will not blithely convert a hostname to an IP address—it will only do so if the program in question is normally allowed to make a socket connection to that host. Otherwise, an untrusted class could be downloaded into your corporate network and determine all the IP addresses that are available on the network behind your firewall. So the getByName() method needs to call the checkConnect() method in order to ensure that the program is allowed to retrieve the information that is being requested.

We see the problem here: the getByName() method keeps calling the checkConnect() method, which in turn keeps calling the getByName() method. In order to prevent this recursion, the checkConnect() method is responsible for setting the inCheck instance variable to true before it starts and then setting it to false when it is finished. Similarly, the getByName() method is responsible for examining this variable (via the return from the getInCheck() method); it does not call the checkConnect() method if a security check is already in progress.

There may be other variations in this cooperation between the security manager and the InetAddress class—other methods of the InetAddress class also use the information from the getInCheck() method to determine whether or not to call the checkConnect() method. But this is the only class where this information is used directly. You can set the inCheck method within other methods of your security manager, but there is no point in doing so.

In 1.2, this variable and method are deprecated. The correct operation to perform in a 1.2-based security manager is to call the AccessController.begin-Privileged() method before calling any method of the InetAddress class, and to call the AccessController.endPrivileged() method after the method invocation returns. In addition, the InetAddress class in 1.2 no longer calls the getInCheck() method.

If you implement a checkConnect() method that calls the InetAddress class and sets the inCheck variable, you must make the checkConnect() method and the getInCheck() methods synchronized. This prevents another thread from directly looking up an IP address at the same time that the security manager has told the InetAddress class not to call the checkConnect() method.

Security Managers and the Class Loader

In addition to the methods of the security manager class that we just examined, a second way by which the security manager can enforce policies is to ask that the class loader for a particular class provide more information on which the security manager may base its decision. This technique requires a coordination between the security manager and the class loader; there is no standard interface by which this information may be obtained (nor is there a limit to the type of information that may be exchanged). The details of the interface are completely at the discretion of the application developer. This technique is useful for both 1.1-based and (to a lesser extent) 1.2-based security managers.

In the last section, we showed an example of the checkWrite() method that threw a security exception only if there was a class loader on the stack; this effectively prevented any class that was loaded from the network from opening a file in order to write to it. A more sophisticated policy would be to allow certain classes loaded over the network to write files, but not other classes. If you recall our example from Chapter 3, XYZ Corporation is using a customized class loader that allows their applications to read classes both from the web server on which the application is hosted and from the centralized administration server. XYZ Corporation might want to establish a security policy whereby classes that are loaded from the administration server can write local files, but other classes cannot. This sort of policy requires some cooperation between the security manager and the class loader—the security manager must ask the class loader for the host the class was loaded from:

```
public void checkWrite(String s) {
    ClassLoader cl = currentClassLoader();
```

```
        if (cl != null) {
            MultiLoader ml = null;
            try {
                ml = (MultiLoader) cl;
            } catch (ClassCastException cce) {
                // This can't happen unless our class loader and our
                // security manager are out of sync
                throw new SecurityException("checkWrite out of sync");
            }
            if (!ml.getTrust(currentLoadedClass()))
                throw new SecurityException("checkWrite");
        }
    }
```

This example only works with a class loader we have defined, since we need a method called getTrust() in the class loader to let us know the origin of the class. That getTrust() method might look like this:

```
    public class MultiLoader extends SecureClassLoader {
        ...
        boolean getTrust(Class c) {
            String name = c.getName();
            if (supportClassesCache.get(name))
                return true;
            return false;
        }
    }
```

Hence, we cast the class loader returned from getClassLoader() to be an instance of MultiLoader. It's easy to keep the class loader and the security manager in sync because the application must install both of them, but it always pays to be sure. We use this class loader to check whether the particular class is to be trusted; the class loader thinks classes that have been loaded from XYZ's support machine are trusted and other classes are not.

This sort of cooperation can be used between the class loader and the security manager to support a variety of requirements—providing different access to classes from different domains, or from different protocols, or anything else the class loader knows about. It just requires that the security manager know about any special interfaces the class loader might have to support these features.

The Class Loader and the Security Manager

The relationship between the security manager and class loader goes both ways— not only is the class loader able to provide additional information about particular classes to the security manager, the class loader is also responsible for calling the security manager to see if particular classes are able to be loaded or defined. We showed the code a class loader uses to do this in Chapter 3.

When a class loader is asked to load a class, it must call the checkPackageAc-cess() method of the security manager so that the security manager can prevent certain classes from being loaded. This is chiefly used to prevent untrusted classes from directly accessing implementation-specific classes. If you ship an application with a set of classes in the com.XYZ package, you can ensure that untrusted classes do not directly call classes in that package by placing the appropriate logic into the checkPackageAccess() method. Java-enabled browsers typically do just that; for example, an applet cannot call any of the classes in the sun package within the HotJava browser.

Additionally, when a class loader is asked to define a class, it must call the check-PackageDefinition() method of the security manager so that the security manager can prevent an untrusted class from defining classes in a particular package. This should be used, for example, to prevent an untrusted class from loading a new class into the java.lang package. Otherwise, an untrusted class could create a class named java.lang.Foo that has access to all the default-protected methods and instance variables of the other classes within the java.lang package.

Implementation Techniques

We'll now turn our attention to implementing security policies. Our goal is to show how to write a security manager—one that can be used in conjunction with the access controller, and one that can stand alone. We'll plug these security managers into our JavaRunner program, and we'll also discuss the implementation of the security manager that comes with the Launcher and how that security manager may be installed.

Utility Classes

In order to make our implementation of the security manger a bit easier, we'll provide a few utility classes.

As we intimated above, there are many times when we want to reject an operation if there is any untrusted class on the stack. In order to simplify this operation, we define this method:

```
private void checkClassLoader(String ask, String ex) {
    // Use the ask string to prompt the user if the operation
    // should succeed
    if (inClassLoader()) {
        throw new SecurityException(ex);
    }
}
```

We've passed a string to this method that allows us to ask the user if the operation in question should be permitted; for example, the application could pop up a dialog window and give the user the opportunity to accept the operation. Whether or not that ability is a good idea is open to debate; we've left it to the reader to provide the logic to implement that feature (if desired).

There are a number of tests we want our security manager to reject if they are attempted directly by an untrusted class, but should succeed if they are attempted indirectly by an untrusted class. For these tests in Java 1.1, we have to rely on the class depth to tell us whether the call originated from an untrusted class or not. We use this method to help us with that task:

```
private void checkClassDepth(int depth, String ask, String ex) {
    int clDepth = classLoaderDepth();
    if (clDepth > 0 && clDepth <= depth + 1) {
        throw new SecurityException(ex);
    }
}
```

Note that we have to add 1 to the class depth for this method to succeed, since calling this method has pushed another method frame onto the stack.

Implementing Network Access

Regardless of the release on which your security manager is based, you typically must write the necessary methods to handle network access, because the default methods of the security manager are usually inadequate. In 1.1, the default behavior for the checkConnect() method is to throw a security violation.

In 1.2, the default behavior for the checkConnect() method is to use the access controller to see if the appropriate entry is in the policy file. This is very useful in some circumstances: we can, for example, specify that all code loaded from *network.xyz.com* can access any other machine in the *xyz.com* domain, but no other machines. But we cannot set up a general rule for the mode of network access we're most accustomed to. We cannot set up a rule saying that code loaded from a particular machine can only make a network connection back to that machine. The problem lies in the fact that we cannot pattern match entries in the policy file; we cannot say something like:

```
grant codeBase http://%template/ {
        permission java.net.SocketPermission "%template", "connect";
};
```

So if we want to implement a security policy where code can only make a connection back to the host from which it was loaded, we must provide a new implementation of the checkConnect() method:

```java
public void checkConnect(String host, int port) {
    try {
        super.checkConnect(host, port);
        return;
    } catch (AccessControlException ace) {
        // continue
    }

    ClassLoader loader = currentClassLoader();
    String remoteHost;

    if (loader == null)
        return;
    if (!(loader instanceof JavaRunnerLoader))
        throw new SecurityException("Class loader out of sync");
    JavaRunnerLoader cl = (JavaRunnerLoader) loader;
    remoteHost = cl.getHost();

    if (host.equals(remoteHost))
        return;

    try {
        AccessController.beginPrivileged();
        InetAddress hostAddr = InetAddress.getByName(host);
        InetAddress remoteAddr = InetAddress.getByName(remoteHost);
        if (hostAddr.equals(remoteAddr))
            return;
    } catch (UnknownHostException uhe) {
        // continue and throw exception
    } finally {
        AccessController.endPrivileged();
    }

    throw new SecurityException(
            "Can't connect from " + remoteHost + " to " + host);
}
```

First, we check our superclass to see if it allows the connection. This is only appropriate for 1.2-based security managers—calling the superclass checks the policy file to see if the connection should be made according to information in that file. If that's true, then we simply want to return: the check should succeed. Otherwise, we continue so we can make sure the destination machine is the same machine we loaded this particular class from. For 1.1, this test must be omitted; the superclass in 1.1 would immediately throw an exception.

If there is no class loader on the stack, we want to permit access to any host, so we simply return. Otherwise, we obtain the hostname the untrusted class was loaded from (via the getHost() method of the class loader) and compare that to the hostname the untrusted class is attempting to contact. If the strings are equal, we're all set and can return. Otherwise, we implement the logic we described earlier by obtaining the IP address for each hostname and comparing the two IP addresses.

Note that the logic here for allowing the InetAddress class to resolve the hostname to an IP address is based on the access controller. For a 1.1-based security manager, you replace the call to the beginPrivileged() method by setting the inCheck variable to true, and replace the call to the endPrivileged() method by setting the inCheck variable to be false. You also need to make this method and the getInCheck() methods synchronized.

This implementation requires yet another change to the class loader we're using. The class loader must now be able to provide us with the name of the host from which a particular class was loaded. Since our class loader is based on a URL, that's an easy method to implement: we simply return the host of the URL:

```
public class JavaRunnerLoader extends SecureClassLoader {
    URL urlBase;
    ... other code from previous examples ...
    String getHost() {
        return urlBase.getHost();
    }
}
```

If you choose to implement a different network security model for your checkConnect() method, there are a few things that you should be aware of:

- The checkConnect() method is frequently called with a port of -1. That usage comes primarily from the methods of the InetAddress class; in order to resolve the name of a machine, you must be able to make a connection to that machine. So if you want to restrict a connection to the privileged ports on your machine (those less than 1024), make sure you test to see that the port is between 0 and 1023, rather than simply less than 1024.

- The host argument passed to the checkConnect() method is frequently an IP address rather than a symbolic hostname. This is an artifact of the way in which the default socket implementation (that is, the PlainSocketImpl class) operates: this class actually generates two calls to the checkConnect() method. The first call contains the actual hostname and a port number of -1 (because the PlainSocketImpl class has called the InetAddress.get-ByName() method), and the second call contains the IP address and the actual port number.

- If you choose to disallow all network access by untrusted classes and you are using a network-based class loader to load classes, you cannot simply write a checkConnect() method that calls the inClassLoader() method and throws an exception if it returns true. The class loader must be allowed to open a socket in order to retrieve additional classes that are referenced by the untrusted class, and such a request will contain the untrusted class on the stack when the call is made. In Java 1.1, you can use the inClass() method to see if the class loader is attempting to open the socket, in which case you should let the operation succeed. In Java 1.2, you can call the beginPrivileged() method of the access controller from within the class loader before it attempts to open the URL.

- There is another checkConnect() method that accepts as arguments the hostname, the port number, and an arbitrary object (a context). Like the similar checkRead() method, this version of the checkConnect() method is never called by the Java API, so the easiest route to take is not to implement it at all. The type of information you might choose to encode within the context could be, for example, the hostname that was retrieved from the current class loader. However, since the security manager is responsible for obtaining the context in the first place, there's no reason why that information cannot be used directly rather than calling this second checkConnect() method.

You may want to implement a similar policy in the checkAccept() method so that a class can only accept a connection from the host from which it was loaded. Since we've just implemented that logic in the checkConnect() method, the easiest way to implement this method is:

```
public void checkAccept(String host, int port) {
    try {
        super.checkAccept(host, port);
        return;
    } catch (AccessControlException ace) {
        // continue
    }
    checkConnect(host, port);
}
```

Network Permissions in the Class Loader

In Java 1.2, there is another way to achieve the network permissions we just outlined. Instead of overriding the checkConnect() method of the security manager, we can arrange for the protection domain of each class to carry with it the permission to open a socket to the host it was loaded from. We can add this permission without regard to the permissions that might be in the policy file.

This implementation requires a change to our class loader:

```
protected Class findLocalClass(String name) {
    . . .
    Policy pol = Policy.getPolicy();
    Permissions p = pol.evaluate(codeSource);
```

```
        p.add(new SocketPermission(
                urlBase.getHost() + ":1024-", "connect"));
        ProtectionDomain pd = new ProtectionDomain(codeSource, p);
        cl = defineClass(name, buf, 0, buf.length, pd, null);
        ...
    }
```

Instead of passing a code source to the defineClass() method, we create a protection domain directly. The protection domain is based on the permissions that come with the code source from the Policy class, but then we explicitly add permission to connect to the host from which we loaded the class.

Implementing Thread Security

Implementing a model of thread security requires that you implement the check-Access() methods as well as implementing the getThreadGroup() method. In 1.1, the checkAccess() methods by default throw a security exception. In 1.2, the default behavior of the security manager is to implement the model we'll describe in this section. Both releases return the thread group of the calling thread for the getThreadGroup() method.

We'll show an example that implements a hierarchical notion of thread permissions which fits well within the notion of the virtual machine's thread hierarchy (see Figure 6-1); this is a model implemented by the SecurityManager class in 1.2. In this model, a thread can manipulate any thread that appears within its thread group or within a thread group that is descended from its thread group. In the example, Program #1 has created two thread groups. The Calc thread can manipulate itself, the I/O thread, and any thread in the Program #1 thread groups; it cannot manipulate any threads in the system thread group or in Program #2's thread group. Similarly, threads within Program #1's thread subgroup #1 can only manipulate threads within that group.

This is a different security model than that which is implemented by the JDK's appletviewer and by some browsers in 1.1. In those models, any thread in any thread group of the applet can modify any other thread in any other thread group of the applet, but threads in one applet are still prevented from modifying threads in another applet or from modifying the system threads. But the model we'll describe fits the thread hierarchy a little better.

Note that this security model does not fit well within the idea of thread permissions and protection domains. An entry in the policy file that grants permission to manipulate threads (that is, a runtime permission with the name "thread") to the classes from which Program #1 is loaded will thus grant Program #1 permission to manipulate any threads in the virtual machine. The 1.2 default security manager does check for this permission and honors it if it is present, but if the permission is not present, the security manager follows the model we're about to describe.

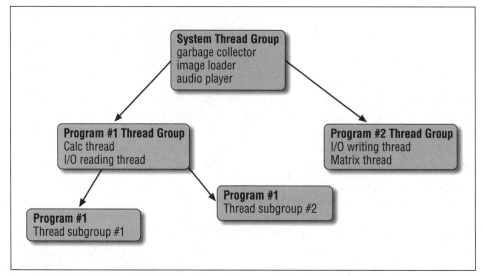

Figure 6-1. A Java thread hierarchy

The key to our model of thread security depends on the getThreadGroup()
method. We can use this method to ensure that each class loader creates its
threads in a new thread group as follows:

- If the program attempts to create a thread in a particular thread group, the
  checkAccess() method can throw a security exception if the thread group in
  question is not a descendant of the thread group that belongs to the class
  loader.

- If the program attempts to create a thread without specifying the thread
  group to which it should belong, we can arrange for the getThreadGroup()
  method to return the class loader's default thread group. This works because
  the constructors of the thread class call the getThreadGroup() method
  directly to obtain the thread group to which a thread should belong.

The simplest way to implement getThreadGroup() is to create a new thread
group for each instance of a class loader. In a browser-type program, this does not
necessarily create a new thread group for each applet, because the same instance
of a class loader might load two or more different applets if those applets share
the same codebase. If we adopt this approach, those different applets will share
the same default thread group. This might be considered a feature. It is also the
approach we'll show; the necessary code to put different programs loaded by the
same class loader into different thread groups is a straightforward extension.

Our getThreadGroup() method, then, looks like this:

```
public ThreadGroup getThreadGroup() {
    ClassLoader loader = currentClassLoader();
    if (loader == null || !(loader instanceof JavaRunnerLoader))
        return super.getThreadGroup();
    JavaRunnerLoader cl = (JavaRunnerLoader) loader;
    return cl.getThreadGroup();
}
```

We want each instance of a class loader to provide a different thread group. The simplest way to implement this logic is to defer to the class loader to provide the thread group. If there is no class loader, we'll use the thread group our   super-class recommends (which, if we've directly extended the SecurityManager class, will be the thread group of the calling thread).

Of course, not every class loader has a getThreadGroup() method, so if the class loader we find isn't of the class that we expect, we again have to defer to our super-class to provide the correct thread group (which, by default, is the thread group of the calling thread). Otherwise, we can ask the class loader, which implies that we need to provide a getThreadGroup() method within that class loader:

```
public class JavaRunnerLoader extends SecureClassLoader {
    private ThreadGroup threadGroup;
    private static int groupNum;
    ...
    ThreadGroup getThreadGroup() {
        if (threadGroup == null)
            threadGroup = new ThreadGroup("JavaRunner ThreadGroup-"
                                    + groupNum++);
        return threadGroup;
    }
}
```

Now we've achieved the first part of our goal: when the program attempts to create a thread without specifying a thread group that it should belong to, the thread is assigned to the desired group. For the second part of our goal, we need to ensure that the checkAccess() method only allows classes from that class loader to create a thread within that thread group (or one of its descendent thread groups).

In order to achieve this second goal, we must implement the checkAccess() methods as follows:

```
public void checkAccess(Thread t) {
    ThreadGroup current = Thread.currentThread().getThreadGroup();
    if (!current.parentOf(t.getThreadGroup()))
        super.checkAccess(t);
}
```

```
public void checkAccess(ThreadGroup tg) {
    ThreadGroup current = Thread.currentThread().getThreadGroup();
    if (!current.parentOf(tg))
            super.checkAccess(tg);
}
```

This logic prevents threads in sibling thread groups from manipulating each other, as well as preventing threads in groups that are lower in the thread hierarchy from manipulating threads in their parent groups. Though that makes it more restrictive than the model employed by the 1.1 JDK, it matches the concept of a thread group hierarchy better than the JDK's model.

There are two caveats with this model. The first has to do with the way in which thread groups are created. When you create a thread group without specifying a parent thread group, the new thread group is placed into the thread hierarchy as a child of the thread group of the currently executing thread. For example, in Figure 6-1, when the Calc thread creates a new thread group, by default that thread group is a child of Program Thread Group #1 (e.g., it could be Program Subgroup #1). Hence, if you start a program, you must ensure that it starts by executing it in the thread group that would be returned by its class loader—that is, the default thread group of the program. That's why we included that logic at the beginning of our JavaRunner example.

The second caveat is that threads may not be expecting this type of enforcement of the thread hierarchy, since it does not match many popular browser implementations. Hence, programs may fail under this model, while they may succeed under a different model.

Implementing Package Access

A final area for which the default security manager is generally inadequate is the manner in which it checks for package access. In 1.2, the security manager looks for a permission of package.access.<package name>, while in 1.1 the security manager rejects all package accesses.

The situation in 1.2 is further complicated by the fact that we're used to using property files to specify which packages to deny access to (e.g., untrusted classes are often denied the ability to use the sun package), but the *java.policy* files only allows us to specify packages we are permitted to access. It would be impossible to know beforehand every package that an application was likely to use, especially when it might define some of them.

For that reason, and also to provide a better migration between releases (and because it's the only way to do it in 1.1), you may want to include the logic to process these old policies within your new security manager. In that way, users will not need to make any changes on their system; in this case, the user will not have to put the appropriate `PropertyPermission` entries into the *java.policy* files by hand.

The `checkPackageAccess()` method is most often used to restrict untrusted classes from directly calling certain packages—e.g., you may not want untrusted classes directly calling the `com.xyz.support` pacakge of your application. Unfortunately, the only way to do that while relying on the access controller and security manager is to rely on the class depth, which we want to avoid.

One solution is to introduce a property for the application that defines packages that the untrusted classes in the application are not allowed to access. HotJava and the `appletviewer` do this by setting properties of the form:

```
package.restrict.access.pkgname = true
```

In the `checkPackageAccess()` method, you can use the parameter to construct this property (substituting for the `pkgname`) and see if the corresponding property is set: if it is, and if the `inClassLoader()` method returns `true`, you can throw the security exception. For our purposes, however, we will allow classes to access any package, and write our `checkPackageAccess()` method like this:

```
public void checkPackageAccess(String pkg) {
}
```

The `checkPackageDefinition()` method is somewhat different—you probably don't want untrusted classes defining things in the java package, for example. So we want to test for that package explicitly. But we also want to respect the permissions for the applications, so the general solution for cases such as this is to first check with the access controller (via the security manager's superclass), and then to implement the original logic:

```
public void checkPackageDefinition(String pkg) {
    if (!pkg.startsWith("java."))
        return;
    try {
        super.checkPackageDefinition(pkg);
        return;
    } catch (AccessControlException ace) {
        // continue
    }
    if (inClassLoader())
        throw new SecurityException("Can't define java classes");
}
```

Note that the name in the test contains the period separator—you don't want an untrusted class to be able to define a class named `java.lang.String`, but you do want it to be able to define a class named `javatest.myClass`. On the other hand, you may or may not want to grant access to classes in the javax package. This method also requires a change to the class loader that we'll show at the end of the chapter.

Establishing a Security Policy in 1.2

We'll now give specific information on how to establish a security policy for 1.2. In Java 1.2, the SecurityManager class is a concrete class—you use it directly, or you may subclass it. The simplest implementation of the SecurityManager class is:

```
public class JavaRunnerManager extends SecurityManager {
}
```

The JavaRunnerManager class inherits the default behavior of the SecurityManager class for all its methods—but it's important to realize that this default behavior is not the behavior we discussed in Chapter 4. The behavior we discussed in that chapter stemmed from the security manager implementations of various popular browsers—that may be the security that is appropriate for your application, but the default behavior for the Security Manager class comes from the *java.policy* files.

The default behavior of the public methods of the SecurityManager class is to call the access controller with an appropriate permission. For example, the implementation of the checkExit() method is:

```
public void checkExit(int status) {
    AccessController.checkPermission(new RuntimePermission("exit"));
}
```

This is why the default security policy for the application can be specified via the *java.policy* files. Table 6-3 lists the methods of the security manager and the permission they construct when they call the access controller.

Table 6-3. The Relationship Between the Security Manager and the Access Controller

Method	Permission
checkCreateClassLoader()	RuntimePermission("createClass-Loader")
checkAccess() [both signatures]	RuntimePermission("thread")
checkExit(int status)	RuntimePermission("exit")
checkExec(String cmd)	FilePermission(cmd, "execute")
checkLink(String lib)	RuntimePermission("loadLibrary." + lib)
checkRead(FileDescriptor fd)	RuntimePermission("fileDe-scriptor.read")

Table 6-3. The Relationship Between the Security Manager and the Access Controller (continued)

Method	Permission
checkRead(String file)	FilePermission(file, "read")
checkRead(String file, Object context)	FilePermission(file, "read");
checkWrite(FileDescriptor fd)	RuntimePermission("fileDescriptor.write")
checkWrite(String file)	FilePermission(file, "write")
checkDelete(String file)	FilePermission(file, "delete")
checkConnect(String h, int p)	*if port == -1* SocketPermission(h, "resolve") *otherwise* SocketPermission(h + ":" + p, "connect")
checkConnect(String h, int p, Object context)	*same as* checkConnect()
checkListen(int port)	*if port == 0* SocketPermission("localhost:1024-","listen") *otherwise* SocketPermission("localhost:" + port, "listen")
checkAccept(String host, int port)	SocketPermission(host + ":" + port, "accept")
checkMulticast() [both signatures]	NetPermission("multicast")
checkPropertiesAccess()	PropertyPermission("*", "read, write")
checkPropertyAccess(String key)	PropertyPermission(key, "read")
checkTopLevelWindow(Object w)	AWTPermission("topLevelWindow")
checkPrintJobAccess()	RuntimePermission("print.queueJob")
checkSystemClipboardAccess()	AWTPermission("systemClipboard")
checkAwtEventQueueAccess()	AwtPermission("eventQueue")
checkPackageAccess(String pkg)	RuntimePermission("package.access." + pkg)
checkPackageDefinition(String pkg)	RuntimePermission("package.define." + pkg)
checkSetFactory()	RuntimePermission("setFactory")
checkMemberAccess(Class c, int which)	RuntimePermission("reflect.declared." + c.getName())

Table 6-3. The Relationship Between the Security Manager and the Access Controller (continued)

Method	Permission
checkSecurityAccess(String action)	SecurityPermission(action)
checkPermission(Permission p)	p (that is, the permission parameter)
checkPermission(Permission p, Object o)	p (that is, the permission parameter)

There are five slight exceptions to the rules laid out in Table 6-3:

- The checkAccess() methods only check for the thread permission if the current thread is not a parent of the target thread, as we discussed previously.

- If the command passed to the checkExec() method is not a fully qualified pathname (that is, if the command will be found by examining the user's PATH variable), the string passed to create the file permission is "<<ALL FILES>>." The domain must have permission to execute all files in the filesystem in this case.

- The methods that use a context expect the context to be an instance of the AccessControlContext class. They then call the checkPermission() method of that context, using the same permission that would normally be used in that call (e.g., a file permission with a read action for the checkRead() method). As we mentioned, these methods are never called by the core API. If the context is not an access control context, then a SecurityException will be thrown.

- The checkTopLevelWindow() method catches the AccessControlException if it is thrown by the access controller. In this case, it returns false. This method does not (by default) throw an exception.

- The checkMemberAccess() method does not call the access controller if the program is inspecting public values (that is, if the which flag is Member.PUBLIC) or if the current class loader is the same class that loaded the target class.

For the most part, it's possible to use the default security manager and the permission mappings we've just identified to support virtually any security policy. But there are certain useful exceptions a security manager will often define:

- Network permissions may want to follow the implementation outlined above.

- Package access and definition permissions may follow the implementation outlined above.

- Exit permissions may be summarily granted to all applications (unless the application is a server that should stick around).

For a complete 1.2-based security manager, then, you typically need to override only the methods involved with these three exceptions. The 1.2-based security manager we'll use for our JavaRunner program looks like this:

```
public class JavaRunnerManager extends SecurityManager {
    public void checkConnect(String host, int port) {
        .. follow implementation given above ..
    }
    public void checkPackageAccess(String pkg) {
        .. follow implementation given above ..
    }
    public void checkPackageDefinition(String pkg) {
        .. follow implementation given above ..
    }
    public void checkExit(int status) {
    }
}
```

Establishing a 1.1 Security Policy

Establishing a security policy in 1.1 is done only by ensuring that the correct security manager is in place. In this section, we're going to discuss how a 1.1-based security manager can be implemented.

The RMI security manager

One of the times a security manager is often used in a Java application is in an RMI server. An RMI server has the capability of loading code from an RMI client located on a remote machine and executing that code on the server—essentially transforming the server (temporarily) into a client.* In essence, the security ramifications of using RMI servers are similar to those of an applet, but in reverse: you now want to protect your server machine from the side effects of untrusted code it got from a client.

In the most common case, you'll want your RMI server to have a simple security model. If the code it's executing was completely loaded from the server, the operation should succeed; if any of the code it's executing was loaded from the client, the operation should fail. Hence, the Java API provides the RMISecurityManager class, which implements just such a policy. In general, the methods of the RMISecurityManager class look like this:

---

* This used to be called "peer computing," although that term has fallen out of favor. But it's a useful concept: just because one machine has to initiate a request shouldn't mean that the roles of client and server have to be immutable.

```
public void checkAccess(Thread t) {
    if (inClassLoader())
        throw new SecurityException("checkAccess");
}
```

You can check the source code (java.rmi.RMISecurityManager) for exact details; this example is a conflation of code found there.

Hence, in the RMI security manager, all local code is trusted and all remote code is untrusted. There are certain methods of this class that have slightly different implementations, however. Because the RMISecurityManager provides a useful basis for a default implementation of your own security manager, we'll list those exceptions here so you can use the RMISecurityManager class and understand where you're starting out.

public void checkPropertyAccess(String key)

An untrusted class can check properties only if a special property is set. If an untrusted class wants to check the property foo.bar, the property foo.bar.stub must be set to true.

public void checkRead(FileDescriptor fd)
public void checkWrite(FileDescriptor fd)

An untrusted class can read or write a file if that file is a socket. Note that the untrusted class still cannot create the socket.

public void checkConnect(String host, int port)

An untrusted class can connect a socket only if called from certain internal RMI classes. If you're using the RMISecurityManager class as the basis for a non-RMI application, the untrusted class is not able to make any connections.

public void checkTopLevelWindow(Object window)

An untrusted class can create a separate window, but it will have the warning banner.

public void checkPackageAccess(String pkg)

An untrusted class can access a package unless the external properties specifically prohibit such access.

public void checkPackageDefinition(String pkg)

An untrusted class can access a package definition unless the external properties specifically prohibit such access.

public void checkSetFactory()

Neither an untrusted class *nor* a trusted class can change a socket factory.

public void checkMemberAccess()

An untrusted class can only check the member access for public members.

A complete 1.1 security manager

In Java 1.1, the SecurityManager class is abstract, so you can't directly instantiate a security manager object. However, none of the methods of Security-Manager is itself abstract, meaning that the simplest implementation of the SecurityManager class is this:

```
public class StrictSecurityManager extends SecurityManager {
}
```

The StrictSecurityManager class inherits the default behavior of the Security-Manager class for all its methods—but once again it's important to realize that this default behavior is not the behavior we discussed earlier in terms of what an untrusted class might or might not be allowed to do. The default behavior of the public methods in the SecurityManager class in 1.1—and hence of the StrictSecurityManager class above—is to deny every operation to every class, trusted or not. Each of the public methods of the SecurityManager class looks similar to this:

```
public void checkAccess(Thread g) {
    throw new SecurityException();
}
```

Thus, if you want to implement your own security manager, you need only override the methods for which you want to provide a more relaxed security policy. If you want to allow (at least some) thread operations, you must override the check-Access() methods; if you do not override those methods, no thread operations will be allowed by any class.

A Null Security Manager

The default security manager class makes you override each method to create a relaxed security policy for that method, but sometimes it might be easier to start with a null security manager: one that provides a completely wide-open policy for every check. You could then override only those methods for which you wanted to tighten the security policy.

The Java API does not provide such a class, but one is available in source form with the Java API source files—if you copy the *SecurityManager.java* file from the API source directory and edit it, you'll find a NullSecurityManager class that implements each method with a wide-open security policy. You can edit out everything but this class, make it a public class, and use it for the basis of your customized security manager. This class was removed from the 1.2 source.

In typical usage, a 1.1-based security manager might want to deny a large number of operations if there is any untrusted class on the stack. These methods might be implemented with the checkClassLoader() method we discussed above. Candidates for this type of check are:

checkAccept()	checkMemberAccess()	checkSecurityAccess()
checkAWTEventQueue-Access()	checkMulticast()	checkSystemClipboardAccess()
checkExit()	checkPrintJobAccess()	
checkListen()	checkSecurityAccess()	

Similarly, there are a number of tests that we want to fail if they are attempted directly by an untrusted class, but that we want to succeed if they are attempted indirectly by an untrusted class. For these tests, we have to rely on the class depth to tell us whether the call originated from an untrusted class or not; we use the checkClassDepth() method to help us with that task. Here are the candidate methods for this test along with the depth that checked for each method:

checkCreateClassLoader()	2	checkLink()	3
checkDelete()	2	checkPropertiesAccess()	2
checkExec()	2	checkPropertyAccess()	2

Finally, there are some methods we must implement with their own logic. Although we've saved these for last, they are the most interesting point of this example, since these are the methods that you'll need to pay the most attention to when you write your own security manager.

Implementing the file access methods

If you are going to implement a security manager, you must determine a policy for reading and writing files and implement that policy in each of the check-Read() and checkWrite() methods. The logic you put into each method is slightly different.

In the case where these methods take a single string argument, the logic is straightforward: the program is attempting to open a file with the given name, and you should either accept or reject that operation. We'll base our decision on the depth of the class loader. Untrusted classes may not directly open a file for reading or writing, but they may cause that to happen through the Java API:

```
public void checkRead(String file) {
    checkClassDepth(2, "Read the file " + file,
                       "Can't read local files");
}
```

Allowing File Access

If you want to write a policy that allows some files on the local machine to be read or written, make sure that you use the `File.getCanonicalPath()` method to find out the actual name of the file before you grant access to that file. If, for example, you want programs to have access to the */tmp* directory on your machine, you want to make sure that access to */tmp/../etc/passwd* is still denied; the program must not be allowed to use the parent directory to jump out of the directory you've allowed. The `getCanon-icalPath()` method removes all references to parent directories, as well as following all symbolic links, shortcuts, and aliases to find out the actual name of the file that's being referenced.

```
public void checkWrite(String file) {
    checkClassDepth(2, "Write the file " + file,
                    "Can't write local files");
}
```

In the case where these methods take a `FileDescriptor` as an argument, the policy is a little harder to define. As far as the Java API is concerned, these methods are only called as a result of calling the `Socket.getInputStream()` or `Socket.getOutputStream()` methods—which means that the security manager is really being asked to determine if the socket associated with the given file descriptor should be allowed to be read or written. By this time, the socket has already been created and has made a valid connection to the remote machine, and the security manager has had the opportunity to prohibit that connection at that time.

What type of access, then, would you prohibit when you implement these methods? It partially depends on the types of checks your security manager made when the socket was created. We'll assume for now that a socket created by an untrusted class can only connect to the site from which the class was loaded, while a socket created by a trusted class can connect to any site. Hence, you might want to prohibit an untrusted class from opening the data stream of a socket created by a trusted class—although if the class was trusted in the first place, you typically want to trust that class's judgement, and if that class passed the socket reference to an untrusted class, the untrusted class should be able to read from or write to the socket.

On the other hand, it is very important to make sure that these methods are actually being called from the socket class. Otherwise, an untrusted class could attempt to pass an arbitrary file descriptor to the `File*Stream` constructor in an attempt to break into your machine.

Typically, then, the only checks you put into this method are to determine that the `FileDescriptor` object is valid and the `FileDescriptor` object does indeed belong to the socket class:

```java
public void checkRead(FileDescriptor fd) {
    if (!inClassLoader())
        return;
    if (!fd.valid() || !inClass("java.net.SocketInputStream"))
        throw new SecurityException("Can't read a file descriptor");
}
public void checkWrite(FileDescriptor fd) {
    if (!inClassLoader())
        return;
    if (!fd.valid() || !inClass("java.net.SocketOutputStream"))
        throw new SecurityException("Can't write a file descriptor");
}
```

Implementing network, thread, and package access

A typical 1.1-based security manager would implement thread, network, and package access as we described above.

Implementing miscellaneous methods

There is one more method of the security manager that we must implement with slightly different rules: the `checkTopLevelWindow()` method. This method uses the standard class depth test for an untrusted class, but it shouldn't throw an exception, so it looks like this:

```java
public boolean checkTopLevelWindow(Object window) {
    if (classLoaderDepth() == 3)
        return false;
    return true;
}
```

Running Secure Applications

In Chapter 1 we showed how `JavaRunner` and the `Launcher` can be used to run a Java application. Now that we have the final piece of the security policy story, we can put everything together and show how the policy can apply to these applications.

The Secure JavaRunner Program

Running a program securely under the auspices of JavaRunner requires that we modify that program to accept a security manager:

```
public class JavaRunner implements Runnable {
    .. other methods are unchanged ..

    public static void main(String args[])
                            throws ClassNotFoundException {
        Class self = Class.forName("JavaRunner");
        System.setSecurityManager(new JavaRunnerManager());
        JavaRunnerLoader jrl = new JavaRunnerLoader(
                            args[0], self.getClassLoader());
        ThreadGroup tg = jrl.getThreadGroup();
        Thread t = new Thread(tg,
                new JavaRunner(jrl, args[1], getArgs(args)));
        t.start();
        try {
            t.join();
        } catch (InterruptedException ie) {
            System.out.println("Thread was interrupted");
        }
    }
}
```

This single-line change installs a security manager for us; the security manager provides the security policy for the target application. Because our security manager defers most of its checks to the access controller, we must have appropriate *java.policy* files somewhere (unless, of course, we have installed a different default Policy class). If these policy files are in the default locations (*$JAVA-HOME/lib/security/java.policy* and *$HOME/.java.policy*), no other steps are necessary. If that file is somewhere else, you must list that file in the *java.security* file as an alternate policy URL.

Note that we cannot use the –usepolicy command-line argument: the –usepolicy command-line argument installs the Launcher's security manager for us, which prevents our security manager from being installed. On the other hand, we could forego the use of the JavaRunnerManager class altogether and use the same security manager that the Launcher uses by specifying the –usepolicy command-line argument.

In Java 1.2, installing this security manager has other ramifications upon the JavaRunner program. Since the JavaRunner class is loaded from the default URL class loader, it is subject to the permissions of the access controller. As a practical matter, this means that one of the *java.policy* files must have certain permissions in it that the JavaRunner program needs: it needs to open sockets (to open the

URLs from which to retrieve the classes), create a class loader, and so on. The simplest way to achieve this is to put the JavaRunner class and its associated class files (the class loader and security manager it uses) into a single directory and grant all permissions to that directory. If, for example, we put those files into the */home/sdo/JavaRunner* directory, we would need to put this entry into a *java.policy* file:

```
grant codeBase "file:/home/sdo/JavaRunner" {
    permission java.security.AllPermission;
};
```

A second change required by the introduction of an access controller–based security manager into this program occurs in the class loader. Remember that the class loader we use—which has just been granted all permissions—is used by other (untrusted) classes to load code. If the JavaRunnerLoader class loader loads the Cat class and the Cat class needs access to the CatFile class, then the JavaRunnerLoader class loader will be asked to load that class. At the time it loads the CatFile class, the Cat class will be on the stack—as will the protection domain associated with that class.

This means that we need to extend the permissions of the class loader so that it will still be able to open the URL and create the socket. This necessitates the following changes to the findLocalClass() method of the class loader:

```
try {
    AccessController.beginPrivileged();
    URL url = new URL(urlBase, urlName + ".class");
    if (printLoadMessages)
        System.out.println("Loading " + url);
    InputStream is = url.openStream();
    buf = getClassBytes(is);
    cl = defineClass(name, buf, 0, buf.length, cs, null);
    return cl;
} catch (Exception e) {
    System.out.println("Can't load " + name + ": " + e);
    return null;
} finally {
    AccessController.endPrivileged();
}
```

The Secure Java Launcher

In 1.2, when you run a program via the command line, no security manager is installed for you and the program has no sandbox (unless one is installed as we did for the JavaRunner program).

However, when you specify the -usepolicy argument on the command line, a default security manager is installed; the effect of that argument is to install the Launcher's security manager. This security manager in turn initializes the access controller—as we mentioned in Chapter 5, the access controller is not initialized until it is first used, and it will not be used until the security manager calls it (unless, of course, your own code calls it). The Launcher's security manager asks the access controller to check for the appropriate permission (that is, the permission that we listed in Table 6-3) with the exceptions that we listed with that table and the additional exception that the checkExit() method always succeeds.

Remember when you use the Launcher that the security provisions only apply to classes that are loaded from the CLASSPATH and not from the Java API.

Summary

Implementing a security manager is a key step in defining a security policy for your own Java applications; the examples presented in this chapter should help you do that effectively. In Java 1.2, you can specify much of the security policy via an external policy file, although there are still instances where you need to write your own security manager in order to achieve specific (but common) policies. In Java 1.1 and previous releases, you need to write your own security manager that implements the security policy you feel is appropriate. Otherwise, your Java application will have no security policy at all.

If you don't feel comfortable running a third-party Java application without a security manager in place, the examples we've provided in this chapter are also key— they provide the cornerstone of the security features that are built into the JavaRunner program.

On the other hand, if you have a secured network and want to expand the parameters of the Java sandbox without resorting to the use and configuration of signed classes (the topic we'll explore for most of the rest of this book), writing your own security manager is also the way to go. For browsers that support it, you can then substitute the new security manager into them, or you can again use the JavaRunner program or Java's Launcher to run the program.

No matter what path you take, the security manager is the most important aspect of the Java sandbox. The methods of the security manager should help you be able to make the appropriate decisions when you implement your own security policies.

7

In this chapter:
- *The Need for Authentication*
- *The Role of Authentication*
- *Cryptographic Engines*

Introduction to Cryptography

So far, we've examined the basic level of Java's security paradigm—essentially, those features that make up the Java sandbox. We're now going to shift gears somewhat and begin our examination of the cryptographic features in the Java security package itself. The Java security package is a set of classes that were added to Java 1.1 (and expanded in 1.2); these classes provide additional layers of security beyond the layers we've examined so far. Although these classes do play a role in the Java sandbox—they are the basis by which Java classes may be signed, and expanding the sandbox based on signed classes is a key goal of Java security—they may play other roles in secure applications.

A digital signature, for example, can authenticate a Java class so that the security policy can allow that class greater latitude in the operations it can perform, but a digital signature is a useful thing in its own right. An HR department may want to use a digital signature to verify requests to change payroll data, an online subscription service might require a digital signature to process a change order, and so on. Thus, while we'll examine the classes of the Java security package from the perspective of what we'll be able to do with a signed class, the techniques we'll show will have broader applicability.

In order to use the classes of the security package, you don't need a deep understanding of cryptographic theory. This chapter will explain the basic concepts of the operations involved, which should be sufficient to understand how to use the APIs involved. On the other hand, one feature of the security package is that different implementations of different algorithms may be provided by third-party vendors. We'll explain how to go about providing such implementations, but it is assumed that readers who are interested in writing such an implementation already understand the mechanics of cryptography. Hence, we won't give any cryptographically valid examples in those sections.

If you already have an understanding of the basics of digital signatures, encryption, and the need for authentication, you can skip this chapter, which provides mainly background information.

The Need for Authentication

We are primarily concerned with one goal of the security package: the ability to authenticate classes that have been loaded from the network. The components of the Java API that provide authentication may have other uses in other contexts (including within your own Java applications), but their primary goal is to allow a Java application (and a Java-enabled browser) to load a class from the network and be assured of two things:

- The identity of the site from which the class was loaded can be verified (author authentication).

- The class was not modified in transit over the network (data authentication).

As we've seen, Java applications typically assume that all classes loaded over the network are untrusted classes, and these untrusted classes are generally given permissions consistent with that assumption. Classes that meet the above two criteria, however, need not necessarily be so constrained. If you walk into your local software store and buy a shrink-wrapped piece of software, you're generally confident that the software will not contain viruses or anything else that's harmful. This is part of the implied contract between a commercial software producer and a commercial software buyer. If you download code from that same software producer's web site, you're probably just as confident that the code you're downloading is not harmful; perhaps it should be given the same access rights as the software you obtained from that company through a more traditional channel.

There's a small irony here, because many computer viruses are spread through commercial software. That's one reason why the fact that a class has been authenticated does not necessarily mean it should be able to access anything on your machine that it wants to. It's also a reason why the fine-grained nature of the access controller is important: if you buy classes from *acme.com*, but only give them access to certain things on your machine, you are still somewhat protected if by mistake *acme.com* includes a virus in their software.

Even if all commercial software were virus free, however, there is a problem with assuming that code downloaded from a commercial site is safe to run on your machine. The problem with that assumption—and the reason that Java by default does not allow that assumption to be made—has to do with the way in which the code you execute makes its way through the Internet. If you load some code from *www.xyz.com* onto your machine, that code will pass through many machines that are responsible for routing the code between your site and XYZ's site. Typically, we like to think that the data that passes between our desktop and *www.xyz.com* enters some large network cloud; it's called a cloud because it contains a lot of details, and the details aren't usually important to us. In this case, however, the details are important. We're very interested to know that the data between our desktop and *xyz.com* passes through, for example, our Internet service provider, two other sites on the Internet backbone, and XYZ's Internet service provider. Such a transmission is shown in Figure 7-1. The two types of authentication that we mentioned above provide the necessary assurance that the data passing through all these sites is not compromised.

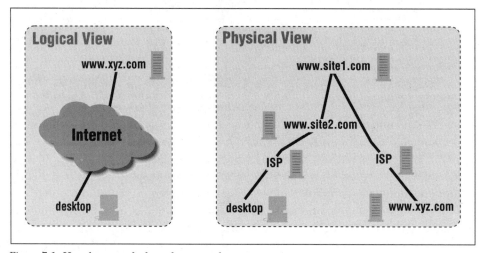

Figure 7-1. How data travels through a network

Author Authentication

First we must prove is that the author of the data is who we expect it to be. When you send data that is destined for *www.xyz.com*, that data is forwarded to *site2*, who is supposed to forward it to *site1*, who should simply forward it to XYZ's Internet service provider. You trust *site1* to forward the data to XYZ's Internet service provider unchanged; however, there's nothing that causes *site1* to fulfill its part of this contract. A hacker at *site1* could arrange for all the data destined for *www.xyz.com* to be sent to the hacker's own machine, and the hacker could send back data through *site2* that looked as if it originated from *www.xyz.com*. The hacker is now successfully impersonating the *www.xyz.com* site. Hence, although the URL in your browser says *www.xyz.com*, you've been fooled: you're actually receiving whatever data the impersonator of XYZ Corporation wants to send to you.

There are a number of ways to achieve this masquerade, the most well-known of which is DNS (or IP) spoofing. When you want to surf to *www.xyz.com*, your desktop asks your DNS server (which is typically your Internet service provider) for the IP address of *www.xyz.com* and you then send off the request to whatever address you receive. If your Internet service provider knows the IP address of *www.xyz.com*, it tells your desktop what the correct address is; otherwise, it has to ask another DNS server (e.g., *site1*) for the correct IP address. If a hacker has control of a machine anywhere along the chain of DNS servers, it is relatively simple for that hacker to send out his own address in response to a DNS request for *www.xyz.com*.

Now say that you surf to *www.xyz.com* and request a Java class (or set of classes) to run a spellchecker for your Java-based word processor. The request you send to *www.xyz.com* will be misaddressed by your machine—your machine will errone-ously send the request to the hacker's machine, since that's the IP address your machine has associated with *www.xyz.com*. Now the hacker is able to send you back a Java class. If that Java class is suddenly trusted (because, after all, it allegedly came from a commercial site), it has access that you wouldn't necessarily approve: perhaps while it's spellchecking your document, it is also searching your hard disk to find the data file of your financial planning software so that it can read that file and send its contents back over the network to the hacker's machine.

Yes, we've made this sound easier than it is—the hacker would have to have inti-mate knowledge of the *xyz.com* site to send you back the classes you requested, and those classes would have to have the expected interface in order for any of their code to be executed. But such situations are not difficult to set up either; if the hackers stole the original class files from *www.xyz.com*—which is usually extremely easy—all they need to do is set themselves up at the right place in the DNS chain.

In the strict Java security model we explored earlier, this sort of situation is possible, but it isn't dangerous. Because the classes loaded from the network are never trusted at all, the class that was substituted by the hackers is not able to damage anything on your machine. At worst, the substituted class does not behave as you expect and may in fact do something quite annoying—like play loud music on your machine instead of spellchecking your document. But the class is not able to do anything dangerous, simply because all classes from the network are untrusted.

In order to trust a class that is loaded from the network, then, we must have some way to verify that the class actually came from the site it said it came from. This authentication comes from a digital signature that comes with the class data—an electronic verification that the class did indeed come from *www.xyz.com*.

Data Authentication

The second problem introduced by the fact that our transmissions to *www.xyz.com* must pass through several hosts is the possibility of snooping. In this scenario, assume that *site2* on the network is under control of a hacker. When you send data to *www.xyz.com*, the data passes through the machine on *site2*, where the hacker can modify it; when data is sent back to you, it travels the same path, which means that the hacker on *site2* can again modify the data.

This lack of privacy in data transmission is one reason you might want data over the network to be encrypted—certainly if the spellchecking software you're using from *www.xyz.com* is something you must pay for, you don't want to send your unencrypted credit card through the network so that *site2* can read it. However, for authentication purposes, encrypting the data is not strictly necessary. All that is necessary is some sort of assurance that the data that has passed through the network has not been modified in transit. This can be achieved by various crypto-graphic algorithms even though the data itself is not encrypted. The simpler path is to use such a cryptographic algorithm (known as a message digest algorithm or a digital fingerprint) instead of encrypting the data.

Encryption Versus Data Authentication

When you send data through a public network, you can use a digital finger-print of that data to ensure that the data was not modified while it was in transit over the network. This fingerprint is sufficient to prevent a snooper from substituting new data (e.g., a new Java class file) for the original data in your transmission.

However, this authentication does not prevent a snooper from reading the data in your transmission; authenticated data is not encrypted data. If you are worried about someone stealing your data, the security provided by data authentication is insufficient. Data authentication prevents writing of data, but not reading of data.

Java only provides authentication and not encryption because of export laws various countries apply to encryption technology. When we discuss the Java Cryptography Extension in Chapter 13, we'll expand upon these restrictions.

Without some cryptographic mechanism in place, the hacker at *site2* has the option of modifying the classes that are sent from *www.xyz.com*. When the classes are read by the machine at *site2*, the hacker could modify them in memory before they are sent back onto the network to be read by *site1* (and ultimately to be read by your machine). Hence, the classes that are sent need to have a digital finger-print associated with them. As it turns out, the digital fingerprint is required to sign the class as well.

Java's Role in Authentication

When Java was first released and touted as being "secure," it surprised many people to discover that the types of attacks we've just discussed were still possible. As we've said, security means many things to many people, but a reasonable argument could be made that the scenarios we've just outlined should not be possible in a secure environment.

The reasons Java did not solve these problems in its first release are varied, but they essentially boil down to one practical reason and one philosophical reason.

The practical reason is that all the solutions we're about to explore depend to a high degree on technologies that are just beginning to become viable. As a practical matter, authentication relies on everyone having public keys available—and as we'll discuss in Chapter 11, that's not necessarily the case. Without a robust mechanism to share public keys, Java had two options:

- Provide no security at all, and allow applets full use of the resources of the user's computer. By now, we know all the possible problems with that route.

- Provide the very strict security that was implemented in 1.0-based versions of Java, with a view toward ways of enhancing that model as technologies evolved. While not the best of all possible worlds, this compromise allowed Java to be adopted much sooner than it would otherwise have been.

On a philosophical level, however, there's another argument: Java shouldn't solve these problems because they are not confined to Java itself. Even if Java classes were always authenticated, that would not prevent the types of attacks we've outlined here from affecting non-Java-related transmissions. If you surf to *www.xyz.com* and that site is subject to DNS spoofing, you'll be served whatever pages the spoofer wants to substitute. If you engage in a standard non-Java, forms-based transmission with *www.xyz.com*, a snooper along the way can steal and modify the data you're sending over the standard HTTP transmission mechanism.

In other words, the attacks we've just outlined are inherent in the design of a public network, and they affect all traffic equally—email traffic, web traffic, ftp traffic, Java traffic, and so on. In a perfect world, solving these problems at the Java level is inefficient, as it means that the same problem must still be solved for all the other traffic on the public network. Solving the problem at the network level, on the other hand, solves the problem once and for all, so that every protocol and every type of traffic are protected.

There are a number of popular technologies that solve this problem in a more general case. If all the traffic between your site and *www.xyz.com* occurs over SSL using an https-based URL, then your browser and the *www.xyz.com* web server will take care of the details of authentication of all web-based traffic, including the

Java-related traffic. That solves the problem at the level of the web browser, but that still is not a complete solution. If the applet needs to open a connection back to *www.xyz.com*, it must use SSL for this communication as well. And we still have other, non-web-related traffic that is not authenticated.

It would be better still to solve this problem at the network level itself. There are many products from various vendors that allow you to authenticate (and encrypt) *all* data between your site and a remote site on the network. Using such a product is really the ideal from a design point of view; in that way, all data is protected, no matter what the source of the traffic is. Either of these solutions makes authentication and fingerprinting of Java classes redundant (and they may offer the benefit that the data is actually encrypted when it passes through the network).

Unfortunately, these solutions lead us back to practical considerations: if it's hard for Java environments to share digital keys and to manage cryptographic technology, it's harder still to depend on the network software to manage this process. So while it might be ideal for this problem to be solved for the network as a whole, it's impractical to expect such a solution. Hence, the Java security package offers a reasonable compromise: it allows you to deploy and use trusted (i.e., authenticated) classes, but their use is not mandated, in case you prefer to employ a broader solution to this problem.

The Role of Authentication

In the preceding discussion, we assumed that you want to load classes from *www.xyz.com* and that you want those classes to be trusted, so that they might have some special permission when they execute on your machine. For example, the spellchecking class might need to open up a local dictionary file to learn how to spellcheck names and other data you customized for the spellchecker.

Do not, however, make the assumption that all classes that are authenticated are therefore to be trusted, or even that all trusted classes should necessarily have the same set of permissions. There's nothing that prevents me from obtaining the necessary information and tools so that I can sign and encrypt all of my classes. When you download those classes, you know with certainty that the classes came from me—they carry my digital signature, and they've been fingerprinted to ensure that they haven't been tampered with.

But that's *all* the information that you know about these classes. In particular, just because the classes were authenticated does not mean that I didn't put a virus into them that's going to erase all the files on your hard disk. And just because you know that a particular Java applet came from me does not mean that you can necessarily track me down when something goes wrong. If you surf to my home page and run my authenticated applet, then surf to *www.sun.com* and run their authenticated applet, then surf to *www.EvilSite.org* and run their authenticated applet, and then two weeks later your hard disk is erased, how will you know which site planted the delayed virus onto your machine? How will you even remember which sites you had visited in the last two weeks (or longer)? If you have an adequate set of backups and other logs, it is conceivable that you might be able to re-create what happened and know at whom to point your finger (and whom to sue), but such a task would be arduous indeed. And if the virus affected your logs, the finger of suspicion might point to the incorrect site.

Hence, the role of authentication of Java classes is not to validate that those classes are trusted or to automatically give those classes special permissions. The role of authentication is to give the user (or, for a corporate network, the system or network administrator) more information on which to base a security policy. A reasonable policy might be that classes that are known to come from *www.SpellChecker.com* can read the user's personal dictionary file—but that doesn't mean they should necessarily be able to read anything else. A reasonable policy would also be that this type of exception to the general rule about permissions given to network classes is only to be granted in very specific cases to only a few well-known sites, and that unknown but authenticated sites are still considered untrusted.

The moral of the story is that authentication does not magically solve any problem; it is merely a tool that can be used in the pursuit of solutions.

Cryptographic Engines

In the next few chapters of this book, we're going to see how Java provides an interface to the algorithms required to perform the sort of authentications we've just talked about. We'll also explore the architecture Java provides for general implementation of these algorithms, including ones (such as encryption) that are not strictly required for authentication. If you're not familiar with the various cryptographic algorithms we've been alluding to so far in this chapter, the next section should sort that all out for you.

Essentially, all cryptographic operations are structured like the diagram in Figure 7-2. Central to this idea is the cryptographic algorithm itself, which is called an engine; the term "algorithm" is reserved to refer to particular implementations of the cryptographic operation. The engine takes some set of input data and (optionally) some sort of key and produces a set of output data. A few points are relevant to this diagram. There are engines that do not require a key as part of their input. In addition, not all cryptographic engines produce symmetric output—that is, it's not always the case that the original text can be reconstructed from the output data. Also, the size of the output is typically not the same as the

size of the input. In the case of message digests and digital signatures, the output
size is a small, fixed-size number of bytes; in the case of encryption engines, the
output size is typically somewhat larger than the input size.

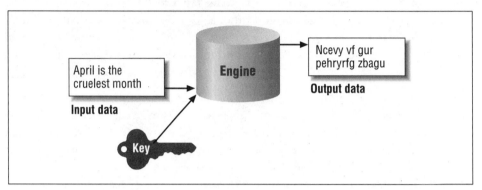

Figure 7-2. A cryptographic engine for encryption

In the Java security package, there are two standard cryptographic engines: a
message digest engine and a digital signature engine. In addition, for some users,
an optional engine is available to perform encryption. Finally, because keys are
central to the use of most of these engines, there is a wide set of classes that
operate on keys, including engines that can be used to generate certain types of
keys. The term "engine" is also used within the security package to refer to other
classes that support these operations.

Message Digests

Message digests are the first cryptographic engines we'll examine. A message
digest is the digital fingerprint we alluded to earlier. Conceptually, a message
digest is a small sequence of bytes that is produced when a given set of data is
passed through the message digest engine. Unlike other cryptographic engines, a
message digest engine does not require a key to operate. It takes a single stream
of data as its input and produces a single output. We call the output a message
digest (or simply a digest, or a hash), and we say that the digest represents the
input data.

The digest that corresponds to a particular set of data does not reflect any information about that data—in particular, there is no way to tell from a digest how
much data it represents, or what the data actually was. A message digest is useful
only when the data it represents is also available. If you want to determine
whether a particular digest represents a particular set of data, you must recalcu-
late the digest and compare the newly calculated digest with the original digest. If

the two are equal, you've verified that the original digest does indeed represent the given set of data.

Data that is fed into a message digest engine is always treated as an ordered set of bytes. If even one byte of the data is altered or absent (or presented out of order), the digest will be different. Hence, a typical message digest algorithm has an internal accumulator that operates on all data fed into the engine. As each byte of data is fed into the engine, it is combined with the data in the accumulator to produce a new value, which is stored in the accumulator to provide input (see Figure 7-3).

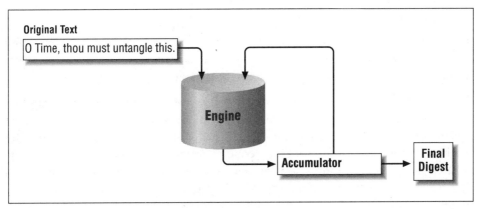

Figure 7-3. The message digest accumulator

As a simple example, consider a message digest algorithm based on the exclusive-or of all the input bytes. The accumulator starts with a value of 0. If the string "O Time, thou must untangle this" is passed to the engine, the engine considers the bytes one at a time.* The first byte, "O", has a value of 0x4f, which will *xor* with the accumulator to provide a value of 0x4f. The next byte, a space (0x20), will *xor* with the accumulator to produce a value of 0x6f. And so on, such that the final result of the accumulator is 0x67.

There are a few differences between this example and a real message digest algorithm. First, standard algorithms typically operate on 4- or 8-byte quantities, so the bytes that are fed into the engine are first grouped into ints or longs, with padding added if the input data is not a multiple of the desired quantity. Second, they produce a digest that is usually 64 or 128 bits long, rather than a single byte;

---

* Don't be confused by the fact that we're dealing in bytes here, when the characters in a Java string are two bytes long. The data passed to the message digest engine is treated as arbitrary binary data—it doesn't matter if the data was originally ASCII (that is, byte-oriented) data, or a Java character string, or a binary class file.

this final digest may be the value left in the accumulator, or it may be the value left in the accumulator subjected to additional operations.

The difference in the output size is one of the crucial differences. At best, the example we just walked through could produce 256 different digests. Any two given inputs have a 1 in 256 chance of producing the same digest, which is clearly not a sufficient guarantee that a digest represents a given set of data. In the example above, the string "O Time, thou must untangle this" produced a digest of 0x67—but so does the string "g". An algorithm that produces a 64-bit digest, on the other hand, produces over 18 quintillion unique digests, so that the odds that two data sequences will produce the same digest are very remote indeed.

This brings us to another of the crucial differences—a successful message digest algorithm must provide an assurance that it is computationally infeasible to find two messages that produce the same digest. This ensures that a new set of data cannot be substituted for the original data so that each produces the same digest.

Note also that a message digest in itself is not a secure entity. A digest is often provided with the data it represents; the recipient of the data then recalculates the digest to make sure that the data was not originally tampered with. But nothing in this scenario prevents someone from modifying both the original data and the digest, since both are transmitted, and since the calculation of the digest is a well-known operation requiring no key. Digests are an important piece of a digital signature, as we'll see in just a bit.

Cryptographic Keys

The second engine we'll look at generates cryptographic keys. Keys are the basis for many cryptographic operations. In its simplest sense, a key is a long string of numbers—not just any string of numbers, but a string of numbers that has very strict mathematical properties. The mathematical properties a key must have vary based on the cryptographic algorithms it is going to be used for, but there's an abstract (logical) set of properties all keys must have. It's this abstract set of properties that we'll see in the Java security package.

In the realm of cryptography, keys can either come alone (in which case they are called secret keys) or in pairs. A key pair has two keys, a public key and a private key. So altogether there are three types of keys—secret, public, and private—but from an algorithmic perspective, there are two types of keys, shared and secret.

When an algorithm requires a secret key, both parties using the algorithm will use the same key. Both parties must agree to keep the key secret, lest the security of the cryptography between the parties be compromised.

The secret key approach suffers from two problems. First, it requires a separate key for every pair of parties that need to send encrypted data. If you want to send your encrypted credit card data to ten different Internet stores, you would need ten different keys. Worse yet, if you operated an Internet store and had millions of customers, you would need literally millions of keys—one per customer. Management of such keys is a very hard problem.

The other problem with this approach is coming up with a method for sharing the keys. It's crucial that the key be kept secret, since anyone with the key can decrypt the data to be shared. Hence, you can't simply send the key over the network without somehow encrypting the key itself; doing so would be tantamount to sending the data itself unencrypted.

For these reasons, most keys in the security package are parts of public key/private key pairs (the exception to this is the encryption engine, which can use any type of key, and which provides a mechanism to share secret keys). Public and private keys can provide asymmetric operation to cryptographic engines. The public key can be used by one party participating in the algorithm, and the private key can be used by the other party.

The usefulness of this type of key pair is that one key can be published to the world. You can email your public key to your friends (and your enemies), you can put it on a global key server somewhere, you can broadcast it on the Internet—as long as you don't lose your private key, you can do anything you like with your public key.

Then, when someone wants to send you some sensitive information, they can use your public key to encrypt the data—and as long as you have kept your private key private, you'll be the only one who is actually able to decrypt the data. Similarly, when you want to send sensitive data to someone, all you need is their public key; when the data has been encrypted with the public key, you know that only the holder of the private key will be able to read what you've sent them. In the area of digital signatures, this key ordering is reversed: you sign a document with your private key, and the recipient of the document needs your public key in order to verify the digital signature.

Public key encryption is not without its key management problems as well, however. When you receive a digitally signed document, you need the public key of the signer of the document. The mechanism to obtain that key is very fluid; there are a number of proposals for centralized key warehouses that would hold public keys and for methods to access those keys, but the infrastructure to make this all a reality is not really in place. Hence, users of public keys have adopted a variety of techniques for obtaining the public keys.

Digital Signatures

The primary engine in the security package (at least as far as authentication goes) is the digital signature engine. Like a real signature, a digital signature is presumed to identify uniquely an entity (that is, an individual or an organization). Like a real signature, a digital signature can be forged, although it's much harder to forge a digital signature than a real signature.* Forging a digital signature requires access to the private key of the entity whose signature is being forged; this is yet another reason why it is important to keep your private keys private. Like a real signature, a digital signature can be "smudged" so that it is no longer recognizable. And because they're based on key certificates, digital signatures have other properties, such as the fact that they can expire.

Digital signatures rely on two things: the ability to generate a message digest, and the ability to encrypt that digest. The entire process is shown in Figure 7-4.

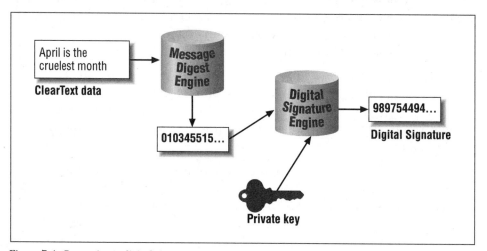

Figure 7-4. Generating a digital signature

The process is as follows:

1. A message digest is calculated that represents the input data.

2. The digest is then encrypted with the private key.

Note that encryption is performed on the digest and not on the data itself. In order to present this signature to another entity, you must present the original data with it—the signature is just a message digest, and, as we mentioned earlier, you cannot reconstruct the input data from the message digest.

---

* On the other hand, a forged digital signature is undetectable, unlike a forged real signature.

Verifying a digital signature requires the same path; the message digest of the original data must be calculated. This digest is then passed through the encryption engine, but this time, the public key of the signer is used. If the digital signature produced by this operation is the same as the digital signature that was presented, the digital signature is deemed valid. Alternately, for some digital signature algorithms, the signed digest could be decrypted with the public key, and the digests compared.

Nothing prevents the signed data from being intercepted. So the data that accompanies the digital signature cannot be sensitive data; the digital signature only verifies that the message came from a particular entity, but it does not actually protect that message.

However, just because someone can snoop the signed data does not mean that it can be tampered with—if the data is altered, it will not produce the same message digest, which in turn will not produce the same digital signature. And it's impossible to change the data, generate a new digest of that data, and then regenerate the digital signature without access to the private key. It is, however, possible to replace one message that was signed by a private key with another message that was signed by that same private key.

Encryption Engines

The final engine we'll discuss handles actual encryption. This engine is part of the Java Cryptography Extension (JCE) rather than the security package itself, and there are various rules on who may and may not obtain the JCE (at least from Sun or other U.S. companies). Encryption engines handle the encryption and decryption of arbitrary data, just as we would expect. An important thing to note is that the encryption engines that are part of the JCE are not used in the generation and verification of digital signatures—digital signatures use their own algorithms to encrypt and decrypt the message digest that are suitable only for manipulating data the size of a message digest. This difference allows the digital signature engine to be exportable, where the encryption engines are not.

Summary

Much of the Java security package is made up of a collection of engines, the basic properties of which we've outlined in this chapter. As a unit, these engines allow us primarily to create digital signatures—a useful notion that authenticates a particular piece of data. One thing that a digital signature can authenticate is a Java class file, which provides the basis for a security manager to consider a class to be trusted (as least to some degree), even though the class was loaded from the network.

The security package, like many Java APIs, is actually a fairly abstract interface that several implementations may be plugged into. Hence, another feature of the security package is its infrastructure to support these differing implementations. In the next chapter, we'll explore the structure of the security package and how it supports these differing implementations; we'll then proceed into how to use the engines of the security package.

8

Security Providers

The cryptographic engines in Java that provide for digital signatures, message digests, and the like are provided as a set of abstract classes in the Java security package. Concrete implementations of these classes are provided by Sun in the JDK, and you also have the option of obtaining third-party implementations of these engines. All of this is made possible through the security provider infrastructure. The provider infrastructure allows concrete implementations of various classes in the security package to be found at runtime, without any changes to the code. In terms of programming, the infrastructure provides a consistent API that can be used by all programs, regardless of who is providing the actual implementation.

Like many other tools discussed in this book, security providers are useful only to developers and users of Java applications. Java-enabled browsers do not implement the security provider infrastructure, nor do they implement any of the cryptographic engines we discuss in the remainder of this book. On the other hand, one of the key features of the Activator—the Java plug-in for Internet Explorer and Netscape Communicator—is that it does implement the entire security provider infrastructure for use within a browser (subject to the restrictions that might be in place by the access controller and security manager). All the features discussed in this chapter are available in both Java 1.1 and 1.2, with some slight differences we'll mention.

In terms of actual programming, the classes we're going to examine in this chapter are rarely used—hence, we will not delve much into programming. For most developers, end users, and administrators, this chapter focuses on the architecture of the security provider, since that gives us the ability to substitute new implementations of the cryptographic engines we'll use in the rest of the book.

Following that discussion, we'll move into the implementation of the architecture, for those readers who are interested in the details.

The Architecture of Security Providers

The security provider abstracts two ideas: engines and algorithms. In this context, "engine" is just another word for operation; there are certain operations the security provider knows about, and in Java, these operations are known as engines. An algorithm defines how a particular operation should be executed. An algorithm can be thought of as an implementation of an engine, but that can lead to confusion, because there may be several implementations of an algorithm.

As a simple example, the Java security package knows about message digests. A message digest is an engine: it is an operation a programmer can perform. The idea behind a message digest is independent of how any particular message digest may be calculated. All message digests share certain features, and the class that abstracts these common features into a single interface is termed an engine. Engines are generally abstract, and are always independent of any particular algorithm.

A message digest may be implemented by a particular algorithm, such as MD5 or SHA. An algorithm is generally provided as a concrete class that extends an abstract engine class, completing the definition of the class. However, there may be many classes that provide a particular algorithm; you may have an SHA class that came with your Java platform, and you may also have obtained an SHA class from a third party. Both classes should provide the same results, but their internal implementations may be vastly different.

Security providers are the glue that manages the mapping between the engines used by the rest of the security package (such as a message digest), the specific algorithms that are valid for those engines (such as an SHA digest), and the specific implementations of that algorithm/engine pair that might be available to any particular Java virtual machine. The goal of the security provider interface is to allow an easy mechanism where the specific algorithms and their implementations can be easily changed or substituted. The security provider allows us to change the implementation of the SHA digest algorithm that is in use, and to introduce a new algorithm to generate a digest.

Hence, a typical programmer only uses the engine classes to perform particular operations. You don't need to worry about the classes that actually perform the computation. The engine classes provide the primary interface to the security package.

Components of the Architecture

The architecture surrounding all of this has these components:

Engine classes

> These classes come with the Java virtual machine as part of the core API.

Algorithm classes

> At the basic level, there is a set of classes that implement particular algorithms for particular engines. A default set of these classes is provided by the supplier of the Java platform, and other third-party organizations (including your own) can supply additional sets of algorithm classes. These classes may implement one or more algorithms for one or more engines; it is not necessary for a set of classes from a particular vendor to implement all possible algorithms or all possible engines. A single algorithm class provides a particular algorithm for a particular engine.

The Provider class

> Each set of algorithm classes from a particular vendor is managed by an instance of the class `Provider`. A provider knows how to map particular algorithms to the actual class that implements the operation.

The Security class

> The `Security` class maintains a list of the provider classes and consulting each in turn to see which operations it supports.

In later chapters, we'll look at the individual algorithms and engines of this architecture; for now, we'll discuss the `Provider` and `Security` classes. These two classes together make up the idea of a security provider.

The security providers rely on cooperation between themselves and the rest of the Java security package in order to fulfill their purpose. The details of this cooperation are handled for us—when we use the `MessageDigest` class to generate a digest, for example, it's the responsibility of the `MessageDigest` class to ask the `Security` class which particular class to use to generate the digest. The `Security` class in turn asks each of the providers whether or not they can supply the desired digest.

So a typical program that wants to use the security package does not interact directly with the security provider. Instead, the security provider provides its usefulness transparently to the programmer and to the end user. An end user, a system administrator, or a developer can configure the security provider; this is a result of the security provider being based on a set of provider classes. While there is a default provider class, the end user or system administrator can replace the default provider with another class. In addition, a user or programmer can augment the default provider class by adding additional provider classes.

When the security package needs to perform an operation, it constructs a string representing that operation and asks the `Security` class for an object that can perform the operation with the given algorithm. For example, the idea of generating a message digest is represented by a particular engine; its name (i.e., `MessageDigest`) is the first component in the request to the security provider. There can be many algorithms that can provide a message digest. SHA-1 and MD5 are the two most common, though we'll explore other possibilities when we look in depth at the corresponding classes that handle digests in Java. So the name of the algorithm (e.g., `MD5`) forms the second component of the string provided to the security class. These components are concatenated into a single string separated by a dot (e.g., `MessageDigest.MD5`).

Six cryptographic engines are supported in the Java security package. In addition, thirteen cryptographic algorithms are common enough to have standard names recognized by the Java security package. However, not every algorithm can be used to perform every operation; the valid combinations Java supports are listed in Table 8-1. Italicized entries are operations that the Java security specification defines as legal, but are not implemented by the default security provider.

Table 8-1. Security Features and Algorithms Expected in the Security API

Engine	Algorithm Name
AlgorithmParameters ★	DSA
AlgorithmParameterGenerator ★	DSA
KeyFactory ★	DSA
KeyPairGenerator	DSA
KeyPairGenerator	*RSA*
MessageDigest	MD5
MessageDigest	SHA-1
MessageDigest	*MD2*
Signature	DSA[a]
Signature	*MD2/RSA*
Signature	*MD5/RSA*
Signature	*SHA-1/RSA*

[a] This becomes SHA/DSA in Java 1.2, though DSA is still accepted.

The names in this table are the strings passed to the security provider in order for it to find the class implementing the operation. In addition, the security provider can be passed certain alias strings that map an alias to one of these valid strings. For example, although the standard name of the secure hash algorithm is SHA-1 (to distinguish it from SHA-0, the first such algorithm, which is now obsolete), this algorithm is often referred to as SHA. So while

```
MessageDigest.SHA-1
```

is a valid string to pass to the security provider, there is a way to construct alias strings so that the alias refers to the original algorithm. Such a string has the form:

```
Alg.Alias.MessageDigest.SHA
```

This string specifies to the security provider that SHA is a valid name for the message digest operation implemented by this provider. We'll see an example of this alias in use when we discuss the Provider class.

A word about the algorithm names in Table 8-1: Though the documentation for the Java security package talks about these algorithm names as the valid names that are supported by Java, that notion is not very helpful. As the entries in italics show, not all pairs of engines and algorithm names are provided by the default JDK. So, even though it's reasonable to ask the Java security package for an engine that provides digital signatures using an RSA algorithm, you won't be successful in obtaining such an engine unless you've installed special software to provide it. Similarly, although these are the supported algorithm names, there's nothing that prevents us from using another name to refer to a new algorithm. If you develop a new algorithm that performs a message digest operation, you can give that algorithm whatever name you like and use that name freely within the Java security package.

As it happens, there are many standard algorithms that have well-known names which are not included in the set of names that the Java security specification defines; there are some six to eight well-known message digest algorithms even though the Java documentation mentions only three of them. Nothing prevents you from using any of these algorithms.

In fact, the default security provider in Sun's provider uses other names for the algorithms it does implement, although those names are undocumented. On the other hand, it is not very useful to have arbitrary names for algorithms; these other names that the Sun provider uses are known as OID names. OID stands for Object IDentifier and is a way that some algorithm names are standardized by the U.S. government. If you're used to dealing with algorithm definitions at that level, rest assured that the Sun provider has aliases for them, but for our purposes, we'll stick with the default names.

Choosing a Security Provider

When the Java virtual machine begins execution, it is responsible for consulting the user's properties in order to determine which security providers should be in place. These properties must be located in the file *$JAVAHOME/lib/security/java.security*. In the reference release of the JDK, this file contains this line (among others):

```
security.provider.1=sun.security.provider.Sun
```

This line tells us that there is at least one provider class that should be consulted, and that class should be an instance of the `sun.security.provider.Sun` class.

Each provider given in this file must be numbered, starting with 1. If you want to use an additional provider, you can edit this file and add that provider at the next number. Say that you obtain a security provider from XYZ Corporation. When you obtain this provider, you are told that the provider's class name is `com.xyz.XYZProvider`; hence, you add this line to the *java.security* file:

```
security.provider.2=com.xyz.XYZProvider
```

Note that there's no reason why the new provider class had to be added at position 2—it would have been perfectly acceptable to add the `XYZProvider` class as `security.provider.1` if the `sun.security.provider.Sun` class were changed to `security.provider.2` (or, alternately, removed altogether). The `Security` class keeps the instances of the providers in an array so that each class is found at the index specified in the *java.security* file. As long as the providers in the *java.security* file begin with 1 and are numbered consecutively, they may appear in any order.

The numbers in this example are significant; when the `Security` class is asked to provide a particular engine and algorithm, it searches the listed providers in order to find the first one that can supply the desired operation. All engine classes use the security class to supply objects. When the message digest engine is asked to provide an object capable of generating SHA message digests, the engine will ask the `Security` class which provider to use. If the first provider in the list can perform SHA message digests, that provider will be used. Otherwise, the second provider is checked, and so on, until there are no providers left (and an exception is thrown) or until a provider that implements the desired operation is found. Hence, the number that follows the `security.provider` string indicates the order in which providers will be searched for particular implementations.

For end users and administrators, that's all there is to adding new security providers. For developers, there is also a programmatic way in which a security provider may be added; we'll explore that when we discuss the interface of the `Security` class. But as we mentioned earlier, the programmatic interface provided by the two classes we're about to discuss is not often needed; you'd need them only if you wanted to supply your own security provider, or if you wanted to inspect or set programmatically the list of existing providers. Otherwise, the classes are interesting only because they are used by the engine classes we'll begin to examine in the next chapter.

The Provider Class

The first class we'll examine in depth is the Provider class (java.security.Provider).

public abstract class Provider extends Properties

> This class forms the basis of the security provider architecture. There is normally a standard subclass that implements a default security feature set; other classes can be installed to implement other security algorithms.

In the core Java API, the Provider class is abstract, and there are no classes in the core Java API that extend the Provider class. The default provider class that comes with the reference JDK is the class Sun in the sun.security.provider package. However, since this class is in the sun package, there's no guarantee that it will be available with every implementation of the Java virtual machine.

In theory, this should not matter. The concepts of the security package will work according to the specification as long as the Java implementation provides an appropriate provider class and appropriate classes to perform the operations a Java program will expect. The exact set of classes a particular program may expect will depend, of course, on the program. In the next section, we'll discuss how different implementations of the Provider class may be loaded and used during the execution of the virtual machine.

Using the Provider Class

The Provider class is seldom used directly by a programmer. This class does contain a number of useful miscellaneous method we'll review here; these methods are generally informational and would be used accordingly.

public String getName()

> Return the name of the provider.

public double getVersion()

> Return the version number of the provider.

public String getInfo()

> Return the info string of the provider.

public String toString()

> Return the string specifying the provider; this is typically the provider's name concatenated with the provider's version number.

As an extension of the Properties class, the Provider class also shares its public interface. Beginning in Java 1.2, the Provider class overrides three of those methods:

public synchronized void clear() ★

> If permission is granted, clear out all entries from the provider.

public synchronized Object put(Object key, Object value) ★

> If permission is granted, add the given property, keyed off the given key.

public synchronized Object remove(Object key) ★

> If permission is granted, remove the object associated with the given key.

Permission to perform these last three options is granted if the checkSecurityAccess() method grants permission based on the argument string Provider.<method name> + getName() where <method name> is clear, put, or remove.

Since the interface to this class is simple, we won't actually show how it is used, although we will use some of these methods later in this chapter. Note also that there is no public constructor for the Provider class—a provider can only be constructed under special circumstances we'll discuss later.

Implementing the Provider Class

If you're going to provide your own set of classes to perform security operations, you must extend the Provider class and register that class with the virtual machine. In this section, we'll explore how to do that. Most of the time, of course, you will not implement your own Provider class—you'll just use the default one, or perhaps install a third-party provider using the techniques that we explore in the next section.

Although the Provider class is abstract, none of its methods are abstract. This means that implementing a provider is, at first blush, simple: all you need do is subclass the Provider class and provide an appropriate constructor. The subclass must provide a constructor, since there is no default constructor within the Provider class. The only constructor available to us is:

protected Provider(String name, double version, String info)

> Construct a provider with the given name, version number, and information string.

Hence, the basic implementation of a security provider is:

```
public class XYZProvider extends Provider {
    public XYZProvider() {
        super("XYZ", 1.0, "XYZ Security Provider v1.0");
    }
}
```

Here we're defining the skeleton of a provider that is going to provide certain facilities based on various algorithms of the XYZ Corporation. Throughout the remainder of this book, we'll be developing the classes that apply to the XYZ's cryptographic methods, but they will be examples only—they lack the rigorous mathematical properties that these algorithms must have. In practice, you might choose to implement algorithms that correspond to the RSA algorithms for the cryptographic engines.

Note that we used a default constructor in this class rather than providing a constructor similar to the one found in the `Provider` class itself. The reason for this has to do with the way providers are constructed, which we'll discuss at the end of this section. When you write a provider, it must provide a constructor with no arguments.

This is a complete, albeit useless, implementation of a provider. In order to add some functionality to our provider, we must put some associations into the provider. The associations will perform the mapping that we mentioned earlier; it is necessary for the provider to map the name of an engine and algorithm with the name of a class that implements that operation. This is why the `Provider` class itself is a subclass of the `Properties` class—so that we can make each of those associations into a property.

The operations that our provider will be consulted about are listed in Table 8-2. In this example, we're going to be providing an SHA-1 algorithm for performing message digests, since that would be needed as part of the signature generation algorithm we want to implement. There's no absolute requirement for this; we could have depended on the default Sun security provider to supply this algorithm for us. On the other hand, there's no guarantee that the default security provider will be in place when our security provider is installed, so it's a good idea for a provider to include all the algorithms it will need.

Table 8-2. Properties Included by Our Sample Provider

Property	Corresponding Class
Signature.SHA-1/XYZ	XYZSignature
KeyPairGenerator.XYZ	XYZKeyPairGenerator
MessageDigest.XYZ	XYZMessageDigest
MessageDigest.SHA-1	SHA1MessageDigest

In order to make these associations from this table, then, our `XYZProvider` class needs to look like this:

```
public class XYZProvider extends Provider {
    public XYZProvider() {
        super("XYZ", 1.0, "XYZ Security Provider v1.0");
```

```
        put("Signature.SHA-1/XYZ", "com.xyz.XYZSignature");
        put("KeyPairGenerator.XYZ", "com.xyz.XYZKeyPairGenerator");
        put("MessageDigest.XYZ", "com.xyz.XYZMessageDigest");
        put("MessageDigest.SHA-1", "com.xyz.SHA1MessageDigest");
        put("Alg.Alias.MessageDigest.SHA", "SHA-1");
    }
}
```

The only properties a provider is required to put into its property list are the properties that match the engine name and algorithm pair with the class that implements that operation. In this example, that's handled with the first four calls to the put() method (but remember too that the provider can implement as few or as many operations as it wants to; it needn't implement more than a single engine with one algorithm, or it can implement dozens of engine/algorithm pairs). Note that the class name is the fully qualified package name of the class.

The provider also has the opportunity to set any other properties that it wants to use. If the provider wants to set aliases (as we've done with the final call to the put() method, using the syntax we showed earlier), it's free to do so. Our example allows the program using this provider to request an SHA message digest in addition to requesting an SHA-1 digest. Doing this for SHA is highly advisable, since that algorithm is typically referred to as SHA rather than SHA-1, but that's the only common case where that aliasing is needed.

A provider can set any other arbitrary properties that it wants as well. For instance, a provider class could set this property:

```
    put("NativeImplementation", "false");
```

if it wanted the classes that use the provider to be able to determine if this particular XYZ implementation uses native methods.* It can also use the convention that certain properties are preceded with the word Alg and contain the algorithm name, like this:

```
    put("Alg.NativeImplementation.XYZ", "false");
```

There's no advantage to setting any additional properties—nothing in the core JDK will use them. They can be set to make the classes that accompany your provider class easier to write—for example, your XYZSignature class might want to inquire which particular providers have a native method implementation of the XYZ algorithm. Whatever information you put into your provider and how your accompanying classes use that information is a design detail that is completely up to you. The Security class will help you manage the information in these proper-

---

* RSA algorithms often use native methods, because there are existing implementations of them that are written in C and have gone through an extensive quality acceptance test that many commercial sites have a level of confidence in. However, many third-party RSA implementations do not use native methods.

ties; this relationship to the Security class is the reason why we used a string value for the NativeImplementation property rather than a Boolean value.

There's one more nonpublic method of the Provider class that is used by the security API:

static Provider loadProvider(String className)
> Instantiate a provider that has as its type the given class. This method is provided mostly for convenience—it simply loads the given class and instantiates it. However, this method also ensures that the loaded class is an instance of the Provider class.

This method creates an instance of a provider. The importance of this method stems from how it performs its task: it creates the instance of the provider object by calling the newInstance() method of the Class class. In order for that operation to succeed, the provider class must therefore have a default constructor—that is, a constructor that requires no arguments. This is why in our example we provided such a constructor and had the constructor hardwire the name, version number, and information string. We could have provided an additional constructor that accepts those values as parameters, but it would never be called, since the only way in which the virtual machine uses providers is to load them via this method.

In the next section, we'll look into the details of how the virtual machine loads those provider classes we want to use.

The Security Class

The Security class (java.security.Security) is responsible for managing the set of provider classes that a Java program can use, and forms the last link in the architecture of the security provider. This class is final, and all its methods are static (except for its constructor, which is private). Like the System and Math classes, then, the Security class can never be created or subclassed; it exists simply to provide a placeholder for methods that deal with the java.security package.

Earlier, we explained how to add entries to the *java.security* file to add new providers to the security architecture. The same feat can be accomplished programmatically via these methods of the Security class:

public static int addProvider(Provider provider)
> Add a new provider into the list of providers. The provider is added to the end of the internal array of providers.

public static int insertProviderAt(Provider provider, int position)

> Add a new provider into the internal array of providers. The provider is added at the specified position; other providers have their index changed if necessary to make room for this provider. Position counting begins at 1.

The notion that these classes are kept in an indexed array is important; when the Security class is asked to provide a particular algorithm for an operation, the array is searched sequentially for a provider that can provide the requested algorithm for the requested operation.

As an example, let's use a modification of the XYZProvider class that we outlined earlier. This class comes with a set of classes to perform generation of key pairs, and it can generate key pairs according to two algorithms: DSA and XYZ. The XYZProvider class, according to an entry added to the *java.security* file, has been added at position 2. Additionally, let's say that our Java program has installed an additional provider class at position 3 called the FooProvider that can generate key pairs and digital signatures according to a single algorithm known as Foo.

Table 8-3. Sample Security Providers

Sun Provider	XYZ Provider	Foo Provider

Signature Engines
    DSA
	Signature Engines
	    XYZ
	    DSA
		Signature Engines
		    Foo

Message Digest Engines
    MD5
	Message Digest Engines
	    XYZ
	    SHA
		Message Digest Engines
		    None

Key Pair Engines
    DSA
	Key Pair Engines
	    XYZ
	    DSA
		Key Pair Engines
		    Foo

This leaves us with the set of provider classes listed in Table 8-3.

Now when our Java program needs to generate a key pair, the security provider is consulted as to which classes will implement the key pair generation we want. If we need to generate a DSA key, the security provider returns to us a class associated with the Sun provider class, since the Sun provider, at position 1, is the first class that says that it can perform DSA key generation. If we had reversed the order of indices in the *java.security* file so that the Sun provider was at position 2 and the XYZ provider was at position 1, a class associated with the XYZ provider would have been returned instead. Similarly, when we request a Foo key pair, a class associated with the Foo provider is returned to us, regardless of what index it occurs at, since that is the only provider class that knows how to perform Foo key generation.

Remember that this is a two-step process. The security class receives a string (like `KeyPairGenerator.DSA`) and locates a class that provides that service (such as `sun.security.provider.Sun`). The Sun class, as a provider class, does not actually know how to generate keys (or do anything else)—it only knows what classes in the Sun security package know how to generate keys. Then the security class must ask the provider itself for the name of the class that actually implements the desired operation. That process is handled by an internal method of the Security class—we'll use that method implicitly over the next few chapters when we retrieve objects that implement a particular engine and algorithm. Before we do that, though, we'll finish looking at the interface of the Security class.

There are a number of other methods in the Security class that provide basic information about the configuration of the security provider.

public static void removeProvider(String name)

> Remove the named provider from the list of provider classes. The remaining providers move up in the array of providers if necessary. If the named provider is not in the list, this method silently returns (i.e., no exception is thrown).

public static Provider[] getProviders()

> Return a copy of the array of providers on which the Security class operates. Note that this is a copy of the array; reordering its elements has no effect on the Security class.

public static Provider getProvider(String name)

> Return the provider with the given name. If the named provider is not in the list held by the Security class, this method returns `null`.

public static String getProperty(String key)

> Get the property of the Security class with the associated key. The properties held in the Security class are the properties that were read from the *java.security* file. In typical usage, one of the properties is `security.provider.1` (as well as any other providers listed in the *java.security* file). Note, however, that properties of this sort may not reflect the actual order of the provider classes: when the `addProvider()`, `insertProviderAt()`, and `removeProvider()` methods are called, the order of the providers changes. These changes are not reflected in the internal property list.
>
> The *java.security* file has a number of other properties within it; these other properties may also be retrieved via this method.

public static String setProperty(String key)

> Set the property of the security class with the associated key.

public static String getAlgorithmProperty(String algName, String propName)

Search all the providers for a property in the form `Alg.propName.algName` and return the first match it finds. For example, if a provider had set the `Alg.NativeImplementation.XYZ` property to the string "false," a call to `getAlgorithmName("XYZ", "NativeImplementation")` returns the string "false" (which is why earlier we used a string value in the provider class).

Here's a simple example, then, of how to see a list of all the security providers in a particular virtual machine:

```
public class ExamineSecurity {
    public static void main(String args[]) {
        try {
            Provider p[] = Security.getProviders();
            for (int i = 0; i < p.length; i++) {
                System.out.println(p[i]);
                for (Enumeration e = p[i].keys(); e.hasMoreElements();)
                    System.out.println("\t" + e.nextElement());
            }
        }
        catch (Exception e) {
            System.out.println(e);
        }
    }
}
```

If we run this program with the 1.2 Sun security provider, we get this output:[*]

```
SUN version 1.2
        Alg.Alias.MessageDigest.SHA
        Alg.Alias.Signature.SHAwithDSA
        Alg.Alias.Signature.1.3.14.3.2.13
        Alg.Alias.Signature.OID.1.2.840.10040.4.3
        Alg.Alias.Signature.SHA-1/DSA
        Alg.Alias.Signature.DSS
        Alg.Alias.Signature.SHA1withDSA
        Alg.Alias.Signature.OID.1.3.14.3.2.13
        AlgorithmParameters.DSA
        KeyFactory.DSA
        Alg.Alias.Signature.1.2.840.10040.4.3
        Alg.Alias.MessageDigest.SHA1
        AlgorithmParameterGenerator.DSA
        Alg.Alias.AlgorithmParameters.1.2.840.10040.4.1
        MessageDigest.MD5
        Alg.Alias.KeyPairGenerator.OID.1.2.840.10040.4.1
        MessageDigest.SHA-1
        Alg.Alias.KeyPairGenerator.OID.1.3.14.3.2.12
```

---

[*] Output is from the beta 3 release of JDK 1.2; there may be slight changes for the FCS security provider.

```
Signature.DSA
Alg.Alias.KeyPairGenerator.1.3.14.3.2.12
Alg.Alias.KeyPairGenerator.1.2.840.10040.4.1
Alg.Alias.Signature.1.3.14.3.2.27
Alg.Alias.Signature.SHA/DSA
KeyPairGenerator.DSA
Alg.Alias.Signature.SHA1/DSA
Alg.Alias.Signature.OID.1.3.14.3.2.27
Alg.Alias.AlgorithmParameters.1.3.14.3.2.12
```

Two things are readily apparent from this example. First, the strings that contain only an engine name and an algorithm implement the expected operations that we listed in Table 8-1. Second, as we mentioned in the section on the `Provider` class, security providers often leverage the fact that the `Provider` class is a subclass of the `Properties` class to provide properties that may make sense only to other classes that are part of the provider package. Hence, the signature algorithm `1.3.14.3.2.13` may make sense to one of the classes in the Sun security provider, but it is not a string that will necessarily make sense to other developers. In fact, those aliases—including the ones that are prefaced by OID—do have meanings within the cryptography standards world, but for our purposes we'll stick with the standard algorithm names that we listed earlier.

The Security Class and the Security Manager

All the public methods of the `Security` class call the `checkSecurityAccess()` method of the security manager. This gives the security manager the opportunity to intervene before an untrusted class affects the security policy of the virtual machine.

Recall that the `checkSecurityAccess()` method accepts a single string parameter. In the case of the methods in the `Security` class, the call that is made looks like this:

```
public static Provider getProvider(String name) {
    SecurityManager sec = System.getSecurityManager();
    if (sec != null)
        sec.checkSecurityAccess("java");
    ... continue to find the provider ...
}
```

The string parameter that is sent to the `checkSecurityAccess()` method has changed between releases of Java; the various methods and the strings they pass to the security manager are listed in Table 8-4.

Table 8-4. Security Checks of the Security Class

Method	1.2 Parameter	1.1 Parameter
`insertProviderAt()`	`Security.insertProvider. +` `provider.getName()`	`java`
`removeProvider()`	`Security.removeProvider. +` `provider.getName()`	`java`
`getProviders()`	– not called –	`java`
`getProvider()`	– not called –	`java`
`getProperty()`	– not called –	`java`
`setProperty()`	`Security.setProperty. + key`	`java`

In typical usage in 1.1, the security manager ignores this string altogether and simply allows all trusted classes to call these methods and prevents all untrusted classes from calling these methods. In 1.2, the security manager constructs a security permission for the given name and calls the access controller to see if the given permission has been granted.

The Architecture of Engine Classes

In the next few chapters, we'll discuss the engine classes that are part of the core Java API. All engine classes share a similar architecture that we'll discuss here.

Most programmers are only interested in using the engine classes to perform their desired operation; each engine class has a public interface that defines the operations the engine can perform. None of this is unusual: it is the basis of programming in Java.

However, the engine classes are designed so that users can employ third-party security providers (using the architecture we've just examined). For programmers who are interested in writing such providers, the engine classes have an additional interface called the security provider interface (SPI). The SPI is a set of abstract methods that a particular engine must implement in order to fulfill its contract of providing a particular operation.

The role of the SPI has changed between Java 1.1 and Java 1.2. In 1.1, the SPI was simply a convention. There were a set of protected, usually abstract, methods in each engine that made up the SPI. By convention, these methods begin with the word "engine"; implementing a 1.1 engine is a matter of implementing each of these protected methods.

In 1.2, the interface of an engine was split between two distinct classes: the engine class itself and the SPI class. For example, in 1.2 there is an engine class called `MessageDigest`, and its SPI class is called `MessageDigestSpi`. For historic reasons, there are differences in various engine classes between the engine class itself and the SPI.

There were three engine classes in 1.1. In 1.2, the SPI class for these classes is a superclass of the engine class; e.g., the `MessageDigest` class extends the `Message-DigestSpi` class. This allows the `MessageDigest` class in 1.2 to have the same interface as it does in 1.1, even though the class hierarchy to which it belongs has changed.

There are three new engine classes in 1.2, and for these classes, the SPI is unrelated to the class itself; e.g., there is a `KeyFactory` class and a `KeyFactorySpi` class, both of which simply subclass the `Object` class. In these cases, the engine class contains an instance of the SPI that it uses to carry out its operations. Table 8-5 summarizes the six core Java engine classes and their corresponding SPI.

Table 8-5. Engine Classes in the Core Java API

Engine	SPI Class	Engine Superclass
AlgorithmParameters ★	AlgorithmParametersSpi	Object
AlgorithmParameterGener-ator ★	AlgorithmParameterGenera-torSpi	Object
KeyFactory ★	KeyFactorySpi	Object
KeyPairGenerator	KeyPairGeneratorSpi	KeyPairGenera-torSpi
MessageDigest	MessageDigestSpi	MessageDigestSpi
Signature	SignatureSpi	SignatureSpi

What this all means is that if you want to implement a security provider under Java 1.2, you would typically extend the SPI. This allows a developer to request a particular engine and receive the correct class according to the following algorithm:

1. The programmer requests an instance of a particular engine that implements a particular algorithm. Engine classes never have public constructors; instead, every engine has a `getInstance()` method that takes the name of the desired algorithm as an argument and returns an instance of the appropriate class.

2. The `Security` class is asked to consult its list of providers and provide the appropriate instance. For example, when the `getInstance()` method of the `MessageDigest` class is called, the `Security` class may determine that the appropriate provider class is called `com.xyz.XYZMessageDigest`.

3. If the retrieved class does not extend the appropriate SPI (e.g., `java.security.MessageDigestSpi` in this case), a `NoSuchAlgorithmException` is generated.

4. An instance of the retrieved class is created and returned to the `getInstance()` method (which in turn returns it to the developer).

For consistency, when you implement any engine class in 1.2, it is always possible to extend the appropriate SPI. However, when you implement one of the three engines that are part of 1.1, it may make more sense to extend the engine class (e.g., the `MessageDigest` class) rather than the SPI (e.g., the `MessageDigestSpi` class). This allows the implementation to be used under both 1.1 and 1.2. An engine class that directly subclasses its SPI in 1.2 cannot be used in 1.1, while an engine class that directly subclasses a Java engine class can be used in both 1.1 and 1.2. That is the convention we'll follow in our examples.

Summary

In this chapter, we've explored the architecture that forms the basis of the Java security API. This architecture is based on the `Security` and `Provider` classes, which together form a set of mappings that allow the security API to determine dynamically the set of classes it should use to implement certain operations.

Implementing a provider is trivial, but implementing the set of classes that must accompany a provider is much harder. We've shown a simple provider class in this chapter. Although we'll show the engine classes in the next few chapters, the mathematics behind designing and implementing a successful cryptographic algorithm are beyond the scope of this book. However, this architecture also allows users and administrators to buy or download third-party implementations of the security architecture and plug those implementations seamlessly into the Java virtual machine; a partial list of available third-party implementations appears in Appendix C.

In the next few chapters, we'll examine the specifics of the engine classes—that is, the operations—that this security provider architecture makes possible. In those chapters, we'll see how the engines are used, and the benefits each engine provides.

9

Message Digests

In this chapter, we're going to look at the API that implements the ability to create and verify message digests. The ability to create a message digest is one of the standard engines provided by the Sun default security provider. You can therefore reasonably expect every Java implementation to create message digests.

Message digests are the simplest of the standard engines that compose the security provider architecture, so they provide a good starting point in our examination of those engines. In addition, message digests provide the first link in creating and verifying a digital signature—the most important goal of the provider architecture. However, message digests are useful entities in their own right, since a message digest can verify that data has not been tampered with—up to a point. As we'll see, there are certain limitations on the security of a message digest that is transmitted along with the data it represents.

Message digests are implemented through a single class:

public abstract class MessageDigest extends MessageDigestSpi
  Implement operations to create and verify a message digest.

In Java 1.1, there is no `MessageDigestSpi` class, and the `MessageDigest` class simply extends `Object`. That difference is important only if you want to implement your own message digest class, which we'll do later in the chapter.

Like all engines in the Java security package, the `MessageDigest` class (`java.security.MessageDigest`) is an abstract class; it defines an interface that all message digests must have, but the implementation details of a particular message digest class are hidden in the private classes that accompany a security provider. This allows a developer to use the message digest class without knowing the details of a message digest implementation by operating on the public methods of the message digest class, and it allows providers of a security package to implement their own message digests by implementing the abstract methods of the class. We'll examine the message class from the perspectives of both developer and implementor in this chapter.

Using the Message Digest Class

For a developer who wants to operate on a message digest, the first step is to obtain an instance of the message digest class. Since the message digest class is abstract, this cannot be done directly; instead, the developer must use one of these methods:

public static MessageDigest getInstance(String algorithm)
public static MessageDigest getInstance(String algorithm, String provider)

> Return an instance of the message digest class that implements the given algorithm. In the first case, the security providers are searched in order following the process we outlined in Chapter 8; otherwise, only the given provider is searched. Valid names for the default Sun security provider are SHA, SHA-1, and MD5. If no provider can be found that implements the given algorithm, a NoSuchAlgorithmException is thrown. If the named provider cannot be found, a NoSuchProviderException is thrown.

Once a message digest object has been obtained, the developer can operate on that object with these methods:

public void update(byte input)
public void update(byte[] input)
public void update(byte[] input, int offset, int length)

> Add the specified data to the digest. The first of these methods adds a single byte to the data, the second adds the entire array of bytes, and the third adds only the specified subset of the array of data.

> These methods may be called in any order and any number of times to add the desired data to the digest. Consecutive calls to these methods append data to the internal accumulation of data over which the digest will be calculated.

public byte[] digest()
public byte[] digest(byte[] input)

> Compute the message digest on the accumulated data (optionally adding the specified data before performing the computation). The resulting digest is returned as a byte array. Once a digest has been calculated, the internal state of the algorithm is reset, so that the object may be reused at this point to create a new message digest.

public int digest(byte[] output, int offset, int len) ★

Compute the message digest on the accumulated data and place the answer into the provided array, starting at the given offset and copying at most `len` bytes. Most implementations do not return a partial digest, so if the amount of space in the buffer (taking into account its offset) is not sufficient to store the digest, a `DigestException` is thrown. This method returns the size of the digest.

public static boolean isEqual(byte digestA[], byte digestB[])

Compare two digests for equality. Two digests are considered equal only if each byte in the first digest is exactly equal to each byte in the second digest and the digests are the same length.

public void reset()

Reset the digest object by discarding all accumulated data and resetting the algorithm that is used to implement the digest. This is equivalent to creating a new instance of the object. In addition, this method throws away any information that the `toString()` method would have printed (see below).

public final String getAlgorithm()

Return the string representing the algorithm name (e.g., SHA).

public String toString()

A string representation of a digest by default contains the name of the class implementing the digest, the words "Message Digest," and the bytes that were returned by a previous call to the `digest()` method. If the `digest()` method has not been called, or if the `reset()` method has been called, then "<incomplete>" is printed instead of the digest. An example string looks like:

```
sun.security.provider.SHA Message Digest \
      <0a808982fee54fd74a86aae72eff7991328ff32b>
```

public Object clone() throws CloneNotSupportedException

Return a clone of the object. Message digest implementations need to implement the `clone()` method because some internal operations on the digest object require a call to the `digest()` method, which resets the digest. These operations are typically done on a clone of the object so that the state of the original object is not changed.

public final int getDigestLength() ★

Return the length of array of bytes that are returned from the `digest()` method. This value is usually constant (i.e., it does not depend on the amount of data that has been sent through the `update()` method).

Let's see an example of how all of this works. As a simple case, let's say that we want to save a simple string to a file, but we're worried that the file might be corrupted when we read the string back in. Hence, in addition to saving the string, we must save a message digest. We do this by saving the serialized string object followed by the serialized array of bytes that constitute the message digest.

In order to save the pieces of data, we use this code:

```
public class Send {
    public static void main(String args[]) {
        try {
            FileOutputStream fos = new FileOutputStream("test");
            MessageDigest md = MessageDigest.getInstance("SHA");
            ObjectOutputStream oos = new ObjectOutputStream(fos);
            String data = "This have I thought good to deliver thee, "+
                "that thou mightst not lose the dues of rejoicing " +
                "by being ignorant of what greatness is promised thee.";
            byte buf[] = data.getBytes();
            md.update(buf);
            oos.writeObject(data);
            oos.writeObject(md.digest());
        } catch (Exception e) {
            System.out.println(e);
        }
    }
}
```

That's all there is to creating a digest of some data. The call to the getInstance() method finds a message digest object that implements the SHA message digest algorithm. After creating our data—which in this case is a simple string—we pass that data to the update() method of the message digest. In practice, this code could be slightly more complicated, since all the data might not be available at once. As far as the message digest object is concerned, though, that situation would just require multiple calls to the update() method instead of a single call (it can also be handled with digest streams, which we'll examine next). Once we've loaded all the data into the object, it is a simple matter to create the digest itself (with the digest() method) and then save our data objects to the file.

Similarly, to retrieve this data we need only read the object back in and verify the message digest. In order to verify the message digest, we must recompute the digest over the data we received and test to make sure the digest is equivalent to the original digest:

```
public class Receive {
    public static void main(String args[]) {
        try {
            FileInputStream fis = new FileInputStream("test");
            ObjectInputStream ois = new ObjectInputStream(fis);
            Object o = ois.readObject();
            if (!(o instanceof String)) {
                System.out.println("Unexpected data in file");
```

```
                          System.exit(-1);
                      }
                      String data = (String) o;
                      System.out.println("Got message " + data);
                      o = ois.readObject();
                      if (!(o instanceof byte[])) {
                          System.out.println("Unexpected data in file");
                          System.exit(-1);
                      }
                      byte origDigest[] = (byte []) o;
                      MessageDigest md = MessageDigest.getInstance("SHA");
                      md.update(data.getBytes());
                      if (MessageDigest.isEqual(md.digest(), origDigest))
                          System.out.println("Message is valid");
                      else System.out.println("Message was corrupted");
                  } catch (Exception e) {
                      System.out.println(e);
                  }
              }
          }
      }
```

Once again, if the data was not available all at once, we would need to make multiple calls to the update() method as the data arrived. We do not, however, need to make sure that calls to the update() methods between the Send and Receive classes match in any sense; that is, if we called the update() method four times in the Send class, we do not need to call the update() method four times (with the same data) in the Receive class—we can call it once, five times, or whatever. The calculation of the digest is unaffected by how the data was placed into the message digest object—as long as the order of the bytes presented to the various calls to the update() methods is the same.

Secure Message Digests

As we stated in Chapter 7, the message digest by itself does not give us a very high level of security. We can tell whether somehow the output file in this example has been corrupted, because the text that we read in won't produce the same message digest that was saved with the file. But there's nothing to prevent someone from changing both the text and the digest stored in the file in such a way that the new digest reflects the altered text.

There are various ways in which a message digest can be made into a Message Authentication Code (MAC), but the Java security API does not provide any standard techniques for doing so. One popular way is to encrypt the message digest using the encryption engine (if one is available to you)—which, in fact, is really a variation of a digital signature.

If we are not able to encrypt the digest, all is not lost; we can also use a passphrase along with the message digest in order to calculate a secure message digest (or MAC). This requires that both the sender and receiver of the data have a shared passphrase that they have kept secret.

Using this passphrase, calculating a MAC requires that we:

1. Calculate the message digest of the secret passphrase concatenated with the data:

```
MessageDigest md = MessageDigest.getInstance("SHA");
String data = "This have I thought good to deliver thee, " +
              "that thou mightst not lose the dues of rejoicing " +
              "by being ignorant of what greatness is promised thee.";
String passphrase = "Sleep no more";
byte dataBytes[] = data.getBytes();
byte passBytes[] = passphrase.getBytes();
md.update(passBytes);
md.update(dataBytes);
byte digest1[] = md.digest();
```

2. Calculate the message digest of the secret passphrase concatenated with the just-calculated digest:

```
md.update(passBytes);
md.update(digest1);
byte mac[] = md.digest();
```

We can substitute this code into our original Send example, writing out the data string and the MAC to the file. Note that we can use the same message digest object to calculate both digests, since the object is reset after a call to the digest() method. Also note that the first digest we calculate is not saved to the file: we save only the data and the MAC. Of course, we must make similar changes to the Receive example; if the MACs are equal, the data was not modified in transit.

As long as we use exactly the same data for the passphrase in both the transmitting and receiving class, the message digests (that is, the MACs) still compare as equal. That gives a certain level of security to the message digest, but it requires that the sender and the receiver agree on what data to use for the passphrase; the passphrase cannot be transmitted along with the text. In this case, the security of the message digest depends upon the security of the passphrase. Normally, of course, you would prompt for that passphrase rather than hardcoding into the source as we've done above.

Message Digest Streams

The interface to the message digest class requires that you supply the data for the digest as a series of single bytes or byte arrays. As we mentioned earlier, this is not always the most convenient way to process data, which may be coming from a file or other input stream. This brings us to the message digest stream classes. These classes implement the standard input and output filter stream semantics of Java streams so that data can be written to a digest stream that will calculate the digest as the data itself is written (or the reverse operation for reading data).

The DigestOutputStream Class

The first of these classes we'll examine is the DigestOutputStream class (java.security.DigestOutputStream). This class allows us to write data to a particular output stream and calculate the message digest of that data transparently as the data passes through the stream:

public class DigestOutputStream extends FilterOutputStream

> Provide a stream that can calculate the message digest of data that is passed through the stream. A digest output stream holds two components internally: the output stream that is the ultimate destination of the data, and a message digest object that computes the data of the stream written to the destination.

The digest output stream is constructed as follows:

public DigestOutputStream(OutputStream os, MessageDigest md)

> Construct a digest output stream that associates the given output stream with the given message digest. Data that is written to the stream is automatically passed to the update() method of the message digest.

In addition to the standard methods available to all output streams, a message digest output stream provides the following interface:

public MessageDigest getMessageDigest()

> Return the message digest associated with this output stream.

public void setMessageDigest(MessageDigest md)

> Associate the given message digest with this output stream. The internal reference to the original message digest is lost, but the original message digest is otherwise unaffected (i.e., if you still hold a reference to the original message digest object, you can still calculate the digest of the data that was written to the stream while that digest was in place).

public void write(int b)

public void write(byte b[], int off, int len)

    Write the given byte or array of bytes to the underlying output stream, and also update the internal message digest with the given data (if the digest stream is marked as on). These methods may throw an IOException from the underlying stream.

public void on(boolean on)

    Turn the message digest stream on or off. When data is written to a stream that is off, the data will be passed to the underlying output stream, but the message digest will not be updated.

Note that this last method does not affect the underlying output stream at all; data is still sent to the underlying stream even if the digest output stream is marked as off. The on/off state only affects whether the update() method of the message digest will be called as the data is written.

We can use this class to simplify the example we used earlier:

```
public class SendStream {
    public static void main(String args[]) {
        try {
            FileOutputStream fos = new FileOutputStream("test");
            MessageDigest md = MessageDigest.getInstance("SHA");
            DigestOutputStream dos = new DigestOutputStream(fos, md);
            ObjectOutputStream oos = new ObjectOutputStream(dos);
            String data = "This have I thought good to deliver thee, "+
                "that thou mightst not lose the dues of rejoicing " +
                "by being ignorant of what greatness is promised thee.";
            oos.writeObject(data);
            dos.on(false);
            oos.writeObject(md.digest());
        } catch (Exception e) {
            System.out.println(e);
        }
    }
}
```

The big change is in constructing the object output stream—we now want to wrap it around the digest output stream so that as each object is written to the file, the message digest will include those bytes. We also want to make sure that we turn off the message digest calculation before we send the digest itself to the file. Turning off the digest isn't strictly necessary in this case, since we don't use the digest object once we've calculated a single digest in this example, but it's good practice to keep the digest on only when strictly required.

Note that there is a subtle difference between the digest produced in this example and the previous example. In the first example, the digest was calculated over just the bytes of the string that we saved to the file. In the second example, the digest was calculated over the serialized string object itself—which includes some information regarding the class definition in addition to the bytes of the string.

The DigestInputStream Class

The symmetric operation to the digest output stream is the DigestInputStream class (java.security.DigestInputStream):

public class DigestInputStream extends FilterInputStream

Create an input stream that is associated with a message digest. When data is read from the input stream, it is also sent to the update() method of the stream's associated message digest.

The digest input stream has essentially the same interface as the digest output stream (with writing replaced by reading). There is a single constructor for the class:

public DigestInputStream(InputStream is, MessageDigest md)

Construct a digest input stream that associates the given input stream with the given message digest. Data that is read from the stream will also automatically be passed to the update() method of the message digest.

The interface provided by the digest input stream is symmetric to the digest output stream:

public MessageDigest getMessageDigest()

Return the message digest that is associated with this output stream.

public void setMessageDigest(MessageDigest md)

Associate the given message digest with this output stream. The internal reference to the original message digest is lost, but the original message digest is otherwise unaffected (e.g., you can still calculate the digest of the data that had been written to the stream while that digest was in place).

public void read(int b)
public void read(byte b[], int off, int len)

Read one or more bytes from the underlying output stream, and also update the internal message digest with the given data (if the digest stream is marked as on). These methods may throw an IOException from the underlying stream.

public void on(boolean on)

Turn the message digest stream on or off. When data is read from a stream that is off, the message digest will not be updated.

Here's how we can use this class to read the file we created with the digest output stream:

```
public class ReceiveStream {
    public static void main(String args[]) {
        try {
            FileInputStream fis = new FileInputStream("test");
            MessageDigest md = MessageDigest.getInstance("SHA");
            DigestInputStream dis = new DigestInputStream(fis, md);
            ObjectInputStream ois = new ObjectInputStream(dis);
            Object o = ois.readObject();
            if (!(o instanceof String)) {
                System.out.println("Unexpected data in file");
                System.exit(-1);
            }
            String data = (String) o;
            System.out.println("Got message " + data);
            dis.on(false);
            o = ois.readObject();
            if (!(o instanceof byte[])) {
                System.out.println("Unexpected data in file");
                System.exit(-1);
            }
            byte origDigest[] = (byte []) o;
            if (MessageDigest.isEqual(md.digest(), origDigest))
                System.out.println("Message is valid");
            else System.out.println("Message was corrupted");
        } catch (Exception e) {
            System.out.println(e);
        }
    }
}
```

Once again, constructing the input stream is a matter of providing a message digest. In this example, we've again turned off the digest input stream after reading the string object in the file. Turning off the stream is strictly required in this case. We want to make sure that the digest we calculate is computed only over the string object and not the stored byte array (that is, the stored message digest).

Implementing a MessageDigest Class

If you want to write your own security provider, you have the option of creating your own message digest engine. Typically, you'd do this because you want to ensure that a particular algorithm like SHA is available regardless of who the default security provider is; if you have a mathematics background, it's conceivable that you might want to implement your own algorithm.

In order to implement a message digest algorithm, you must provide a concrete subclass of the MessageDigest class. This essentially entails providing an implementation of most of the public methods we've just looked at. Although the public methods are not declared abstract, they typically do nothing more than call an internal (protected) method to accomplish their task.

The MessageDigest class exists in both Java 1.1 and 1.2, which is why it extends its SPI (see Chapter 8). For our example, we'll directly subclass the MessageDigest class so that the resulting example will work under both releases, but remember that in 1.2 you have the option of extending the MessageDigestSpi class directly.

There is a single constructor in the MessageDigest class that is available to implementors:

protected MessageDigest(String name)
> Construct a message digest object. Classes that extend the MessageDigest class must call this constructor, as this is the only constructor in the class. As we'll see, however, the constructor of the subclass must take no arguments.

In order to write a message digest class, you must implement each of the following methods:

protected abstract void engineUpdate(byte input)
protected abstract void engineUpdate(byte[] input, int offset, int len)
> Add the given bytes to the data over which the digest will be calculated. Note that there is no method in this list that accepts simply an array of bytes; the update(byte[] b) method in the base class simply uses an offset of 0 and a length equal to the entire array.

protected abstract byte[] engineDigest()
> Calculate the digest over the accumulated data, resetting the internal state of the object afterwards. Note that there is no corresponding method that accepts an array of bytes as an argument; the digest() method in the base class simply calls the engineUpdate() method if needed before calling the engineDigest() method.

protected int engineDigest(byte buf[], int offset, int len) ★
> Calculate the digest, placing the output into the buf array (starting at the given offset and proceeding for len bytes) and returning the length of the calculated digest. The default implementation of this method simply calls the engineDigest() method and then copies the result into buf. The buffer passed to this method always has sufficient length to hold the digest, since if the buffer had been too short the digest() method itself would have thrown an exception.

protected abstract void engineReset()

 Reset the internal state of the engine, discarding all accumulated data and resetting the algorithm to an initial condition.

protected int engineGetDigestLength() ★

 Return the digest length that is supported by this implementation. Unlike most of the protected methods in this class, this method is not abstract; it does not need to be overridden. However, the default implementation simply returns 0. If 0 is returned by this method, the getDigestLength() method attempts to create a clone of the digest object, calculate its digest, and return the length of the calculated digest. If a digest implementation does not override this method and does not implement the Cloneable interface, the getDigestLength() method will not operate correctly.

Each of these methods corresponds to a public method we just looked at, with the name of the public method preceded by the word "engine". The public methods that do not have a corresponding method in this list are fully implemented in the base class and do not need to be implemented in the message digest subclass.

We'll show a simple implementation of a message digest class here. This implementation is based on a hash algorithm that produces a 4-byte output. As bytes are accumulated by this algorithm, they are stored into a 4-byte value (that is, an int); when this value has all four bytes filled, it is XOR-ed to another integer that accumulates the hash.

```
package com.xyz;

public class XYZMessageDigest extends MessageDigest
                              implements Cloneable {
    private int hash;
    private int store;
    private int nBytes;

    public XYZMessageDigest() {
        super("XYZ");
        engineReset();
    }

    public void engineUpdate(byte b) {
        switch(nBytes) {
            case 0:
                store =  (b << 24) & 0xff000000;
                break;
            case 1:
                store |= (b << 16) & 0x00ff0000;
                break;
            case 2:
                store |= (b <<  8) & 0x0000ff00;
```

```
                    break;
                case 3:
                    store |= (b <<  0) & 0x000000ff;
                    break;
            }
        nBytes++;
        if (nBytes == 4) {
            hash = hash ^ store;
            nBytes = 0;
            store = 0;
        }
    }

    public void engineUpdate(byte b[], int offset, int length) {
        for (int i = 0; i < length; i++)
            engineUpdate(b[i + offset]);
    }

    public void engineReset() {
        hash = 0;
        store = 0;
        nBytes = 0;
    }

    public byte[] engineDigest() {
        while (nBytes != 0)
            engineUpdate((byte) 0);
        byte b[] = new byte[4];
        b[0] = (byte) (hash >>> 24);
        b[1] = (byte) (hash >>> 16);
        b[2] = (byte) (hash >>>  8);
        b[3] = (byte) (hash >>>  0);
        engineReset();
        return b;
    }
}
```

The implementation of this class is simple, which isn't surprising given the fact that the algorithm itself is too simple to be considered an effective digest algorithm. The major points to observe are:

- The name of the class (XYZMessageDigest) and the name of the algorithm that it implements (XYZ) must match one of the strings in the provider package for this class to be found. Hence, in our provider class in Chapter 8, we included this property:

```
put("MessageDigest.XYZ", "com.xyz.XYZMessageDigest");
```

- Our constructor calls the only constructor available to us, and the string "XYZ" that we pass to that constructor takes on significance—it's the name of

the algorithm we've implemented in this class. This in turn becomes the
name that is registered in the security provider architecture; it must match
the name of the algorithm we registered in our provider.

- In order for the getDigestLength() method to function, we chose to implement the Cloneable interface instead of overriding the engineGetDi-
  gestLength() method. Since there are no embedded objects in this class, we
  do not need to override the clone() method. The default implementation of
  that method (a shallow copy) is sufficient for this class.

- The engineUpdate() methods accumulate bytes of data until an integer has
  been accumulated, at which point that integer can be XOR-ed into the saved
  state held in the hash instance variable.

- The engineDigest() method converts the hash instance variable into a byte
  array and returns that to the programmer. Note that the engineDigest()
  method is responsible for resetting the internal state of the algorithm. In addition, the engineDigest() method is responsible for padding the data so that
  it is a multiple of four bytes (the size of a Java integer). This type of data padding is a common feature of message digest calculation.

- The engineReset() method initializes the algorithm to its initial state.

Once we have an implementation of a message digest, we must install it into the
security provider architecture. If we use the XYZProvider class from Chapter 8, we
can change our Send class above to use our new digest algorithm:

```
public class SendXYZ {
    public static void main(String args[]) {
        try {
            Security.addProvider(new XYZProvider());
            FileOutputStream fos = new FileOutputStream("test.xyz");
            MessageDigest md = MessageDigest.getInstance("XYZ");
            ObjectOutputStream oos = new ObjectOutputStream(fos);
            String data = "This have I thought good to deliver thee, "+
                "that thou mightst not lose the dues of rejoicing " +
                "by being ignorant of what greatness is promised thee.";
            byte buf[] = data.getBytes();
            md.update(buf);
            oos.writeObject(data);
            oos.writeObject(md.digest());
        } catch (Exception e) {
            System.out.println(e);
        }
    }
}
```

Similar changes to the Receive class will allow us to accept the message that we've
saved to the file *test.xyz*.

Summary

In this chapter, we've explored the first link in creating an authenticated and secure system: the message digest. The facility to calculate a message digest is straightforward and easy to use; the facility to write our own message digest class is equally straightforward.

The message digest by itself gives us some comfort about the state of the data it represents, but it does not give us a completely secure system. If we have a shared passphrase, we can construct a secure message digest (that is, a Message Authentication Code), but there are no easy means to share that passphrase. A MAC is similiar to a digital signature (where digital keys replace the passphrase); in the next few chapters, we'll continue our exploration of the API to provide the necessary components of a digital signature, beginning with an exploration of the keys required to create a digital signature.

10

Keys and Certificates

In this chapter, we discuss the classes in the Java security package that handle keys and certificates. Keys are a necessary component of many cryptographic algorithms—in particular, keys are required to create and verify digital signatures. The keys we're going to discuss in this chapter are public keys and private keys, since those are the keys most often used in a digital signature. Secret keys—used for encryption algorithms—are discussed in Chapter 13. We defer that discussion because secret keys do not come with standard Java implementations; they come only with the Java Cryptography Extension.

We also cover the implementation of certificates in this chapter. Certificates are used to authenticate keys; when keys are transmitted electronically, they are often embedded within certificates.

Keys and certificates are normally associated with some person or organization, and the way in which keys are stored, transmitted, and shared is an important topic in the security package. Management of keys is left for the next chapter, however; right now, we're just concerned about the APIs that implement keys and certificates. As usual, we'll show how a programmer interacts with keys and certificates, as well as how you might implement your own versions of each.

The classes and engines we discuss in this chapter are outlined in Figure 10-1. There are two engines that operate on keys:

- The KeyPairGenerator class generates keys from scratch. With no input (or, possibly, input to initialize it to a certain state), the generator can produce one or more pairs of keys.

- The KeyFactory class translates between key objects and their external representations, which may be either a byte array or a key specification; this translation goes both ways.

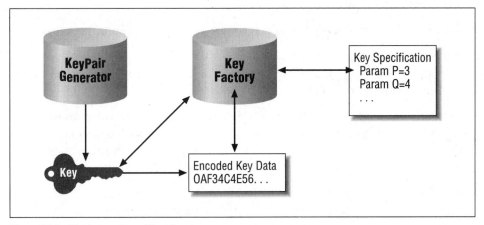

Figure 10-1. The interaction of key classes

There are a number of classes and interfaces we'll discuss to facilitate support for Figure 10-1; in addition to the engine classes themselves, there are several classes and interfaces that represent the key objects and the key specifications (the encoded key data is always an array of bytes). In an effort to provide the complete story, we'll delve into the details of all of these classes; for the most part, however, the important operations that most developers will need are:

- The ability to create a new pair of keys from scratch using the key pair generator
- The ability to export a key, either as a parameter specification or as a set of bytes, and the corresponding ability to import that data in order to create a key

This means that, for the most part, the data objects we explore in this chapter—the Key classes and interfaces as well as the various KeySpec classes (key specification classes)—can be treated by most programmers as opaque objects. We'll show their complete interface (which you might be curious about, and which is absolutely needed if you're writing your own security provider), but we'll try not to lose sight of the two goals of this chapter.

Also note that the idea of the key factory and key specifications is available only with Java 1.2. In Java 1.1, you can get the encoded key data directly from a key, but that's a one-way operation.

Keys

Let's start with the various classes that support the notion of keys within Java.

The Key Interface

The concept of a key is modeled by the Key interface (`java.security.Key`):

public interface Key extends Serializable
> Model the concept of a single key. Because keys must be transferred to and from various entities, all keys must be serializable.

As we discussed in Chapter 8, there might be several algorithms available for generating (and understanding) keys, depending on the particular security providers that are installed in the virtual machine. Hence, the first thing a key needs to be able to tell us is what algorithm generated it:

public String getAlgorithm()
> Return a string describing the algorithm used to generated this key; this string should be the name of a standard key generation algorithm.

We listed the standard algorithm names for key generation in Chapter 8, but with the default provider with the JDK, this string is always DSA.

When a key is transferred between two parties, it is usually encoded as a series of bytes; this encoding must follow a format defined for the type of key. Keys are not required to support encoding—in which case the format of the data transferred between the two parties in a key exchange is either obvious (e.g., simply the serialized data of the key) or specific to a particular implementation. Keys tell us the format they use for encoding their output with this method:

public String getFormat()
> Return a string describing the format of the encoding the key supports.

For DSA keys produced by the Sun security provider, this format is always PKCS#8 for private keys and X.509 for public keys. The encoded data of the key itself is produced by this method:

public byte[] getEncoded()
> Return the bytes that make up the particular key in the encoding format the key supports. The encoded bytes are the external representation of the key in binary format.

Those are the only methods that a key is guaranteed to implement (other than methods of the `Object` class, of course; most implementations of keys override many of those methods). In particular, you'll note that there is nothing in the key interface that says anything about decoding a key. We'll say more about that later.

There are two additional key interfaces in the Java security API:

public interface PublicKey extends Key
public interface PrivateKey extends Key

These interfaces contain no additional methods. They are used simply for type convenience. A class that implements the `PublicKey` interface identifies itself as a public key, but it contains no methods that are different from any other key.

DSA keys

The keys supported by the Sun security provider are built around the DSA algorithm. DSA-generated keys are important enough to have several interfaces built around them; these interfaces enhance your ability to work with these specific types of keys. These interfaces are necessary because DSA keys have certain pieces of information that are not reflected in the default key interfaces: the DSA algorithm-specific parameters p, q, and g that are used to generate the keys. Knowledge of these variables is abstracted into the `DSAParams` interface (`java.security.interfaces.DSAParams`):

```
public interface DSAParams {
    public BigInteger getP();
    public BigInteger getQ();
    public BigInteger getG();
}
```

Keys that are generated by DSA will typically implement the `DSAKey` interface (`java.security.interfaces.DSAKey`):

public interface DSAKey
    Provide DSA-specific information about a key.

Implementing this interface serves two purposes. First, it allows the programmer to determine if the key is a DSA key by checking its type. The second purpose is to allow the programmer to access the DSA parameters using this method in the `DSAKey` interface:

public DSAParams getParams()
    Return the DSA parameters associated with this key.

These methods and interfaces allow us to do specific key manipulation like this:

```
public void printKey(Key k) {
    if (k instanceof DSAKey) {
        System.out.println("key is DSA");
        System.out.println("P value is " +
                        ((DSAKey) k).getParams().getP());
    }
    else System.out.println("key is not DSA");
}
```

The idea of a DSA key is extended even further by these two interfaces (both of which are in the java.security.interfaces package):

public interface DSAPrivateKey extends DSAKey
public interface DSAPublicKey extends DSAKey

These interfaces allow the programmer to retrieve the additional key-specific values (known as *y* for public keys and *x* for private keys in the DSA algorithm):

```
public void printKey(DSAKey k) {
    if (k instanceof DSAPublicKey)
        System.out.println("Public key value is " +
                                    ((DSAPublicKey) k).getY());
    else if (k instanceof DSAPrivateKey)
        System.out.println("Private key value is " +
                                    ((DSAPrivateKey) k).getX());
    else System.out.println("Bad key implementation");
}
```

DSA keys are often used in the Java world (and elsewhere in cryptography), and if you know you're dealing with DSA keys, these interfaces can be very useful. In particular, if you're writing a security provider that provides an implementation of DSA keys, you should ensure that you implement all of these interfaces correctly. For most programmers, however, keys are opaque objects, and the algorithm-specific features of DSA keys are not needed.

The KeyPair Class

There are no classes in the core JDK that implement any of the Key interfaces. However, there is one concrete class, the KeyPair class (java.security.KeyPair), that extends the abstraction of keys:

public final class KeyPair
    Model a data object that contains a public key and a private key.

The KeyPair class is a very simple data structure class, containing two pieces of information: a public key and a private key. When we need to generate our own keys (which we'll do next), we'll need to generate both the public and private key at once. This object will contain both of the necessary keys. If you're not interested in generating your own keys, this class may be ignored.

The KeyPair class contains only two methods:

public PublicKey getPublic()
public PrivateKey getPrivate()
    Return the desired key from the key pair.

A key pair object is instantiated through a single constructor:

public KeyPair(PublicKey pub, PrivateKey priv)
> Create a key pair object, initializing each member of the pair.

In theory, a key pair should not be initialized without both members of the pair being present; there is nothing, however, that prevents us from passing null as one of the keys. Similarly, there are no security provisions within the KeyPair class that prevent the private key from being accessed—no calls to the security manager are made when the getPrivate() method is invoked. Hence the KeyPair class should be used with caution.

The KeyPairGenerator Class

Generation of public and private keys is one of the standard engines that can be provided by a Java security provider. This operation is provided by the KeyPair-Generator class (java.security.KeyPairGenerator):

public abstract class KeyPairGenerator
> Generate and provide information about public/private key pairs.
>
> In Java 1.1, this class extends only the Object class; in Java 1.2, this class extends the KeyPairGeneratorSpi class (java.security.KeyPairGenera-torSpi). As is usual with this architecture, some of the methods we're going to use are methods of the KeyPairGenerator class in Java 1.1 and methods of the KeyPairGeneratorSpi class in 1.2; for the developer, the end result is the same.

Generating a key pair is a very time-consuming operation. Fortunately, it does not need to be performed often; much of the time, we obtain keys from a key management system rather than generating them. However, when we establish our own key management system in the next chapter, we'll need to use this class; it is often easier to generate your own keys from scratch rather than use a key management system as well.

Using the KeyPairGenerator Class

Like all engine classes, the KeyPairGenerator is an abstract class for which there is no implementation in the core API. However, it is possible to retrieve instances of the KeyPairGenerator class via these methods:

public static KeyPairGenerator getInstance(String algorithm)
public static KeyPairGenerator getInstance(String algorithm, String provider)
> Find the implementation of the engine that generates key pairs with the named algorithm. The algorithm should be one of the standard API algorithm

names; if an appropriate implementation cannot be found, this method throws a NoSuchAlgorithmException.

The first format of this method searches all available providers according to the rules we outlined in Chapter 8. The second method searches only the named provider, throwing a NoSuchProviderException if that provider has not been loaded.

These methods search the providers that have been registered with the security provider interface for a key pair generator that supports the named algorithm. In the Sun security provider, this method allows us to retrieve the key pair generator that generates keys using the DSA algorithm.

Once we have the key pair generator, we can invoke any of the following methods on it:

public String getAlgorithm()

Return the name of the algorithm that this key pair generator implements (e.g., DSA).

public void initialize(int strength)
public abstract void initialize(int strength, SecureRandom random)

Initialize the key pair generator to generate keys of the given strength. The idea of strength is common among key pair generator algorithms; typically it means the number of bits that are used as input to the engine to calculate the key pair, but the actual meaning may vary between algorithms.

Most key algorithms restrict on the values that are valid for strength. In the case of DSA, the strength must be between 512 and 1024 and it must be a multiple of 64. If an invalid number is passed for strength, an InvalidParameterException will be thrown.

Key pairs typically require a random number generator to assist them. You may specify a particular random number generator if desired; otherwise, a default random number generator (an instance of the SecureRandom class) is used.

In Java 1.2, the second of these methods is inherited from the KeyPairGeneratorSpi class.

public void initialize(AlgorithmParameterSpec params) ★
public void initialize(AlgorithmParameterSpec params, SecureRandom random) ★

Initialize the key pair generator using the specified parameter set (which we'll discuss a little later). By default, the first method simply calls the second method with a default instance of the SecureRandom class; the second method, by default, will throw an UnsupportedOperationException. The second of these methods is inherited from the KeyPairGeneratorSpi class.

public abstract KeyPair generateKeyPair()

public final KeyPair genKeyPair() ★

> Generate a key pair, using the initialization parameters previously specified. A `KeyPairGenerator` object can repeatedly generate key pairs by calling one of these methods; each new call generates a new key pair. The `genKeyPair()` method simply calls the `generateKeyPair()` method.

> In Java 1.2, the `generateKeyPair()` method is inherited from the SPI.

Using these methods, generating a pair of keys is very straightforward:

```
KeyPairGenerator kpg = KeyPairGenerator.getInstance("DSA");
kpg.initialize(512);
KeyPair kp = kpg.generateKeyPair();
```

According to the Java documentation, you are allowed to generate a key pair without initializing the generator; in this situation, a default strength and random number generator are to be used. However, this feature does not work with the Sun security provider in 1.1: a `NullPointerException` is thrown from within the `generateKeyPair()` method. Since it is possible that third-party providers may behave similarly, it is always best to initialize the key pair generator.

We'll show what to do with these keys in the next chapter, when we discuss the topic of key management.

Generating DSA Keys

The abstraction provided by the key pair generator is usually all we need to generate keys. However, sometimes the particular algorithm needs additional information to generate a key pair. When a DSA key pair is generated, default values for p, q, and g are used; in the Sun security provider, these values are pre-computed to support strength values of 512 and 1024. Precomputing these values greatly reduces the time required to calculate a DSA key. Third-party DSA providers may provide precomputed values for additional strength values.

It is possible to ask the key generator to use different values for p, q, and g if the key pair generator supports the `DSAKeyPairGenerator` interface (`java.security.interfaces.DSAKeyPairGenerator`):

public interface DSAKeyPairGenerator

> Provide a mechanism by which the DSA-specific parameters of the key pair engine can be manipulated.

There are two methods in this interface:

public void initialize(int modlen, boolean genParams, SecureRandom random)

> Initialize the DSA key pair generator. The modulus length is the number of bits used to calculate the parameters; this must be any multiple of 8 between

512 and 1024. If genParams is true, then the p, q, and g parameters will be generated for this new modulus length; otherwise, a precomputed value will be used (but precomputed values in the Sun security provider are available only for modlen values of 512 and 1024). If the modulus length is invalid, this method throws an InvalidParameterException.

public void initialize(DSAParams params, SecureRandom random)

Initialize the DSA key pair generator. The p, q, and g parameters are set from the values passed in params. If the parameters are not correct, an InvalidParameterException is generated.

As with the DSAKey interface, a DSA key pair generator implements the DSAKeyPairGenerator interface for two purposes: for type identification, and to allow the programmer to initialize the key pair generator with the desired algorithm-specific parameters:

```
KeyPairGenerator kpg = KeyPairGenerator.getInstance("DSA");
if (kpg instanceof DSAKeyPairGenerator) {
    DSAKeyPairGenerator dkpg = (DSAKeyPairGenerator) kpg;
    dkpg.initialize(512, true, new SecureRandom());
}
else kpg.initialize(512);
```

In sum, this interface allows us to use the generic key pair generator interface while providing an escape clause that allows us to perform DSA-specific operations.

Implementing a Key Pair Generator

If you want to implement your own key pair generator—either using a new algorithm or, more typically, a new implementation of a standard algorithm—you need to create a concrete subclass of the KeyPairGenerator class. In Java 1.2, you may create a subclass of the KeyPairGeneratorSpi class instead; in this case, the SPI is the superclass of the engine class.

To construct a key pair generator, there is a single protected method at your disposal:

protected KeyPairGenerator(String name)

Construct a key pair generator that implements the given algorithm.

As with the other engines in the security API, there is no default constructor available within the engine class. When the key pair generator is constructed, it must pass the name of the algorithm that it implements to its superclass so that the algorithm name may be correctly registered with the Security class.

There are two abstract public methods of the key pair generator (or its SPI) that we must implement in our key pair generator: the initialize() method and the generateKeyPair() method. For this example, we'll generate a simple key pair that could be used for a simple rotation-based encryption scheme. In this scheme, the key serves as an offset that we add to each ASCII character—hence, if the key is 1, an encryption based on this key converts the letter a to the letter b, and so on (the addition is performed with a modulus such that z will map to a). To support this encryption, then, we need to generate a public key that is simply a number between 1 and 25; the private key is simply the negative value of the public key.

We must also define a class to represent keys we're implementing.* We can do that with this class:

```
public class XYZKey implements Key, PublicKey, PrivateKey {
    int rotValue;

    public String getAlgorithm() {
        return "XYZ";
    }

    public String getFormat() {
        return "XYZ Special Format";
    }

    public byte[] getEncoded() {
        byte b[] = new byte[4];
        b[3] = (byte) ((rotValue << 24) & 0xff);
        b[2] = (byte) ((rotValue << 16) & 0xff);
        b[1] = (byte) ((rotValue <<  8) & 0xff);
        b[0] = (byte) ((rotValue <<  0) & 0xff);
        return b;
    }
}
```

The only data value our key class cares about is the value to be used as the index; for simplicity, we've made it a simple instance variable accessible only by classes in our package. Because this example is simple, we can use the same class as the interface for the public and the private key; normally, of course, public and private keys are not symmetric like this.

With these pieces in place, we're ready to define our key pair generation class:

```
public class XYZKeyPairGenerator extends KeyPairGenerator {
    SecureRandom random;

    public XYZKeyPairGenerator() {
```

---

* This is true even if you're implementing the DSA algorithm—the classes the Sun security provider uses to represent keys are not in the java package, so they are unavailable to us. So even if you're implementing DSA, you must still define classes that implement all the DSA interfaces we looked at earlier.

```
        super("XYZ");
    }

    public void initialize(int strength, SecureRandom sr) {
        random = sr;
    }

    public KeyPair generateKeyPair() {
        int rotValue = random.nextInt() % 25;
        XYZKey pub = new XYZKey();
        XYZKey priv = new XYZKey();
        pub.rotValue = rotValue;
        priv.rotValue = -rotValue;
        KeyPair kp = new KeyPair(pub, priv);
        return kp;
    }
}
```

As a last step, we must install this class using the security provider architecture that we examined in Chapter 8. Now obtaining a new key pair for the XYZ algorithm is as simple as substituting the string XYZ for the algorithm name in the example we gave earlier for DSA key pair generation.

The KeyFactory Class

Although there are times when you'll generate your own keys, they are more often obtained electronically. The final engine and related set of classes we'll examine show us how to import and export keys. The source or destination of these keys is not specified by any of these classes—you may have read the data from a file, or from a socket, or you may have typed it in manually. The classes in this section merely enable you to convert a key object to a known external representation and to perform the reverse conversion.

Key factories are available only in Java 1.2. Exporting keys in 1.1 is simple: the encoded bytes of the key can be obtained and transmitted in any manner that is convenient. But importing keys in 1.1 is very difficult, because there is no way to take the encoded bytes and produce a key from them. As a fallback measure, you can serialize a key object to export it and then deserialize that data to import the key, although that's not something we generally recommend (see "Keys, Certificates, and Object Serialization" later in this chapter).

There are two external representations by which a key may be transmitted—by its encoded format, or by the parameters that were used to generate the key. Either of these representations may be encapsulated in a key specification, which is used to interact with the KeyFactory class (java.security.KeyFactory) that actually imports and exports keys:

public class KeyFactory ★

Provide an infrastructure for importing and exporting keys according to the specific encoding format or parameters of the key.

Using the KeyFactory class

The `KeyFactory` class is an engine class, which provides the typical method of instantiating itself:

public static final KeyFactory getInstance(String alg) ★
public static final KeyFactory getInstance(String alg, String provider) ★

Create a key factory capable of importing and exporting keys that were generated with the given algorithm. The class that implements the key factory comes from the named provider or is located according to the standard rules for provider engines. If a key factory that implements the given algorithm is not found, a `NoSuchAlgorithmException` is generated. If the named provider is not found, a `NoSuchProviderException` is generated.

A key factory presents the following public methods:

public final Provider getProvider() ★

Return the provider that implemented this particular key factory.

public final PublicKey generatePublic(KeySpec ks) ★
public final PrivateKey generatePrivate(KeySpec ks) ★

These methods are used to import a key: they create the key based on the imported data that is held in the key specification object. If the key cannot be created, an `InvalidKeySpecException` is thrown.

public final KeySpec getKeySpec(Key key, Class keySpec) ★

This method is used to export a key: it creates a key specification based on the actual key. If the key specification cannot be created, an `InvalidKeySpecException` is thrown.

public final Key translateKey(Key key) ★

Translate a key from an unknown source into a key that was generated from this object. This method can be used to convert the type of a key that was loaded from a different security provider (e.g., a DSA key generated from the XYZ provider—type `com.XYZ.DSAPrivateKey`—could be converted to a DSA key generated from the Sun provider—type `sun.security.provider.DSAPrivateKey`). If the key cannot be translated, an `InvalidKeyException` is generated.

public final String getAlgorithm() ★

Return the algorithm this key factory supports.

We'll defer examples of these methods until we discuss the `KeySpec` class later.

Implementing a Key Factory

Like all engines, the key factory depends on a service provider interface class: the KeyFactorySpi class (java.security.KeyFactorySpi):

public abstract class KeyFactorySpi ★

Provide the set of methods necessary to implement a key factory that is capable of importing and exporting keys in a particular format.

However, since the KeyFactory class did not exist in 1.1, its SPI is unrelated in the class hierarchy. Implementing a key factory therefore requires that we subclass the SPI rather than subclassing the KeyFactory class directly. The KeyFactorySpi class is required to implement a key factory because the KeyFactory class contains only this constructor:

protected KeyFactory(KeyFactorySpi keyFacSpi, Provider provider, String algorithm)

Construct a key factory based on the given factory service provider class that is implemented by the given provider and that provides keys of the given algorithm.

This constructor is called by the Security class itself; all we need to do is ensure that the class we register with the security provider interface is a subclass of the KeyFactorySpi class.

The KeyFactorySpi class contains the following methods; since each of these methods is abstract, our class must provide an implementation of all of them:

protected abstract PublicKey engineGeneratePublic(KeySpec ks) ★
protected abstract PrivateKey engineGeneratePrivate(KeySpec ks) ★

Generate of the public or private key. Depending on the key specification, this means either decoding the data of the key or regenerating the key based on specific parameters to the key algorithm. If the key cannot be generated, an InvalidKeyException should be thrown.

protected abstract KeySpec engineGetKeySpec(Key key, Class keySpec) ★

Export the key. Depending on the key class specification, this means either encoding the data (e.g., by calling the getEncoded() method) or saving the parameters that were used to generate the key. If the specification cannot be created, an InvalidKeySpecException should be thrown.

protected Key engineTranslateKey(Key key) ★

Perform the actual translation of the key. This is typically performed by translating the key to its specification and back. If the key cannot be translated, an InvalidKeyException should be thrown.

Although we show how to use a key factory later, we won't show how to implement one; the amount of code involved is large and relatively uninteresting. However, the online examples do contain a sample key factory implementation if you're interested in seeing one.

Key Specifications

Importing and exporting a key are based on classes that implement the KeySpec interface (java.security.spec.KeySpec):

public interface KeySpec ★
> Identify a class as one that is able to hold data that can be used to generate a key.

The KeySpec interface is an empty interface; it is used for type identification only. This interface in turn forms the basis of two interfaces, each of which handles one method of importing a key.

The EncodedKeySpec class

Earlier, we mentioned that the Key class must provide a getEncoded() method for the key that outputs a series of bytes in a format specific to the type of key; this format is generally part of the specification for the key algorithm. For DSA keys, for example, the encoding format might be PKCS#8 or X.509. An encoded key specification holds the encoded data for a key and is defined by the EncodedKey-Spec class (java.security.spec.EncodedKeySpec):

public abstract class EncodedKeySpec implements KeySpec ★
> Provide an object to hold the encoded data of a key.

An encoded key specification can be operated on via these methods:

public abstract byte[] getEncoded() ★
> Return the actual encoded data held by the object.

public abstract String getFormat() ★
> Return the string that represents the format of the encoded data (e.g., PKCS#8).

There are two core classes that provide a concrete implementation of this class (both of which are in the java.security.spec package):

public class PKCS8EncodedKeySpec extends EncodedKeySpec ★
public class X509EncodedKeySpec extends EncodedKeySpec ★
> Provide an implementation of the encoded key specification. The PCKS8 encoded key specification is used for DSA private keys, and the X509 encoded key specification is used for DSA public keys.

Both of these classes are constructed by passing in the encoded data:

public PKCS8EncodedKeySpec(byte data[]) ★
public X509EncodedKeySpec(byte data[]) ★

Construct an encoded key specification object that holds the given encoded data. The format of the data is not checked for validity. The input data is saved within the object to be returned via the getEncoded() method.

Taken together, the methods of these classes allow us to import and export keys. Keys are exported via the getEncoded() method, and they are imported by constructing an object based on the encoded bytes.

The AlgorithmParameterSpec interface

In addition to their encoded format, keys are typically able to be specified by providing the parameters to the algorithm that produced the key. Specifying keys in this manner is a function of the AlgorithmParameterSpec interface (java.security.spec.AlgorithmParameterSpec):

public interface AlgorithmParameterSpec ★

Provide an infrastructure for specifying keys based on the parameters used to generate them.

Like the KeySpec interface, this interface provides no methods and is used only for type identification. The DSAParameterSpec class (java.security.spec.DSAParameterSpec) is the single core class that implements this interface:

public class DSAParameterSpec implements AlgorithmParameterSpec, DSAParams ★

Provide a class that holds the parameters used to generate a DSA key.

As we mentioned earlier, there are three parameters that are common to all DSA keys: *p*, *q*, and *g*. Hence, an instance of this class can be constructed as follows:

public DSAParameterSpec(BigInteger p, BigInteger q, BigInteger g) ★

Create an object that holds the common parameters used to generate a DSA key.

The only methods of this class are used to retrieve those parameters:

public BigInteger getP() ★
public BigInteger getQ() ★
public BigInteger getG() ★

Return the parameter held by the specification object.

While those three parameters are common to every DSA key, a DSA public key has an additional parameter (*y*) and a DSA private key has a different additional parameter (x). Hence, to represent a DSA key fully requires one of these classes (both of which are in the `java.security.spec` package):

public class DSAPublicKeySpec implements KeySpec ★
public class DSAPrivateKeySpec implements KeySpec ★
   Provide an object to hold all parameters of a DSA public or private key.

Instances of these classes are constructed by providing all parameters:

public DSAPublicKeySpec(BigInteger y, BigInteger p, BigInteger q, BigInteger g) ★
public DSAPrivateKeySpec(BigInteger x, BigInteger p, BigInteger q, BigInteger g) ★
   Create an object that holds all the parameters used to generate a DSA key.

This final parameter can be retrieved via a class-specific method (`getX()` or `getY()` as appropriate).

Once again, these classes in total allow us to export keys (via the various `get*()` methods) and to import keys via the constructors.

A Key Factory Example

As we mentioned at the beginning of this section, the prime reason for key factories is that they give us the ability to import and export keys. Exporting a key specification is typically done by transmitting the individual data elements of the key specification (those individual elements vary by the type of key). Importing a key specification typically involves constructing the specification with the transmitted elements as parameters to the constructor.

Here's an example using a DSA algorithmic parameter specification. We'll look first at exporting a key:

```
public class Export {
    public static void main(String args[]) {
        try {
            KeyPairGenerator kpg = KeyPairGenerator.getInstance("DSA");
            kpg.initialize(512, new SecureRandom());
            KeyPair kp = kpg.generateKeyPair();
            Class spec = Class.forName(
                        "java.security.spec.DSAPrivateKeySpec");
            KeyFactory kf = KeyFactory.getInstance("DSA");
            DSAPrivateKeySpec ks = (DSAPrivateKeySpec)
                               kf.getKeySpec(kp.getPrivate(), spec);
            FileOutputStream fos = new FileOutputStream("exportedKey");
            ObjectOutputStream oos = new ObjectOutputStream(fos);
            oos.writeObject(ks.getX());
            oos.writeObject(ks.getP());
            oos.writeObject(ks.getQ());
            oos.writeObject(ks.getG());
```

```
            } catch (Exception e) {
                e.printStackTrace();
            }
        }
    }
```

Two items are interesting in this code. First, one argument to the getKeySpec() method is a class object, requiring us to construct the class object using the forName() method (a somewhat unusual usage). Then, once we have the key specification itself, we have to figure out how to transmit the specification. Since in this case, the specification is an algorithmic specification, we chose to write out the individual parameters from the specification.* If we had used an encoded key specification, we simply would have written out the byte array returned from the getEncoded() method.

We can import this key as follows:

```
public class Import {
    public static void main(String args[]) {
        try {
            FileInputStream fis = new FileInputStream("exportedKey");
            ObjectInputStream ois = new ObjectInputStream(fis);
            DSAPrivateKeySpec ks = new DSAPrivateKeySpec(
                        (BigInteger) ois.readObject(),
                        (BigInteger) ois.readObject(),
                        (BigInteger) ois.readObject(),
                        (BigInteger) ois.readObject());
            KeyFactory kf = KeyFactory.getInstance("DSA");
            PrivateKey pk = kf.generatePrivate(ks);
            System.out.println("Got private key");
        } catch (Exception e) {
            e.printStackTrace();
        }
    }
}
```

This example is predictably symmetric to exporting a key.

Certificates

When you are given a public and private key, you often need to provide other people with your public key. If you sign a digital document (using your private key), the recipient of that document will need your public key in order to verify your digital signature.

---

* The DSAPrivateKeySpec class—like all key specification classes—is not serializable itself. But for reasons that we'll discuss later, it's better not to serialize key classes that are to be imported into another Java VM anyway.

The inherent problem with a key is that it does not provide any information about the identity to which it belongs; a key is really just a sequence of seemingly arbitrary numbers. If I want you to accept a document that I digitally signed, I could mail you my public key, but you normally have no assurance that the key (and the original email) came from me at all. I could, of course, digitally sign the e-mail so that you knew that it came from me, but there's a circular chain here—without my public key, you cannot verify the digital signature. You would need my public key in order to authenticate the public key I've just sent you.

Certificates solve this problem by having a well-known entity (called a certificate authority, or CA) verify the public key that is being sent to you. A certificate can give you the assurance that the public key in the certificate does indeed belong to the entity that the certificate authority says it does. However, the certificate only validates the public key it contains: just because Fred sends you his public key in a valid certificate does not mean that Fred is to be trusted; it only means that the public key in question does in fact belong to Fred.

In practice, the key may not belong to Fred at all; certificate authorities have different levels at which they assess the identity of the entity named in the certificate. Some of these levels are very stringent and require the CA to do an extensive verification that Fred is who he says he is. Other levels are not stringent at all, and if Fred can produce a few dollars and a credit card, he is assumed to be Fred. Hence, one of the steps in the process of deciding whether or not to trust the entity named in the certificate includes the level at which the certificate authority generated the certificate. Each certificate authority varies in its approach to validating identities, and each publishes its approach to help you understand the potential risks involved in accepting such a certificate.

A certificate contains three pieces of information (as shown in Figure 10-2):

- The name of the entity for whom the certificate has been issued. This entity is referred to as the subject of the certificate.

- The public key associated with the subject.

- A digital signature that verifies the information of the certificate. The certificate is signed by the issuer of the certificate.

Because the certificate carries a digital signature of the certificate authority, we can verify that digital signature—and if the verification succeeds, we can be assured that the public key in the certificate does in fact belong to the entity the certificate claims (subject to the level at which the CA verified the subject).

We still have a bootstrapping problem here—how do we obtain the public key of the certificate authority? We could have a certificate that contains the public key of the certificate authority, but who is going to authenticate *that* certificate?

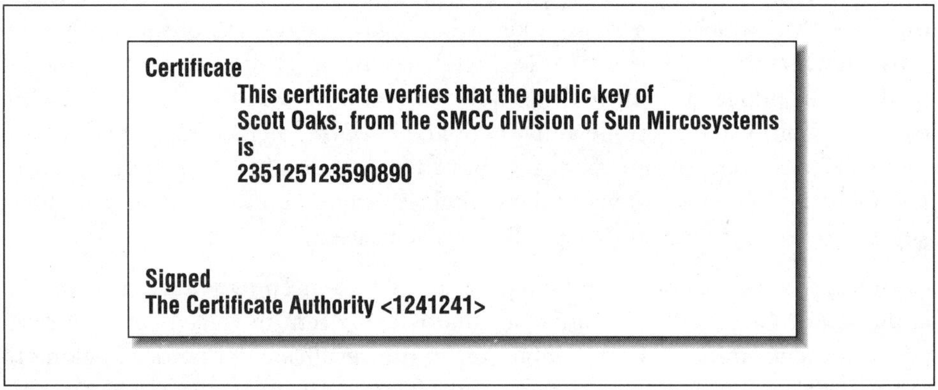

```
Certificate
        This certificate verfies that the public key of
        Scott Oaks, from the SMCC division of Sun Mircosystems
        is
        235125123590890



Signed
The Certificate Authority <1241241>
```

Figure 10-2. Logical representation of a certificate

This bootstrapping problem is one reason why key management (see Chapter 11) is such a hard topic. Most Java-enabled browsers solve this problem by providing the public keys for certain well-known certificate authorities along with the browser. This has worked well in practice, though it clearly is not an airtight solution (especially when the browser is downloaded from some site on the Internet—theoretically, the certificates that come with the browser could be tampered with as they are in transit). Although there are various proposals to strengthen this model, for now we will assume that the certificate of at least one well-known certificate authority is delivered along with the Java application. This situation allows me to mail you a certificate containing my public key; if the certificate is signed by a certificate authority you know about, you are assured that the public key actually belongs to me.

There are many well-known certificate authorities—and therein lies another problem. I may send you a certificate that is signed by the United States Post Office, but that certificate authority may not be one of the certificate authorities you recognize. Simply sending a public key in a certificate does not mean that the recipient of the public key will accept it. A more important implication of this is that a key management system needs to be prepared to assign multiple certificates to a particular individual, potentially one from each of several certificate authorities.

Another implication of this profusion of certificate authorities is that certificates are often supplied as a chain. Let's say that you have the certificate of the U.S. Post Office certificate authority, and I want to send you my certificate that has been generated by the Acme Certificate company. In order for you to accept this certificate, I must send you a chain of certificates: my certificate (certified by the Acme Certificate company), and a certificate for the Acme Certificate company (certified by the U.S. Post Office). This chain of certificates may be arbitrarily long.

The last certificate in this chain—that is, the public key for a certificate authority—is generally stored in a certificate that is self-signed: the certificate authority has signed the certificate that contains its own public key. Self-signed certificates tend to crop up frequently in the Java world as well, since the tools that come with the JDK will create self-signed certificates. The certificates are intended to be submitted to a certificate authority, who will then return a CA-signed certificate. But there's no reason why the certificate itself can't be used as a valid certificate. Whether or not you want to accept a self-signed certificate is up to you, but it obviously carries certain risks.

Finally, for all this talk of certificates, you have to consider whether or not they are actually necessary to support your application. If you'll generally be receiving signed items from people you do not know (e.g., a signed JAR file from a web site), then they are absolutely necessary. On the other hand, large-scale computer installations often consider using certificates to authenticate and validate their employees; this results in a computer system that has much better internal security than one that relies solely on passwords. But it is not the certificate that generates the security advantage, it is the use of public key cryptography. The computer installation can achieve the same level of security without using a certificate infrastructure.

Consider the security necessary to support XYZ Corporation's payroll application. When an employee wants to view her payroll statements, she must submit a digitally signed request to do so. Hence, XYZ should distribute to each employee a private key to be used to create the digital signature. XYZ can also store the employee's public keys in a database; when a request comes that claims to be from a particular employee, the payroll server can simply examine the database to obtain that employee's public key and verify the signature. No certificate is required in this case—and in general, no certificate is required when the recipient of the digital signature is already known to have the public key of the entity that signed the data. For applications within a corporation, this is almost always the case.

We issue this caveat about certificates being necessary because certificate support in Java (even in Java 1.2) is not fully complete—while it is possible to set up your own certificate authority to distribute the certificates for your company, it's very hard to write the necessary code to do that in Java (at present). Hence, we'll focus our discussion of the certificate API on accepting (i.e., validating) existing certificates.

Certificate: Class or Interface

There's an unfortunate ambiguity in Java's use of the term "certificate." In Java 1.1, an interface called `java.security.Certificate` was introduced and used by the `javakey` utility and by the `appletviewer` when they used signed classes. The `Certificate` interface was implemented by platform-specific classes.

In Java 1.2, there is a new class called `java.security.cert.Certificate`. This class is the preferred class for all interactions with certificates, and is used by the utilities provided with the 1.2 JDK. The `java.security.Certificate` interface has been deprecated starting with Java 1.2.

One problem where this manifests itself is with `import` statements. If you import the following packages:

```
import java.security.*;
import java.security.cert.*;
```

the compiler will be unable to reconcile the definition of `Certificate`. When dealing with certificates, you'll either need to refer to them by their fully qualified name or only import those classes in the security package that you explicitly need.

In the main text of this book, whenever we talk about a certificate object, we mean an instance of the `java.security.cert.Certificate` class (or one of its subclasses). Except for some examples in Appendix B, we will not show usage of the `Certificate` interface.

The Certificate Class

There are many formats that a certificate can take (depending on the cryptographic algorithms used to produce the certificate). Hence, the Java API abstracts the generic notion of a certificate with the `Certificate` class (`java.security.cert.Certificate`):

public abstract class Certificate ★

Provide the necessary (and very basic) operations to support a certificate.

Like many classes in the Java security package, the `Certificate` class is abstract; it relies upon application-specific classes to provide its implementation. In the case of the JDK, there are classes in the `sun` package that implement certain certificate formats (but more about that in just a bit).

There are three essential operations that you can perform upon a certificate:

public abstract byte[] getEncoded() ★

>   Return a byte array of the certificate. All certificates must have a format in
>   which they may be transmitted as a series of bytes, but the details of this
>   encoding format are specific to the type of the certificate. If the encoding
>   cannot be generated, a `CertificateEncodingException` is thrown.

public abstract void verify(PublicKey pk) ★
public abstract void verify(PublicKey pk, String provider) ★

>   Verify that the certificate is valid. In order to verify a certificate, you must
>   have the public key of the certificate authority that issued it; a valid certificate
>   is one in which the signature of the certificate authority is valid. A valid certifi-
>   cate does not imply anything about the trustworthiness of the certificate
>   authority or the subject to which the certificate belongs; it merely means that
>   the signature in the certificate is valid for the supplied public key. If the certifi-
>   cate is invalid, this method throws a `CertificateException`.
>
>   The signature is verified according to the digital signature details we'll
>   examine in Chapter 12. The process of creating an object to verify the digital
>   signature as well as the actual verification of the signature may thrown a
>   `NoSuchProviderException`, a `NoSuchAlgorithmException`, an `Invalid-`
>   `KeyException`, or a `SignatureException`.

public abstract PublicKey getPublicKey() ★

>   Extract the public key from the certificate—that is, the key that belongs to the
>   subject the certificate vouches for.

These are the basic operations that are valid for any certificate. Notice that while
we can encode a certificate into a byte array in order to transmit the certificate,
there is nothing in the basic API that allows us to create a certificate from such a
byte array. In fact, there's no practical way to instantiate a certificate object at all;
the `Certificate` class is usually used as a base class from which individual certificate types are derived. Fortunately, the next class allows us to both import and
export certificates.

The X509Certificate Class

As we mentioned, there are many certificate formats that could be in use by a key
management system; one of the most common of these is the X509 format. X509
has gone through a few revisions; the version supported by the Java API is version
3. This format is an ANSI standard for certificates, and while there are PGP and
other certificate formats in the world, the X509 format is dominant. This is the
only format of certificate for which Java provides a standard API; if you want to
support another certificate format, you must implement your own subclass of
`Certificate`.

The X509Certificate class (java.security.cert.X509Certificate) is defined as follows:

public abstract class X509Certificate extends Certificate implements X509Extension ★
    Provide an infrastructure to support X509 version 3 formatted certificates.

The X509Certificate class looks like an engine class, but it is slightly different. Instead of relying upon its implementation to be provided in the security provider infrastructure, it relies upon an implementation that is specified directly in the *java.security* file itself. The JDK comes with a particular implementation that appears in the default *java.security* file as:

```
cert.provider.x509=sun.security.x509.X509CertImpl
```

You may write or purchase your own implementation of this class and substitute that class in the *java.security* file.

Like the engine classes, an instance of this class is created by the getInstance() method:

public static final X509Certificate getInstance(InputStream is) ★
public static final X509Certificate getInstance(byte[] data) ★
    Create an X509 certificate based on the encoded data to be read from the given input stream or byte array. If the certificate cannot be created from the data in the input stream or array, a CertificateException is generated.

There is no getInstance() method that instantiates an empty certificate: certificates in this API must always be instantiated based on existing data. In other words, we can use the certificate API to import a certificate, but we cannot use it to create a certificate from scratch.* The standard X509 implementation requires that the data to be read is encoded in a format known as DER (for Definite Encoding Rules).

An X509 certificate has a number of properties that are not shared by its base class:

- A start and end date: An X509 certificate is valid only for a certain period of time, as specified by these dates.

- A version: Various versions of the X509 standard exist; the default implementation of this class supports version 3 of the standard.

- A serial number: Each certificate that is issued by a certificate authority must have a unique serial number. The serial number is only unique for a particu-

---

* This is a primary reason why we won't get into the issues involved in writing your own certificate authority for your local enterprise.

lar authority, so that the combination of serial number and certificate authority guarantee a unique certificate.

- The distinguished name* of the certificate authority.

- The distinguished name of the subject represented by the certificate.

These properties can be retrieved with the following set of methods:

public abstract void checkValidity() ★
public abstract void checkValidity(Date d) ★

Check that the specified date (or today if no date is specified) is within the
start and end dates for which the certificate is valid. If the specified date is
before the start date of the certificate, a `CertificateNotYetValidException`
is thrown; if it is after the end date of the certificate, a `Certifi-
cateExpiredException` is thrown.

public abstract int getVersion() ★

Return the version of the X509 specification that this certificate was created
with. For the Sun implementation, this will be version 3.

public abstract BigInteger getSerialNumber() ★

Return the serial number of the certificate.

public abstract Principal getIssuerDN() ★

Extract the distinguished name of the certificate authority from the certificate
and use that name to instantiate a principal object.

public abstract Principal getSubjectDN() ★

Extract the distinguished name of the subject entity in the certificate and use
that name to instantiate a principal object.

public abstract Date getNotBefore() ★

Return the first date on which the certificate is valid.

public abstract Date getNotAfter() ★

Return the date after which the certificate is invalid.

From a programmatic view, these are the most useful of the attributes of a certificate. If your X509 certificate is contained in the file *sdo.cer*, you could import and
print out information about the certificate as follows:

```
public class PrintCert {
    public static void main(String args[]) {
        try {
            FileInputStream fr = new FileInputStream("sdo.cer");
            X509Certificate c = X509Certificate.getInstance(fr);
            System.out.println("Read in the following certificate:");
```

---

* See the sidebar "What's in a Name?" in Chapter 11 for an explanation of distinguished names.

```
            System.out.println("\tCertificate for: " +
                                    c.getSubjectDN());
            System.out.println("\tCertificate issued by: " +
                                    c.getIssuerDN());
            System.out.println("\tThe certificate is valid from " +
                        c.getNotBefore() + " to " + c.getNotAfter());
            System.out.println("\tCertificate SN# " +
                                    c.getSerialNumber());
            System.out.println("\tGenerated with " +
                                    c.getSigAlgName());
        } catch (Exception e) {
            e.printStackTrace();
        }
    }
}
```

Running this program would produce the following output:

```
Read in the following certificate:
    Certificate for:
        CN=Scott Oaks, OU=SMCC, O=Sun Microsystems, L=NY, S=NY, C=US
    Certificate issued by:
        CN=Scott Oaks, OU=SMCC, O=Sun Microsystems, L=NY, S=NY, C=US
    The certificate is valid from Sun Oct 19 11:40:24 EDT 1997 to
        Sat Jan 17 10:40:24 EST 1998
    Certificate SN# 3895020084
    Generated with SHA1withDSA
```

Importing and Exporting Certificates

The input data to the X509Certificate class must be a certificate that is encoded in DER format. This encoding is specified by the X509 standard, so obtaining a certificate with that encoding is not normally a problem. Hence, a certificate can usually be imported into your program using the code in the example we just showed.

Often, however, you'll obtain a certificate that is in RFC 1421 format. In this case, the 8-bit bytes that comprise the DER-encoded certificate have been transformed into 7-bit ASCII characters; this facilitates the transmission of the certificate over some public networks (and through some mail systems) that are unable to transmit 8-bit binary data. In addition, the certificate will begin with the string:

```
-----BEGIN CERTIFICATE-----
```

and conclude with the string:

```
-----END CERTIFICATE-----
```

The ASCII-encoded data will appear between these two string delimiters.

The translation from 8-bit to 7-bit data (and back to 8-bit data) is defined by RFC 1521 and is referred to as Base64 encoding. In this encoding scheme, each 3 bytes of 8-bit data are turned into 4 bytes of 7-bit data from a specified character set. There are many third-party Java classes that perform this manipulation, so we'll not repeat it here. Assuming that you have a class to perform the decoding, you could read in an RFC 1421 certificate as follows:

```
String s;
BufferedReader br = new BufferedReader(new FileReader("sdo.cer"));
while ((s = br.readLine()) != null &&
            !s.equals("-----BEGIN CERTIFICATE-----"))
    continue;
if (s == null)
    throw new IOException("Malformed certificate");
StringBuffer buf = new StringBuffer();
while ((s = br.readLine()) != null) &&
            !s.equals("-----END CERTIFICATE-----"))
    buf.append(s);
if (s == null)
    throw new IOException("Malformed Certificate");
Base64Decoder dec = new Base64Decoder();
byte data[] = dec.decode(buf.toString());
X509Certificate c = X509Certificate.getInstance(data);
```

Exporting of certificates is predictably symmetric: to produce a DER-encoded certificate, you simply call the getEncoded() method on the certificate and write out the bytes. To produce an RFC 1421 format certificate, you print out the beginning delimiter, followed by the DER-encoded data that has been run through a Base64 encoder, followed by the ending delimiter.

Advanced X509Certificate Methods

There are a number of other methods of the X509Certificate class. For the purposes of this book, these methods are not generally useful; they enable you to perform more introspection on the certificate itself. We'll list these methods here simply as a matter of record.

public abstract byte[] getTBSCertificate() ★

Get the DER-encoded TBS certificate. The TBS certificate is the body of the actual certificate; it contains all the naming and key information held in the certificate. The only information in the actual certificate that is not held in the TBS certificate is the name of the algorithm used to sign the certificate and the signature itself.

The TBS certificate is used as the input data to the signature algorithm when the certificate is signed or verified.

public abstract byte[] getSignature() ★

> Get the raw signature bytes of the certificate. These bytes could be used to verify the signature explicitly (e.g., using the methods we'll describe in Chapter 12) instead of relying upon the verify() method to do so.

public abstract String getSigAlgName() ★

> Return the name of the algorithm that was used to sign the certificate. For the Sun implementation, this will always be SHA1withDSA.

public String getSigAlgOID() ★

> Return the OID of the signature algorithm used to produce the certificate.

public abstract byte[] getSigAlgParams() ★

> Return the DER-encoded parameters that were used to generate the signature. In general, this will return null, since the parameters are usually specified by the certificate authority's public key.

public abstract byte[] getIssuerUniqueID() ★

> Return the unique identifier for the issuer of the certificate. The presence of a unique identifier for each issuer allows the names to be reused, although in general it is recommended that certificates not make use of the unique identifier.

public abstract byte[] getSubjectUniqueID() ★

> Return the unique identifier for the subject of the certificate (again, this is unused in general).

public abstract BitSet getKeyUsage() ★

> Return the key usage extension, which defines the purpose of the key: the key may be used for digital signing, nonrepudiation, key encipherment, data encipherment, key agreement, certificate signing, and more. The key usage is an extension to the X509 specification and need not be present in all X509 certificates.

public abstract int getBasicConstraints() ★

> An X509 certificate may contain an optional extension that identifies whether the subject of the certificate is a certificate authority. If the subject is a CA, this extension returns the number of certificates that may follow this certificate in a certification chain.

Revoked Certificates

Occasionally, a certificate authority needs to revoke a certificate it has issued—perhaps the certificate was issued under false pretenses, or maybe the user of the certificate has engaged in illegal conduct using the certificate. Under circumstances such as these, the expiration date attached to the certificate is insufficient protection; the certificate must be immediately invalidated.

This invalidation occurs as the result of a CRL—a certificate revocation list. Certificate authorities are responsible for issuing certificate revocation lists that contain (predictably) a list of certificates the authority has revoked. Validators of certificates are required to consult this list before accepting the validity of a certificate.

Unfortunately, the means by which an authority issues a CRL is one of those areas that is in flux, and while the interfaces to support revoked certificates have been established, they are not completely integrated into most certificate systems. In particular, the validate() method of the Certificate class does not automatically consult any CRL. The CRL itself is typically obtained in an out-of-band fashion (just as the certificates of the authority were obtained); once you have a CRL, you can check to see if a particular certificate in which you are interested is on the list.

While the notion of revoked certificates in not necessarily specific to an X509 certificate, the Java implementation is. Revoked certificates themselves are represented by the RevokedCertificate class (java.security.cert.Revoked-Certificate):

public abstract class RevokedCertificate implements X509Extension ★
Provide a framework for revoked certificate objects. The revoked certificate is tied to the notion of an X509 certificate because it is based upon an X509 serial number. There are no public concrete implementations of this class; they are instantiated and provided by the X509CRL class (see below).

The methods of this class are simple and are based upon the fields present in a revoked X509 certificate:

public abstract BigInteger getSerialNumber() ★
Return the serial number of the revoked certificate.

public abstract Date getRevocationDate() ★
Return the date on which the certificate was revoked.

public abstract boolean hasExtensions() ★
Indicate whether the implementation of the class has any X509 extensions.

Revoked certificates are generated by the X509CRL class (java.security.cert.X509CRL):

public abstract class X509CRL implements X509Extension ★
Provide the support for an X509-based certificate revocation list.

Like the X509Certificate class, the X509CRL class may be provided by a third party; its Sun implementation is provided by this entry in the *java.security* file:

```
crl.provider.x509=sun.security.x509.X509CRLImpl
```

Instances of this class are therefore generated by the getInstance() method:

public static final X509CRL getInstance(byte[] data) ★
public static final X509CRL getInstance(InputStream is) ★

Create a CRL based on the given input data. The format of the input data is defined by the X509 standard and is DER-encoded; in logical terms, the input stream contains a series of revoked certificates (corresponding to the above class) and the signature of the certificate authority who issued the CRL. An error in parsing the data may result in a CRLException or an X509ExtensionException.

Once the class has been instantiated, you may operate upon it with these methods. As you can see, there is a strong synergy between the methods that are used to operate upon an X509 certificate and those used to operate upon a CRL:

public abstract void verify(PublicKey pk) ★
public abstract void verify(PublicKey pk, String sigProvider) ★

Verify that the signature that accompanied the CRL is valid (based on the standard signature verification we'll look at in Chapter 12). The public key should be the public key of the certificate authority that issued the CRL.

An error in the underlying signature object may generate a NoSuchAlgorithmException, a NoSuchProviderException, an InvalidKeyExcep-tion, or a SignatureException.

public abstract boolean isRevoked(BigInteger serialNumber) ★

Indicate whether or not the certificate with the given serial number has been revoked (that is, is present in the given CRL).

public abstract int getVersion() ★

Return the version of the CRL. The present version of the X509 CRL specification is 2.

public abstract Principal getIssuerDN() ★

Extract the distinguished name of the issuer of the CRL and return a principal object that contains that name.

public abstract Date getThisUpdate() ★

Extract and return the date when the authority issued this CRL.

public abstract Date getNextUpdate() ★

Extract and return the date when the authority expects to issue its next CRL. This value may not be present in the CRL, in which case null is returned.

public abstract RevokedCertificate getRevokedCertificate(BigInteger sn) ★

Instantiate and return a revoked certificate object based on the given serial number. If the serial number is invalid, a CRLException is thrown.

public abstract Set getRevokedCertificates() ★

Instantiate a revoked certificate object for each certificate in the CRL and return the set of those objects. This method may throw a `CRLException`.

public abstract byte[] getEncoded() ★

Return the DER-encoded CRL itself. This method may throw a `CRLException`.

public abstract byte[] getTBSCertList() ★

Return the DER-encoded TBS certificate list—that is, all the data that came with the CRL aside from the name of the algorithm used to sign the CRL and the digital signature itself. This data can be used to verify the signature directly. Parsing of the underlying data may throw a `CRLException` or an `X509ExtensionException`.

public abstract byte[] getSignature ★

Return the actual bytes of the signature.

public abstract String getSigAlgName() ★

Return the name of the signature algorithm that was used to sign the CRL.

public abstract String getSigAlgOID() ★

Return the OID string of the signature algorithm that was used to sign the CRL.

public abstract byte[] getSigAlgParams() ★

Return the DER-encoded algorithms used in the signature generation. This generally returns `null`, as those parameters (if any) usually accompany the authority's public key.

When all is said and done, the point of the `CRL` class (and the revoked certificate class) is to provide you with the tools necessary to see if a particular certificate has been invalidated. This checking is up to your application to perform; you might choose to implement it as follows:

```java
public Certificate importCertificate(byte data[])
                                throws CertificateException {
    X509Certificate c = null;
    try {
        c = X509Certificate.getInstance(data);
        Principal p = c.getIssuerDN();
        PublicKey pk = getPublicKey(p);
        c.verify(pk);
        InputStream crlFile = lookupCRLFile(p);
        X509CRL crl = X509CRL.getInstance(crlFile);
        BigInteger bi = c.getSerialNumber();
        if (crl.isRevoked(bi))
            throw new CertificateException("Certificate revoked");
    } catch (NoSuchAlgorithmException nsae) {
        throw new CertificateException("Can't verify certificate");
```

```
        } catch (NoSuchProviderException nspe) {
            throw new CertificateException("Can't verify certificate");
        } catch (SignatureException se) {
            throw new CertificateException("Can't verify certificate");
        } catch (InvalidKeyException ike) {
            throw new CertificateException("Can't verify certificate");
        } catch (CRLException ce) {
            // treat as no crl
        } catch (X509ExtensionException xee) {
            // treat as no crl
        }
        return c;
    }
```

This method encapsulates importing a certificate and checking its validity. It is passed the DER-encoded data of the certificate to check (this data must have been read from a file or other input stream, as we showed earlier). Then we consult the certificate to find out who issued it, obtain the public key of the issuer, and validate the certificate. Before we return, however, we obtain the latest CRL of the issuing authority and ensure that the certificate we're checking has not been revoked; if it has been, we throw a CertificateException.

We've glossed over two details in this method: how we obtain the public key of the authority that issued the certificate, and how we get the CRL list associated with that authority. Implementing these methods is the crux of a key/certificate management system, and we'll show some ideas on how to implement the key lookup in Chapter 11. Obtaining the CRL is slightly more problematic, since you must have access to a source for the CRL data. Once you have that data, however, it's trivial to create the CRL via the getInstance() method.

Keys, Certificates, and Object Serialization

Before we conclude this chapter, a brief word on object serialization, keys, and certificates. Keys and certificates are often transmitted electronically, and a reasonable mechanism for transmitting them between Java programs is to send them as serialized objects. In theory—and, most of the time, in practice—this is a workable solution. If you modify some of the examples in this chapter to save and restore serialized keys or certificates, that will certainly work in a testing environment.

A problem arises, however, when you send these serialized objects between virtual machines that have two different security providers. Let's take the case of a DSA public key. When you create such a key with the Sun security provider, you get an instance of the sun.security.provider.DSAPublicKey class. When you create such a key with a third-party security provider, you may get an instance of the com.xyz.XYZPublicKey class. Although both public keys are extensions of the PublicKey class, they cannot be interchanged by object serialization. Serializing a public key created with the Sun security provider requires that the sun.security.provider.DSAPublicKey class be used, and deserialization creates an object of that type, no matter what security providers the deserializing virtual machine has installed. Whether or not the Sun security provider has been installed in the destination virtual machine is irrelevant. The process of deserializing the object uses that class if it is available, and deserialization fails if that class is not available.

Hence, while they are serializable objects, keys and certificates should only be transmitted as encoded data. For keys, you also have the option of transmitting the data contained in the key specification as we did earlier; the key specification classes are not serializable themselves, so you still have to rely on transmitting only the data that those objects contain.

This rule applies not only to keys and certificates that stand alone, but also to classes that embed one of those objects. Take, for example, this class:

```
public class Message implements Serializable {
    String msg;
    X509Certificate cert;
    byte signature[];
}
```

If you want to send an object of this class to a remote virtual machine (or save the object to a file), you should override the writeObject() and readObject() methods of the class so that when it is transmitted, the certificate is transmitted only as its encoded data and not as an instance of the sun.security.x509.X509CertImpl class. We'll do just that in Chapter 12.

Summary

Keys are a basic feature of any cryptographic system; they provide one of the inputs required to produce a digital signature (as well as other potential cryptographic operations). In this chapter, we looked at the basic classes that implement the notion of a key within the Java security package.

Keys are closely tied to the notion of certificates; a certificate contains a public key as well as an assurance from some known entity that the public key belongs to a specific entity. In a general sense, there are a great many things you can do with certificates, but for our purposes, we're interested in certificates only from the perspective of the certificate's user—that is, we want to be able to import and verify a certificate, but we're not too interested in creating our own certificates or in becoming a certificate authority.

Given that the operations we want to perform on keys and certificates are simple—importing and exporting those certificates—you'd expect that we could leave our discussion of keys for the time being. Unfortunately, the topic of finding a key for a particular entity (which is really just a case of importing a key) is a particularly troublesome topic, which we'll examine in the next chapter.

11

Key Management

In this chapter, we're going to discuss key management, and the facilities in Java that enable key management. The problem of key management turns out to be a hard one to solve: there is no universally accepted approach to key management, and although many features in Java (and on the Internet) are available to assist with key management, all key management techniques remain very much works in progress.

The fluidity of key management is evident in the progress of Java itself. Key management with the 1.1 API is very different from key management in 1.2. Further complicating this picture is the fact that no Java-enabled browser (including HotJava, but not including the Java Activator) uses the technique for key management that comes with the JDK. Each requires keys to be kept in a different key database, and each uses a different technique to store and retrieve keys from that application-specific database. Key management remains application-specific.

In this chapter, we'll discuss the basic features of Java that are available for key management, including the default key management features of the JDK. We'll conclude with an example of implementing your own key management system. The key management features we're going to discuss apply primarily to Java 1.2. If you must implement a key management system under Java 1.1, you'll need to use the IdentityScope class as discussed in Appendix B. However, the Identity-Scope class itself, while not officially deprecated, has been pretty much replaced by the classes we are going to explore in this chapter.

Overview of Key Management

Keys are important to Java's security model because they allow us to create or verify a digital signature. In the sandbox model, we usually think of the use of digital signatures in the context of a signed JAR file. When a JAR file is signed, we are assured that the classes contained in that file were actually provided by the entity (the person or corporation) that signed the JAR file. This allows us to grant privileges to the signed classes because we know that the classes have not been forged by a third party. Of course, digital signatures have many other uses in a particular application.

We'll discuss the details of digital signatures in Chapter 12. For now, it's enough to know that a digital signature is created with a private key, then transferred electronically (along with the data it signed). When the digital signature is received, it must be verified, which requires a public key that corresponds to the private key that generated the signature.

The purpose of a key management system is two-fold. When you need to digitally sign something, the key management system must provide your private key for the code that creates the digital signature. When you need to verify a digital signature, the key management system must provide the public key that will be used for verification. A key management system may encompass other operations (it may, for example, provide information about the degree to which a particular individual should be trusted), but it exists primarily to serve up keys.

Hence, there are three elements of a key management system:

Keys

> The keys in a key management system can be used for several cryptographic operations, but in general we will use them to sign data, such as a JAR file. An entity in the key management database can have no keys, a public key, or both a public key and a private key.

Certificates

> Certificates are used to verify that the association between a public key and an entity is valid. Verification of a digital signature requires the public key that belongs to the entity that created the digital signature; a certificate verifies that the public key itself has not been forged and does indeed belong to the desired identity.

Identities

> Identities are an abstraction of individuals, companies, or any other entity that might have a key. The purpose of a key management system is to associate identities with their keys. This association must be stored somewhere; we refer to the database in which these associations are stored as the key database or the keystore.

Java 1.1 comes with a key management system that is based upon the javakey utility. Javakey has several limitations; in particular, it stores public and private keys in the same, unprotected location (often called an identity database). This allows anyone with access to the javakey database to determine all the keys that were stored in the file. Since access is required to obtain your own private key to generate your own digital signature, this essentially gives all users access to each other's keys. This problem was a limitation of the javakey utility itself. It's possible to use the 1.1 classes to write a key database in such a way that your private key is held separately from a group of public keys (see Appendix B).

The javakey utility was an interim solution to the key management problem; it is no longer available. In 1.2, javakey has been replaced by a new utility called keytool. Keytool is a much better tool, in that individual private and public keys can be stored in the same database, and retrieval of each key can be made subject to a password. The keytool database is often referred to as the keystore.

Unfortunately, the default implementation of the keytool database still has certain limitations; in particular, it is difficult to share the keys in a keytool database among a widely dispersed group of people (like all the employees of XYZ Corporation). We can, however, use the framework that the keytool database uses to create a key management system that has whatever features we require.

That framework is the ultimate goal of this chapter. First, however, we must discuss the last of the APIs that make up the necessary parts of a key management system: identities.

Identities

You probably noticed in Chapter 10 that none of the key classes had any notion of whom the key belonged to. Keys are really just an arbitrary-appearing series of bytes. The set of classes we'll examine now deal with the notion of identity: the entity to which a key belongs. An identity can represent an individual or a corporation (or anything else that can possess a public or a private key).

The classes we'll examine in this section were originally designed to support the 1.1 javakey utility. In 1.2, these classes still provide a useful abstraction for the entity that holds a set of keys, but they play a far less important role in a keytool-based key management system than they did in a javakey-based one.

Principals

Classes that are concerned with identities and key management in the Java security package generally implement the Principal interface (java.security.Principal):

public interface Principal

> Provide an interface that supports the notion of an entity. In particular, principals have a name, but little else.

There is a single method that implementors of the `Principal` interface must implement:

public String getName()

> Return the name of the principal. This is typically an X.500 distinguished name, but it may be any arbitrary name.

The only idea that the `Principal` interface abstracts is that principals have a name. The Java documentation claims that a principal is anything that can have an identity, but don't be confused by that statement; the word "identity" is being overloaded in this context. The `Identity` class we're about to introduce is a principal, but there are classes implementing the `Principal` interface that are unrelated to the `Identity` class.

Further confusion about this interface can arise because there are two principal objects in Java 1.2: the `java.security.Principal` interface (introduced in 1.1), and the `org.omg.CORBA.Principal` class (introduced in 1.2). These classes are unrelated, and we'll discuss only the `java.security.Principal` interface throughout this book.

The name that is stored in a principal is often an X.500 distinguished name (DN). That is particularly true when a principal is used in certain certificates (like X509 certificates); it is not an absolute requirement by any means.

There are other methods listed in the `Principal` interface—namely, the `equals()`, `toString()`, and `hashCode()` methods. There's no reason for those methods to be listed in the `Principal` interface, since every class already inherits those methods from the `Object` class. If you implement the `Principal` interface, the only method you must implement is the `getName()` method. You should make sure that the other methods of the `Principal` interface are implemented correctly—but you should ensure that these methods of the `Object` class are implemented correctly for all your classes, not just those that implement the `Principal` interface.

The Identity Class

Now we'll look at the primary class used to encapsulate an entity that has a public key, the `Identity` class (`java.security.Identity`):

public class Identity implements Principal, Serializable

> Implement an identity—an entity that has a public key. In 1.1, this class is abstract.

What's in a Name?

X509 certificates (and many other ANSI standards) make use of the idea of a distinguished name (usually referred to as a DN). The distinguished name of an individual includes these fields:

Common Name (CN)
> The (full) common name of the individual

Organizational Unit (OU)
> The unit the individual is associated with

Organization (O)
> The organization the individual is associated with

Location (L)
> The city where the individual is located

State (S)
> The state/province where the individual is located

Country (C)
> The country where the individual is located

The DN specification allows other fields as well, although these are the fields used internally in Java. The organization that is associated with an individual is typically the company the individual works for, but it can be any other organization (and of course, you may not be associated with an organization under a variety of circumstances).

The idea behind a DN is that it limits to some extent name duplication. There are other Scott Oakses in the world, but only one who has a DN of:

```
CN=Scott Oaks, OU=SMCC, O=Sun Microsystems, L=NY,
S=NY, C=US
```

On the other hand, this is not absolute; there are many non-unique DNs.

An identity object holds only a public key; private keys are held in a different type of object (the signer object, which we'll look at a little later). Hence, identity objects represent the entities in the world who have sent you their public keys in order for you to verify their identity.

In 1.1, the Identity class is an abstract class that contains no abstract methods; in 1.2 it is concrete. For compatibility, then, we typically subclass the Identity class in order to create an identity object. Although you're not required to, you'll want to override certain methods if you implement a subclass of the Identity class.

An identity contains five pieces of information:

- A name—the name of the identity; this satisfies the `Principal` interface that the identity implements.

- A public key.

- An optional information string describing the identity.

- An optional identity scope. Identities can be aggregated into a collection, which is called an identity scope. This feature is primarily used to support the `javakey` utility; it is not used in Java 1.2.

- A list of certificates that vouch for the identity..

Identities and Identity Scopes

In 1.1, an identity was closely tied to the notion of an identity scope. The idea behind this was that the `javakey` utility needed the ability to operate on a collection of identities (all the identities in the `javakey` database). Hence, the introduction of the `IdentityScope` class (`java.security.IdentityScope`).

The `IdentityScope` class is similar to other container classes. It has add- and remove-based methods and a way to enumerate its elements. It also provides methods to search the identity scope for a particular name, certificate, or public key. But the architecture of this class is somewhat complicated, since the `IdentityScope` class extends the `Identity` class, allowing for the idea of nested (as well as disjoint) identity scopes.

The real purpose of the `IdentityScope` class was to support the 1.1 `javakey` database; as `javakey` was replaced by `keytool`, this class became much less useful. In general, we'll ignore the idea of identity scopes altogether and assume that identities exist independent of a scope.

Details of the identity scope class will be given in Appendix B.

Note that the default implementation of an identity object carries with it no notion of trustworthiness. You're free to add that feature to your own identity class, though typically that information is held elsewhere (e.g., in the policy database we examined in Chapter 5).

Using the identity class

If you want to use an identity object, you have the following methods at your disposal:

public final String getName()
> Return the name of the identity.

public final IdentityScope getScope()
> Return the identity scope to which the identity belongs.

public PublicKey getPublicKey()
> Return the public key associated with the identity.

public void setPublicKey(PublicKey key) throws KeyManagementException
> Set the public key associated with the identity to the given public key. This replaces any previous public key as well as any previous certificates associated with this identity. If the public key is already associated with another identity in the identity scope to which this identity belongs, a `KeyManagementException` is thrown. The implementation of this method in the base class does not actually check the identity scope to see if the key already exists in another identity; it's up to the concrete subclass to provide this functionality.

public String getInfo()
> Return the information string associated with the identity.

public void setInfo(String info)
> Set the information string in the identity, replacing any existing information string.

public void addCertificate(java.security.cert.Certificate certificate) ★
public void addCertificate(java.security.Certificate certificate) ☆
> Add the given certificate to the list of certificates in the identity. If the identity has a public key and that public key does not match the public key in the certificate, a `KeyManagementException` is thrown. If the identity does not have a public key, the public key in the certificate becomes the public key for the identity. Like the `setPublicKey()` method, this should generate a `KeyManagementException` if this conflicts with another key in the identity scope, but the implementation in the base class doesn't automatically provide that.

public void removeCertificate(java.security.cert.Certificate) ★
public void removeCertificate(java.security.Certificate certificate) ☆
> Remove the given certificate from the list of certificates in the identity. If the given certificate isn't in the identity's list of certificates, no exception is thrown.

public java.security.cert.Certificate[] getCertificates() ★
public java.security.Certificate[] certificates() ☆

> Return a copy of the array of certificates held in the identity. The array itself
> is a copy of what is held by the object, but the certificate objects themselves
> are not.

public final boolean equals(Object id)

> Test if the given identity is equal to the current object. Identities are consid-
> ered equal if they are in the same scope and have the same name. Otherwise,
> they are considered equal if the identityEquals() method returns true. By
> default, identities in different scopes are considered equal by the identi-
> tyEquals() method if they have the same name and the same public key.

If you have an identity object, those are the methods you can invoke on that
object. There are three ways to obtain an identity object—via the getIdentity()
method of the IdentityScope class, by implementing your own subclass of the
Identity class, or (in 1.2 only) by directly constructing an identity object. In
typical Java programs, the IdentityScope class is unused (at least in 1.2); all identities that we use in this book are ones we construct ourselves.

Implementing an Identity class

An application that wants to work with identities will typically provide its own identity class. A typical implementation of the Identity class is trivial:

```
public class XYZIdentity extends Identity {
    public XYZIdentity(String name) throws KeyManagementException {
        super(name);
    }
}
```

Because all of the methods in the Identity class are fully implemented, our class
need only construct itself. Here are the constructors in the Identity class that we
have the option of calling:

protected Identity()

> Construct an unnamed identity. This constructor is not designed to be used
> directly; it is provided for use by object serialization only.

public Identity(String name)

> Construct an identity object that does not belong to an identity scope.

public Identity(String name, IdentityScope scope) throws KeyManagementException

> Construct an identity object that belongs to the given scope. A KeyManage-
> mentException is thrown if the given name already exists in the identity
> scope.

public Identity(String name, String info, Certificate c[], PublicKey pk) ★
    Construct an identity object with the given name, information string, list of certificates, and public key.

We've chosen in this example only to implement the second of these constructors.

Other than the constructor, we are not required to implement any methods in our class. If you are implementing an identity within an identity scope, there are methods that you'll need to override in order to get the expected semantics.

Our identity class has one other option available to it, and that is the ability to determine when two identities will compare as equal (via the `equals()` method). The `equals()` method itself is `final`, and it will claim that two identities are equal if they exist in the same scope and have the same name. If either of those tests fails, however, the `equals()` method relies on the following method to check for equality:

protected boolean identityEquals(Identity id)
    Test for equality between the given identity and this identity. The default behavior for this method is to return `true` if the identities have the same name and the same key.

If your identity class has other information, you may want to override this method to take that other information into account.

The Identity class and the security manager

The identity class uses the `checkSecurityAccess()` method of the security manager to prevent many of its operations from being performed by untrusted classes. This mechanism has changed somewhat between 1.1 and 1.2; Table 11-1 lists the methods of the `Identity` class that make this check and the argument they pass to the `checkSecurityAccess()` method.

Table 11-1. Methods in the Identity Class that Call the Security Manager

Method	Argument in 1.2	Argument in 1.1
`setPublicKey()`	`Identity.setPublicKey`	`set.public.key`
`setInfo()`	`Identity.setInfo`	`set.info`
`addCertificate()`	`Identity.addCertificate`	`add.certificate`
`removeCertificate()`	`Identity.removeCertificate`	`remove.certificate`
`toString()`	– not used –	`print`

In 1.1, the argument to the `checkSecurityAccess()` method is constructed from four pieces of information: the name of the class that is providing the implementation of the identity class, the string listed in the table above, the name of the

particular identity in question (that is, the string returned by the getName() method), and the name of the class that implements the identity scope to which the identity belongs (if any). For example, in 1.1, a call to the setPublicKey() method of our example class XYZIdentity would end up passing the string XYZIdentity.set.public.key.sdo to the checkSecurityAccess() method.

In common implementations of the security manager in 1.1, this string is ignored, and trusted classes are typically allowed to work with identities, while untrusted classes are not. In 1.2, the default implementation of the security manager will create a security permission object (with the name set as the string given in Table 11-1) and see if that permission has been granted by the access controller.

Signers

An identity has a public key, which can be used to verify the digital signature of something signed by the identity. In order to create a digital signature, we need a private key. An identity that carries with it a private key is modeled by the Signer class (java.security.Signer):

public abstract class Signer extends Identity
> A class to model an entity that has both a public key and a private key. Since this is a subclass of the Identity class, the public key comes from the implementation of that class, and a signer class needs only to be concerned with the private key.

The Signer class is fully implemented even though it is declared as abstract; an implementation of the Signer class need not implement any methods.

Using the Signer class

A signer is used just like an identity, with these additional methods:

public PrivateKey getPrivateKey()
> Return the private key of the signer.

public final void setKeyPair(KeyPair pair)
> Set both the public and private key of the signer. Since public and private keys must match in order to be used, this class requires that in order to set the private key, the public key must be set at the same time. If only one key is present in the key pair, an InvalidParameterException is thrown. The act of setting the public key might generate a KeyManagementException (a subclass of KeyException, which this method throws).

Except for these two operations, a signer is identical to an identity.

Implementing a signer

Signers are trivial to implement, given that none of their methods are abstract. Hence, it is simply a matter of calling the appropriate constructor:

```
public class XYZSigner extends Signer {
    public XYZSigner(String name) throws KeyManagementException {
        super(name);
    }
}
```

Note an unfortunate problem here: if you've added additional logic to your identity subclass, your signer subclass cannot use that logic. Your own signer subclass must extend Java's Signer class, not your own identity subclass.

Signers and the security manager

In addition to the security checks that will be made as part of the methods of the Identity class, the signer class calls the checkSecurityAccess() method of the security manager in the following cases with the strings in Table 11-2.

Table 11-2. Methods of the Signer Class That Call the Security Manager

Method	Parameter in 1.2	Parameter in 1.1
getPrivateKey()	Signer.getPrivateKey	get.private.key
setKeyPair()	Signer.setKeyPair	set.private.keypair

As with the Identity class, in 1.1 the actual string passed to the security manager is preceded with the name of the class, and the name of the identity is appended to the class along with the name of the identity's scope.

The KeyStore Class

Now that we understand the pieces that make up a key management system, we can look at the topic of key management itself. From an administrative perspective, the primary tool that provides key management for Java 1.2 is the keytool utility. Keytool operates upon a file (or other storage system) containing a set of private keys and certificates for those keys. The keytool file contains a set of entries; each entry may have the following attributes:

- An alias. This is a name you can use to reference the entity in the database. For example, an alias for my entry might be sdo, or ScottOaks.

- One or more certificates that vouch for the identity of the entry. These certificates also provide the public key for the entry.

- Optionally, a private key. If present, the private key can be protected by a password.

We'd be tempted to call the entries in this database identities, but that's potentially confusing: the entries stored in the keytool database are not instances of the Identity class (although we could create an identity object based on the information retrieved from the database).

Figure 11-1 shows the role of the keytool database in the creation and execution of a signed JAR file. The jarsigner utility consults the keytool database for the private key of the entity that is signing the JAR file. Once the signed JAR file is produced, it is placed on a web server, where it can be downloaded into an appletviewer or other Java-enabled browser.* When the JAR file is read on the remote system, the keytool database is consulted in order to retrieve the public key of the entity that signed the JAR file so that the JAR file's signature can be verified.

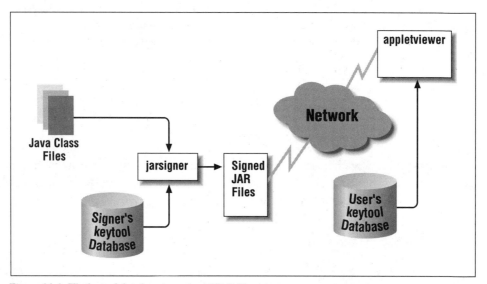

Figure 11-1. The keytool database in a signed JAR file

Note that the two keytool databases in this example are (probably) separate databases, on separate machines. They probably have completely different entries as well—even for the entry that represents the signer. The signer's entry in her own database must have the private key of the signer, while the signer's entry in the user's database needs only a certificate (public key) for the signer. However, the *keytool* database could (in this and all examples) be a shared database—but more

---

* As we mentioned, however, Netscape Navigator, Internet Explorer, and HotJava at present all use a different key management system than the keytool database, so the appletviewer is the best example here.

about that later. The default keytool database is the file *.keystore* that is held in the user's home directory.

The class that implements the keytool database is the `KeyStore` class (`java.security.KeyStore`):

public abstract class KeyStore ★

> Represent a set of private keys, aliases (entities), and their corresponding certificates. A keystore object is typically one that has been read in from disk; that is, the keystore object is an in-memory representation of the keytool database.

Although they share the features of a provider interface, keystores are not part of the security provider interface. Instead, they are installed by modifying the *java.security* property file directly; the default Sun keystore implementation is listed in the *java.security* file as:

```
keystore=sun.security.tools.JavaKeyStore
```

Just like classes that are implemented through the provider interface, a keystore object is returned from the `getInstance()` method:

public static final KeyStore getInstance() ★

> Return an instance of `KeyStore` that was given by the class named in the *java.security* file. This method throws a `KeyStoreException` if it gets an error.

When the keystore object is created, it is initially empty. Although the `getInstance()` method has constructed the object, it is not expected that the object's constructor will read in a keystore from any particular location. The interaction between the keystore object and the keytool database comes via these two methods:

public abstract void load(InputStream is, String password) ★

> Initialize the keystore from the data provided over the given input stream. The integrity of the keystore is typically protected by using a message digest: when the keystore is stored, a message digest that represents the data in the keystore is also stored. Before the digest is created, the password is added to the digest data; this means that the digest cannot be re-created from a tampered keystore without knowledge of the password. The password for this method can be `null`, in which case the keystore is loaded and not verified.

> This use of the password is a property of the Sun implementation of the `KeyStore` class; the password could be used for anything else (including encrypting the entire keystore) if you were to write your own implementation. To call this parameter a password is somewhat misleading (although that's what the `javadoc` documentation calls it), since Sun's implementation lets you read the entire keystore without it. The Sun implementation of the

KeyStore class requires another password to access each private key in the keystore, so this isn't a potential security hole; all you're reading is public certificates.

You cannot require a password for load() to succeed, since the Sun implementation of the Policy class calls this method without a password when it constructs the information needed for the access controller. You may, of course, provide your own implementation of the Policy class that provides a password if desired.

In the Sun implementation, if the class required to support the underlying message digest is not available, a NoSuchAlgorithmException is thrown. An error in reading the data results in an IOException, and generic format errors in the data result in a CertificateException.

public abstract void store(OutputStream os, String password) ★

Store the keystore to the given output stream. The password is typically included in a digest calculation of the keystore; this digest is then written to the output stream as well (but again, your own implementation of this class could use the password differently).

The Sun implementation of this method may throw an IOException if the output stream cannot be read, a NoSuchAlgorithmException if the class used to create the digest cannot be found, or a CertificateException if the keystore object contains a certificate that cannot be parsed.

There is no default file that holds the keystore. Within the core Java API, the only class that opens the keystore is PolicyFile, and that opens the keystore that is listed in the *java.policy* file. The tools that use the keystore (the jarsigner and keytool tools) allow you to use a command-line argument to specify the file that contains the keystore; by default, that file is *.keystore* in the user's home directory. This is the convention your own programs will need to use. If your application needs to open the keystore (for example, to obtain a private key to sign an object), it should provide either a command-line argument or a property to specify the name of the file to open. By convention, we'll use the *.keystore* file in the user's home directory in our examples.

While we mentioned that the keystore may not be encrypted, the private keys themselves typically are encrypted so that if someone gains access to the keystore file, they do not have access to the private keys in that file without the password used to encrypt those keys. If you provide a keystore implementation that supplies keys from a protected location, you do not necessarily need to store the private keys in encrypted format. When private keys are delivered over the network, you probably want to make sure that the transmission of those keys is encrypted so that no one can snoop the network and discover the private key.

A keystore is arranged in terms of alias names. Aliases are arbitrarily assigned to an entry; while the name embedded in the certificate for a particular entry may be a long, complicated, distinguished name, the alias for that entry can provide a shorter, easier-to-remember name. There are a number of simple methods in the KeyStore class that deal with these alias names:

public abstract Date getCreationDate(String alias) ★
> Return the date on which the entry referenced by the given alias was created.

public abstract void deleteEntry(String alias) ★
> Delete the entry referenced by the given alias from the keystore.

public abstract Enumeration aliases() ★
> Return an enumeration of all the aliases in the keystore.

public abstract boolean containsAlias(String alias) ★
> Indicate whether the keystore contains an entry referenced by the given alias.

public abstract int size() ★
> Return the number of entries/aliases in the keystore.

Note that this list has a method to delete an entry but not one to create an entry—creating an entry in the keystore depends upon the type of entry you want to create.

The keystore holds two types of entries: certificate entries and key entries. The dichotomy between these two entries is one we explored earlier when we looked at the Identity and Signer classes. A certificate entry is an entry that contains only a public key (encapsulated in a certificate) and can be used only to verify a digital signature, while a key entry is an entry that contains both a private and a public key and can be used to create and to verify a digital signature. Hence, you may think of a key entry as a signer and a certificate entry as an identity, although those classes are not used in the keystore interface (they may be used in the keystore implementation).

There are two basic differences between key entries and certificate entries:

- A key entry contains a private key, while a certificate entry does not.

- A key entry may contain a chain of certificates that verifies it, while a certificate entry contains a single certificate.

For a given alias, you can determine what type of entry it represents via these two methods:

public abstract boolean isKeyEntry(String alias) ★
public abstract boolean isCertificateEntry(String alias) ★
> Indicate whether the given alias represents a key entry or a certificate entry.

For a given alias, you cannot retrieve an object that represents the entire entry. You may use these methods to retrieve information about the entry represented by an alias:

public abstract PrivateKey getPrivateKey(String alias, String password) ★

Return the private key for the entry associated with the given alias. For a certificate entry, this method returns null. An UnrecoverableKeyException is thrown if the key cannot be retrieved (e.g., if the key has been damaged).

Retrieving a private key typically requires a password; this may or may not be the same password that was used to read the entire keystore. This allows private keys to be stored encrypted so they cannot be read without the appropriate password. If the class that provides encryption cannot be found, this method throws a NoSuchAlgorithmException.

public abstract Certificate[] getCertificateChain(String alias) ★

Return the certificate chain that verifies the entry associated with the given alias, which must represent a key entry. For an alias that represents a certificate entry, this method returns null.

public abstract Certificate getCertificate(String alias) ★

Return the certificate associated with the given alias. If the alias represents a key entry, the certificate returned is the user's certificate (that is, the first certificate in the entry's certificate chain); certificate entries have only a single certificate.

public abstract String getCertificateAlias(Certificate cert) ★

Return the alias that corresponds to the entry that matches the given certificate (using the equals() method of certificate comparison). If no matches occur, null is returned.

Finally, in order to create or modify an entry, you may use one of these methods. All of these methods create a new entry if the given alias does not exist:

public abstract void setKeyEntry(String alias, byte privateKey[], Certificate chain[]) ★
public abstract void setKeyEntry(String alias, PrivateKey pk, String password, Certificate chain[]) ★

Assign the given private key and certificate chain to the key entry represented by the given alias, creating a new key entry if necessary. Any previous private key and certificate chain for this entry are lost; if the previous entry was a certificate entry, it now becomes a key entry.

A KeyStoreException is thrown if the key entry cannot be encrypted by the internal encrypting algorithm of the keystore. In the Sun implementation, when the key is passed in as a series of bytes, it is not encrypted—in this case, you are expected to have performed the encryption yourself.

public abstract void setCertificateEntry(String alias, Certificate c) ★

Assign the given certificate to the certificate entry represented by the given alias. If an entry for this alias already exists and is a key entry, a KeyStoreException is thrown. Otherwise, if an entry for this alias already exists, it is overwritten.

These are the basic methods by which we can manage a keystore. We'll see examples of many of these methods throughout the rest of this book; for now, let's look at a simple example that looks up a given entry in the keystore:

```java
public class KeyStoreLookup {
    public static void main(String args[]) {
        try {
            KeyStore ks = KeyStore.getInstance();
            String fname = System.getProperty("user.home") +
                             File.separator + ".keystore";
            FileInputStream fis = new FileInputStream(fname);
            ks.load(fis, null);
            if (ks.isKeyEntry(args[0])) {
                System.out.println(args[0] +
                            " is a key entry in the keystore");
                System.out.println("The private key for " + args[0] +
                        " is " + ks.getPrivateKey(args[0], args[1]));
                Certificate certs[] = ks.getCertificateChain(args[0]);
                if (certs[0] instanceof X509Certificate) {
                    X509Certificate x509 = (X509Certificate) certs[0];
                    System.out.println(args[0] + " is really " +
                        x509.getSubjectDN());
                }
                if (certs[certs.length - 1] instanceof
                                X509Certificate) {
                    X509Certificate x509 = (X509Certificate)
                                certs[certs.length - 1];
                    System.out.println(args[0] + " was verified by " +
                        x509.getIssuerDN());
                }
            }
            else if (ks.isCertificateEntry(args[0])) {
                System.out.println(args[0] +
                            " is a certificate entry in the keystore");
                Certificate c = ks.getCertificate(args[0]);
                if (c instanceof X509Certificate) {
                    X509Certificate x509 = (X509Certificate) c;
                    System.out.println(args[0] + " is really " +
                        x509.getSubjectDN());
                    System.out.println(args[0] + " was verified by " +
                        x509.getIssuerDN());
                }
            }
```

```
            else {
                System.out.println(args[0] +
                        " is unknown to this keystore");
            }
        } catch (Exception e) {
            e.printStackTrace();
        }
    }
}
```

This program expects two arguments: the name of the entity in the keystore for which information is desired, and the password that was used to encrypt the private key.

There are a number of points to pick out from this example. First, note that we constructed the keystore using the convention we mentioned earlier—the *.keystore* file in the user's home directory.

After we've read in the data, the first thing we do is determine if the entry that we're interested in is a key entry or a certificate entry—mostly so that we can handle the certificates for these entries differently. In the case of a key entry, we obtain the entire certificate chain, and use the first entry in that chain to print out the Distinguished Name (DN) for the entry, while the last entry in the chain is used to print out the DN for the last certificate authority in the chain. For a certificate entry, our task is simpler: there is a single certificate, and we simply print out its information.

A Key Management Example

The Sun implementation of the `keytool` utility is useful in many circumstances where users have disjoint databases. In Figure 11-1 we showed just such an example, and we mentioned that this example was set up in such a way that the code signer and the end user could have different key databases.

This is not to say, however, that those two databases could not have been the same database—that is, one that is shared by the signer and the end user. Since access to the private key of the signer is protected by a password, the signer and the end user are able to share a single database without concern that the end user may obtain access to the signer's private key (assuming that she keeps her password secret, of course). In the case of a corporate network, this flexibility is important, since an enterprise may want to maintain a single database that contains the private keys of all of its employees as well as the certificates of all known external entities.

We could have these users share the keystore by using the appropriate filename in the application and the *java.policy* files. But sharing the keytool database by a file is somewhat inefficient. If the global file is on a machine in New York and is referenced by a user in Tokyo, you'll want to use a better network protocol to access it than a file-based protocol. In addition, the `load()` method reads in the entire file. If there are 10,000 users in your corporate keystore database, you shouldn't need to read each entry into memory to find the one entry you are interested in using.

Hence, for many applications, you'll want to provide your own implementation of the `KeyStore` class. We'll show a very simple example here as a starting point for your own implementations. For the payroll application being deployed by XYZ Corporation, a database containing each employee in the corporation is necessary. The HR department could set up its own keystore for this purpose, but a similar keystore will be needed by the finance department to implement its 401K application; a better solution is to have a single keystore that is shared between all departments of XYZ Corporation.

In this case, the question becomes how best to share this keystore. A single global file would be too large for programs to read into memory and too unwieldy for administrators to distribute to all locations of XYZ Corporation. A better architecture is shown in Figure 11-2. Here, the application uses the security provider architecture to instantiate a new keystore object (of a class that we'll sketch out below). Unknown to the users of this object, the keystore class uses RMI (or CORBA, or any other distributed computing protocol) to talk to a remote server, which accesses the 10,000 employee records from a database set up for that purpose.

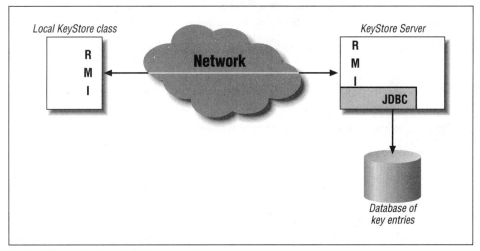

Figure 11-2. A distributed keystore example

Without getting bogged down in the details of the network and database programming required for this architecture, let's look at how the KeyStore class itself would be designed.

Many of the methods of our new class are simple passthroughs to the remote server. If the handle to the remote server is held in the instance variable rks, a typical method looks like this:

```
public Date getCreationDate(String alias) {
    return rks.getCreationDate(alias);
}
```

The methods that could be implemented in this manner are:

```
getPrivateKey()
getCertificateChain()
getCertificate()
getCreationDate()
aliases()
containsAlias()
size()
isKeyEntry()
isCertificateEntry()
getCertificateAlias()
```

On the other hand, many methods should probably throw an exception—especially those methods that are designed to alter the keystore. In an architecture such as this one, changes to the keystore should probably be done through the database itself—or at least through a different server than the server used by all employees in the corporation. So many functions may look simply like this:

```
public void setKeyEntry(String alias, PrivateKey key,
                        String passphrase, Certificate chain[])
                    throws KeyStoreException {
    throw new KeyStoreException("Can't change the keystore");
}
```

Methods that could be implemented in this manner are:

```
setKeyEntry()
setCertificateEntry()
deleteEntry()
store()
```

Note that we did not include the load() method in the above list. The load() method is useful to us, because it allows the application to require a password from the user before a connection to the remote server can be made. This differs slightly from normal programming for this class. Typically, the load() method is called with the input stream from which to read the keystore. In this case, the `load()` method is expected to be called with a `null` input stream, and sets up the connection to the remote server itself:

```
public void load(InputStream is, String password)
        throws IOException, NoSuchAlgorithmException,
            CertificateException {
    rks = Naming.lookup("rmi://KSServer/DistributedKeyServer");
    if (!rks.authenticate(password)) {
        rks = null;
        throw new IOException("Incorrect password");
    }
}
```

Since the keystore database in this architecture cannot be written through the server, there is some question as to whether a password should be required to access the keystore at all (since there are individual passwords on the private keys). Every employee will potentially have access to the password (unless it is embedded into the application itself); you can decide if a password really adds security in that case. If no password is desired, the `load()` method could be empty and the connection to the remote server could be made in the constructor.

On the server side, implementation of the required methods is simply a matter of making appropriate database calls:

```
public int size() {
    int sz = -1;
    try {
        Connection conn = connectToDatabase();
        Statement st = conn.createStatement();
        boolean restype = st.execute("select count(*) from entries");
        if (restype) {
            ResultSet rs = st.getResultSet();
            sz = Integer.parseInt(rs.getString(1));
        }
        st.cancel();
    } catch (Exception e) {
        ...
    }
    finally {
        return sz;
    }
}
```

This architecture works well because it allows the passwords for each of the private keys to be held in the database itself, so retrievals of private keys can easily test the password via a simple string comparison. Implementations of file-based keystores are more problematic: if the file is readable by the user, obviously the password cannot be stored in the file as a simple string. File-based keystores must store their passwords and their private keys in encrypted form, perhaps using the encryption APIs we'll examine in Chapter 13. Assuming that the database machine is secured, such encryption is not required in this architecture.

Encrypting Private Keys

In this section, we've discussed the need for private keys to be stored encrypted whenever those keys are stored in a location that is generally accessible to other users. The Sun implementation of the `KeyStore` class does this using an internal algorithm to perform the encryption.

The strength of this encryption is limited; because it is part of the standard Sun distribution, the encryption must be weak enough to be exportable from the United States. "Weak" is a relative term in this context; it still requires some effort for the encryption to be broken, but it can be done.

In your own `KeyStore` class, if you need to encrypt the private keys you'll want to use the strongest form of encryption that is suitable for your situation. If you're a multinational organization, this encryption will not be very strong, and you're better off storing your private keys on a private database as we've described here.

There are unlimited possibilities in the implementation of a keystore. One technique might be to create a floppy for each employee that contains only that employee's entry and to write a keystore class that looks for key entries from the file on the floppy and for certificate entries from a global file somewhere.* This type of implementation is very simple. The new keystore can contain two instances of the Sun `KeyStore` class that have read in both files, and it can use object delegation to implement all of its methods.

Note that this type of two-tiered system is really the ideal. If the private keys are transmitted over the network, as in our previous case, then internal spies on the network might snoop the password used to retrieve the key or the private key that is sent back. If the private key is held locally, however, and only the public keys are retrieved from the remote key store, you have a much better implementation.

---

* Of course, we don't want to use a floppy for this—we want to use a Java-enabled smart card, though of course we don't all have smart card readers on our computers. At least, not yet...

Installing a KeyStore Class

In order to use an alternate keystore implementation, the *java.security* file must be updated to set the keystore property, like this:

```
keystore=DistributedKeyStore
```

If necessary, you'll need to establish a convention by which the input stream that is opened for the load() method is created—unless your keystore does not require one at all (as, for example, our RMI-based keystore would not).

The Policy class uses the keystore in a predictable manner. Given this entry in the *java.policy* file:

```
grant CodeBase "http://piccolo/", signedBy "sdo" {
    ...
}
```

the Policy class uses the keystore to look up the alias for sdo, retrieve sdo's public key, and use that public key to verify any signature that comes from the site *piccolo*. Remember, however, that the Sun implementation of the Policy class requires an entry in the *java.policy* file that specifies the URL from which to load the keystore.

Summary

In this chapter we examined the key management facilities of Java. Key management revolves around keys and certificates—ideas we've already discussed—but it also depends upon the notion of an identity—an individual or a corporation—and the idea that a particular identity can be certified.

Key management in Java can be handled either programmatically with the standard Java API or with the key management tool keytool. Keytool itself is a good example of how the programming API can be used, although there are some trade-offs involved here; for example, loading a large keystore is not necessarily the most appropriate choice for a thin-client application. Fortunately, the security package gives us the necessary tools to implement our own keystore when that is appropriate.

For all the time we've spent on them, keys are not interesting by themselves. They are interesting for what they allow us to do, which among other things includes the ability to operate on a digital signature. In the next chapter, we'll look at digital signatures, their relationship to keys, and the operations that keys and digital signatures enable us to perform.

12

Digital Signatures

In the previous few chapters, we've examined various aspects of Java's security package with an eye toward the topics of this chapter: the ability to generate and to verify digital signatures. We've now reached the fruits of that examination. In this chapter, we'll explore the mechanisms of the digital signature.

The use and verification of digital signatures is another standard engine that is included in the security provider architecture. Like the other engines we've examined, the classes that implement this engine have both a public interface and an SPI for implementors of the engine.

In the JDK, the most common use of digital signatures is to create signed classes; users have the option of granting additional privileges to these signed classes using the mechanics of the access controller. In addition, a security manager and a class loader can use this information to change the policy of the security manager; this technique is quite useful in 1.1. Hence, we'll also show an example that reads a signed JAR file.

The Signature Class

Operations on digital signatures are abstracted by the `Signature` class (`java.security.Signature`):

public abstract class Signature extends SignatureSpi

> Provide an engine to create and verify digital signatures. In Java 1.1, there is no `SignatureSpi` class, and this class simply extends the `Object` class.

The Sun security provider includes a single implementation of this class that generates signatures based on the DSA algorithm.

Using the Signature Class

As with all engine classes, instances of the Signature class are obtained by calling one of these methods:

public static Signature getInstance(String algorithm)
public static Signature getInstance(String algorithm, String provider)

> Generate a signature object that implements the given algorithm. If no provider is specified, all providers are searched in order for the given algorithm as discussed in Chapter 8; otherwise, the system searches for the given algorithm only in the given provider. If an implementation of the given algorithm is not found, a NoSuchAlgorithmException is thrown. If the named security provider cannot be found, a NoSuchProviderException is thrown.

> Beginning in 1.2, if the algorithm string is "DSA", the string "SHA/DSA" is substituted for it. Hence, implementors of this class that provide support for DSA signing must register themselves appropriately (that is, with the message digest algorithm name) in the security provider.

Once a signature object is obtained, the following methods can be invoked on it:

public void final initVerify(PublicKey publicKey)

> Initialize the signature object, preparing it to verify a signature. A signature object must be initialized before it can be used. If the key is not of the correct type for the algorithm or is otherwise invalid, an InvalidKeyException is thrown.

public final void initSign(PrivateKey privateKey)

> Initialize the signature object, preparing it to create a signature. A signature object must be initialized before it can be used. If the key is not of the correct type for the algorithm or is otherwise invalid, an InvalidKeyException is thrown.

public final void update(byte b)
public final void update(byte[] b)
public final void update(byte b[], int offset, int length)

> Add the given data to the accumulated data the object will eventually sign or verify. If the object has not been initialized, a SignatureException is thrown.

public final byte[] sign()

> Create the digital signature, assuming that the object has been initialized for signing. If the object has not been properly initialized, a SignatureException is thrown. Once the signature has been generated, the object is reset so that it may generate another signature based on some new data (however, it is still initialized for signing; a new call to the initSign() method is not required).

public final boolean verify(byte[] signature)

Test the validity of the given signature, assuming that the object has been initialized for verification. If the object has not been properly initialized, then a `SignatureException` is thrown. Once the signature has been verified (whether or not the verification succeeds), the object is reset so that it may verify another signature based on some new data (no new call to the `initVerify()` method is required).

public final String getAlgorithm()

Get the name of the algorithm this object implements.

public String toString()

A printable version of a signature object is composed of the string "`Signature object:`" followed by the name of the algorithm implemented by the object, followed by the initialized state of the object. The state is either `<not initialized>`, `<initialized for verifying>`, or `<initialized for signing>`. However, the Sun DSA implementation of this class overrides this method to show the parameters of the DSA algorithm instead.

public final void setParameter(String param, Object value) ☆
public final void setParameter(AlgorithmParameterSpec param) ★

Set the parameter of the signature engine. In the first format, the named parameter is set to the given value; in the second format, parameters are set based on the information in the `param` specification.

In the Sun implementation of the DSA signing algorithm, the only valid `param` string is `KSEED`, which requires an array of bytes that will be used to seed the random number generator used to generate the k value. There is no way to set this value through the parameter specification, which in the Sun implementation always returns an `UnsupportedOperationException`.

public final Object getParameter(String param) ☆

Return the named parameter from the object. The only valid string for the Sun implementation is `KSEED`.

public final Provider getProvider() ★

Return the provider that supplied the implementation of this signature object.

It is no accident that this class has many similarities to the `MessageDigest` class; a digital signature algorithm is typically implemented by performing a cryptographic operation on a private key and the message digest that represents the data to be signed. For the developer, this means that generating a digital signature is virtually the same as generating a message digest; the only difference is that a key must be presented in order to operate on a signature object. This difference is important, however, since it fills in the hole we noticed previously: a message digest can be altered along with the data it represents so that the tampering is unnoticeable. A signed message digest, on the other hand, can't be altered without knowledge of the key that was used to create it. The use of a public key in the digital signature algorithm makes the digital signature more attractive than a message authentication code, in which there must be a shared key between the parties involved in the message exchange.

Let's take our example from Chapter 9 where we saved a message and its digest to a file; we'll modify it now to save the message and the digital signature. We can create the digital signature like this:

```
public class Send {
    public static void main(String args[]) {
        String data;
        data = "This have I thought good to deliver thee, " +
                "that thou mightst not lose the dues of rejoicing " +
                "by being ignorant of what greatness is promised thee.";

        try {
            FileOutputStream fos = new FileOutputStream("test");
            ObjectOutputStream oos = new ObjectOutputStream(fos);
            KeyStore ks = KeyStore.getInstance();
            ks.load(new FileInputStream(
                            System.getProperty("user.home") +
                            File.separator + ".keystore"), null);
            PrivateKey pk = ks.getPrivateKey(args[0], args[1]);

            Signature s = Signature.getInstance("DSA");
            s.initSign(pk);

            byte buf[] = data.getBytes();
            s.update(buf);
            oos.writeObject(data);
            oos.writeObject(s.sign());
        } catch (Exception e) {
            e.printStackTrace();
        }
    }
}
```

This example puts together many of the examples from the past few chapters. In order to create the digital signature we must accomplish the following:

1. Obtain the private key that is used to sign the data. Here we're using the conventional keystore database (*$HOME/.keystore*) and the command-line arguments to obtain the alias and password of the private key we want to use.

2. Obtain a signing object via the getInstance() method and initialize it. Since we're creating a signature in this example, we use the initSign() method for initialization.

3. Pass the data to be signed as a series of bytes to the update() method of the signing object. Multiple calls could be made to the update() method even though in this example we only need one.

4. Obtain the signature by calling the sign() method. We save the signature bytes and write them to a file with the data so that the data and the signature can be retrieved at a later date.

Reading the data and verifying the signature are similar:

```
public class Receive {
    public static void main(String args[]) {
        try {
            String data = null;
            byte signature[] = null;
            FileInputStream fis = new FileInputStream("test");
            ObjectInputStream ois = new ObjectInputStream(fis);
            Object o = ois.readObject();
            try {
                data = (String) o;
            } catch (ClassCastException cce) {
                System.out.println("Unexpected data in file");
                System.exit(-1);
            }
            o = ois.readObject();
            try {
                signature = (byte []) o;
            } catch (ClassCastException cce) {
                System.out.println("Unexpected data in file");
                System.exit(-1);
            }
            System.out.println("Received message");
            System.out.println(data);

            KeyStore ks = KeyStore.getInstance();
            ks.load(new FileInputStream(
                    System.getProperty("user.home") +
                    File.separator + ".keystore"), args[1]);

            Certificate c = ks.getCertificate(args[0]);
            PublicKey pk = c.getPublicKey();
            Signature s = Signature.getInstance("DSA");
            s.initVerify(pk);
            s.update(data.getBytes());
            if (s.verify(signature)) {
                System.out.println("Message is valid");
```

```
            }
            else System.out.println("Message was corrupted");
        } catch (Exception e) {
            System.out.println(e);
        }
    }
}
```

The process of verifying the signature still requires four steps. The major differences are that in step two, we initialize the signing object for verification by using the initVerify() method, and in step four, we verify (rather than create) the existing signature by using the verify() method. Note that we still have to know who signed the message in order to look up the correct key—but more about that a little later.

The SignedObject Class

In our last example, we had to create an object that held both the data in which we are interested and the signature for that data. This is a common enough requirement that Java provides the SignedObject class (java.security.SignedObject) to encapsulate an object and its signature:

public final class SignedObject implements Serializable ★

Encapsulate an object and its digital signature. The encapsulated object must be serializable so that a serialization of a signed object can do a deep copy of the embedded object.

Signed objects are created with this constructor:

public SignedObject(Serializable o, PrivateKey pk, Signature engine) ★

Create a signed object based on the given object, signing the serialized data in that object with the given private key and signature object. The signed object contains a copy of the given object; this copy is obtained by serializing the object parameter. If this serialization fails, an IOException is thrown.

It's very important to realize that this constructor makes, in effect, a copy of its parameter; if you create a signed object based on a string buffer and later change the contents of the string buffer, the data in the signed object remains unchanged. This preserves the integrity of the object encapsulated with its signature.

Here are the methods we can use to operate on a signed object:

public Object getContent() ★

Return the object embedded in the signed object. The object is reconstituted using object serialization; an error in serialization may cause either an IOException or a ClassNotFoundException to be thrown.

public byte[] getSignature() ★
> Return the signature embedded in the signed object.

public String getAlgorithm() ★
> Return the name of the algorithm that was used to sign the object.

public boolean verify(PublicKey pk, Signature s) ★
> Verify the signature within the embedded object with the given key and signature engine. The signature engine parameter may be obtained by calling the `getInstance()` method of the `Signature` class. The underlying signature engine may throw an `InvalidKeyException` or `SignatureException`.

We'll use this class in examples later in this chapter.

Signing and Certificates

In the previous examples, we specified on the command line the name of the entity that we assumed generated the signature in the file. This was necessary because the file contained only the actual signature of the entity and the data that was signed; it did not contain any information about who the signer actually is. That's fine for an example, but it is not always appropriate in a real application. We could have asked the user for the name of the entity that was supposed to have signed the data, but that course is fraught with potential errors:

- The user could have no idea what names are in the keystore of the application. Especially in a corporate environment, users may not know what data the keystore database might contain.

- The user could get the name of the keystore alias wrong. Say that the application asks the user to enter the name of the signer; the user, knowing that the data came from me, may enter "sdo" as the alias of the identity.

  What the user may not remember is that when the keystore was first created, she received a public key from the San Diego Oil company; that public key was entered into the keystore with the alias "sdo." When my identity was added to the keystore, a different alias had to be chosen, so my public key was added with the alias "ScottOaks." But that was a long time ago, now forgotten, and because I use the sdo moniker all over my writings, the user assumes that I am the sdo in the keystore. And so the wrong alias will be chosen, and the signature verification will fail when it should have succeeded.

For these reasons, it makes more sense to include the public key with the signature and the signed data. This allows the application to find the identity based on the unique public key in order to determine who the signer of the data is.

We could do that by simply sending the encoded public key with the signature and data. A better solution, however, would be to send the certificate that verifies the public key. That way, if the public key is not found in the database, the credentials of the certificate can be presented to the user, and the user can have the opportunity to decide on the fly if the particular entity should be trusted.

Although an embedding of signature, data, and certificate is very common, the SignedObject class does not include the capability to contain a certificate. So we'll use the SignedObject class in this example, but we'll still need an object that contains the signed object and the certificate. We'd like to do this by extending the SignedObject class, but since that class is final we're forced to adopt this approach:

```
public class Message implements Serializable {
    SignedObject object;
    transient Certificate certificate;

    private void writeObject(ObjectOutputStream out)
                                    throws IOException {
        out.defaultWriteObject();
        try {
            out.writeObject(certificate.getEncoded());
        } catch (CertificateEncodingException cee) {
            throw new IOException("Can't serialize object " + cee);
        }
    }

    private void readObject(ObjectInputStream in)
                        throws IOException, ClassNotFoundException {
        in.defaultReadObject();
        try {
            byte b[] = (byte []) in.readObject();
            X509Certificate x509 = X509Certificate.getInstance(
                                new ByteArrayInputStream(b));
            certificate = x509;
        } catch (CertificateException ce) {
            throw new IOException("Can't de-serialize object " + ce);
        }
    }
}
```

We've made the certificate variable in this class transient and have explicitly serialized and deserialized it using its external encoding. As we discussed in Chapter 10, whenever we have an embedded certificate or key, we must follow a procedure like this to ensure that the receiving party is able to deserialize the class.

As it turns out, the X509 certificate implementation that comes with the JDK (that is, the sun.security.x509.X509CertImpl class) also overrides the writeObject() and readObject() methods, so if we serialize a certificate explicitly, the encoded data is written to or read from the file. It is not sufficient to rely upon that, however—if we use the default serialization methods for the Message class, a reference to the sun.security.x509.X509CertImpl class is embedded into the serialized stream. A user with another security provider (and hence a different implementation of the X509Certificate class) would not be able to deserialize the stream because there is no access to the Sun implementation of the X509Certificate class. Explicitly serializing and deserializing the certificate as we've done here avoids embedding any reference to the provider class and makes the data file more portable.

When we save the message to the file, we now have to make sure that we save a certificate with it. Other than that, changes to the class are minor:

```java
public class SendObject {
    public static void main(String args[]) {
        try {
            FileOutputStream fos = new FileOutputStream("test.obj");
            ObjectOutputStream oos = new ObjectOutputStream(fos);
            KeyStore ks = KeyStore.getInstance();
            ks.load(new FileInputStream(
                    System.getProperty("user.home") +
                    File.separator + ".keystore"), args[1]);

            Certificate certs[] = ks.getCertificateChain(args[0]);
            PrivateKey pk = ks.getPrivateKey(args[0], args[1]);
            Message m = new Message();
            m.object = new SignedObject(
               "This have I thought good to deliver thee, " +
               "that thou mightst not lose the dues of rejoicing " +
               "by being ignorant of what greatness is promised thee.",
                        pk, Signature.getInstance("DSA"));
            m.certificate = certs[0];
            oos.writeObject(m);
        } catch (Exception e) {
            System.out.println(e);
        }
    }
}
```

Retrieving the data is now more complicated, since we must verify both the signature in the signed object and the identity of the authority that signed the embedded certificate:

```java
public class ReceiveObject {
    private static void verifySigner(Certificate c, String name)
                                    throws CertificateException {
        Certificate issuerCert = null;
        X509Certificate sCert = null;
        KeyStore ks = null;
```

```
    try {
        ks = KeyStore.getInstance();
        ks.load(new FileInputStream(
                    System.getProperty("user.home") +
                    File.separator + ".keystore"), null);
    } catch (Exception e) {
        throw new CertificateException("Invalid keystore");
    }

    String signer = ks.getCertificateAlias (c);
    if (signer != null) {
            System.out.println("We know the signer as " + signer);
            return;

        }

    for (Enumeration al = ks.aliases(); al.hasMoreElements(); ) {
        String s = (String) al.nextElement();
        try {
            sCert = (X509Certificate) ks.getCertificate(s);
        } catch (Exception e) {
            continue;
        }
        if (name.equals(sCert.getSubjectDN().getName())) {
            issuerCert = sCert;
            break;
        }
    }
    if (issuerCert == null) {
        throw new CertificateException("No such certificate");
    }
    try {
        c.verify(issuerCert.getPublicKey());
    } catch (Exception e) {
        throw new CertificateException(e.toString());
    }
}

private static void processCertificate(X509Certificate x509)
                                throws CertificateParsingException {
    Principal p;
    p = x509.getSubjectDN();
    System.out.println("This message was signed by " +
                    p.getName());
    p = x509.getIssuerDN();
    System.out.println("This certificate was provided by " +
                    p.getName());
    try {
        verifySigner(x509, p.getName());
```

```
    } catch (CertificateException ce) {
        System.out.println("We don't know the certificate signer");
    }
    try {
        x509.checkValidity();
    } catch (CertificateExpiredException cee) {
        System.out.println("That certificate is no longer valid");
    } catch (CertificateNotYetValidException cnyve) {
        System.out.println("That certificate is not yet valid");
    }
}

public static void main(String args[]) {
    try {
        FileInputStream fis = new FileInputStream("test.obj");
        ObjectInputStream ois = new ObjectInputStream(fis);
        Object o = ois.readObject();
        if (o instanceof Message) {
            Message m = (Message) o;
            System.out.println("Received message");
            processCertificate((X509Certificate) m.certificate);
            PublicKey pk = m.certificate.getPublicKey();
            if (m.object.verify(pk, Signature.getInstance("DSA"))) {
                System.out.println("Message is valid");
                System.out.println(m.object.getObject());
            }
            else System.out.println("Message signature is invalid");
        }
        else System.out.println("Message is corrupted");
    } catch (Exception e) {
        e.printStackTrace();
    }
}
}
```

We've seen most of this code in previous chapters; in particular, the processCer-
tificate() method uses the standard certificate methods to extract and print
information about the certificate. The new code for us is primarily in the verify-
Signer() method, where we search the entire keystore for a name that matches
the issuer of the certificate that was sent to us. If we find a match, we use the corresponding public key to verify the certificate we received.

This method shows yet another need for an alternate implementation of the
KeyStore class—if you have to search the entire list of keys for a matching certificate like this, you clearly don't want to perform a linear search each time. An
alternate keystore could provide a more efficient means of searching for
certificates.

Signed Classes

One of the primary applications of digital signatures in Java is to create and verify signed classes. Signed classes allow the expansion of Java's sandbox in two different ways:

- The policy file can insist that classes coming from a particular site be signed by a particular entity before the access controller will grant that particular set of permissions. In the policy file, such an entry contains a signedBy directive:

```
grant signedBy "sdo", codeBase "http://piccolo.East.Sun.COM/" {
        java.io.FilePermission "-", "read,write";
}
```

    This entry allows classes that are loaded from *piccolo.East.Sun.COM* to read and write any local files under the current directory only if the classes have been signed by sdo.

- The security manager can cooperate with the class loader in order to determine whether or not a particular class is signed; the security manager is then free to grant permissions to that class based on its own internal policy. This technique is far more important in Java 1.1, since most Java 1.2 security managers simply defer decisions to the access controller.

In this section, we'll explore the necessary components behind this expansion of the Java sandbox. This example in the rest of the section fills in the remaining details of the JavaRunner program by showing us how to use a signed class.

There are three necessary ingredients to expand the Java sandbox with signed classes:

- A method to create the signed class. The jarsigner utility is used for this (see Appendix A).

- A class loader that knows how to understand the digital signature associated with the class. The URLClassLoader class knows how to do this, but we'll show an example of how to do that for our JavaRunnerLoader class as well.

- A security manager or access controller that grants the desired permissions based on the digital signature. The default access controller will do this for us; we'll show how the security manager might do this directly.

Reading Signed JAR Files

Signed classes in the Java-browser world are typically delivered as signed JAR files; there are various tools (javakey for Java 1.1 and jarsigner for Java 1.2) that can take an ordinary JAR file and attach a digital signature to it. A signed JAR file has three special elements:

- A manifest (MANIFEST.MF), containing a listing of the files in the archive that have been signed, along with a message digest for each signed file.

- A signature file (XXX.SF, where XXX is the name of the entity that signed the archive) that contains signature information. The data in this file is comprised of message digests of entries in the manifest file.

- A block file (XXX.DSA, where XXX is the name of the entity that signed the archive and DSA is the name of the signature algorithm used to create the signature). The block file contains the actual signature data in a format known as PKCS7.

There are many advantages to this format, not the least of which is that the PKCS7 block file (that is, the signature itself) is a standard format for external signatures. Unfortunately, the necessary classes to create PKCS7 blocks are not part of Java's public API; if you want to be able to write a signed JAR file, you'll need to write the classes to create the signature block yourself.

However, we can read a signed JAR file using the core API. This means that the class loader we've been using for the JavaRunner program can be modified to read a standard JAR file and associate the digital signature of that archive with the classes it loads.

We'll enhance the JarLoader class loader that we first developed in Chapter 3 in order to read the signature. For reference, we'll show the entire class again here, although only the highlighted portions of it have changed (it also contains some methods that we added in Chapter 6):

```
public class JarLoader extends SecureClassLoader {
    private URL urlBase;
    public boolean printLoadMessages = true;
    Hashtable classArrays;
    Hashtable classIds;
    static int groupNum = 0;
    ThreadGroup threadGroup;

    public JarLoader(String base, ClassLoader parent) {
        super(parent);
        try {
            if (!(base.endsWith("/")))
                base = base + "/";
            urlBase = new URL(base);
            classArrays = new Hashtable();
            classIds = new Hashtable();
        } catch (Exception e) {
            throw new IllegalArgumentException(base);
        }
    }
```

```
private byte[] getClassBytes(InputStream is) {
    ByteArrayOutputStream baos = new ByteArrayOutputStream();
    BufferedInputStream bis = new BufferedInputStream(is);
    boolean eof = false;
    while (!eof) {
        try {
            int i = bis.read();
            if (i == -1)
                eof = true;
            else baos.write(i);
        } catch (IOException e) {
            return null;
        }
    }
    return baos.toByteArray();
}

protected Class findLocalClass(String name) {
    String urlName = name.replace('.', '/');
    byte buf[];
    Class cl;

    SecurityManager sm = System.getSecurityManager();
    if (sm != null) {
        int i = name.lastIndexOf('.');
        if (i >= 0)
            sm.checkPackageDefinition(name.substring(0, i));
    }

    buf = (byte[]) classArrays.get(urlName);
    if (buf != null) {
        Object ids[] = (Object []) classIds.get(urlName);
        CodeSource cs = getCodeSource(urlBase, ids);
        cl = defineClass(name, buf, 0, buf.length, cs, ids);
        return cl;
    }

    try {
        AccessController.beginPrivileged();
        URL url = new URL(urlBase, urlName + ".class");
        if (printLoadMessages)
            System.out.println("Loading " + url);
        InputStream is = url.openConnection().getInputStream();
        buf = getClassBytes(is);
        CodeSource cs = getCodeSource(urlBase, null);
        cl = defineClass(name, buf, 0, buf.length, cs, null);
        return cl;
    } catch (Exception e) {
```

```java
            System.out.println("Can't load " + name + ": " + e);
            return null;
        } finally {
            AccessController.endPrivileged();
        }
    }

    public void readJarFile(String name) {
        URL jarUrl = null;
        JarInputStream jis;
        JarEntry je;

        try {
            jarUrl = new URL(urlBase, name);
        } catch (MalformedURLException mue) {
            System.out.println("Unknown jar file " + name);
            return;
        }
        if (printLoadMessages)
            System.out.println("Loading jar file " + jarUrl);

        try {
            jis = new JarInputStream(
                        jarUrl.openConnection().getInputStream());
        } catch (IOException ioe) {
            System.out.println("Can't open jar file " + jarUrl);
            return;
        }

        try {
            while ((je = jis.getNextJarEntry()) != null) {
                String jarName = je.getName();
                if (jarName.endsWith(".class"))
                    loadClassBytes(jis, jarName, je);
                // else ignore it; it could be an image or audio file
                jis.closeEntry();
            }
        } catch (IOException ioe) {
            System.out.println("Badly formatted jar file");
        }
    }

    private void loadClassBytes(JarInputStream jis,
                                String jarName, JarEntry je) {
        if (printLoadMessages)
            System.out.println("\t" + jarName);
        BufferedInputStream jarBuf = new BufferedInputStream(jis);
        ByteArrayOutputStream jarOut = new ByteArrayOutputStream();
        int b;
```

```
                    try {
                        while ((b = jarBuf.read()) != -1)
                            jarOut.write(b);
                        String className = jarName.substring(0, jarName.length() -
        6);
                        classArrays.put(className, jarOut.toByteArray());
                        Object ids[] = je.getIdentities();
                        if (ids != null)
                            classIds.put(className, ids);
                    } catch (IOException ioe) {
                        System.out.println("Error reading entry " + jarName);
                    }
                }


            public void checkPackageAccess(String name) {
                SecurityManager sm = System.getSecurityManager();
                if (sm != null)
                    sm.checkPackageAccess(name);
            }


            ThreadGroup getThreadGroup() {
                if (threadGroup == null)
                    threadGroup = new ThreadGroup(
                                    "JavaRuner ThreadGroup-" + groupNum++);
                return threadGroup;
            }


            String getHost() {
                return urlBase.getHost();
            }
        }
```

Interestingly enough, all the details of the digital signature are handled for us by the classes in the jar package. All that we're left to do is obtain the array of signers when we read in each JAR entry and then use that array of signers when we construct the code source we use to define the class. Remember that each file in a JAR file may be signed by a different group of identities and that some may not be signed at all. This is why we must construct a new code source object for each signed class that was in the JAR file.

The Signed JAR File and Security Policies

The last item in our examination of signed JAR files involves the security policy and its interaction with the signed JAR file. In the case where the security policy is completely determined by the access controller, the class loader has already done all our work for us; the access controller depends on each class to have an appro-

priate code source, and permissions for that code will be completely defined in
the policy file.

In Java 1.1, the mechanism is different; we can't use the JAR classes to parse a
signed JAR file, and we can't use the defineClass() method to set the signers for
a particular signed class. The first of these problems is harder to overcome; it
requires that you implement the equivalent of the java.util.jar package. We've
presented all the background information you'd need to do that, but it is a lot of
code to write (so we won't). The second of these problems means that your class
loader must define a class as follows:

```
if (isSecure(urlName)) {
    cl = defineClass(name, buf, 0, buf.length);
    if (ids != null)
        setSigners(cl, ids);
}
else cl = defineClass(name, buf, 0, buf.length);
```

The isSecure() method in this case must base its decision on information
obtained from reading the manifest of the JAR file and verifying the signature
that is contained in the signature file. The array of ids will need to be created by
constructing instances of the Identity class to represent the signer of the class.

The reason for setting the signers in this way is to allow the security manager to
retrieve those signatures easily. When the security manager does not defer all
permissions to the access controller—and, hence, in all Java 1.1 programs—the
security manager will need to take advantage of signed class information to base
its decisions. This is typically done by programming the security manager to
retrieve the keys that were used to sign a class via the getSigners() method. This
allows the security manger to function with any standard signature-aware class
loader. The security manager could then do something like this:

```
public void checkAccess(Thread t) {
    Class cl = currentLoadedClass();
    if (cl == null)
        return;
    Identity ids[] = (Identity[]) cl.getSigners();
    for (int i = 0; i < ids.length; i++) {
        if (isTrustedId(ids[i]))
            return;
    }
    throw new SecurityException("Can't modify thread states");
}
```

The key to this example is writing a good isTrustedId() method. A possible
implementation is to use the information stored in the keystore (for 1.2) or identity database (for 1.1) to grant a level of trust to an entity; such an implementation
requires that you have a non-default implementation of these databases. Alter-

nately, your application could hardwire the public keys of certain entities (like the public key of the HR group of XYZ corporation) and use that information as the basis of its security decisions.

Implementing a Signature Class

Now that we've seen how to use the Signature class, we'll look at how to implement our own class. The techniques we'll see here should be very familiar from our other examples of implementing an engine in the security provider architecture. In particular, since in 1.2 the Signature class extends its own SPI, we can implement a single class that extends the Signature class.

To construct our subclass, we must use the following constructor:

protected Signature(String algorithm)
> This is the only constructor of the Signature class, so all subclasses of this class must use this constructor. The string passed to the constructor is the name that will be registered with the security provider.

Once we've constructed our engine object, we must implement the following methods in it:

protected abstract void engineInitVerify(PublicKey pk)
> Initialize the object to prepare it to verify a digital signature. If the public key does not support the correct algorithm or is otherwise corrupted, an InvalidKeyException is thrown.

protected abstract void engineInitSign(PrivateKey pk)
> Initialize the object to prepare it to create a digital signature. If the private key does not support the correct algorithm or is otherwise corrupted, an InvalidKeyException is thrown.

protected abstract void engineUpdate(byte b)
protected abstract void engineUpdate(byte b[], int off, int len)
> Add the given bytes to the data that is being accumulated for the signature. These methods are called by the update() methods; they typically call the update() method of a message digest held in the engine. If the engine has not been correctly initialized, a SignatureException is thrown.

protected abstract byte[] engineSign()
> Create the signature based on the accumulated data. If there is an error in generating the signature, a SignatureException is thrown.

protected abstract boolean engineVerify(byte b[])
> Return an indication of whether or not the given signature matches the expected signature of the accumulated data. If there is an error in validating the signature, a SignatureException is thrown.

protected abstract void engineSetParameter(String p, Object o) ☆
protected abstract void engineSetParameter(AlgorithmParameterSpec p) ★

> Set the given parameters, which may be algorithm-specific. If this parameter does not apply to this algorithm, this method should throw an `InvalidParameterException`.

protected abstract Object engineGetParameter(String p) ☆

> Return the desired parameter, which is algorithm-specific. If the given parameter does not apply to this algorithm, this method should throw an `InvalidParameterException`.

In addition to those methods, there are a few protected instance variables that keep track of the state of the signature object—whether it has been initialized, whether it can be used to sign or to verify, and so on:

protected final static int UNINITIALIZED
protected final static int SIGN
protected final static int VERIFY
protected int state

> These variables control the internal state of signature object. The state is initially UNITIALIZED; it is set to SIGN by the `initSign()` method and to VERIFY by the `initVerify()` method.

These variables are not normally used by the subclasses of `Signature`, since the logic to maintain them is already implemented in the `Signature` class itself.

Here is an implementation of a signature class. Note that the `XYZSign` class depends on other aspects of the security architecture—in this example, the message digest engine to create an SHA message digest, and the DSA key interfaces to handle the public and private keys. This is very typical of signature algorithms—even to the point where the default name of the algorithm reflects the underlying components. The actual encryption of the message digest will use a simple XOR-based algorithm (so that we can, as usual, avoid the mathematics involved with a secure example).

```java
public class XYZSign extends Signature implements Cloneable {
    private DSAPublicKey pub;
    private DSAPrivateKey priv;
    private MessageDigest md;

    public XYZSign() throws NoSuchAlgorithmException {
        super("XYZSign");
        md = MessageDigest.getInstance("SHA");
    }

    public void engineInitVerify(PublicKey publicKey)
                            throws InvalidKeyException {
```

```
        try {
            pub = (DSAPublicKey) publicKey;
        } catch (ClassCastException cce) {
            throw new InvalidKeyException("Wrong public key type");
        }
    }


    public void engineInitSign(PrivateKey privateKey)
                                    throws InvalidKeyException {
        try {
            priv = (DSAPrivateKey) privateKey;
        } catch (ClassCastException cce) {
            throw new InvalidKeyException("Wrong private key type");
        }
    }


    public void engineUpdate(byte b) throws SignatureException {
        try {
            md.update(b)';
        } catch (NullPointerException npe) {
            throw new SignatureException("No SHA digest found");
        }
    }


    public void engineUpdate(byte b[], int offset, int length)
                                    throws SignatureException {
        try {
            md.update(b, offset, length);
        } catch (NullPointerException npe) {
            throw new SignatureException("No SHA digest found");
        }
    }


    public byte[] engineSign() throws SignatureException {
        byte b[] = null;
        try {
            b = md.digest();
        } catch (NullPointerException npe) {
            throw new SignatureException("No SHA digest found");
        }
        return crypt(b, priv);
    }


    public boolean engineVerify(byte[] sigBytes)
                                    throws SignatureException {
        byte b[] = null;
        try {
            b = md.digest();
        } catch (NullPointerException npe) {
            throw new SignatureException("No SHA digest found");
```

```
        }
        byte sig[] = crypt(sigBytes, pub);
        return MessageDigest.isEqual(sig, b);
    }

    public void engineSetParameter(String param, Object value) {
        throw new InvalidParameterException("No parameters");
    }

    public void engineSetParameter(AlgorithmParameterSpec aps) {
        throw new InvalidParameterException("No parameters");
    }

    public Object engineGetParameter(String param) {
        throw new InvalidParameterException("No parameters");
    }

    public void engineReset() {
    }

    private byte[] crypt(byte s[], DSAKey key) {
        DSAParams p = key.getParams();
        int rotValue = p.getP().intValue();
        byte d[] = rot(s, (byte) rotValue);
        return d;
    }

    private byte[] rot(byte in[], byte rotValue) {
        byte out[] = new byte[in.length];
        for (int i = 0; i < in.length; i++) {
            out[i] = (byte) (in[i] ^ rotValue);
        }
        return out;
    }
}
```

Like all implementations of engines in the security architecture, this class must have a constructor that takes no arguments, but it must call its superclass with its name. The constructor also is responsible for creating the instance of the underlying message digest using whatever algorithm this class feels is important. It is interesting to note that this requires the constructor to specify that it can throw a NoSuchAlgorithmException (in case the SHA algorithm can't be found).

The keys for this test algorithm are required to be DSA public and private keys. In general, the correspondence between an algorithm and the type of key it requires is very strong, so this is a typical usage. Hence, the two engine initialization methods cast the key to make sure that the key has the correct format. The engine initialization methods are not required to keep track of the state of the signature object—that is, whether the object has been initialized for signing or for verifying. That logic, since it is common to all signature objects, is present in the generic initialization methods of the Signature class itself.

The methods that update the engine can simply pass their data to the message digest, since the message digest is responsible for providing the fingerprint of the data that this object is going to sign or verify. Hence, the only interesting logic in this class is that employed by the signing and verification methods. Each method uses the message digest to create the digital fingerprint of the data. Then, to sign the data, the digest must be encrypted or otherwise operated upon with the previously defined private key—this produces a unique digest that could only have been produced by the given data and the given private key. Conversely, to verify the data, the digest must be decrypted or otherwise operated upon with the previously defined public key; the resulting digest can then be compared to the expected digest to test for verification.

Clearly, the security of this algorithm depends on a strong implementation of the signing operations. Our example here does not meet that definition—we're simply XORing every byte of the digest with a byte obtained from the parameters used to generate the keys. This XOR-encryption provides a good example, since it's both simple and symmetric; a real digital signature implementation is much more complex.

These engine signing and verification methods are also responsible for setting the internal state of the engine back to an initialization state, so that the same object can be used to sign or verify multiple signatures. In this case, no other work needs to be done for that; the message digest object itself is already reset once it creates its digest, and there is no other internal state inside the algorithm that needs to be reset. But if there were another state, it would need to be reset in those methods.

Summary

We've now completed our look at the basic engines that comprise the default security architecture on the Java platform. The digital signatures we've examined in this chapter form the pinnacle of that architecture, since they are the mechanism by which the parameters of the Java security sandbox can be extended: a digital signature gives the user the assurance that particular Java classes were provided by known entities. The user is then free to adopt a security policy for those classes based on the user's assessment of the trustworthiness of the entity that provided the classes.

The digital signature engine is interesting also because it requires the use of the other engines we've looked at in earlier chapters—the message digest engine to generate the fingerprint of the data that the digital signature will sign, and the key pair engine (and its related classes) to provide the necessary keys to feed into this engine. In sum, then, the engines provided with Java can really be thought of as having a single purpose: creating and verifying digital signatures. A digital signature thus becomes the basis of the advanced Java security model.

Important as digital signatures are, however, they do not complete what many people would expect from a security provider, in that the data communicated with a digital signature is itself not encrypted. This data is therefore vulnerable to being read by anyone. In the next chapter, we'll delve into an optional engine that can be loaded into the Java virtual machine—the engine to provide encryption of arbitrary streams of data. Although that engine cannot be used universally, it does provide (in those situations where it can be used) this last piece of security.

13

Encryption

In this chapter, we'll examine the Java Cryptography Extension, which provides (among other things) an engine to perform encryption of arbitrary data. This engine allows developers to send and receive encrypted streams of data over the network or through a filesystem (subject to some export restrictions we'll also discuss).

The encryption engine we'll discuss in this chapter does not come with the JDK. Information in this chapter is based on the early access 1.2 release of the Java Cryptography Extension (JCE); because it is an early access release, the information is subject to change when JCE is officialy released (tentatively scheduled for mid-1998). The JCE introduces four new engine classes to the Java security architecture—one to perform encryption, and three that handle keys for encryption—and it comes with a new security provider to implement those classes. We'll discuss all of these features in this chapter.

Export Restrictions

Use of the JCE is strictly limited by the export restrictions of the U.S. government. Sun Microsystems is headquartered in the United States, so the export of the JCE is controlled by the U.S. government. Because this implementation is capable of strong encryption, the only countries where it may be used are the United States and Canada.

There are ongoing legal challenges to this position as well as increasing negotiations with the U.S. government to change this policy; at the same time, there are increasing efforts to prohibit the use of this technology even within the United States. The official policy regarding export of encryption software has changed a few times over the past few years and is likely to change frequently in the next few years as various parties attempt to reach a coherent policy. Right now, the U.S. government will grant an exemption for certain types of companies to use encryption in their global business; what will happen in the future is anyone's guess.

In addition, the U.S. is not the only government that is hostile to the use of encryption, and encryption software can face import restrictions as well as export restrictions. In France, for example, it is illegal to import the JCE without a license. Other countries have regulations for cryptography, but in most cases they are less onerous than those of the United States. However, it is always wise to check your local policies to be sure (see Appendix C for resources to find more information about these limitations).

According to the letter of the restrictions, technical information regarding the JCE also cannot be exported except in the form of published books such as this one (because the book is protected by the first amendment to the U.S. Constitution). This has not prevented several companies and groups outside the United States from reimplementing the JCE encryption APIs, with the result that there are now several third-party security providers that include their own implementations of the JCE and are available outside the United States (the list of third-party security providers in Appendix C includes some of these implementations).

Many of the popular algorithms that are used by the encryption engine (and some of the other cryptographic engines that we've looked at) are patented algorithms, which also restricts their use. RSA Data Security, Inc., holds a patent in the U.S. on several algorithms involving RSA encryption and digital signatures; Ascom System AG in Switzerland holds both U.S. and European patents on the IDEA method of performing encryption. If you live in a country where these patents apply, you cannot use these underlying algorithms without paying a license to the patent holder. In particular, this means that many of the third-party security providers and third-party implementations of the JCE cannot be used within the United States because of patents held by RSA (although some of them have reached a licensing agreement with RSA Data Security, Inc.—again, it is best to check with the provider to see what restrictions might apply).

For at least the time being, then, Java programmers are faced with the following restrictions on use of the JCE:

- The JCE must be procured separately from the JDK. The official JCE from Sun may only be procured by citizens of the United States and Canada, but third-party implementations of the JCE may be obtainable elsewhere.

- Electronic documentation of the JCE is subject to the same restriction. In practice, the restriction about electronic documentation of encryption techniques—which applies to many things other than the JCE—is rarely enforced and widely violated.

- Code that uses the APIs we are going to discuss in this chapter and that was developed inside the United States or Canada may not be distributed electronically outside the United States and Canada. Hence, if you are a resident of the United States or Canada, you cannot use these APIs to develop applets that you put on the Internet, or to develop applications that you send outside the United States and Canada.

  Since no browser currently implements the JCE, the impact of this restriction on browsers is somewhat muted. However, some third-party implementations of the JCE will be compatible with popular browsers; these third-party implementations could be downloaded and installed manually by the user, who could then use cryptography only in applets that were developed outside the United States and Canada or that are available only on private networks wholly within the United States and Canada.

  This restriction also means that, unlike the other examples in this book, the examples in this chapter may not be downloaded from the O'Reilly ftp site.

- Questions about these APIs cannot be answered via email (although this is another rule that applies in general to encryption algorithms and is—again, at least presently—rarely enforced in the general case).

These APIs, then, will typically be used:

- To develop applications for use on a private intranet that is located wholly within the United States and Canada. XYZ Corporation may want to use this technology for their payroll application; without this technology, although payroll data may only be retrieved upon a valid signed request, that data is still shipped over the network unencrypted, where an inside corporate spy could snoop the wire and obtain the data.

  With the APIs we'll discuss in this chapter, we could encrypt the payroll data as it is passed over the network. This completes the security protection that such an application really needs. We are assured that the payroll data is only being sent to an authorized user, and we are assured that no one can decode the data while it is in transit.

- By developers outside the United States, who are effectively in a much better position to take advantage of them than are their U.S. counterparts. These developers, however, will be dependent upon third-party implementations of the JCE.

You'll notice that this is the only part of this book where we've discussed export restrictions. Somewhat surprisingly, that is because this is the only instance in which the export restrictions of the U.S. government apply. Encryption of arbitrary data is considered a weapons-grade munition, but message digests and digital signatures are not. Hence, the APIs that allow us to calculate a message

---

Encryption and Weaponry

The prohibitions we've been discussing here occur because strong encryption is considered by the U.S. government to be a munitions-grade weapon. While this position is often questioned, it comes from a long tradition in computer science.

During WWII, the Allies waged a successful and pivotal campaign in the Atlantic against the Axis navy. The success of this campaign was greatly due to the work of Alan Turing, who with his colleagues broke the German encryption algorithm known as Enigma. Turing was also one of the founding fathers of modern computer science, much of which was based on the work he developed in service to his country during the war.

Ironically, the reward that Turing reaped for his efforts was that some years after the war, he was arrested and forced to undergo harmful chemical treatments because he was gay. There's an odd parallel here: many of the harsh restrictions that are presently placed on encryption technology make no more sense in a world with a global Internet than did England's persecution of Alan Turing in the 1950s. But the links between encryption and military security run deep and are not likely to be broken anytime soon.

---

digest and a digital signature are freely exportable, but the APIs that allow us to encrypt and decrypt data are not.

Note also that the restriction here is not only on the algorithms that perform encryption, but on the APIs themselves. Like other engines we've examined, the encryption engine allows us to plug in any arbitrary algorithm to perform the encryption. This includes a weak encryption algorithm (that is, one that can be broken) that by itself would be exportable. But since the API allows a strong encryption algorithm to be used as well, the export restrictions apply to the API itself, even if the strong encryption implementation is not provided. Hence, the JCE may not be exported in its present form.

The Sun Security Provider in the JCE

The JCE follows the same security provider infrastructure as does the rest of the Java security architecture; the JCE comes with an additional security provider that includes implementations of the engines of the JCE. In normal use, this security provider supplements the default security provider of the JDK; the security provider within the JCE contains implementations only of the engines of the JCE.

Hence, to use the Sun JCE security provider, you need to add the SunJCE class (com.sun.crypto.provider.SunJCE) to your *java.security* file like this:

```
security.provider.2=com.sun.crypto.provider.SunJCE
```

Alternately, you may use the addProvider() or insertProviderAt() methods of the Security class. You may, of course, insert this provider at any position in the list of providers.

There are four new engine classes in the JCE: the Cipher, KeyAgreement, KeyGenerator, and SecretKeyFactory engines. Table 13-1 lists the engines and algorithms that are provided by the SunJCE security provider. In addition to implementations of the new engines, the SunJCE security provider gives us a key factory and a key pair generator for Diffie-Hellman (DH) keys. As always, there may be additional algorithm names in third-party security providers. Also note that the algorithm name for the cipher engine may be more complex than we've shown here.

Table 13-1. Engine Classes of the JCE

Engine Name	Algorithm
Cipher	DES
Cipher	DESede
Cipher	PBEWithMD5AndDES
KeyAgreement	DH
KeyFactory	DH
KeyGenerator	DES
KeyGenerator	DESede
KeyPairGenerator	DH
SecretKeyFactory	DES
SecretKeyFactory	DESede
SecretKeyFactory	PBE

Key Types in the JCE

The JCE introduces many new types of keys. Some of these are new types of public and private keys that extend our previous exploration of keys, and some of these are a new type of key: a secret key.

The new public and private key types are defined in the javax.crypto.interfaces package of the JCE as new interfaces:

public interface DHKey
public interface DHPrivateKey extends DHKey, PrivateKey
public interface DHPublicKey extends DHKey, PublicKey

> This set of interfaces defines keys suitable for use in Diffie-Hellman algorithms. In the SunJCE provider, they are used for the key agreement engine.

public interface RSAPrivateKey extends PrivateKey
public interface RSAPrivateKeyCrt extends PrivateKey
public interface RSAPublicKey extends PublicKey

> This set of interfaces defines keys suitable for use in RSA algorithms. However, in the SunJCE provider, there are no classes that model these keys, nor any RSA-based implementations. The interfaces are defined here more for the convenience of third-party implementors of the JCE than for use by the SunJCE provider.*

Like their DSA-based counterparts (the DSAKey, DSAPublicKey, and DSAPrivateKey classes), these interfaces all have specific methods to retrieve the values of certain parameters of the key. Since they are all keys, they support a byte-encoded format as well. For our purposes, however, we'll treat their data as opaque objects. The Diffie-Hellman keys are used in the key agreement protocol we discuss later in this chapter.

Secret Keys

The new type of key in the JCE is a secret key. A secret key is a key that is shared between two parties in a cryptographic operation.

Until now, we've used public key/private key pairs for all our operations. For instance, the digital signature algorithms we explored in Chapter 12 all depended on public key cryptography to alter the message digest of the data they signed. These algorithms chose to use public key encryption because it simplified the way in which keys were exchanged, as well as reducing the number of keys that needed to be exchanged between parties. It is possible to use public and private key pairs to perform encryption of data using the APIs in this chapter; because two different keys are involved, this type of encryption is called asymmetric encryption.

Cryptographic algorithms can also implement symmetric operations, in which case only a single key is necessary. In symmetric encryption, the same key that was originally used to encrypt the data can also be used to decrypt the data. Hence, for these encryption algorithms, only a single key is necessary. This single key is

---

* However, third-party implementors of other parts of the security package—e.g., digital signatures—may also choose to provide RSA-based algorithms and will also need RSA key types independent of the Java Cryptography Extension.

also called a secret key, since the key itself must be kept secret by the parties who are exchanging the encrypted data. Anyone who has access to the key and to the encrypted data also has access to the data.

The key used by the encryption engine—whether it is used by a symmetric or an asymmetric encryption algorithm—is still an instance of the class java.security.Key. Just as there were interfaces that identified types of keys as public (PublicKey) or private (PrivateKey), there is a new SecretKey interface (javax.crypto.SecretKey) that is used by symmetric keys:

public interface SecretKey extends Key

Identify a class as being a symmetric key. Like other extensions of the Key interface, this interface has no methods and is used strictly for type identification.

As usual, there are no classes in the javax package that implement this interface, though some are provided in the sun package. A simple implementation of this interface must include the usual methods that are in the Key interface:

```
public class XORKey implements SecretKey {
    byte value;

    public XORKey(byte b) {
        value = b;
    }

    public String getAlgorithm() {
        return "XOR";
    }

    public String getFormat() {
        return "XOR Special Format";
    }

    public byte[] getEncoded() {
        byte b[] = new byte[1];
        b[0] = value;
        return b;
    }
}
```

Unlike public and private keys, secret keys are not associated with identities and are not integrated into a key management system. Secret keys must therefore be managed with different techniques, which we'll examine at the end of this chapter.

Secret Key Engines

In the JCE, there are new ways to generate keys. Since the existing key engines only operate on public and private keys, the JCE introduces two new engines that can operate on secret keys. Note also in Table 13-1 that the SunJCE security provider implements a new algorithm to generate key pairs for Diffie-Hellman key agreement; that algorithm uses the standard KeyPairGenerator class we explored in Chapter 10.

The KeyGenerator Class

The first engine we'll look at is the KeyGenerator class (javax.crypto.Key-Generator); this class is used to generate secret keys. This class is very similar to the KeyPairGenerator class except that it generates instances of secret keys instead of pairs of public and private keys:

public class KeyGenerator

> Generate instances of secret keys for use by a symmetric encryption algorithm.

The KeyGenerator class is an engine within the JCE. As such, it has all the hallmarks of a cryptographic engine. It has a complementary SPI and a set of public methods that are used to operate upon it, and its implementation must be registered with the security provider.

Using the KeyGenerator class

Like other engine classes, the KeyGenerator class does not have any public constructors. An instance of a KeyGenerator is obtained by calling one of these methods:

public static final KeyGenerator getInstance(String algorithm)
public static final KeyGenerator getInstance(String algorithm, String provider)

> Return an object capable of generating secret keys that correspond to the given algorithm. These methods use the standard rules of searching the list of security providers in order to find an object that implements the desired algorithm. If the generator for the appropriate algorithm cannot be found, a NoSuchAlgorithmException is thrown; if the named provider cannot be found, a NoSuchProviderException is thrown.

Once an object has been obtained with these methods, the generator must be initialized by calling one of these methods:

public final void init(SecureRandom sr)
public final void init(AlgorithmParameterSpec aps)
public final void init(AlgorithmParameterSpec aps, SecureRandom sr)

Initialize the key generator. Like a key pair generator, the key generator needs a source of random numbers to generate its keys (in the second method, a default instance of the SecureRandom class will be used). In addition, some key generators can accept an algorithm parameter specification to initialize their keys (just as the key pair generator); however, for the DES-style keys generated by the SunJCE security provider, no algorithm parameter specification may be used.

A key generator does not have to be initialized explicitly, in which case it is initialized internally with a default instance of the SecureRandom class. However, it is up to the implementor of the engine class to make sure that this happens correctly; it is better to be sure your code will work by always initializing your key generator.

A secret key can be generated by calling this method:

public final SecretKey generateKey()

Generate a secret key. A generator can produce multiple keys by repeatedly calling this method.

There are two additional methods in this class, both of which are informational:

public final String getAlgorithm()

Return the string representing the name of the algorithm this generator supports.

public final Provider getProvider()

Return the provider that was used to obtain this key generator.

In the next section, we'll show the very simple code needed to use this class to generate a secret key.

Implementing a KeyGenerator class

Implementing a key generator requires implementing its corresponding SPI. Like all engines that are not available in Java 1.1, the SPI for the KeyGenerator class is unrelated in the class hierarchy to the KeyGenerator class itself, and the class that we register with the security provider must extend the KeyGeneratorSpi class (javax.crypto.KeyGeneratorSpi):

public abstract class KeyGeneratorSpi

This class forms the service provider interface class for the KeyGenerator class.

There are three protected methods of this class that we must implement if we want to provide an SPI for a key generator:

protected abstract SecretKey engineGenerateKey()

> Generate the secret key. This method should use the installed random number generator and (if applicable) the installed algorithm parameter specification to generate the secret key. If the engine has not been initialized, it is expected that this method will initialize the engine with a default instance of the SecureRandom class.

protected abstract void engineInit(SecureRandom sr)
protected abstract void engineInit(AlgorithmParameterSpec aps, SecureRandom sr)

> Initialize the key generation engine with the given random number generator and, if applicable, algorithm parameter specification. If the class does not support initialization via an algorithm parameter specification, or if the specification is invalid, an InvalidAlgorithmParameterException should be thrown.

Hence, a complete implementation might look like this:

```
public class XORKeyGenerator extends KeyGeneratorSpi {
    SecureRandom sr;

    public void engineInit(SecureRandom sr) {
        this.sr = sr;
    }

    public void engineInit(AlgorithmParameterSpec ap, SecureRandom sr)
                    throws InvalidAlgorithmParameterException {
        throw new InvalidAlgorithmParameterException(
            "No parameters supported in this class");
    }

    public SecretKey engineGenerateKey() {
        if (sr == null)
            sr = new SecureRandom();

        byte b[] = new byte[1];
        sr.nextBytes(b);
        return new XORKey(b[0]);
    }
}
```

Keys, of course, are usually longer than a single byte. However, unlike a public key/private key pair, there is not necessarily a mathematical requirement for generating a symmetric key. Such a requirement depends on the encryption algorithm the key will be used for, and some symmetric encryption algorithms require a key that is just an arbitrary sequence of bytes.

The SecretKeyFactory Class

The second engine that we'll look at is the `SecretKeyFactory` class (`javax.crypto.SecretKeyFactory`). Like the `KeyFactory` class, this class can convert from algorithmic or encoded key specifications to actual key objects and can translate key objects from one implementation to another. Unlike the `KeyFactory` class, which can only operate on public and private keys, the `Secret-KeyFactory` class can operate only on secret keys:

public class SecretKeyFactory

> Provide an engine that can translate between secret key specifications and secret key objects (and vice versa). This allows for secret keys to be imported and exported in a neutral format.

The interface to the `SecretKeyFactory` class is exactly the same at a conceptual level as the interface to the `KeyFactory`. At a programming level, this means that while most of the methods between the two classes have the same name and perform the same operation, they may require slightly different parameters: a secret key, rather than a public or private key. In addition, instead of methods to generate public or private keys, the `SecretKeyFactory` class contains this method:

public final SecretKey generateSecret(KeySpec ks)

> Generate the secret key according to the given specification. If the specification is invalid, an `InvalidKeySpecException` is thrown.

Because of its similarity to the `KeyFactory` class, we won't show an example of how to use it; you may use examples from Chapter 10 and simply substitute this new method.

Secret key specifications

The specifications used to import and export secret keys depend on the underlying algorithm that generated the secret key. As a result, the JCE provides twelve new key specifications that deal with the new keys the JCE provides:

public class DESKeySpec implements KeySpec
public class DESParameterSpec implements AlgorithmParameterSpec

> These classes provide the encoded and algorithmic parameter specifications for DES keys.

public class DESedeKeySpec implements KeySpec

> This class provides the encoded specification for DESede keys. Note that there is no corresponding parameter specification for this algorithm.

public class DHGenParameterSpec implements AlgorithmParameterSpec
public class DHParameterSpec implements AlgorithmParameterSpec

> These classes implement algorithm specifications for Diffie-Hellman keys.

public class DHPrivateKeySpec implements KeySpec
public class DHPublicKeySpec implements KeySpec

These classes implement the encoded key specifications for Diffie-Hellman keys.

public class PBEKeySpec implements KeySpec
public class PBEParameterSpec implements AlgorithmParameterSpec

These classes implement the encoded and algorithm key specifications for the password-based cipher algorithm (the PKCS#5 standard).

public class RSAPrivateKeySpec implements KeySpec
public class RSAPrivateKeyCrtSpec extends RSAPrivateKeySpec implements KeySpec
public class RSAPublicKeySpec implements KeySpec

These classes implement the encoded key specifications for RSA keys.

We typically treat the values contained in these specifications as opaque values. Table 13-2 lists the methods for each class needed to import and export each of these key specifications. As usual for key specifications, exporting a specification involves transmitting the individual data elements of the class, while importing a specification involves constructing the specification with the correct values.

Table 13-2. Importing and Exporting Values from the Key Specification Classes

Key Specifications	Methods to Export Data	Methods to Import Data
DESKeySpec	byte[] getKey()	DESKeySpec(byte[] buf) DESKeySpec(byte[] buf, int offset)

DESParameterSpec	byte[] getIV()	DESParameterSpec(
		    byte[] buf)
		DESParameterSpec(
		    byte[] buf, int
		offset)

DESedeKeySpec	byte[] getKey()	DESedeKeySpec(byte[] buf) DESedeKeySpec(byte[] buf, int offset)

DHGenParameter-
Spec
	int getPrimeSize()
	int getExponentSize()
		DHGenParameterSpec(
		    int primeSize,
		    int exponentSize)

DHParameterSpec	BigInteger getP()
	BigInteger getG()
	int getL()
		DHParameterSpec(
		    BigInteger p,
		    BigInteger g)
		DHParameterKeySpec(
		    BigInteger p,
		    BigInteger g,
		    int l)

Table 13-2. Importing and Exporting Values from the Key Specification Classes (continued)

Key Specifications	Methods to Export Data	Methods to Import Data

DHPrivateKeySpec	BigInteger getX()
	BigInteger getP()
	BigInteger getG()
	int getL()
		DHPrivateKeySpec(
		    BigInteger x,
		    BigInteger p,
		    BigInteger g)
		DHPrivateKeySpec(
		    BigInteger x,
		    BigInteger p,
		    BigInteger g, int l)

DHPublicKeySpec	BigInteger getY()
	BigInteger getP()
	BigInteger getG()
	int getL()
		DHPublicKeySpec(
		    BigInteger x,
		    BigInteger p,
		    BigInteger g)
		DHPublicKeySpec(
		    BigInteger x,
		    BigInteger p,
		    BigInteger g, int l)

PBEKeySpec	String getPassword()	PBEKeySpec(String pw)
PBEParameterSpec	int getIterationCount() byte[] getSalt()	PBEParameterSpec(byte[] salt, int count)

RSAPrivateKey-
Spec
	BigInteger getModulus()
	BigInteger getPrivate-
	Exponent()
		RSAPrivateKeySpec(
		    BigInteger mod,
		    BigInteger exp)

RSAPrivateKey-
CrtSpec
	BigInteger getCrtCoef-
	ficient()
	BigInteger getPrimeEx-
	ponentP()
	BigInteger getPrimeEx-
	ponentQ()
	BigInteger getPrimeP()
	BigInteger getPrimeQ()
	BigInteger getPublicEx-
	ponent()
		RSAPrivateKeyCrtSpec(
		    BigInteger mod,
		    BigInteger publicExp,
		    BigInteger privateExp,
		    BigInteger primeP,
		    BigInteger primeQ,
		    BigInteger primeExpP,
		    BigInteger primeExpQ,
		    BigInteger crtCoeff)

RSAPublicKeySpec	BigInteger getModulus()
	BigInteger getPublicEx-
	ponent()
		RSAPublicKeySpec(
		    BigInteger mod,
		    BigInteger exp)

The secret key factory SPI

Like all engines, the secret key engine is implemented via an SPI; if you want to implement your own secret key factory you must extend the SecretKeyFactorySpi class (javax.crypto.SecretKeyFactorySpi):

public abstract class SecretKeyFactorySpi

> This class is the SPI for the `SecretKeyFactory` class. As this class is only available as an extension to 1.2, the SPI is unrelated to the engine class; providers must extend this class directly to provide a secret key factory.

Implementation of this class follows the implementation of a key factory SPI, except that the methods of this class must operate upon secret keys rather than public or private keys. If you want to implement a secret key factory SPI, you can use the sample key factory SPI as a model.

Encrypting Data

In this section, we'll look at the engine that performs encryption within the JCE. This engine is called the `Cipher` class (`javax.crypto.Cipher`); it provides an interface to encrypt and decrypt data either in arrays within the program or as that data is read or written through Java's stream interfaces:

public class Cipher implements Cloneable

> Perform encryption and decryption of arbitrary data, using (potentially) a wide array of encryption algorithms.

Like all security engines, the cipher engine implements named algorithms. However, the naming convention for the cipher engine is different, in that cipher algorithms are compound names that can include the name of the algorithm along with the name of a padding scheme and the name of a mode. Padding schemes and modes are specified by names—just like algorithms. In theory, just as you may pick a new name for an algorithm, you may specify new names for a padding scheme or a mode, although the SunJCE security provider specifies several standard ones.

Modes and padding schemes are present in the `Cipher` class because that class implements what is known as a block cipher; that is, it expects to operate on data one block (e.g., 8 bytes) at a time. Padding schemes are required in order to ensure that the length of the data is an integral number of blocks.

Modes are provided to further alter the encrypted data in an attempt to make it harder to break the encryption. For example, if the data to be encrypted contains a number of similar patterns—repeated names, or header/footer information, for example—any patterns in the resulting data may aid in breaking the encryption. Different modes of encrypting data help prevent these sorts of attacks. Depending upon the mode used by a cipher, it may need to be initialized in a special manner when the cipher is used for decryption. Some modes require initialization via an initialization vector.

Modes also enable a block cipher to behave as a stream cipher; that is, instead of requiring a large, 8-byte chunk of data to operate upon, a mode may allow data to be processed in smaller quantities. So modes are very important in stream-based operations, where data may need to be transmitted one or two characters at a time.

The modes specified by the SunJCE security provider are:

ECB

> This is the electronic cookbook mode. ECB is the simplest of all modes; it takes a simple block of data (8 bytes in the SunJCE implementation, which is standard) and encrypts the entire block at once. No attempt is made to hide patterns in the data, and the blocks may be rearranged without affecting decryption (though the resulting plaintext will be out of order). Because of these limitations, ECB is recommended only for binary data; text or other data with patterns in it is not well-suited for this mode.

> ECB mode can only operate on full blocks of data, so it is generally used with a padding scheme.

> ECB mode does not require an initialization vector.

CBC

> This is the cipher block chaining mode. In this mode, input from one block of data is used to modify the encryption of the next block of data; this helps to hide patterns (although data that contains identical initial text—such as mail messages—will still show an initial pattern). As a result, this mode is suitable for text data.

> CBC mode can only operate on full blocks of data (8-byte blocks in the SunJCE implementation), so it is generally used with a padding scheme.

> CBC mode requires an initialization vector for decryption.

CFB

> This is the cipher-feedback mode. This mode is very similar to CBC, but its internal implementation is slightly different. CBC requires a full block (8 bytes) of data to begin its encryption, while CFB can begin encryption with a smaller amount of data. So this mode is suitable for encrypting text, especially when that text may need to be processed a character at a time. By default, CFB mode operates on 8-byte (64-bit) blocks, but you may append a number of bits after CFB (e.g., CFB8) to specify a different number of bits on which the mode should operate. This number must be a multiple of 8.

> CFB requires that the data be padded so that it fills a complete block. Since that size may vary, the padding scheme that is used with it must vary as well. For CFB8, no padding is required, since data is always fed in an integral number of bytes.

CFB mode requires an initialization vector for decryption.

OFB

This is the output-feedback mode. This mode is also suitable for text; it is used most often when there is a possibility that bits of the encrypted data may be altered in transit (e.g., over a noisy modem). While a 1-bit error would cause an entire block of data to be lost in the other modes, it only causes a loss of 1 bit in this mode. By default, OFB mode operates on 8-byte (64-bit) blocks, but you may append a number of bits after OFB (e.g., OFB8) to specify a different number of bits on which the mode should operate. This number must be a multiple of 8.

OFB requires that the data be padded so that it fills a complete block. Since that size may vary, the padding scheme that is used with it must vary as well. For OFB8, no padding is required, since data is always fed in an integral number of bytes.

OFB mode requires an initialization vector for decryption.

PCBC

This is the propagating cipher block chaining mode. This mode is popular in a particular system known as Kerberos; if you need to speak to a Kerberos version 4 system, this is the mode to use. However, this mode has some known methods of attack, and Kerberos version 5 has switched to using CBC mode. Hence, PCBC mode is no longer recommended.

PCBC mode requires that the input be padded to a multiple of 8 bytes.

PCBC mode requires an initialization vector for decryption.

The padding schemes specified by the SunJCE security provider are:

PKCS5Padding

This padding scheme ensures that the input data is padded to a multiple of 8 bytes.

NoPadding

When this scheme is specified, no padding of input is done. In this case, the number of input bytes presented to the encryption cipher must be a multiple of the block size of the cipher; otherwise, when the cipher attempts to encrypt or decrypt the data, it generates an error.

Remember that these uses of mode and padding are specific to the SunJCE security provider. The modes and padding schemes are based upon accepted standards and are thus likely to be implemented in this manner by third-party security providers as well, but you should check your third-party provider documentation to be sure.

The mode and padding scheme specified for decryption must match the mode and padding scheme specified for encryption, or the decryption will fail.

Using the Cipher Class

In order to obtain an instance of the Cipher class, we call one of these methods:

public static Cipher getInstance(String algorithmName)
public static Cipher getInstance(String algorithmName, String provider)

> Obtain a cipher engine that can perform encryption and decryption by implementing the named algorithm. The engine is provided by the given security provider, or the list of installed security providers is searched for an appropriate engine.
>
> If an implementation of the given algorithm cannot be found, a NoSuchAlgorithmException is thrown. If the named provider cannot be found, a NoSuchProviderException is thrown.
>
> The algorithm name passed to the getInstance() method may either be a simple algorithm name (e.g., DES), or it may be an algorithm name that specifies a mode and padding in this format: algorithm/mode/padding (e.g., DES/ECB/PKCS5Padding). If the mode and padding are not specified, they default to an implementation-specific value; in the SunJCE security provider, the mode defaults to ECB and padding defaults to PKCS5.

Once you've obtained a cipher object, you must initialize it. An object can be initialized for encryption or decryption, but in either case, you must provide a key. If the algorithm is a symmetric cipher, you should provide a secret key; otherwise, you should provide a public key to encrypt data and a private key to decrypt data (in fact, the key must match the algorithm type: a DES cipher must use a DES key, and so on). Initialization is achieved with one of these methods:

public final void init(int op, Key k)
public final void init(int op, Key k, AlgorithmParameterSpec aps)
public final void init(int op, Key k, AlgorithmParameterSpec aps, SecureRandom sr)
public final void init(int op, Key k, SecureRandom sr)

> Initialize the cipher to encrypt or decrypt data. If op is Cipher.ENCRYPT_MODE, the cipher is initialized to encrypt data; if op is Cipher.DECRYPT_MODE, the cipher is initialized to decrypt data. (In practice, other values will initialize the cipher for encryption rather than generating an exception; this is arguably a bug in the early-access implementation of the JCE.)
>
> These calls reset the engine to an initial state, discarding any previous data that may have been fed to the engine. Hence, a single cipher object can be used to encrypt data and then later to decrypt data.

Many algorithm modes we discussed earlier require an initialization vector to be specified when the cipher is initialized for decrypting. In these cases, the initialization vector must be passed to the init() method within the algorithm parameter specification; the DESParameterSpec class is typically used to do this for DES encryption.

In the SunJCE security provider, specifying an initialization vector for a mode that does not support it will eventually lead to a NullPointerException. Failure to specify an initialization vector for a mode that requires one will generate incorrect decrypted data.

After an engine has been initialized, it must be fed data. There are two sets of methods to accomplish this. The first set can be used any number of times:

public final byte[] update(byte[] input)
public final byte[] update(byte[] input, int offset, int length)
public final int update(byte[] input, int offset, int length, byte[] output)
public final int update(byte[] input, int offset, int length, byte[] output, int outOffset)

Encrypt or decrypt the data in the input array (starting at the given offset for the given length, if applicable). The resulting data is either placed in the given output array (in which case the size of the output data is returned) or returned in a new array. If the cipher has not been initialized, an Illegal-StateException is thrown.

If the length of the data passed to this method is not an integral number of blocks, any extra data is buffered internally within the cipher engine; the next call to an update() or doFinal() method processes that buffered data as well as any new data that is just being provided.

If the given output buffer is too small to hold the data, a ShortBufferException is thrown. The required size of the output buffer can be obtained from the getOutputSize() method. A ShortBufferException does not clear the state of the cipher: any buffered data is still held, and the call can be repeated (with a correctly sized buffer) with no ill effects.

This second set of methods should only be called once:

public final byte[] doFinal()
public final int doFinal(byte[] output, int offset)
public final byte[] doFinal(byte[] input)
public final byte[] doFinal(byte[] input, int offset, int length)
public final int doFinal(byte[] input, int offset, int length, byte[] output)
public final int doFinal(byte[] input, int offset, int length, byte[] output, int outOffset)

Encrypt or decrypt the data in the input array as well as any data that has been previously buffered in the cipher engine. This method behaves exactly the same as the update() method, except that this method signals that all data has been fed to the engine. If the engine is performing padding, the padding scheme will be used to process the pad bytes (i.e., add padding bytes for encryption and remove padding bytes for decryption). If the cipher engine is not performing padding and the total of all processed data is not a multiple of the mode's block size, an `IllegalBlockSizeException` is thrown.

These methods throw an `IllegalStateException` or a `ShortBufferException` in the same circumstances as the `update()` methods.

In order to initialize some ciphers for decryption, you need to specify an initialization vector; this initialization vector must be the same vector that was used when the cipher was initialized for encryption. For encryption, you may specify the initialization vector, or you may use a system-provided initialization vector. In order to retrieve this vector for later use (e.g., to send it to someone who will eventually need to decrypt the data), you may use this method:

public final byte[] getIV()
Return the initialization vector that was used to initialize this cipher. If a system-provided initialization vector is used, that vector is not available until after the first call to an `update()` or `doFinal()` method.

In order to preallocate an output buffer for use in the `update()` and `doFinal()` methods, you must know its size, which is returned from this method:

public final int getOutputSize(int inputLength)
Return the output size for the next call to the `update()` or `doFinal()` methods, assuming that one of those methods is called with the specified amount of data. Note that the size returned from this call includes any possible padding that the `doFinal()` method might add. A call to the `update()` method may actually generate less data than this method would indicate, because it will not create any padding.

Finally, there are two miscellaneous methods of this class:

public final Provider getProvider()
Return the provider class that defined this engine.

public final int getBlockSize()
Get the block size of the mode of the algorithm that this cipher implements.

Let's put this all together into a simple example:

```
public class CipherTest {
    public static void main(String args[]) {
        try {
            KeyGenerator kg = KeyGenerator.getInstance("DES");
            Cipher c = Cipher.getInstance("DES/CBC/PKCS5Padding");
            Key key = kg.generateKey();
```

```
            c.init(Cipher.ENCRYPT_MODE, key);
            byte input[] = "Stand and unfold yourself".getBytes();
            byte encrypted[] = c.doFinal(input);
            byte iv[] = c.getIV();

            DESParameterSpec dps = new DESParameterSpec(iv);
            c.init(Cipher.DECRYPT_MODE, key, dps);
            byte output[] = c.doFinal(encrypted);
            System.out.println("The string was ");
            System.out.println(new String(output));
        } catch (Exception e) {
            e.printStackTrace();
        }
    }
}
```

We've reused the single engine object to perform both the encryption and the decryption. Since DES is a symmetric encryption algorithm, we generated a single key that is used for both operations. Within the try block, the second block of code performs the encryption:

1. We initialize the cipher engine for encrypting.

2. We pass the bytes we want to encrypt to the doFinal() method. Of course, we might have had any number of calls to the update() method preceding this call, with data in any arbitrary amounts. Since we've specified a padding scheme, we don't have to worry about the size of the data we pass to the doFinal() method.

3. Finally, we save the initialization vector the system provided to perform the encryption. Note that this step would not be needed for ECB mode.

Performing the decryption is similar:

1. First, we initialize the cipher engine for decrypting. In this case, however, we must provide an initialization vector to initialize the engine in order to get the correct results (again, this would be unnecessary for ECB mode).

2. Next, we pass the encrypted data to the doFinal() method. Again, we might have had multiple calls to the update() method first.

In typical usage, of course, encryption is done in one program and decryption is done in another program. In the example above, this entails that the initialization vector and the encrypted data must be transmitted to a receiver; this may be done via a socket or a file or any other convenient means. There is no security risk in transmitting the initialization vector, as it has the same properties as the rest of the encrypted data.

An alternate choice to using an initialization vector, by the way, is simply to generate a dummy block of data at the beginning of the data to be encrypted, and to throw away the first block of data that results from decryption. Using that technique, the cipher that is used for decryption needs to be initialized only with the secret key; we'll use this technique a little later.

In this example, we used the PKCS5 padding scheme to provide the necessary padding. This is by far the simplest way. If you want to do your own padding—if, for example, you're using a CFB32 mode for some reason—you need to do something like this:

```
Cipher c = Cipher.getInstance("DES/CFB32/NoPadding");
c.init(Cipher.ENCRYPT_MODE, desKey);
int blockSize = c.getBlockSize();
byte b[] = "This string has an odd length".getBytes();
byte padded[] = new byte[b.length + blockSize - (b.length % blockSize)];
System.arraycopy(b, 0, padded, 0, b.length);
for (int i = 0; i < blockSize - (b.length % blockSize); i++)
    padded[b.length + i] = 0;
byte output[] = c.doFinal(padded);
```

The problem with this code is that when the data is decrypted, there is no indication of how many bytes should be discarded as padding. PKCS5 and other padding schemes solve this problem by encoding that information into the padding itself.

The NullCipher Class

The JCE includes one subclass of the Cipher class: the NullCipher class (javax.crypto.NullCipher). This class performs no encryption. Data passes through the null cipher unchanged, and no padding or blocking is performed (the getBlockSize() method will return 1). Unlike a traditional cipher engine, instances of the NullCipher class must be constructed directly:

```
Cipher c = new NullCipher();
```

This class can be used to test the logic of your program without actually encrypting or decrypting the data.

Cipher Algorithms

The SunJCE security provider supports three cipher algorithms:

• *DES*, the Data Encryption Standard algorithm, a standard that has been adopted by various organizations, including the U.S. government. There are known ways to attack this encryption, though they require a lot of computing power to do so; despite widespread predictions about the demise of DES, it continues to be used in many applications and is generally considered secure. The examples in this chapter are mostly based on DES encryption.

- *DESede*, also known as triple-DES or multiple-DES. This algorithm uses multiple DES keys to perform three rounds of DES encryption or decryption; the added complexity greatly increases the amount of time required to break the encryption. It also greatly increases the amount of time required to encrypt and to decrypt the data.

  From a developer's perspective, DESede is equivalent to DES; only the algorithm name passed to the key generator and cipher engines is different. Although DESede requires multiple keys, these keys are encoded into a single secret key. Hence, the programming steps required to use DESede are identical to the steps required to use DES.

- *PBEWithMD5AndDES*, the password-based encryption defined in PKCS#5. This algorithm entails using a password, a byte array known as *salt*, and an iteration count along with an MD5 message digest to produce a DES secret key; this key is then used to perform DES encryption or decryption. PKCS#5 was developed by RSA Data Security, Inc., primarily to encrypt private keys, although it may be used to encrypt any arbitrary data.

  From a developer's perspective, this algorithm requires some special programming to obtain the key. A password-based cipher cannot be initialized without special data that is passed via the algorithm specification. This data is known as the salt and iteration count. Hence, a password-based cipher is initialized as follows:

```
String password = "Come you spirits that tend on mortal thoughts";
byte[] salt = { (byte) 0xc9, (byte) 0x36, (byte) 0x78, (byte) 0x99,
                (byte) 0x52, (byte) 0x3e, (byte) 0xea, (byte) 0xf2 };
PBEParameterSpec paramSpec = new PBEParameterSpec(salt, 20);
PBEKeySpec keySpec = new PBEKeySpec(password);
SecretKeyFactory kf = SecretKeyFactory.getInstance("PBEWithMD5AndDES");
SecretKey key = kf.generateSecret(keySpec);
Cipher c = Cipher.getInstance("PBEWithMD5AndDES");
c.init(Cipher.ENCRYPT_MODE, key, paramSpec);
```

The rationale behind this system is that is allows the password to be shared verbally (or otherwise) between participants in the cipher; rather than coding the password as we've done above, the user would presumably enter the password. Since these types of passwords are often easy to guess (a string comparison of the above password against the collected works of Shakespeare would guess the password quite easily, despite its length), the iteration and salt provide a means to massage the password into something more secure. The salt itself should be random, and the higher the iteration count, the more expensive a brute-force attack against the key becomes (though it also takes longer to generate the key itself).

Of course, despite the presence of the salt and iteration, the password chosen in the method should not be easy to guess in the first place: it should contain special characters, not be known quotes from literature, and follow all the other usual rules that apply to selecting a password.

Implementing the Cipher Class

s in all 1.2-based engines, the SPI for the `Cipher` class is a separate class: the `CipherSpi` class (`javax.crypto.CipherSpi`):

public abstract class CipherSpi
> The SPI for the `Cipher` class. This class is responsible for performing the encryption or decryption according to its internal algorithm. Support for various modes or padding schemes must be handled by this class as well.

There is very little intelligence in the `Cipher` class itself; virtually all of its methods are simply passthough calls to corresponding methods in the SPI. The one exception to this is the `getInstance()` method, which is responsible for parsing the algorithm string and removing the mode and padding strings if present. If it finds a mode and padding specification, it calls these methods of the SPI:

public abstract void engineSetMode(String s)
> Set the mode of the cipher engine according to the specified string. If the given mode is not supported by this cipher, a `NoSuchAlgorithmException` should be thrown.

public abstract void engineSetPadding(String s)
> Set the padding scheme of the cipher engine according to the specified string. If the given padding scheme is not supported by this cipher, a `NoSuch-PaddingException` should be thrown.

Remember that the mode and padding strings we looked at earlier are specific to the implementation of the `SunJCE` security provider. Hence, while ECB is a common mode specification, it is completely at the discretion of your implementation whether that string should be recognized or not. If you choose to implement a common mode, it is recommended that you use the standard strings, but you may use any naming convention that you find attractive. The same is true of padding schemes.

Complicating this matter is the fact that there are no classes in the JCE that assist you with implementing any mode or padding scheme. So if you need to support a mode or padding scheme, you must write the required code from scratch.

The remaining methods of the SPI are all called directly from the corresponding methods of the `Cipher` class:

public abstract int engineGetBlockSize()

Return the number of bytes that comprise a block for this engine. Unless the cipher is capable of performing padding, input data for this engine must total a multiple of this block size (though individual calls to the `update()` method do not necessarily have to provide data in block-sized chunks).

public abstract byte[] engineGetIV()

Return the initialization vector that was used to initialize the cipher. If the cipher was in a mode where no initialization vector was required, this method should return `null`.

public abstract int engineGetOutputSize(int inputSize)

Return the number of bytes that the cipher will produce if the given amount of data is fed to the cipher. This method should take into account any data that is presently being buffered by the cipher as well as any padding that may need to be added if the cipher is performing padding.

public void engineInit(int op, Key key, SecureRandom sr)
public void engineInit(int op, Key key, AlgorithmParameterSpec aps, SecureRandom sr)

Initialize the cipher based on the `op`, which will be either `Cipher.ENCRYPT_MODE` or `Cipher.DECRYPT_MODE`. This method should ensure that the key is of the correct type and throw an `InvalidKeyException` if it is not (or if it is otherwise invalid), and use the given random number generator (and algorithm parameters, if applicable) to initialize its internal state. If algorithm parameters are provided but not supported or are otherwise invalid, this method should throw an `InvalidAlgorithmParameterException`.

public abstract byte[] engineUpdate(int input[], int offset, int len)
public abstract int engineUpdate(int input[], int offset, int len, byte[] output, int outOff)

Encrypt or decrypt the input data. The data that is passed to these methods will is not necessarily an integral number of blocks. It is the responsibility of these methods to process as much of the input data as possible and to buffer the remaining data internally. Upon the next call to an `engineUpdate()` or `engineDoFinal()` method, this buffered data must be processed first, followed by the input data of that method (and again leaving any leftover data in an internal buffer).

public abstract byte[] engineDoFinal(int input[], int offset, int len)
public abstract int engineDoFinal(int input[], int offset, int len, byte[] output, int outOff)

Encrypt or decrypt the input data. Like the `update()` method, this method must consume any buffered data before processing the input data. However, since this is the final set of data to be processed, this method must make sure that the total amount of data has been an integral number of blocks; it should not leave any data in its internal buffers.

If the cipher supports padding (and padding was requested through the engineSetPadding() method), this method should perform the required padding; an error in padding should cause a BadPaddingException to be thrown. Otherwise, if padding is not being performed and the total amount of data has not been an integral number of blocks, this method should throw an IllegalBlockSizeException.

Using our typical XOR strategy of encryption, here's a simple implementation of a cipher engine:

```java
public class XORCipher extends CipherSpi {
    byte xorByte;

    public void engineInit(int i, Key k, SecureRandom sr)
                    throws InvalidKeyException {
        if (!(k instanceof XORKey))
            throw new InvalidKeyException("XOR requires an XOR key");
        xorByte = k.getEncoded()[0];
    }

    public void engineInit(int i, Key k, AlgorithmParameterSpec aps,
                SecureRandom sr) throws InvalidKeyException,
                        InvalidAlgorithmParameterException {
        throw new InvalidAlgorithmParameterException(
            "Algorithm parameters not supported in this class");
    }

    public byte[] engineUpdate(byte in[], int off, int len) {
        return engineDoFinal(in, off, len);
    }

    public int engineUpdate(byte in[], int inoff, int length,
                        byte out[], int outoff) {
        for (int i = 0; i < length; i++)
            out[outoff + i] = (byte) (in[inoff + i] ^ xorByte);
        return length;
    }

    public byte[] engineDoFinal(byte in[], int off, int len) {
        byte out[] = new byte[len - off];
        engineUpdate(in, off, len, out, 0);
        return out;
    }

    public int engineDoFinal(byte in[], int inoff, int len,
                        byte out[], int outoff) {
```

```
        return engineUpdate(in, inoff, len, out, outoff);
    }

    public int engineGetBlockSize() {
        return 1;
    }

    public byte[] engineGetIV() {
        return null;
    }

    public int engineGetOutputSize(int sz) {
        return sz;
    }

    public void engineSetMode(String s)
                    throws NoSuchAlgorithmException {
        throw new NoSuchAlgorithmException("Unsupported mode " + s);
    }

    public void engineSetPadding(String s)
                    throws NoSuchPaddingException {
        throw new NoSuchPaddingException("Unsupported padding " + s);
    }
}
```

The bulk of the work of any cipher engine will be in the `engineUpdate()` method, which is responsible for actually providing the ciphertext or plaintext. In this case, we've simply XORed the key value with every byte, a process that works both for encryption as well as decryption. Because the work done by the `engine-Update()` method is so symmetric, we don't need to keep track internally of whether we're encrypting or decrypting; for us, the work is always the same. For some algorithms, you may need to keep track of the state of the cipher by setting an internal variable when the `engineInit()` method is called.

Similarly, because we can operate on individual bytes at a time, we didn't have to worry about padding and buffering internal data. Such an extension is easy, using the code we showed earlier that uses the modulus operator to group the input arrays into blocks.

To use this class, we would need to add these two lines to the `XYZProvider` class we developed in Chapter 8:

```
put("Cipher.XOR", "XORCipher");
put("KeyGenerator.XOR", "XORKeyGenerator");
```

Then it is a simple matter of installing the XOR security provider and getting an instance of this cipher engine:

```
Security.addProvider(new XYZProvider());
KeyGenerator kg = KeyGenerator.getInstance("XOR");
Cipher c = Cipher.getInstance("XOR");
```

Note that "XOR" is the only valid algorithm name for this implementation since we do not support any modes or padding schemes.

Cipher Streams

In the Cipher class we just examined, we had to provide the data to be encrypted or decrypted as multiple blocks of data. This is not necessarily the best interface for programmers: what if we want to send and receive arbitrary streams of data over the network? It would often be inconvenient to get all the data into buffers before it can be encrypted or decrypted.

The solution to this problem is the ability to associate a cipher object with an input or output stream. When data is written to such an output stream, it is automatically encrypted, and when data is read from such an input stream, it is automatically decrypted. This allows a developer to use Java's normal semantics of nested filter streams to send and receive encrypted data.

The CipherOutputStream Class

The class that encrypts data on output to a stream is the CipherOutputStream class (javax.crypto.CipherOutputStream):

public class CipherOutputStream extends FilterOutputStream
Provide a class that will encrypt data as it is written to the underlying stream.

Like all classes that extend the FilterOutputStream class, constructing a cipher output stream requires that an existing output stream has already been created. This allows us to use the existing output stream from a socket or a file as the destination stream for the encrypted data:

public CipherOutputStream(OutputStream outputStream, Cipher cipher)
Create a cipher output stream, associating the given cipher object with the existing output stream. The given cipher must already have been initialized, or an IllegalStateException will be thrown.

The output stream may be operated on with any of the methods from the Filter-OutputStream class—the write() methods, the flush() method, and the close() method, which all provide the semantics you would expect. Often, of course, these methods are never used directly—for example, if you're sending text data over a socket, you'll wrap a cipher output stream around the socket's output stream, but then you'll wrap a print writer around that; the programming interface then becomes a series of calls to the print() and println() methods. You can use any similar output stream to get a different interface.

It does not matter if the cipher object that was passed to the constructor does automatic padding or not—the CipherOutputStream class itself does not make that restriction. As a practical matter, however, you'll want to use a padding cipher object, since otherwise you'll be responsible for keeping track of the amount of data passed to the output stream and tacking on your own padding.

Usually, the better alternative is to use a byte-oriented mode such as CFB8. This is particularly true in streams that are going to be used conversationally: a message is sent, a response received, and then another message is sent, etc. In this case, you want to make sure that the entire message is sent; you cannot allow the cipher to buffer any data internally while it waits for a full block to arrive. And, for reasons we're just about to describe, you cannot call the flush() method in this case either. Hence, you need to use a streaming cipher (or, technically, a block cipher in streaming mode) in this case.

When the flush() method is called on a CipherOutputStream (either directly, or because the stream is being closed), the padding of the stream comes into play. If the cipher is automatically padding, the padding bytes are generated in the flush() method. If the cipher is not automatically padding and the number of bytes that have been sent through the stream is not a multiple of the cipher's block size, then the flush() method (or indirectly the close() method) throws an IllegalBlockSizeException (note that this requires that the IllegalBlockSizeException be a runtime exception).

If the cipher is performing padding, it is very important not to call the flush() method unless it is immediately followed by a call to the close() method. If the flush() method is called in the middle of processing data, padding is added in the middle of the data. This means the data does not decrypt correctly. Remember that certain output streams (especially some types of PrintWriter streams) flush automatically; if you're using a padding cipher, don't use one of those output streams.

We can use this class to write some encrypted data to a file like this:

```
public class Send {
    public static void main(String args[]) {
        try {
            KeyGenerator kg = KeyGenerator.getInstance("DES");
            kg.init(new SecureRandom());
            SecretKey key = kg.generateKey();
            SecretKeyFactory skf = SecretKeyFactory.getInstance("DES");
            Class spec = Class.forName("javax.crypto.spec.DESKeySpec");
            DESKeySpec ks = (DESKeySpec) skf.getKeySpec(key, spec);
            ObjectOutputStream oos = new ObjectOutputStream(
```

```
                        new FileOutputStream("keyfile"));
          oos.writeObject(ks.getKey());
          oos.close();

          Cipher c = Cipher.getInstance("DES/CFB8/NoPadding");
          c.init(Cipher.ENCRYPT_MODE, key);
          CipherOutputStream cos = new CipherOutputStream(
                        new FileOutputStream("ciphertext"), c);
          PrintWriter pw = new PrintWriter(
                        new OutputStreamWriter(cos));
          pw.print("XXXXXXXX");
          pw.println("Stand and unfold yourself");
          pw.close();
        } catch (Exception e) {
          System.out.println(e);
        }
      }
    }
```

There are two steps involved here. First, we must create the cipher object, which means that we must have a secret key available. The problem of secret key management is a hard one to solve; we'll discuss it a little farther along. For now, we're just going to save the key object to a file that can later be read by whomever needs the key. Note that we've gone through the usual steps of writing the data produced by the secret key factory so that the recipient of the key need not use the same provider we use.

After we generate the key, we must create the cipher object, initialize it with that key, and then use that cipher object to construct our output stream. Once the data is sent to the stream, we close the stream, which flushes the cipher object, performs any necessary padding, and completes the encryption.

Note that in this example, we've sent 8 arbitrary bytes before the real data. We've done this instead of getting the initialization vector from the cipher and transmitting the initialization vector (as we did in the earlier example); we'll have to remember to discard the first 8 bytes when we read the data later. Because of the possibility that someone might recognize a pattern in these bytes, this method is slightly less secure, but it is clearly more convenient (and it would be more secure if we didn't pick such an obvious pattern).

In this case, we've chosen to use CFB8 mode, so there is no need for padding. But in general, this last step is important: if we don't explicitly close the PrintWriter stream, when the program exits, data that is buffered in the cipher object itself will not get flushed to the file. The resulting encrypted file will be unreadable, as it won't have the correct amount of data in its last block.*

The CipherInputStream Class

The output stream is only half the battle; in order to read that data, we must use the CipherInputStream class (javax.crypto.CipherInputStream):

public class CipherInputStream extends FilterInputStream
> Create a filter stream capable of decrypting data as it is read from the underlying input stream.

A cipher input stream is constructed with this method:

public CipherInputStream(InputStream is, Cipher c)
> Create a cipher input stream that associates the existing input stream with the given cipher. The cipher must previously have been initialized.

All the points we made about the CipherOutputStream class are equally valid for the CipherInputStream class. You can operate on it with any of the methods in its superclass, although you'll typically want to wrap it in something like a buffered reader, and the cipher object that is associated with the input stream needs to perform automatic padding or use a mode that does not require padding (in fact, it must use the same padding scheme and mode that the output stream that is sending it data used).

The CipherInputStream class does not directly support the notion of a mark. The markSupported() method returns false unless you've wrapped the cipher input stream around another class that supports a mark.

Here's how we could read the data file that we created above:

```
public class Receive {
    public static void main(String args[]) {
        try {
            ObjectInputStream ois = new ObjectInputStream(
                    new FileInputStream("keyfile"));
            DESKeySpec ks = new DESKeySpec((byte[]) ois.readObject());
            SecretKeyFactory skf = SecretKeyFactory.getInstance("DES");
            SecretKey key = skf.generateSecret(ks);
            ois.close();

            Cipher c = Cipher.getInstance("DES/CFB8/NoPadding");
            c.init(Cipher.DECRYPT_MODE, key);
            CipherInputStream cis = new CipherInputStream(
                    new FileInputStream("ciphertext"), c);
            cis.read(new byte[8]);
            BufferedReader br = new BufferedReader(
                    new InputStreamReader(cis));
```

---

* Closing the output stream is necessary whenever the stream performs buffering, but it is particularly important to remember in this context.

```
            System.out.println("Got message");
            System.out.println(br.readLine());
        } catch (Exception e) {
            System.out.println(e);
        }
    }
}
```

In this case, we must first read the secret key from the file where it was saved, and then create the cipher object initialized with that key. Then we can create our input stream and read the data from the stream, automatically decrypting it as it goes.

SSL Encryption

In the world of the Internet, data encryption is often achieved with SSL—the Secure Socket Layer protocol. These sockets use encryption to encrypt data as it is written to the socket and to decrypt that data as it is read from the socket.

SSL encryption is built into many popular web browsers and web servers; these programs depend on SSL to provide the necessary encryption to implement the https protocol. For Java applet developers who want to use SSL, there are three options:

1. Use the URL class.

   The URL class can be used to open a URL that the applet can read data from. If the URL is a POST URL, the applet can send some initial data before it reads the data. On browsers that will support it, you can specify an https protocol when the URL is constructed, in which case the data exchanged by the applet and the remote web server will be encrypted. Note that this is not supported by the JDK itself.

   There are a few limitations with this method. First, the data exchange is limited to the web server and the applet using the single request-response protocol of HTTP. Data cannot be streamed in this way, and you must write an appropriate back-end cgi-bin script, servlet, or other program to process the data. Second, not all browsers support the https protocol, and those that do support https may not support a Java applet opening an https URL. On the other hand, this will tunnel data through a firewall, which is one of the main reasons why it is used.

2. Use an SSLSocket class.

   There are a number of vendors who supply SSLSocket and SSLServerSocket classes that extend the Socket and ServerSocket classes; these classes provide all the semantics of their java.net counterparts with the additional feature that the data they exchange is encrypted with the SSL algorithm.

These classes are generally subject to import and export restrictions; in particular, Sun's `SSLSocket` and `SSLServerSocket` classes (which come with the Java Server product) cannot be exported, and certain countries will not allow these implementations to be imported. There are SSL implementations that have been written outside the United States, so they have fewer restrictions (but they may contain implementations of RSA that may not be used within the United States).

3. Use an RSA-based security provider.

   The `Cipher` class that we examined above has the ability to support RSA encryption. Many third-party security providers will have RSA implementations; some of these are listed in Appendix C.

For now, none of these solutions is completely attractive. The technique of using URLs is well known and demonstrated in any book on Java network programming, but suffers from the limitations we discussed above. The SSL-based `Socket` classes have a known interface and are simple to use, but suffer from availability questions (although no more than the JCE itself).

Symmetric Key Agreement

When we discussed public and private key pairs, we talked about the bootstrapping issue involved with key distribution: the problem of obtaining the public key of a trusted certificate authority. In the case of key pairs, keeping the private key secret is of paramount importance. Anyone with access to the private key will be able to sign documents as the owner of the private key; he or she will also be able to decrypt data that is intended for the owner of the private key. Keeping the private key secret is made easier because both parties involved in the cryptographic transfer do not need to use it.

With the symmetric key we introduced in this chapter, however, the bootstrapping issue is even harder to solve because both parties need access to the same key. The question then becomes how this key can be transmitted securely between the two parties in such a way that only those parties have access to the key.

One technique to do this is to use traditional (i.e., nonelectronic) means to distribute the key. The key could be put onto a floppy disk, for example, and then mailed or otherwise distributed to the parties involved in the encryption. Or the key could be distributed in paper format, requiring the recipient of the key to type in the long string of hex digits (the password-based encryption algorithm makes this easier, of course). This is the type of technique we used in the section on cipher data streams. In those examples, the key was saved in a file that was created when the ciphertext was generated (although the key could have been pregenerated, and the `Send` class could have also read it from a file).

Another technique is to use public key/private key encryption to encrypt the symmetric key, and then to send the encrypted key over the network. This allows the key to be sent electronically and then to be used to set up the desired cipher engine. This is a particularly attractive option, because symmetric encryption is usually much faster than public key encryption. You can use the slower encryption to send the secret key, and then use the faster encryption for the rest of your data. This option requires that your security provider implement a form of public key encryption (which the SunJCE security provider does not).

The final option is to use a key agreement algorithm. Key agreement algorithms exchange some public information between two parties so they each can calculate a shared secret key. However, they do not exchange enough information that eavesdroppers on the conversation can calculate the same shared key.

In the JCE, these algorithms are represented by the KeyAgreement class (javax.crypto.KeyAgreement):

public class KeyAgreement

Provide an engine for the implementation of a key agreement algorithm. This class allows for two cooperating parties to generate the same secret key while preventing parties unrelated to the agreement from generating the same key.

As an engine class, this class has no constructors, but it has the usual method to retrieve instances of the class:

public final KeyAgreement getInstance(String algorithm)
public final KeyAgreement getInstance(String algorithm, String provider)

Return an instance of the KeyAgreement class that implements the given algorithm, loaded either from the standard set of providers or from the named provider. If no suitable class that implements the algorithm can be found, a NoSuchAlgorithmException is generated; if the given provider cannot be found, a NoSuchProviderException is generated.

The interface to this class is very simple (much simpler than its use would indicate, as our example will show):

public final void init(AlgorithmParameterSpec aps)
public final void init(AlgorithmParameterSpec aps, SecureRandom sr)
public final void init(SecureRandom sr)

Initialize the key agreement engine. The parameter specifications will vary depending upon the underlying algorithm implemented by the agreement engine; if the parameters are invalid, of the incorrect class, or not supported, an InvalidAlgorithmParameterException is generated.

public final Key doPhase(int phase, Key key)

> Execute a phase of the key agreement protocol. Key agreement protocols usually require a set of operations to be performed in a particular order. Each operation is represented in this class by a particular phase. Phases must be executed in order. If the phase number is incorrect, an `IllegalStateException` is thrown. Phases usually require a key to succeed. If the provided key is not supported by the key agreement algorithm, is incorrect for the current phase, or is otherwise invalid, an `InvalidKeyException` is thrown.

> The number of phases, along with the types of keys they require, vary drastically from key agreement algorithm to algorithm. Your security provider must document the order of calls and arguments to this method.

public final byte[] generateSecret()
public final int generateSecret(byte[] secret, int offset)

> Generate the bytes that represent the secret key; these bytes can then be used to create a `SecretKey` object. The type of that object will vary depending upon the algorithm implemented by this key agreement. The bytes are either returned from this argument or placed into the given array (starting at the given offset). In the latter case, if the array is not large enough to hold all the bytes a `ShortBufferException` is thrown. If all phases of the key agreement protocol have not been executed, an `IllegalStateException` is generated.

> After this method has been called, the engine is reset and may be used to generate more secret keys (starting with a new set of calls to the `doPhase()` method).

public final String getAlgorithm()

> Return the name of the algorithm implemented by this key agreement object.

public final Provider getProvider()

> Return the provider that implemented this key agreement.

Despite its simple interface, using the key agreement engine can be very complex. The SunJCE security provider implements one key agreement algorithm: Diffie-Hellman key agreement. This key agreement is based on the following protocol:

1. Alice (the first party in the exchange) generates a Diffie-Hellman public key/private key pair.

2. Alice transmits the public key and the algorithm specification of the key pair to Bob (the second party in the exchange).

3. Bob uses the algorithm specification to generate his own public and private keys; he sends the public key to Alice.

4. Alice uses her private key and Bob's public key to create a secret key. In the `KeyAgreement` class, this requires two phases: one that uses her private key and one that uses her public key.

5. Bob performs the same operations with his private key and Alice's public key. Due to the properties of a Diffie-Hellman key pair, this generates the same secret key Alice generated.

6. Bob and Alice convert their secret keys into a DES key.

7. Alice uses that key to encrypt data that she sends to Bob.

8. Bob uses that key to decrypt data that he reads.

These last two steps, of course, are symmetric: both Bob and Alice can encrypt as well as decrypt data with the secret key. They can both send and receive data as well.

Nothing in this key agreement protocol prevents someone from impersonating Bob—Alice could exchange keys with me, I could say that I am Bob, and then Alice and I could exchange encrypted data. So even though the transmissions of the public keys do not need to be encrypted, they should be signed for maximum safety.

This algorithm works because of the properties of the Diffie-Hellman public key/private key pair. These keys are not suitable for use in an encryption algorithm; they are used only in a key agreement such as this.

Here's how a key agreement might be implemented:

```
public class DHAgreement implements Runnable {
    byte bob[], alice[];
    boolean doneAlice = false;
    byte[] ciphertext;

    BigInteger aliceP, aliceG;
    int aliceL;

    public synchronized void run() {
        if (!doneAlice) {
            doneAlice = true;
            doAlice();
        }
        else doBob();
    }

    public synchronized void doAlice() {
        try {
            // Step 1:  Alice generates a key pair
            KeyPairGenerator kpg = KeyPairGenerator.getInstance("DH");
            kpg.initialize(1024);
```

```java
KeyPair kp = kpg.generateKeyPair();

// Step 2:  Alice sends the public key and the
//       Diffie-Hellman key parameters to Bob
Class dhClass = Class.forName(
                    "javax.crypto.spec.DHParameterSpec");
DHParameterSpec dhSpec = (
                (DHPublicKey) kp.getPublic()).getParams();
aliceG = dhSpec.getG();
aliceP = dhSpec.getP();
aliceL = dhSpec.getL();
alice = kp.getPublic().getEncoded();
notify();

// Step 4 part 1:  Alice performs the first phase of the
//       protocol with her private key
KeyAgreement ka = KeyAgreement.getInstance("DH");
ka.doPhase(1, kp.getPrivate());

// Step 4 part 2:  Alice performs the second phase of the
//       protocol with Bob's public key
while (bob == null) {
    wait();
}
KeyFactory kf = KeyFactory.getInstance("DH");
X509EncodedKeySpec x509Spec = new X509EncodedKeySpec(bob);
PublicKey pk = kf.generatePublic(x509Spec);
ka.doPhase(2, pk);

// Step 4 part 3:  Alice can generate the secret key
byte secret[] = ka.generateSecret();

// Step 6:  Alice generates a DES key
SecretKeyFactory skf = SecretKeyFactory.getInstance("DES");
DESKeySpec desSpec = new DESKeySpec(secret);
SecretKey key = skf.generateSecret(desSpec);

// Step 7:  Alice encrypts data with the key and sends
//       the encrypted data to Bob
Cipher c = Cipher.getInstance("DES/ECB/PKCS5Padding");
c.init(Cipher.ENCRYPT_MODE, key);
ciphertext = c.doFinal(
                "Stand and unfold yourself".getBytes());
notify();
} catch (Exception e) {
    e.printStackTrace();
}
}
```

```java
public synchronized void doBob() {
    try {
        // Step 3:  Bob uses the parameters supplied by Alice
        //       to generate a key pair and sends the public key
        while (alice == null) {
            wait();
        }
        KeyPairGenerator kpg = KeyPairGenerator.getInstance("DH");
        DHParameterSpec dhSpec = new DHParameterSpec(
                        aliceP, aliceG, aliceL);
        kpg.initialize(dhSpec);
        KeyPair kp = kpg.generateKeyPair();
        bob = kp.getPublic().getEncoded();
        notify();

        // Step 5 part 1:  Bob uses his private key to perform the
        //       first phase of the protocol
        KeyAgreement ka = KeyAgreement.getInstance("DH");
        ka.doPhase(1, kp.getPrivate());

        // Step 5 part 2:  Bob uses Alice's public key to perform
        /        the second phase of the protocol.
        KeyFactory kf = KeyFactory.getInstance("DH");
        X509EncodedKeySpec x509Spec =
                    new X509EncodedKeySpec(alice);
        PublicKey pk = kf.generatePublic(x509Spec);
        ka.doPhase(2, pk);

        // Step 5 part 3:  Bob generates the secret key
        byte secret[] = ka.generateSecret();

        // Step 6:  Bob generates a DES key
        SecretKeyFactory skf = SecretKeyFactory.getInstance("DES");
        DESKeySpec desSpec = new DESKeySpec(secret);
        SecretKey key = skf.generateSecret(desSpec);

        // Step 8:  Bob receives the encrypted text and decrypts it
        Cipher c = Cipher.getInstance("DES/ECB/PKCS5Padding");
        c.init(Cipher.DECRYPT_MODE, key);
        while (ciphertext == null) {
            wait();
        }
        byte plaintext[] = c.doFinal(ciphertext);
        System.out.println("Bob got the string " +
                    new String(plaintext));
    } catch (Exception e) {
        e.printStackTrace();
    }
}
```

```
public static void main(String args[]) {
    DHAgreement test = new DHAgreement();
    new Thread(test).start();// Starts Alice
    new Thread(test).start();// Starts Bob
}
}
```

In typical usage, of course, Bob and Alice would be executing code in different classes, probably on different machines. We've shown the code here using two threads in a shared object so that you can run the example more easily (although beware: generating a Diffie-Hellman key is an expensive operation, especially for a size of 1024; a size of 128 will be better for testing). Our second reason for showing the example like this is to make explicit the points at which the protocol must be synchronized: Alice must wait for certain information from Bob, Bob must wait for certain information from Alice, and both must perform the operations in the order specified. Once the secret key has been created, however, they may send and receive encrypted data at will.

Otherwise, despite its complexity, this example merely reuses a lot of the techniques we've been using throughout this book. Keys are generated, they are transmitted in neutral (encoded) format, they are re-formed by their recipient, and both sides can continue.

Sealed Objects

The final class in the JCE that we'll investigate is the SealedObject class (javax.crypto.SealedObject). This class is very similar to the SignedObject class we examined in Chapter 12, except that the stored, serialized object is encrypted rather than signed:

public class SealedObject

A class that can embed within it a serializable object in an encrypted form.

Constructing a sealed object is achieved as follows:

public SealedObject(Serializable obj, Cipher c)

Construct a sealed object. The sealed object serializes the given object to an embedded byte array, effectively making a copy of the object. It then uses the given cipher to encrypt the embedded byte array. If the object is unable to be serialized, an IOException is thrown; an error in encrypting the byte array results in an IllegalBlockSizeException. If the cipher object has not been initialized, an IllegalStateException is generated.

To retrieve the object, we use this method:

public Object getObject(Cipher c)

Decrypt the embedded byte array and deserialize it, returning the reconstituted object. The cipher must have been initialized with the same mode and key as the cipher that was passed to the constructor when the object was first created, otherwise a `BadPaddingMethodException` or an `IllegalBlockSize-Exception` is thrown. If the cipher was not initialized, an `IllegalStateException` is generated; failure to find the serialized class results in a `ClassNotFoundException`, and generic deserialization errors results in an `IOException`.

These are the only two operations that may be performed upon a sealed object. Just keep in mind that the embedded object in this class is a serialized instance of the original object: the technique the object uses to perform serialization may affect the resulting object that is retrieved from the sealed object. This class can help us prevent someone from tampering with our serialized object, but the reconstituted object may be lacking transient fields or other information (depending, of course, on the implementation of the object itself).

Summary

In this chapter, we explored the final engine of the Java security package—the encryption engine. The encryption engine is part of the Java Cryptography Extension (JCE). Due to export limitations, the JCE from Sun is available only within the United States and Canada. Third-party implementations of the JCE are available elsewhere. No matter where you get it from, the JCE must be obtained separately from the rest of the Java platform.

The encryption engine performs encryption of arbitrary chunks or streams of data according to various algorithms. Though support for RSA and other popular algorithms is possible within the provider architecture, the SunJCE security provider supplies only DES encryption. DES encryption has a different requirement for keys than the other cryptographic engines we've examined—DES encryption depends on both parties in the cryptographic exchange using the same key. Hence the JCE also provides a new key type known as a secret key (or symmetric key), as well as an engine to generate these keys.

Secret keys pose an interesting distribution problem—they cannot be distributed electronically unless the secret key itself is encrypted. This problem is often solved by relying on public key encryption to deliver the encrypted key, after which the symmetric key can be used to create the type of cipher that we've discussed in this chapter. The JCE also includes support for key agreement protocols to accomplish key sharing, one of which (the Diffie-Hellman key agreement protocol) is implemented in the SunJCE security provider.

The encryption engine finally provides what many people envision as the ultimate goal in security: the ability to send arbitrary encrypted data streams in a conversational manner across the network. Although its use is limited by governmental restrictions, it provides the last piece of the Java security puzzle that we outlined at the beginning of this book.

A

Security Tools

In this appendix, we'll discuss the tools that come with the JDK that allow developers, end users, and system administrators to deal with the security aspects of the Java platform. These tools are only available in Java 1.2, since they primarily deal with operations that require the support of 1.2.* As Java's security model advances, these tools have become primary interfaces to establishing a secure sandbox for Java applications.

To a lesser extent, these tools have become an interface for establishing a secure sandbox for Java applets as well. However, as we've seen, not all the security features of the Java platform have yet been uniformly adopted by all browsers. In part, it is a problem with logistics. As this book went to press, Java 1.2 was still a beta release. Clearly it will take some time before these new features can be propagated to browsers. Part of the problem, though, lies in the fact that Java applications (and Java browsers) ultimately decide upon their own security features.

This last fact is true of your own applications as well: you can certainly use the keytool utility that comes with the JDK to manage your public key/private key databases. But if it is appropriate, you may want to replace (or at least supplement) the keytool with your own key management tool that handles some of the situations we discussed in Chapter 11.

---

* The javakey utility in 1.1 can be used to sign JAR files and to operate like the keytool; that utility is obsolete in 1.2. In fact, the signed JAR files and identity database that javakey produces cannot be read by 1.2 utilities at all.

The keytool

In Chapter 11 we discussed the KeyStore class, which provides an interface to a key management system. The Java platform comes with a tool—keytool—that provides an administrative interface to that class. Keytool allows end users and system administrators to add, delete, and modify entries in the keystore (provided that they have sufficient permissions, of course).

When we discussed the KeyStore class, we mentioned that it had some limitations that may lead you to write your own implementation of that class. The good news is that if you write such a class, you may still use keytool to administer your set of keys. Since keytool uses the standard interface provided by the KeyStore class, it will be (mostly) compatible with any new class that you install into that interface (we'll remind you how to do that at the end of this appendix). However, there are some exceptions to this: keytool itself places some restrictions upon the algorithms that may be used to support particular keys.

Before we examine the workings of keytool, let's review a few objects that we talked about in Chapter 11. When we discussed the KeyStore class, we defined the following terms:

keystore

> The keystore is the file that actually holds the set of keys; keytool operates on this file. In other implementations of the KeyStore class, the keystore may not be a file—the keys in that implementation may be held in a database or some other structure. Regardless, we refer to the set of keys on disk (or wherever they are located) as the keystore.
>
> In keytool, this file is called *.keystore* and is held in the directory specified by the property user.home. On Unix systems, this directory defaults to the user's home directory (e.g., *$HOME*); on Windows systems, this directory defaults to the concatenation of the HOMEDRIVE and HOMEPATH environment variables (e.g., *C:*).

alias

> An alias is a shortened, keystore-specific name for an entity that has a key in the keystore. I choose to store my public and private key in my local keystore under the alias "sdo"; if you have a copy of my public key, you may use that alias, or you may use another alias (like "ScottOaks"). The alias used for a particular entity is completely up to the discretion of the individual who first enters that entity into the keystore.

DN (distinguished name)

> The distinguished name for an entity in the keystore is a subset of its full X.500 name. This is a long string; for example, my DN is:
>
> ```
> CN=Scott Oaks, OU=SMCC, O=Sun Microsystems, L=New York, S=NY, C=US
> ```

DNs are used by certificate authorities to refer to the entities to whom they supply a certificate. Hence, unlike an alias, the DN for a particular key is the same no matter what keystore it is located in: if I send you my public key, it will have the DN encoded in the public key's certificate.

However, nothing prevents me from having two public keys with different DNs (I might have one for personal use that omits references to my place of employment). And there is no guarantee that two unrelated individuals will not share the same DN (in fact, you can count on this type of namespace collision to occur).

key entries and certificate entries

There are two types of entries in the keystore: key entries and certificate entries. A key entry is an entry that has a private key as well as a corresponding public key. The public key in this case is embedded in a certificate, and there is a chain of certificates that vouch for the public key.

A certificate entry, on the other hand, does not contain a private key; it contains only a public key held in a certificate. In addition, there is only a single certificate associated with this entry.

With that in mind, we'll look at the various commands that keytool provides. At present, keytool only has a command-line interface; we'll look at the typical commands that add, modify, list, and delete entries in the keystore.

Global Options to keytool

Keytool implements a number of global options—options that are available to most of its commands. We'll list these as appropriate for each command, but here's an explanation of what they do:

-alias alias

Specify the alias the operation should apply to (e.g., -alias sdo). The default for this value is "mykey."

-dname distinguishedName

Specify the distinguished name. There is no default for this value, and if you do not specify it on the command line, you will be prompted to enter it when it is needed. Letting keytool prompt you is generally easier, since the tool will prompt for the name one field at a time. Otherwise, you must enter the entire name in one quoted string, e.g.:

```
-dname \
"CN=Scott Oaks, OU=SMCC, O=Sun Microsystems, L=New York, S=NY, C=US"
```

-keypass password

> Specify the password used to protect the entire keystore. Access to any element in the keystore requires this global password (programmatically, this is the password that is passed to the `load()` method of the `KeyStore` class). If this password is not provided on the command line, you will be prompted for it. This is generally more secure than typing it on a command line or in a script where others might see it. Passwords must be at least six characters long.

> Note that even though the `KeyStore` class allows you to read entries from the keystore without this password, `keytool` does not.

-keystore filename

> Specify the name of the file that holds the keystore (programmatically, this file will be opened and passed as the input stream argument to the `load()` method of the `KeyStore` class). The default value of this is the *.keystore* file described above.

-storepass password

> Specify the password used to protect a particular entry's private key. This is usually not (and should not be) the same as the global password. There should be a different password for each private key that is specific to that entry. This allows the keystore to be shared among many users. If this password is not provided on the command line, you will be prompted for it, which is generally the more secure way to enter this password.

-v

> Verbose—print some information about the operations `keytool` is performing.

Adding a Certificate Entry

In order to add a certificate entry to the database, you use this command:

-import

> Import a certificate into the database. This command either creates a new certificate entry or imports a certificate for an existing key entry. This command supports the following options:

> *-alias alias*
> *-keypass keypass*
> *-keystore keystore*
> *-storepass storepass*
> *-v*
> *-file inputFile*

>> The file containing the certificate that is being imported. The certificate must be in RFC 1421 format. The default is to read the data from `System.in`.

-noprompt

> Do not prompt the user about whether or not the certificate should be accepted.

When you import a certificate, the information contained in that certificate is printed out; this information includes the distinguished names of the issuer and the principal, and the fingerprint of the certificate. Well-known certificate authorities will publish their fingerprints (on the Web, in trade papers, and elsewhere). It is very important for you to verify the displayed fingerprint with the published fingerprint in order to verify that the certificate does indeed belong to the principal named in the certificate.

Let's say that I have a certificate for the ACME certificate authority in the file *amce.cer*. I can import it with this command:

```
piccolo% keytool -import -alias acme -file acme.cer
Enter keystore password:   ******
Owner: CN=ACME, OU=ACME CA Services, O=ACME Inc., L=New York, S=NY,
C=US
Issuer: CN=ACME, OU=ACME CA Services, O=ACME Inc., L=New York, S=NY,
C=US
Serial Number: 34cbd057
Valid from: Sun Jan 25 18:52:55 EST 1998 until: Sat Apr 25 19:52:55
EDT 1998
Certificate Fingerprints:
    MD5:   51:4E:52:2C:1B:14:38:52:DB:30:5D:46:A9:46:FF:BB
    SHA1:  9F:B2:18:4A:63:8B:F8:EB:A6:A0:56:DB:C7:1B:B3:CC:F5:4B:BA:72
Trust this certificate? [no]:  yes
```

After typing in the command, keytool prints the given names, serial number, and fingerprints, and asks for verification before it actually enters the certificate into the keystore. After receiving a yes answer, the entry is made.

Adding a Key Entry

To add a key entry to the database (that is, an entry containing a private key), use this command:

-genkey

> Generate a key pair and add that entry to the keystore. This command supports these options:
>
> *-alias alias*
> *-dname DN*
> *-keypass keypass*
> *-keystore keystore*

-storepass storepass
-keyalg AlgorithmName

> Use the given algorithm to generate the key pair. For the default Sun security provider, the name must be DSA, which is also the default value for this option. Despite the presence of this option, you cannot really specify another algorithm name, nor, for that matter, can you use a non-Sun DSA provider. Internally, `keytool` expects the key generator to produce keys that belong to a specific class in the sun package.

-keysize keysize

> Use the given keysize to initialize the key pair generator. The default value for this option is 1024. Since the key is a DSA key, the value must be between 512 and 1024 and be a multiple of 64.

-sigalg signatureAlgorithm

> Specify the signature algorithm that will be used to create the self-signed certificate; this defaults to SHA-1/DSA, which is supported by the Sun security provider. Like the key algorithm, this option is not particularly useful at present, since you cannot use your own security provider classes to implement the signature.

-validity nDays

> Specify the number of days for which the self-signed certificate should be valid. The default value for this option is 90 days.

The key entry that is created in this manner has the generated private key. In addition, the public key is placed into a self-signed certificate; that is, a certificate that identitifies the holder of the public key (using the distinguished name argument) and is signed by the holder of the key itself. This is a valid certificate in all senses, although other sites will probably not accept the certificate since it is not signed by a known certificate authority (CA). But the self-signed certificate can be used to obtain a certificate from a CA.

In order to use this self-signed certificate to obtain a certificate from a CA, you must first generate a certificate signing request (CSR). The CSR contains the distinguished name and public key for a particular alias and is signed using the private key of the alias; the CA can then verify that signature and issue a certificate verifying the public key. CSRs are generated with this option:

-csr

> Generate a certificate signing request. This command supports the following options:
>
> *-alias alias*
> *-keypass keypass*
> *-keystore keystore*
> *-storepass storepass*

-*v*

-*sigalg signatureAlgorithm*

> Use the given algorithm to sign the CSR. This option is not presently useful, as the internal design of `keytool` only supports SHA-1/DSA signatures created by the Sun security provider.

-*file outputFile*

> Store the CSR in the given file. The format of the CSR is defined in PKCS#10. The default is to write the CSR to `System.out`.

Once you have the CSR in a file, you must send it to the CA of your choice. Different CAs have different procedures for doing this, but all of them will send you back a certificate they have signed that verifies the public key you have sent to them. There are a few different formats in which the CA will send back a certificate; the only format that is presently supported by `keytool` is RFC 1421 (so you should use a CA that supports this format, of course). You must also use a CA for whom you have a certificate entry (but the CA will often send you its self-signed certificate anyway).

Once you've received the file containing the new certificate, you can import it into the keystore using the `-import` command we discussed previously.

Here's an example of how all these commands can be used to create an entry with a private key and a certified public key. First, we must create the entry:

```
piccolo% keytool -genkey -alias sdo
Enter keystore password:  ******
What is your first and last name?
  [Unknown]:  Scott Oaks
What is the name of your organizational unit?
  [Unknown]:  SMCC
What is the name of your organization?
  [Unknown]:  Sun Microsystems
What is the name of your City or Locality?
  [Unknown]:  New York
What is the name of your State or Province?
  [Unknown]:  NY
What is the two-letter country code for this unit?
  [Unknown]:  US
Is <CN=Scott Oaks, OU=SMCC, O=Sun Microsystems, L=New York, S=NY,
C=US> correct?
  [no]:  yes

Enter key password for <sdo>
        (RETURN if same as keystore password):  ******
```

At this point, we now have an entry for sdo in the keystore. That entry has a self-signed certificate; note that we had the tool prompt us for all the entries that comprise the DN rather than attempting to type it all in on the command line. The next step is to generate the CSR:

```
piccolo% keytool -csr -alias sdo -file sdoCSR.cer
Enter keystore password:  ******
```

The file *sdoCSR.cer* contains the CSR which must now be sent to a CA. Note that we must send the CSR to an authority for whom we already have a certificate entry—that is, for whom we already have a public key. Otherwise, when the response to the CSR comes, we will be unable to verify the signature of the CA that issued the new certificate.

When the response does come, we must save it to a file. If we save it to the file *sdo.cer*, we can import it with this command:

```
piccolo% keytool -import -file sdo.cer -alias sdo
Enter keystore password:  ******
```

Assuming that the certificate is valid, this imports the new certificate into the keystore. The certificate is invalid if the public key for sdo does not match the previously defined public key in the database, or if the certificate was issued by an authority for whom we do not possess a public key, or if the certificate signature is invalid (which would be the case if data in the certificate had been modified in transit).

The state of the sdo entry in the keystore has changed during this example:

- After the first command, the sdo entry has a single certificate; that certificate is issued by sdo.

- After the import command, the sdo entry has two certificates in its certificate chain: the first certificate is issued by Acme and has a principal of sdo; the second certificate is Acme's self-signed certificate (a copy of the one that was imported when the Acme certificate entry was created).

In programmatic terms, the getCertificateChain() method of the KeyStore class will return an array of one and two elements, respectively, for these cases.

Modifying Keystore Entries

There is no practical way to modify a certificate entry in the keystore. You may delete an existing entry and add a new one if required.

There is one command that can modify the data within a key entry:

-selfcert

> Change the certificate chain associated with the target key entry. Any previous certificates (including ones that may have been imported from a valid certificate authority) are deleted and replaced with a new self-signed certificate; this

certificate can be used to generate a new CSR. The public and private keys associated with the alias are unchanged, but you may specify a new value for the DN on the command line. Hence, one use for this command is to change the DN for a particular entry.

This command supports the following options:

-alias alias
-dname DN
-keypass keypass
-keystore keystore
-storepass storepass
-sigalg algorithmName

> Use the given algorithm to generate the signature in the self-signed certificate; as in other cases, this option only supports the DSA algorithm no matter what algorithms may be supported by your security provider.

-validity nDays

> The number of days for which the self-signed certificate is valid. The default is 90 days.

The *-selfcert* command is often used with this command, which can create a copy of the original entry before the DN is changed:

-keyclone

> Clone the target entry. The cloned entry will have the same private key and certificate chain as the original entry. This command supports the following options:

-alias alias
-keypass keypass
-keystore keystore
-storepass storepass
-v
-dest newAlias

> The new alias name of the cloned entry. If this is not specified, you will be prompted for it.

-new newPassword

> The new password for the cloned entry. If this is not specified, you will be prompted for it.

To change the password associated with a particular key entry, use this command:

-keypasswd

> Change the password for the given key entry. This command supports the following options:

-alias alias
-keystore keystore
-storepass storePassword
-keypass originalPassword
-new newPassword

> Specify the new password for the entry. If this option is not supplied, you will be prompted for the new password.

Deleting Keystore Entries

There is a single command to delete either a key entry or a certificate entry:

-delete

> Delete the entry of the specified alias. If a certificate entry for a certificate authority is deleted, there is no effect upon key entries that have been validated by the authority. This command supports the following options:

-alias alias
-keystore keystore
-storepass storepass
-v

Examining Keystore Data

If you want to examine one or more entries in the keystore, you may use the following commands:

-list

> List (to `System.out`) one or more entries in the keystore. If an alias option is given to this command, only that alias will be listed; otherwise, all entries in the keystore are listed. This command supports the following options:

-alias alias
-keystore keystore
-storepass storepass
-v
-rfc

> When displaying certificates, display them in RFC 1421 standard. This option is incompatible with the *-v* option.

-export

> Export the certificate for the given alias to a given file. The certificate is exported in RFC 1421 format. If the target alias is a certificate entry, that certificate is exported. Otherwise, the first certificate in the target key entry's

certificate chain will be exported. This command supports the following options:

-alias alias
-keystore keystore
-storepass storepass
-v
-file outputFile
> The file in which to store the certificate. The default is to write the certificate to `System.out`.

-printcert
> Print out a certificate. The input to this command must be a certificate in RFC 1421 format; this command will display that certificate in readable form so that you may verify its fingerprint. Unlike all other commands, this command does not use the keystore itself, and it requires no keystore passwords to operate. It supports the following options:

-v
-file certificateFile
> The file containing the RFC 1421 format certificate. The default is to read the certificate from `System.in`.

Miscellaneous Commands

There are two remaining commands. The first allows you to change the global password of the keystore:

-storepasswd
> Change the global password of the keystore. This command supports the following options:

-keystore keystore
-storepass storepass
-v
-new newPassword
> The new global password for the keystore. If you do not specify this value, you will be prompted for it.

Finally, you can get a summary of all commands with this command:

-help
> Print out a summary of the usage of `keytool`.

The jarsigner Tool

The next tool we'll look at is the jarsigner tool; this tool creates signed JAR files. The jarsigner tool uses the information in a keystore to look up information about a particular entity and uses that information either to sign or to verify a JAR file. As we discussed in the section on keytool, the keystore that jarsigner uses is subject to the KeyStore class that has been installed into the virtual machine; if you have your own keystore implementation, jarsigner will be able to use it. Similarly, if you use the standard keystore implementation, but hold the keys in a file other than the default *.keystore* file, jarsigner will allow you to use that other file as well.

A signed JAR file is identical to a standard JAR file except that a signed JAR file contains two additional entries:

- *SIGNER.SF*—A file containing an SHA message digest for each class file in the archive. The digest is calculated from the three lines in the manifest for the class file. The base of this name (SIGNER) varies; it is typically based upon the alias of the keystore entry used to sign the archive.

- *SIGNER.DSA*—A file containing the digital signature of the .SF file. The base of this name matches the first part of the .SF file; the extension is the algorithm used to generate the signature. This file also contains the certificate of the entity that signed the archive.

  The algorithm used to generate the signature depends upon the type of the key found in the keystore: if the key is a X509 (DSA) key, a DSA signature will be generated. If the key is an RSA key, an RSA signature will be generated (assuming you have installed a security provider capable of producing such signatures). If you have a keystore that contains other types of keys, jarsigner will be unable to use them to sign the JAR file.

These entries are held in the META-INF directory of the JAR file.

Creating a Signed JAR File

The simplest command to sign a JAR file is:

```
piccolo% jarsigner xyz.jar sdo
```

This command takes the existing JAR file *xyz.jar* and signs it using the private key of the given alias (sdo). The private key is obtained by searching for the given alias from the default keystore (which will be the *.keystore* file in the user.home directory unless a command-line argument is given). The signature files in this example will be named *SDO.SF* and *SDO.DSA* and will be added to the existing JAR file.

A JAR file can be signed by any number of entities simply by executing this command multiple times with different aliases. Each act of signing the JAR file creates a new set of *.SF* and *.DSA* files in the archive.

There are a number of options that can be used in conjunction with this command:

-keystore keystore

Specify the filename that the `KeyStore` class should use as the keystore.

-storepass storepass

Specify the global password that should be used to open the keystore. If this value is not provided, you will be prompted for it (which, as always, is the more secure way to enter a password).

-keypass password

Specify the password for the key entry of the given alias. If this value is not provided, you will be prompted for it.

-sigfile file

Specify the base name to be used for the *.SF* and *.DSA* files. The default for this value is the alias specified on the command line translated to all upper-case letters (e.g., *SDO* in the example above). If the alias name has more than eight letters, only the first eight letters are used. The file argument in this option can only contain uppercase letters, the digits 0–9, and an underscore; it must contain eight or fewer letters.

-signedjar file

Write the signed JAR file to the named file instead of adding the signature entries to the existing JAR file.

-verbose

Print out information as `jarsigner` progresses.

Verifying a JAR File

In the process of verifying a JAR file, `jarsigner` will use the public key of the certificate embedded in the JAR file to verify that the signature is valid. The simplest command to verify a JAR file is:

```
piccolo% jarsigner -verify xyz.jar
jar verified.
```

If the signature in the JAR file is not valid, `jarsigner` will produce this output:

```
jar is unsigned. (signatures missing or not parsable)
```

Verification accepts the following options:

-sigfile file

Use the given base name to look up the *.SF* and *.DSA* files. This option is useful when the JAR file has been signed by multiple entities.

-verbose

Provide verbose output for the verification, indicating for each file if it was signed and whether or not the signer of the file has been found in the keystore. Sample output from this command might appear like this:

```
piccolo% jarsigner -verify -verbose xyz.jar

        402 Mon Jan 26 19:25:52 EST 1998 META-INF/SDO.SF
       1395 Mon Jan 26 19:25:52 EST 1998 META-INF/SDO.DSA
smk     596 Sat Jan 24 22:18:22 EST 1998 XYZKey.class
smk     814 Sat Jan 24 22:17:46 EST 1998 XYZKeyPairGenerator.class
smk    1155 Sat Jan 24 21:56:40 EST 1998 XYZProvider.class
smk     900 Sat Jan 24 22:11:22 EST 1998 XYZSignature.class

  s = signature was verified
  m = entry is listed in manifest
  k = at least one certificate was found in keystore

jar verified.
```

Note the legend for each file that is printed by this command. We know if the file was signed, whether or not it was listed in the JAR file's manifest, and whether or not the signer of the file was found in the keystore.

In the vast majority of cases, the information for each file will be the same: JAR files are usually signed all at once by the same person. However, there's nothing to prevent someone from adding a new class to a signed JAR file (in which case the class would appear as unsigned), or for a JAR file to contain multiple signers (some of whom may have signed some of the classes, while others may have signed only a few of the classes).

In order to determine whether the certificate was found in the keystore, jarsigner opens the default instance of the KeyStore class and loads it. Note that no password is required for this operation. As we mentioned in Chapter 11, reading the public information out of the keystore does not require a password (at least in the Sun implementation of the KeyStore class).

-ids

In conjunction with the -verbose option, print out the distinguished name and alias of the certificate (if any) that is found with each class. With this option, the output for a particular class looks like this:

```
smk     900 Sat Jan 24 22:11:22 EST 1998 XYZSignature.class
```

```
CN=Scott Oaks, OU=SMCC, O=Sun Microsystems, L=NY, S=NY, C=US (sdo)
```

In this case, the class was signed by the given distinguished name; the name of the alias associated with the certificate is shown in parentheses (sdo).

This option has no effect unless the −verbose option is specified.

-keystore keystore

Use the given file as the name of the keystore to load. The default for this option is to use the *.keystore* file in the directory specified by the user.home property. This name is only used for the −verbose option to look up the certificates of the signer.

The policytool

The last security-related tool that comes with the Java platform is policytool. This tool allows you to manage entries in a *java.policy* file. Unlike the other tools we've discussed, policytool is a graphical tool. As such, it has no command-line options or arguments.

When you first start policytool, you see a blank window with two pull-down menus: File and Edit. Initially, there are no policy entries loaded into this tool; if you want to work on an existing policy file, the first thing you must do is choose the Open command from the File menu. Otherwise, you can add new entries and create a new file containing those entries. Whichever method you choose, keep in mind that policytool is designed to operate on a single policy file.

When you've completed editing the entries for a policy file, you can save your changes. Under the File menu, you can use the Save or Save As command to overwrite the file you loaded or to save your changes to a new file.

Managing Policy Codebases

The initial screen for this tool displays the name of the currently loaded policy file (which is blank if no file has been loaded); the name of the keystore referenced within this file; buttons to add, edit, or remove policy entries; and a list of the current set of policy entries. In this context, a policy entry is the URL from which classes will be loaded; that is, a codebase or a code source. Hence, a single policy entry may contain many individual permissions. In Figure A-1 we've loaded the default *java.policy* file, which has one policy entry: an entry that grants permissions to all codebases.

Note that the keystore entry for this file is *.keystore*. You can change that value through an option under the Edit menu.

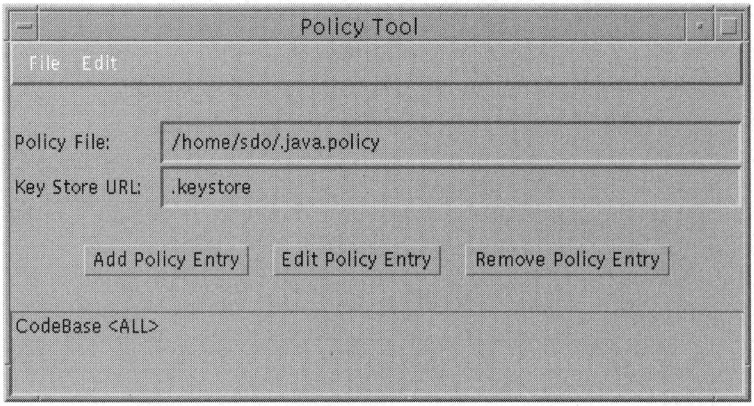

Figure A-1. policytool loaded with one policy entry

You can add new codebases to this file by selecting the Add Policy Entry button; when you add a policy entry, you are allowed to specify a URL and a signer (both of which are optional). The entry for the signer should be an alias in the keystore; if you enter a signer who is not in the keystore, you'll get a warning, but the operation will continue.

You may delete codebases by selecting one and pressing the Remove Policy Entry button. Selecting a codebase and pressing the Edit Policy Entry button allows you to edit the specific set of permissions for a codebase.

Managing Permissions

When you press the Edit Policy Entry button, you get a window similar to that shown in Figure A-2. This window lists all permissions that are associated with the given codebase, and provides the opportunity to add or remove individual permissions.

When you add permissions for a particular codebase, you have the option of adding only a subset of the standard Java permissions: AWT permissions, file permissions, property permissions, net permissions, runtime permissions, and socket permissions. If you have your own permission class (e.g., the XYZPayrollPermission class), you will not be able to add XYZ payroll permissions to the file using policytool. Policytool is designed (at least at present) to work only with the standard set of Java permissions. To add instances of other permission classes—including your own—you need to edit the file manually.

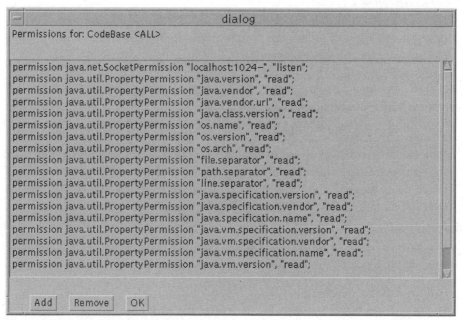

Figure A-2. A set of permissions for a codebase

Managing Certificate Entries

Policytool also allows you to perform some rudimentary operations on the default keystore (again, using whatever KeyStore class implementation has been installed into your Java platform). Under the Edit menu, there are options to add and remove public key aliases. These public key aliases are certificate entries in the keystore. In order to add an alias, you must specify a name for the alias and the name of a file containing a certificate (in RFC 1421 format) to import for that alias; you may remove an alias simply by name.

Files to Administer by Hand

There are two security-related files in the Java platform that must be modified by hand (rather than by a tool). We've talked about these files throughout the book, but for reference, we'll discuss the files and the information they hold.

The java.security File

The *java.security* file must be in the *$JAVAHOME/lib/security* directory. This file is consulted for the following information:

A list of security providers

You may have any number of entries in this file that specify a security provider that should be installed into the virtual machine. By default, there is one security provider specified by this entry:

```
security.provider.1=sun.security.provider.Sun
```

You may specify additional security providers by listing their full class name in this file. Make sure that all security providers are numbered consecutively starting with 1; additional providers can be added before the Sun provider as long as the number assigned to the Sun provider is adjusted accordingly (or the Sun provider could be removed altogether). Remember that this list of providers is consulted when the virtual machine first starts, but that programs with sufficient permissions may add and delete providers from this list.

A KeyStore class implementation

You must have an entry in this file that lists the class that should be used to provide the keystore. By default, that class is listed as:

```
keystore=sun.security.tools.JavaKeyStore
```

If you change the class listed in this entry, the new class will be instantiated whenever a keystore object is required. There can be only one keystore entry in this file.

A Policy class implementation

You must have an entry in this file that lists the class that should be used to provide the implementation of the `Policy` class. By default, that class is listed as:

```
policy.provider=java.security.PolicyFile
```

If you change the class listed in this entry, the new class will be instantiated when the policy object is required (i.e., when the permissions for a given codebase are first used). There can be only one policy entry in this file.

The names of the default policy files

When the default implementation of the `Policy` class reads in permissions, it will read them from the URLs listed as this set of properties:

```
policy.url.1=file:${java.home}/lib/security/java.policy
policy.url.2=file:${user.home}/.java.policy
```

You may specify any number of files in this manner, but the list must start at 1 and be numbered consecutively. The set of permissions will be the aggregate of all permissions found in these URLs.

Remember that these URLs contain only global permissions. You may also specify on the command line a file containing policies with the –usepolicy argument. If the name following the -usepolicy argument begins with an equals sign, the URLs listed in the *java.security* file are ignored:

```
-usepolicy:/globals/java.policy
```

adds the policies in the */globals/java.policy* file to the set of policies in force, but:

```
-usepolicy:=/globals/java.policy
```

sets the policy only to the entries contained in the */globals/java.policy* file. The -usepolicy argument also initializes a security manager for an application, so you may use it by itself if you want to use only the files listed in the *java.security* file.

Other implementations of the `Policy` class may or may not use these properties.

Whether or not property substitution is allowed

The ability to make property substitutions for entries in the *java.security* file or in the *java.policy* file depends on this entry:

```
policy.expandProperties=true
```

Whether or not the -usepolicy argument can be used

The ability to use the -usepolicy argument depends on this entry:

```
policy.allowSystemProperty=true
```

The name of the class to provide X509 certificates

When the `X509Certificate` class is asked to return a certificate (via its `getInstance()` method), it creates an instance of the class named in this property:

```
cert.provider.x509=sun.security.x509.X509CertImpl
```

The name of the class to provide X509 certificate revocation lists

When the `X509CRL` class is asked to return a certificate revocation list (via its `getInstance()` method), it creates an instance of the class named in this property:

```
crl.provider.x509=sun.security.x509.X509CRLImpl
```

The java.policy File

In many cases, you'll use `policytool` to modify the entries in a *java.policy* file (or create a new one). However, if you need to add custom permissions to this file that aren't supported by `policytool`, you must edit it by hand.

The format of the *java.policy* file is as follows:

```
keystore "<keystore_url>";

grant [signedBy "<signer1[, signer2]>"] [codeBase "<URL>"] {
    permission <classname> ["<name>"] [, "<actions>"]
                    [, signedBy "<signer1[, signer2]>"];
    ...
```

```
};
...
```

Items in square brackets are optional. Items in angled brackets are replaced by specific information, e.g., a signer must be a valid alias in the keystore. Within a grant block, there may be any number of permissions, and within a file, there may be any number of grant blocks.

For example, here are some typical entries in the *java.policy* file:

```
grant {
    permission java.util.PropertyPermission "java.version", "read";
}

grant signedBy "sdo", codeBase "http://piccolo/" {
    permission java.io.FilePermission "${/}tmp${/}-", "read, write,
delete";
    permission XYZPayrollPermission "*", "read, write";
}

grant codeBase "http://www.sun.com" {
    permission java.io.FilePermission "${/}tmp${/}-", "read";
    permission java.io.FilePermission "${/}tmp${/}-",
                "read, write, delete", signedBy "sdo";
}
```

In the first block, permission is given to code that comes from any location to access the `java.version` property. The second block grants permissions (including a custom XYZ payroll permission) to any code that is loaded from the site *piccolo* and that is signed by sdo. The third block grants permission to any code that is loaded from *www.sun.com* to read files in the */tmp* directory (or any of its subdirectories); if that code is signed by sdo, it is allowed to read, write, and delete such files.

B

Identity-Based Key Management

In Java 1.1, the primary tool that was used for key management was `javakey`, which is based heavily on the `Identity` and `IdentityScope` classes. The keytool utility that comes with 1.2 is a better way to implement key management, and the `KeyStore` class on which `keytool` is based is definitely more flexible than the classes on which `javakey` is based. In addition, the javakey database uses some classes and interfaces that have been deprecated in 1.2—primarily the `java.security.Certificate` interface. As a result, it is not possible to upgrade a javakey-based identity database to a keystore-based one.

Nonetheless, for developers who are still using 1.1, a key management system based upon the `Identity` and `IdentityScope` classes is the only possible solution. In this appendix, we'll show how these classes can be used for key management. All of the techniques we'll discuss in this appendix have a complementary technique in key management with the `KeyStore` class. In particular, although the `Identity` class is used in certain limited situations in 1.2, the `IdentityScope` class and the identity database that it represents are not needed in 1.2 (as we'll see, it is almost impossible even to use the identity database in 1.2).

Identity Scopes

The database that an identity is held in is an identity scope. There can be multiple identity scopes in a Java program, though typically there is only a system identity scope. By default, the system identity scope for all Java programs is read from a file; this file is the database that `javakey` operates on. But the architecture of an identity scope can be more complex than a single scope.

As Figure B-1 shows, multiple identity scopes can be nested, or they can be disjoint. This is because an identity scope may itself be scoped—that is, just like an identity can belong to a particular scope, an identity scope can belong to another scope.

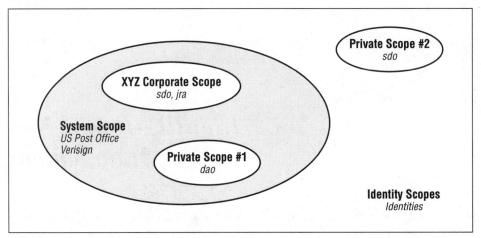

Figure B-1. Identity scopes

This architecture is not as useful as it might seem, since the identity scope class does not give any particular semantics to the notion of a nested identity scope. If you search the system scope in the figure for sdo's identity, you may or may not find it, depending on how the system identity scope is implemented. That's because there's no requirement that an identity scope recursively search its enclosed scopes for any information. And the default identity scope does not do such a recursive search.

This is not to prevent you from writing identity scope classes that use such semantics—indeed, writing such a scope is the goal of this appendix.

The idea of an identity scope, of course, is to hold one or more unique identities. However, possible implementations of an IdentityScope class (java.security.IdentityScope) are conceivably more complicated than that because of the definition of this class:

public abstract class IdentityScope extends Identity
> Implementations of this class are responsible for storing a set of identities and for performing certain operations on those identities.

Hence, an identity scope is also an identity. That means that an identity scope might have a name and a public key, which gives you the ability to model an identity database in very different ways. Conceivably, you might want an identity scope for an organization that contains all the identities of individuals within that organization. Rather than having a separate identity for the organization itself, the organization's identity can be subsumed by the identity scope. Since the organization itself also needs a name and a public key, this type of model might offer some flexibility over the alternative: a model that just has a list of identities, some of which are individuals and one of which is the organization.

However, we'll ignore that possibility for now, and just explore the identity scope class with a view to its simplest use: as a holder of one or more identities.

Using the IdentityScope Class

The IdentityScope class is an abstract class, and there are no classes in the core JDK that extend the IdentityScope class. Like other classes in the security package, instances of it may be retrieved by a static method (albeit with a different name than we've been led to expect):

public static IdentityScope getSystemScope()
> Return the default identity scope provided by the virtual machine. For javakey, this is the identity scope held in the *identitydb.obj* file in the user's home directory (or an alternate file specified in the *java.security* property file).

Once you have retrieved the system's default scope (or any other identity scope), you can operate on it with the following methods:

public abstract int size()
> Return the number of identities that are held in this scope. By default, this does not include the number of nested identities in other scopes that are held in this scope.

public abstract Identity getIdentity(String name)
> Return the identity object associated with the corresponding name.

public abstract Identity getIdentity(Principal principal)
> Using the principal's name, return the identity object associated with the corresponding principal.

public abstract Identity getIdentity(PublicKey key)
> Return the identity object associated with the corresponding public key.

public abstract void addIdentity(Identity identity)
> Add the given identity to this identity scope. A KeyManagementException is thrown if the identity has the same name or public key as another identity in this scope.

public abstract void removeIdentity(Identity identity)
> Remove the given identity from this identity scope. A KeyManagementException is thrown if the identity is not present in this scope.

public abstract Enumeration identities()
> Return an enumeration of all the identities in this scope.

For the most part, using these methods is straightforward. For example, to list all the identities in the default identity database, we need only find the system identity scope and enumerate it:

```
public class Test {
    public static void main(String args[]) {
        try {
            IdentityScope is = IdentityScope.getSystemScope();
            System.out.println(is);
            Enumeration e = is.identities();
            while (e.hasMoreElements()) {
                Identity id = (Identity) e.nextElement();
                System.out.println(id);
            }
        } catch (Exception ex) {}
    }
}
```

There is one exception to this idea of simplicity, however. An identity scope is typically persistent—the javakey database is in a local persistent file, and you could write your own scope that was saved in a file, a database, or some other storage. However, you'll notice that there are no methods in the IdentityScope class that allow you to save the database for a particular scope. Hence, we could add a new identity to the system identity scope like this:

```
IdentityScope is = IdentityScope.getSystemScope();
Identity me = somehowCreateIdentity("sdo");
try {
    is.addIdentity(me);
} catch (KeyManagementException kme) {}
```

That adds an sdo identity to the system identity scope for the current execution of the virtual machine, but unless we can somehow save that scope to the *identitydb.obj* file, the sdo identity will be lost when we exit the virtual machine. Unfortunately, there are no public methods to save the identity scope.

As an aside, we'll note that the *identitydb.obj* file just happens to be the serialized version of an IdentityScope object—to save the database, we need only open an ObjectOutputStream and write the is instance variable to that output stream. Changes in the definition of the Identity class between 1.1 and 1.2, however, make this database incompatible between these releases: you cannot deserialize a 1.1-based identity scope object in a 1.2 program.

There's another point here that we must mention: the JDK's notion of the system identity scope expects to hold identity objects that are instances of a particular class that exists only in the sun package. This means that we can't actually write a fully correct somehowCreateIdentity() method—we can create identities, but they will not be of the exact class that the system identity scope expects. This can affect some of the operations of the javakey database, since some of those operations are dependent on properties of the Sun implementation of an identity that are not in the generic idea of an identity. When we write our own identity-based database at the end of this appendix, that will no longer be a problem (but we won't be able to use the javakey utility on that database, either).

Writing an Identity Scope

We'll now implement our own identity scope, which will be one of the classes that we'll use at the end of this appendix to put together an identity-based key management database. We'll write a generic identity scope that implements the notion that its identities are held in a file:

```
public class XYZFileScope extends IdentityScope {
    private Hashtable ids;
    private static String fname;

    public XYZFileScope(String fname) throws KeyManagementException {
        super("XYZFileScope");
        this.fname = fname;
        try {
            FileInputStream fis = new FileInputStream(fname);
            ObjectInputStream ois = new ObjectInputStream(fis);
            ids = (Hashtable) ois.readObject();
        } catch (FileNotFoundException fnfe) {
            ids = new Hashtable();
        } catch (Exception e) {
            throw new KeyManagementException(
                        "Can't load identity database " + fname);
        }
    }

    public int size() {
        return ids.size();
    }

    public Identity getIdentity(String name) {
        Identity id;
        id = (Identity) ids.get(name);
        return id;
    }

    public Identity getIdentity(PublicKey key) {
        if (key == null)
            return null;
        Identity id;
        for (Enumeration e = ids.elements(); e.hasMoreElements(); ) {
            id = (Identity) e.nextElement();
```

```
            PublicKey k = id.getPublicKey();
            if (k != null && k.equals(key))
                return id;
        }
        return null;
    }

    public void addIdentity(Identity identity)
                        throws KeyManagementException {
        String name = identity.getName();
        if (getIdentity(name) != null)
            throw new KeyManagementException(
                        name + " already in identity scope");

        PublicKey k = identity.getPublicKey();
        if (getIdentity(k) != null)
            throw new KeyManagementException(
                        name + " already in identity scope");
        ids.put(name, identity);
    }

    public void removeIdentity(Identity identity)
                            throws KeyManagementException {
        String name = identity.getName();
        if (ids.get(name) == null)
            throw new KeyManagementException(
                        name + " isn't in the identity scope");
        ids.remove(name);
    }

    public Enumeration identities() {
        return ids.elements();
    }

    public void save() {
        try {
            FileOutputStream fos = new FileOutputStream(fname);
            ObjectOutputStream oos = new ObjectOutputStream(fos);
            oos.writeObject(ids);
        } catch (Exception e) {
            System.out.println(e);
            throw new RuntimeException("Can't save id database");
        }
    }
}
```

Let's delve into the implementation of this class. First, there are two instance variables. The ids variable will hold the identities themselves; we've decided to hold the identities in a hashtable so that we can easily search them based on a key. That key will be their name, which makes locating identities in this scope by name very easy (but notice that locating them by public key is harder). The second variable, fname, is the name of the file that will hold the persistent copy of this identity scope.

There are three constructors in the IdentityScope class that are available to us:

protected IdentityScope()
> Construct an unnamed identity scope. This constructor is not designed to be used by programmers; it is provided only so that an identity scope may be subject to object serialization.

public IdentityScope(String name)
public IdentityScope(String name, IdentityScope scope)
> Construct an identity scope with the given name. If an identity scope is speci-fied, the new identity scope will be scoped within the specified scope; otherwise, the new identity scope will have no scope associated with it (like Private Scope #2 in figure Figure B-1). A KeyManagementException will be thrown if an identity or identity scope with the desired name already exists in the given scope.

In our case, we've chosen only to provide our identity scope with a name. After calling the appropriate superclass constructor, our class opens up the stored version of the identity database and reads it in. Like the default javakey imple-mentation, we've chosen the simple expedient of object serialization to a persistent file to provide our storage. If the file isn't found, we create an empty identity scope.

We've provided a simple save() method that serializes the private database out to the same file that we read it in from; this method has a package protection so that it will only be accessible by the code we develop. The remaining methods in our class are all methods we are required to implement, because they are methods that are abstract in our superclass. Because we're storing identities in a hashtable, their implementations are usually simple:

- The size() method can simply return the size of the hashtable.

- The getIdentity(name) method can simply use the name as the lookup key into the hashtable.

- The getIdentity(key) method is the most complex method, although only slightly: it merely needs to enumerate the identities and test each one individ-ually to see if the keys match.

- The addIdentity() method can search to make sure that the name and pub-lic key of the new identity are unique and then simply store the identity into the hashtable with the name as its key.

- The `removeIdentity()` method can just tell the hashtable to remove the identity with the appropriate key.

- The `identities()` method can just return the hashtable enumeration.

There is one remaining protected method of the `IdentityScope` class:

protected static void setSystemScope(IdentityScope scope)
    Set the system identity scope to be the given scope.

We haven't used this method in this example, but it is one that we'll rely on later when we extend this example. This method replaces the system identity database. Replacing the system database makes things easier for developers. When developers need to operate on identities, they expect to access those identities through the system database. Now that our class is the system database, we can return identities whether they exist in the user's private key database or in the shared public key database.

IdentityScope and the Security Manager

Like the `Identity` class, the `IdentityScope` class uses the `checkSecurityAccess()` method of the security manager to protect many of its operations from being performed by untrusted classes. This method is called by the `setSystemScope()` method (with an argument of "set.system.scope" in 1.1 and an argument of "IdentityScope.setSystemScope" in 1.2); no other methods of the `IdentityScope` class call this method by default.

However, in the default identity scope implemented in the sun package in 1.1, in the following situations, these methods call the `checkSecurityAccess()` method with the given string:

- When the `getIdentity()` method would return a signer—that is, an identity that has a private key ("get.signer")

- When the `addIdentity()` and `removeIdentity()` methods are called ("add.identity" and "remove.identity", respectively)

- When the database is written to a file via object serialization ("serialize.identity.database")

When we implemented the abstract methods of our `IdentityScope` class, we probably should have made the decision to let the security manager override the ability of an untrusted (or other) class to perform these operations. Hence, a better implementation of the `getIdentity()` method would be:

```
public Identity getIdentity(String name) {
    Identity id;
    id = (Identity) ids.get(name);
```

```
        if (id instanceof Signer) {
            SecurityManager sec = System.getSecurityManager();
            if (sec != null)
                sec.checkSecurityAccess("get.signer");
        }
        return id;
    }
```

Key Management in an Identity Scope

We're now going to put together the identity scope with the information about the identity class we touched upon in Chapter 11 to produce another key management system. One of the primary limitations of the default identity scope is that it's based upon a single file. If you're in a corporation, you may want to have an identity scope that encompasses the public keys of every employee in the corporation—but you can't afford to put the private keys of the employees in that database. Every employee needs read access to the database to obtain his or her own key; there's no practical way with a single identity scope to prevent these users from reading each other's private keys.

Hence, in this example, we're going to develop an identity scope that provides for the architecture shown in Figure B-2.

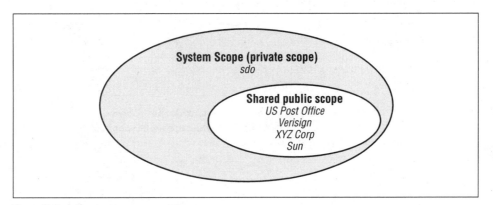

Figure B-2. A key management architecture

There are two simple goals to this example:

- There should be a central database (identity scope) managed by the system administrators of the XYZ Corporation. This database will hold the public keys of all identities that are used in the system, along with a security level that is assigned to each identity.

- Each user should have a private database that holds the user's private key. The user's private key will be certified by the XYZ Corporation itself, so this private database will need to have the public key of the XYZ Corporation. We'll make this scope the system scope so that it can encapsulate the knowledge that there are two scopes in use; to a program, it will appear as only a single scope.

This architecture allows a program to access the user's private key, but not anyone else's private key; it also allows the corporation to set security policies for classes that are signed by particular entities.

There's a certain schizophrenic approach that a system administrator must take in order to use a system like the one we're describing here. Many of the operations that are provided by javakey cannot be duplicated by a standard Java program. Hence, we must always rely on javakey to perform certain operations (like importing a 1.1-based certificate), and then we need to convert from the javakey database to our own database.

We must implement three classes for this example: an identity class, a signer class, and a shared identity scope class (which will be based upon the XYZFileScope class that we showed above).

Implementing an Identity Class

First, let's look at an implementation of the identity class:

```
public class XYZIdentity extends Identity {
    private int trustLevel;

    protected XYZIdentity() {
    }

    public XYZIdentity(String name, IdentityScope scope)
                            throws KeyManagementException {
        super(name, scope);
        scope.addIdentity(this);
        trustLevel = 0;
    }

    public void setPublicKey(PublicKey key)
                            throws KeyManagementException {
        IdentityScope is = getScope();
        Identity i = is.getIdentity(key);
        if (i != null && !equals(i))
            throw new KeyManagementException("Duplicate public key");
        super.setPublicKey(key);
    }

    public void addCertificate(Certificate cert)
                            throws KeyManagementException {
```

```
        Identity i = getScope().getIdentity(cert.getPublicKey());
        if (i != null && !equals(i))
            throw new KeyManagementException("Duplicate public key");
        super.addCertificate(cert);
    }

    public int getTrust() {
        return trustLevel;
    }

    void setTrust(int x) {
        if (x < 0 || x > 10)
            throw new IllegalArgumentException("Invalid trust level");
        trustLevel = x;
    }

    public String toString() {
        return super.toString() + " trust level: " + trustLevel;
    }
}
```

We've chosen in this class to ensure that an identity always belongs to a scope and so we only provided one constructor. There's a somewhat confusing point here, however. Constructing an identity as part of a scope does not automatically add that identity to the scope. That logic is required either in the constructor (as we've done), or the design of the class will require that the developer using the class explicitly assigns the identity to the scope later. The former case is probably more useful; make sure to assign your identities inside their constructors.

Other than the constructor, we're not required to implement any other methods in our identity class. However, we've chosen to override the setPublicKey() and addCertificate() methods so that those methods throw an exception when an identity is to be assigned a public key that already exists in the identity scope. You'll recall that when we first introduced the Identity class, we mentioned that this logic was not present. Adding that logic is a simple matter of checking to see if the public key in question is already in the identity scope.

Finally, we've introduced a variable in our identity to determine the level of trust that we place in this identity. This is similar to the binary option that javakey gives us as to whether an identity is trusted or not; in our version, we allow the identity to have a level of trust. A trust level of 3 might indicate that the identity is fully trusted and hence should have access to all files; a level of 2 might indicate that the identity should be allowed access only to files in the user's temporary directory; a level of 1 might indicate that the identity should never be allowed to access a local file. The point is, the notion of trust associated with an identity is completely up to the programmer to decide—you're free to assign whatever semantics you like for this (or any other value), or to dispense with such an idea altogether. The idea behind this variable is that the security manager might use it (or other such information) to determine an appropriate security policy.

Implementing a Signer Class

Implementing the Signer class that we require follows virtually the same process:

```java
public class XYZSigner extends Signer {
    private int trustLevel;

    public XYZSigner(String name, IdentityScope scope)
                                throws KeyManagementException {
        super(name, scope);
        scope.addIdentity(this);
    }

    public void setPublicKey(PublicKey key)
                                throws KeyManagementException {
        IdentityScope scope = getScope();
        if (scope != null) {
            Identity i = getScope().getIdentity(key);
            if (i != null && !equals(i))
                throw new KeyManagementException(
                            "Duplicate public key");
        }
        super.setPublicKey(key);
    }

    public void addCertificate(Certificate cert)
                                throws KeyManagementException {
        IdentityScope scope = getScope();
        if (scope != null) {
            Identity i = getScope().getIdentity(cert.getPublicKey());
            if (i != null && !equals(i))
                throw new KeyManagementException(
                            "Duplicate public key");
        }
        super.addCertificate(cert);
    }

    public int getTrust() {
        return trustLevel;
    }

    void setTrust(int x) {
        if (x < 0 || x > 10)
            throw new IllegalArgumentException("Invalid trust level");
        trustLevel = x;
    }
```

```
    public String toString() {
        return super.toString() + " trust level: " + trustLevel;
    }
}
```

We do not need to provide an overridden method for the setKeyPair() method of the Signer class to ensure that a duplicate private key is not inserted into the identity scope. Since we can only insert a private key with a public key, and since there is a one-to-one correspondence between such keys, we know that if the public keys are unique, the private keys are unique as well.

A Shared System Identity Scope

In the architecture we're examining, there are two identity scopes:

- The private scope. This scope will hold one and only one instance of XYZ-Signer. This signer will represent the user who owns that particular database.

- The public scope. This scope will hold several instances of XYZIdentity, but no signers—since it is to be shared, we don't want it to contain any private keys.

Each of these scopes will be an instance of the XYZFileScope that we showed earlier. To combine them, we'll create another identity scope that holds a reference to both scopes:

```
public class XYZIdentityScope extends IdentityScope {
    private transient IdentityScope publicScope;
    private transient IdentityScope privateScope;

    public XYZIdentityScope() throws KeyManagementException {
        super("XYZIdentityScope");
        privateScope = new XYZFileScope("/floppy/floppy0/private");
        publicScope = new XYZFileScope("/auto/shared/sharedScope");
        setSystemScope(this);
    }

    public int size() {
        return publicScope.size() + privateScope.size();
    }

    public Identity getIdentity(String name) {
        Identity id;
        id = privateScope.getIdentity(name);
        if (id == null)
            id = publicScope.getIdentity(name);
        return id;
    }
```

```java
public Identity getIdentity(PublicKey key) {
    Identity id;
    id = privateScope.getIdentity(key);
    if (id == null)
        id = publicScope.getIdentity(key);
    return id;
}

public void addIdentity(Identity identity)
                            throws KeyManagementException {
    throw new KeyManagementException(
            "This scope does not support adding identities");
}

public void removeIdentity(Identity identity)
                            throws KeyManagementException {
    throw new KeyManagementException(
            "This scope does not support removing identities");
}

class XYZIdentityScopeEnumerator implements Enumeration {
    private boolean donePrivate = false;
    Enumeration pubEnum = null, privEnum = null;

    XYZIdentityScopeEnumerator() {
        pubEnum = publicScope.identities();
        privEnum = privateScope.identities();
        if (!privEnum.hasMoreElements())
            donePrivate = true;
    }

    public boolean hasMoreElements() {
        return pubEnum.hasMoreElements() ||
                privEnum.hasMoreElements();
    }

    public Object nextElement() {
        Object o = null;
        if (!donePrivate) {
            o = privEnum.nextElement();
            if (!privEnum.hasMoreElements())
                donePrivate = true;
        }
        else o = pubEnum.nextElement();
        if (o == null)
            throw new NoSuchElementException(
                    "XYZIdentityScopeEnumerator");
        return o;
    }
```

```
    }

    public Enumeration identities() {
        return new XYZIdentityScopeEnumerator();
    }
}
```

The idea behind this class is that it is going to hold identities containing private keys, and that those private keys should be held somewhere safe. For this example, we're assuming that the private identity scope database will be stored on a floppy disk somewhere—that way, a user can move the identity scope around with her, and the private key won't be left on a disk where some malicious person might attempt to retrieve it.

This class is completely tailored to a Solaris machine, since we've hardwired the name of the private file to a file on the default floppy drive of a Solaris machine, and we've hardwired the name of the public file to a file that can be automounted on the user's machine. On other machines, the name of the floppy drive will vary, and a complete implementation of this class would really require that filename to be a property. The property can be set to the appropriate value for the hardware on which the Java virtual machine is running. The public database probably shouldn't even be a file; it should be held on a remote machine somewhere and accessed via RMI or another technique. We'll leave those enhancements as an exercise for the reader.

Now that we have the two scopes we're interested in, completing the implementation is a simple matter of:

- Setting this identity scope to be the system identity scope. This allows the developer to use the standard methods we've already seen to extract information from this scope.

- Overriding the getIdentity() and identities() methods so that they operate on both included identity scopes. Remember that often identity scopes are disjoint; in this case, however, it makes sense for there to be a single interface to the two identity scopes.

- Overriding the addIdentity() and removeIdentity() methods to prevent them from changing the underlying identity databases. We'll see how to manipulate the individual database in the next section.

Creating Identities

The XYZ Corporation is concerned about two sorts of identities: identities from corporations and individuals outside the corporation, and identities of employees. The latter must all have private keys in order for the employees to be able to sign documents and will be instances of the XYZSigner class; the former need only public keys and will be instances of the XYZIdentity class.

In order to create these identities, we're going to rely on the facilities provided by javakey to do the bulk of the work for us, then we're going to read the generic entity out of the javakey database and turn it into an XYZ-based entity. This allows us to import or create certificates for these identities, which is something that only javakey can do in Java 1.1.

When a new employee comes to the XYZ Corporation, we must generate a private identity database for that employee on a floppy that can be given to the employee. As a first step, however, we must create the employee in a standard javakey database so that the employee can be given a certificate to accompany her identity. Once we've got the employee into the javakey database, here's the code we use to convert the javakey entry into the XYZIdentityScope we just examined:

```
public class NewEmployee {
    public static void main(String args[]) {
        try {
            IdentityScope is = IdentityScope.getSystemScope();
            Signer origSigner = (Signer) is.getIdentity(args[0]);

            System.out.println(
                    "Please insert the floppy for " + args[0]);
            System.out.print("Press enter when ready:  ");
            System.in.read();
            XYZFileScope privateScope =
                    new XYZFileScope("/floppy/floppy0/private");
            XYZSigner newSigner = new XYZSigner(args[0], privateScope);
            KeyPair kp = new KeyPair(origSigner.getPublicKey(),
                                    origSigner.getPrivateKey());
            newSigner.setKeyPair(kp);
            newSigner.setInfo(origSigner.getInfo());
            Certificate certs[] = origSigner.certificates();
            for (int i = 0; i < certs.length; i++)
                newSigner.addCertificate(certs[i]);
            newSigner.setTrust(Integer.parseInt(args[1]));
            privateScope.save();

            XYZFileScope sharedScope =
                    new XYZFileScope("/auto/shared/sharedScope");
            XYZIdentity newId = new XYZIdentity(args[0], sharedScope);
            newId.setPublicKey(origSigner.getPublicKey());
            newId.setInfo(origSigner.getInfo());
            certs = origSigner.certificates();
            for (int i = 0; i < certs.length; i++)
                newId.addCertificate(certs[i]);
            newId.setTrust(Integer.parseInt(args[1]));
```

```
            sharedScope.save();
        } catch (Exception e) {
            System.out.println(e);
        }
    }
}
```

This program is then run with the name of the employee as an argument. When the program is run, two things happen:

1. The correct private key database is created and written to the floppy. The private key database has the signing identity of the new employee loaded into it.

2. The shared public database is opened, and the identity of the new employee is added to it.

In both cases, it was necessary to read the existing data out of the entity read from the javakey database and convert that data into an XYZ-based class. We could have used the existing object (a subclass of the Identity or Signer class), but that would not have allowed us to associate a level of trust with these entities in our database. After the program has run, both databases have the desired entity, with the desired set of keys.

When the system administrator for the XYZ Corporation receives a public key (and a certificate) for an entity that is not going to be a signer within the XYZ Corporation, a similar procedure would need to be followed to enter the certificate into the javakey database, and then extract out the new identity and update only the shared identity scope. Code to do that would be very similar to the code shown above.

Summary

In this appendix, we've shown an example of an identity-based key management system. Such a system is the only choice for key management for developers in Java 1.1. In the realm of Java 1.2, such a system is fairly limited: the keystore-based key management systems are more flexible and are better integrated into the Java API.

The identity-based key management system does have one advantage: it allows the retrieval of identity objects from the database, while the keystore-based system only allows for retrieval of keys and certificates. This means that an identity-based system can embed within it other information about an entity (including, for example, a level of trust associated with that individual); this other information is available to users of the database in a straightforward way.

C

Security Resources

Books are very useful for learning some things, and hopefully you've gotten some benefit from the one you're holding in your hand. However, for some types of information, the Internet remains the better choice. In this appendix, we'll list and discuss various network resources that relate to Java and security.

One reason why this information is better found on the Internet is because it is subject to rapid change. The APIs we've discussed may remain fairly stable (despite the big changes in many of them between 1.1 and 1.2), but the information to be found in these resources is more dynamic.

Security Bugs

Early in my computer science career, I handed in an exam that ended up receiving a lower grade than I had expected.* As part of the exam, I was asked to write an algorithm, prove that it was correct, and then provide an implementation of the algorithm.

While my algorithm and its accompanying proof were completely correct, my implementation received a failing grade. This was a rather dispiriting result: I had come up with a solution and proved that the solution was correct. But the "real" solution—the implementation—was still flawed.

Such is the potential problem with implementing a security model. A lot of design and analysis has gone into Java's default security model, and hopefully you'll put your own effort into making your own applications secure. But no matter how sound the design of a security model, in the end it is the implementation that matters.

---

* Okay, that was not an unusual event for me...

In this section, we'll discuss some past bugs in Java's security implementation and list some common resources for finding out about and fixing present bugs.

Few issues in the Java world receive more attention than security bugs; report of a new bug is guaranteed to produce a flurry of activity. As a result, readers of the trade press often have the idea that Java is riddled with security bugs, or that it isn't secure to begin with. This is not the case. While some important bugs in Java's security implementation have been reported, the impact of these bugs has (at least until now) been minimal.

Bugs that are reported against Java's security model fall into one of five categories:

1. Reports that are not bugs, but that arise from a lack of understanding of Java's security model

   There are two types of very common bugs in this category: applets that perform annoying tasks, and applets that seem to break out of the sandbox. The former category includes applets that take lots of CPU time or otherwise consume many resources. As we mentioned at the outset of this book, such attacks are annoying but are not security attacks.

   The latter category often involves bugs that hinge upon someone having installed a local class file (or worse, a local native library); as we know by now, these local class files are treated as trusted classes. When one of these local classes is able to read (or remove) files on your disk, contact a machine on your local network, or engage in some other potentially malicious behavior, word goes out that Java is not secure, or at best has bugs in its security model.

   The lesson to learn from these reports is this: no computer security model is a substitute for vigilant practices by the end user. If your policy is never to run shareware programs downloaded from the Internet, then your policy should be never to install local classes on your system. And while newer versions of browsers, along with the ability in 1.2 to run applications in a secure environment, help to mitigate the potential danger of installing a local class file, such features will never obviate the need for users and system administrators to understand and work with the security model. There may be real bugs in the Java implementation—but don't assume that all reports you hear about the sandbox being broken fall into that category.

2. Bugs that are misclassified; that is, actual bugs that are reported as being security bugs when they are not

   As we've seen, security is pervasive in the Java platform—the bytecode verifier, the class loader, the security manager, and the compiler all have aspects of security to them. Hence, bugs in these areas are often considered security bugs even when they are not. For example, a bug in the bytecode verifier is usually assumed to be a security bug, even if it is not; if the verifier doesn't accept a particular construct that it should accept, for example, no security concerns arise.

3. Web-related bugs that are not Java-specific

Often, security problems on the Internet are associated with Java without any direct cause. In particular, bugs related to JavaScript™ and to ActiveX often fall into this category.

When the first reports of ActiveX security bugs were circulated, there was a lot of discussion about "active content"; the assertion in many quarters was that the security problems that plagued ActiveX were inherent in any active content system. This assertion attempted to place Java in the same light as ActiveX since both were active content systems. The reality is that Java and ActiveX have very different security models.

Similarly, bugs about JavaScript are often confused with bugs about Java, in part because of the name. It is probably well known by this point, but it doesn't hurt to reiterate: JavaScript and Java are completely different technologies produced by separate companies (Netscape and Sun, respectively). The two technologies are complementary in many ways, but they are fundamentally different from a security perspective.

Finally, Java is not immune to security problems that plague the Web in general. Data that is sent between sites among Java applets and servers can be snooped just like data that is sent via HTTP can be snooped (unless the Java traffic is using SSL or another encryption technique). A hacker that sets up a site to impersonate *XYZ.com* will be able to serve Java applets just as it is able to serve HTML.

4. Bugs in third-party trusted classes

When you install third-party classes, it is possible that one of them may breach the security model that you think is in place: it may provide a mechanism for an untrusted class to open a file, for example, based upon the permissions normally given to the third-party class.

Complicating this factor is the manner in which these classes are often installed: they are often put into a directory and the user's CLASSPATH is globally set to include those classes. Now untrusted classes will be able to access the third-party classes.

5. Bugs in the Java implementation

There have been several well-publicized bugs that do involve Java's security implementation; as with any large computer system, there are bound to be others.

This last point should not minimized—there have been and will be bugs in the Java security implementation. But the potential for bugs and their potential impact must be weighed against the potential benefits of using Java. I know of one corporation where Java is not allowed to be used for any internal project. This site is not worried about employees doing malicious things to other employees, and they filter out Java class files at their corporate firewall, but developers at this company are still not permitted to use Java for any internal project due to security concerns.

When I asked about this policy, I was told that this corporation had "zero-tolerance" for security problems, and the mere risk of a Java security bug was enough for them to forbid the use of Java. Of course, this site that had zero-tolerance for security problems had a floppy disk drive on every one of their desktop computers, and users routinely took files to and from the office via floppy disks. The potential for a virus being spread by floppy disk drive (which is very real) was outweighed for them by the benefit of their users doing work at home. Meanwhile, the thought that Java would somehow spontaneously corrupt their isolated network was, for them, enough to outweigh any of the potential benefits they saw to using Java within their extremely distributed, heterogeneous network. Assessing the security of a platform always involves assessing the potential risks and the potential rewards, though apparently that is sometimes hard to do.

Java Security Bugs

One of the ways to assess the potential impact of Java security bugs is to understand the bugs that have occurred to date and their relative impact. The fact that all these bugs have been fairly minor and quickly fixed is of some comfort. That is not to say that a future bug won't be more devastating or harder to fix; the point here is really to shed light on the bugs that have been found.

The bugs we'll discuss in this section all have another property: attacks based on these bugs were very hard to construct. In fact, attacks based on these bugs never made it out onto the Internet or other networks; the bugs were all reported by various researchers, and often even the researchers had difficulty in constructing an attack against them.

Here's a chronology of security bugs that have been found in Java through March 1998:

DNS spoofing

    In February 1996, the first Java security bug was posted. It involved a DNS spoofing scenario in which an applet could make a connection to a third-party host other than the one from which it was loaded. Such an attack required access by the attacker to a DNS server that was used by the user and knowledge of the IP address of the third-party machine. DNS spoofing is a general problem (i.e., this bug falls into category 3 in our above list), but Java was fixed in 1.0.1 to circumvent this scenario.

Class loader implementation bug

In March 1996, a bug was found that allowed an applet to load a class referenced by an absolute pathname. This bug was fixed in 1.0.1.

Verifier implementation bug

In March 1996, a bug was discovered that took advantage of an implementation error in the bytecode verifier. An attack via this bug needed to be very sophisticated, but it did allow the applet to perform any operation (delete a file, write a file, etc.) on the user's machine. This bug was fixed in 1.0.2.

URL name resolution attack

In April 1996, a bug related to an obscure network configuration was reported. This bug required that the user's machine be running in a DNS domain that it was not registered to and that the attacker's machine be running in that same DNS domain. This bug was fixed in 1.0.2.

Class loader bug

In May 1996, a bug in the class loader was discovered that allowed two applets loaded in different class loaders to exploit a way of casting between different classes with the same distinct name. This bug was fixed in 1.1.

Verifier implementation bug

In March 1997, Sun discovered a bug in the implementation of the verifier. Exploiting this bug would have required knowledge of the bug itself as well as writing Java bytecodes by hand. This bug was fixed in 1.1.1.

Class signing bug

A bug in the getSigners() method of the Class class was discovered in April 1997. This bug allowed code signed by one entity to be treated as if were signed by a different entity (possibly with more access to the user's machine). This bug was fixed in 1.1.2.

Verifier implementation bug

A bug that could allow the VM to crash in the bytecode verifier was discovered in May 1997; this bug was fixed in 1.1.2.

Illegal type casting

A bug related to illegal type casting was reported in June 1996. This bug allowed an applet to undermine the typing system of Java. This bug was fixed in 1.1.3.

Tracking Security Bugs

The nature of tracking security bugs makes it impossible to track them through a book such as this; we're sure that the above list is already out of date. Hence, the better way to track security issues with Java's implementation is to check periodically the following resources on the Web.

An important point to realize about these sites and the bugs we've just listed is that much of the research on security implementation bugs occurs outside of Sun. Sun's approach to Java security is to achieve security by openness—that is, the more people who can examine the platform for implementation bugs, the better that implementation will become. This is one reason why the JDK source code is freely available for noncommercial purposes.

http://java.sun.com/sfaq/chronology.html
> This page lists the known bugs in the security implementation (the above list was culled from this page). New bugs and their fixes are reported here first.

http://www.cert.org/
> The CERT organization tracks security-related bugs for all types of computer systems, including Java implementations. Java-related security bugs are often published as CERT advisories.

http://www.cs.princeton.edu/sip/
> Many of the bugs in Java's security implementation have been discovered as a result of work done at Princeton's Security Internet Programming (SIP) group. This page summarizes their work, including several of the bugs that were listed above.
>
> Work at SIP is funded by many companies, including Sun itself.

news://comp.security.announce
> This newsgroup tracks security-related announcements about all systems, including Java.

http://kimera.cs.washington.edu/
> This research group is also responsible for finding some of the bugs that were listed above.

http://www.alw.nih.gov/Security/security-advisories.html
> This site has links to several services that publish advisories when Java (and other) security-related bugs are discovered.

Third-Party Security Providers

There is an increasing number of third-party security providers for both the standard Java Cryptography Architecture and for the Java Cryptography Extension. A partial list of these security providers follows. Note that most of them are based outside the United States. As we discussed in Chapter 13, this frees some restrictions and places other restrictions upon their use: the non-U.S. implementations of the JCE are freed from the export restrictions of the U.S. government (but may still be subject to other export and import restrictions). However, these packages may be subject to patent restrictions—especially within the United States if they include RSA or RC4 forms of cryptography (even if the package originated outside the United States), and within the U.S. and Europe if they include IDEA encryption.

The following list is not exclusive: new providers will certainly have been written in the time this book has been published, and the algorithms provided by each entry in the list are subject to change. In addition to the listed engines, these packages will all provide the necessary key classes and engines to support the algorithms in the package.

- Baltimore Technologies (*http://www.baltimore.ie/jcrypto.htm*)

  The J/Crypto product of Baltimore Technologies in Ireland furnishes a security provider for the standard JCA that includes implementations of the following engines:

  Message digests: MD5 and SHA
  Digital signatures: DSA and RSA/SHA

  In addition, J/Crypto provides a JCE-compatible replacement that includes the following engines:

  Cipher: DES, DESede, RSA, RC4, PBE
  Key agreement: Diffie-Hellman

- IAIK-JCE (*http://kopernikus.iaik.tu-graz.ac.at/JavaSecurity/index.htm*)

  This package from the Institute for Applied Information Processing and Communications in Austria (IAIK) comes with a security provider that performs the following:

  Digital signatures: RSA/MD5 and RSA/SHA
  Message digests: MD5 and SHA
  Certificate and CRL classes: X509

  While IAIK must be purchased for commercial use, it is free for noncommercial use.

  IAIK also provides a JCE-compatible replacement that includes the following engines:

  Cipher: DES, DESede, IDEA, RC2, RC4

- JCP Computer Services LTD (*http://www.jcp.co.uk/products/index.html*)

  The JCP Crypto product of JCP Computer Services LTD in the United Kingdom furnishes a security provider that includes implementations of the following engines:

  Message digests: MD5 and SHA
  Digital signatures: RSA/MD5 and RSA/SHA

  JCP Crypto also comes with a JCE replacement that includes implementations of the following:

  Cipher: DES, DESede, IDEA, RSA, RC4

- Systemics LTD (*http://www.systemics.com/software/cryptix-java/*)

  The Cryptix package from Systemics LTD in the United Kingdom furnishes a security provider that includes implementations of the following engines:

  Message digest: Haval, MD2, MD4, MD5, RIPE-MD128, RIPE-MD160, SHA
  Digital signature: RSA with MD2, MD4, MD5 and SHA, El Gamal

  In addition, Cryptix supplies a replacement for the JCE that includes the following:

  Cipher: Blowfish, CAST 5, DES, DESede, IDEA, Loki, RC2, RC4, Safer, Speed,
  *   Square, El Gamal*

  Cryptix is freely available.

- RSA Data Security, Inc. (*http://www.rsa.com/rsa/products/jsafe/*)

  The JSafe product from RSA Data Security in the United States furnishes a security provider that implements the following:

  Message digest: MD5, SHA
  Digital signature: RSA/MD5, RSA/SHA

  In addition, JSafe has a JCE-security provider that implements the following:

  Cipher: DES, DESede, RC2, RC4, RC5
  Key agreement: Diffie-Hellman

  Since RSA is the holder of the patents for these algorithms in the United States, they are able to sell licenses for this technology within the U.S. Note that unlike the other items listed in this section, the JCE security provider is just that; it requires the official JCE from Sun. The remaining JCE packages come with their own JCE implementation.

Security References

Finally, here is a number of white papers and other references that are of general interest:

http://java.sun.com/security/
> This is the main index site for all security-related features of the JDK. In particular, this page has links to security white papers, API and tool documentation, security specifications, and more. This site also has links to many of the other sites we've listed here.

http://java.sun.com/sfaq/
> This is the Frequently Asked Questions page for Java security. This page primarily addresses what applets can and cannot do.

http://java.sun.com/products/jdk1.2/docs/guide/security/security-spec.html
> This document is the specification for the 1.2 Java security architecture; it provided invaluable background for this book. When you download the JDK 1.2 documentation, this document can be found at *$JAVA-HOME/docs/guide/security/spec/security-spec.html*.

http://www.users.zetnet.co.uk/hopwood/papers/compsec97.html
> This document gives an interesting perspective on the topic of authentication, and in particular whether Java's techniques for authentication are secure.

http://www.doc.gov/
> The Department of Commerce of the U.S. government. The Commerce Department governs and publishes the export restrictions of encryption and can grant exceptions for exporting encryption technology.

http://www.crypto.com/
> The Export Policy Resource page contains a number of links and other references to sites concerned with the U.S. government encryption policies.

Bruce Schneier. Applied Cryptography. *John Wiley & Sons, New York, NY. 1996*
> Okay, it is not a web site, but this book is another invaluable reference for details of all the cryptographic topics of this book (Mr. Schneier's web site, for the library-impaired, is *http://www.counterpane.com/*).

Jonathan Knudsen. Java Cryptography. *O'Reilly & Associates, Sebastopol, CA. 1998*
> For a discussion of implementing cryptographic algorithms in Java with a series of excellent examples, check out this book.

D

Quick Reference

This appendix contains a quick-reference guide to the classes that we have discussed in this book. The primary focus is on classes that are in the java.security package and its sub-packages, as well as the javax.crypto extension package. Accordingly, the classes listed in this appendix are organized by their primary package. Of course, there are a number of security-related classes—such as the various permission classes—that do not belong to one of these packages; these are listed in the "Miscellaneous Packages" section at the end of this appendix. Information in this appendix is based only on Java 1.2.

Package java.security

Class java.security.AccessControlContext

An access control context allows the access controller to substitute a different context (that is, a different set of protection domains) than the context provided by the stack of the current thread. This class might be used by a server thread to determine if a particular calling thread should be allowed to perform particular operations.

Class Definition

```
public final class java.security.AccessControlContext
    extends java.lang.Object {

    // Constructors
    public AccessControlContext(ProtectionDomain[]);
```

```
// Instance Methods
public void checkPermission(Permission);
public boolean equals(Object);
public int hashCode();
}
```

See also: AccessController

Class java.security.AccessController

The access controller is responsible for determining whether or not the current thread can execute a given operation. This decision occurs in the checkPermission() method and is based upon all the protection domains that are on the stack of the calling thread and the set of permissions that have been granted to those protection domains. The access controller is heavily used by the security manager to enforce a specific security policy, and it may be used by arbitrary code to enforce an application-specific security policy as well.

Class Definition

```
public final class java.security.AccessController
    extends java.lang.Object {

    // Class Methods
    public static native void beginPrivileged();
    public static native void beginPrivileged(AccessControlContext);
    public static void checkPermission(Permission);
    public static native void endPrivileged();
    public static AccessControlContext getContext();
}
```

See Also: Permission, ProtectionDomain, Policy

Class java.security.AlgorithmParameterGenerator

This engine class is used to generate algorithm-specific parameters, which may then be turned into algorithm parameters specifications to be used to initialize other engine classes. In normal usage, those engines can be initialized directly via the same init() methods that exist in this class; hence, this class is little used.

Class Definition

```
public class java.security.AlgorithmParameterGenerator {

    // Constructors
    protected AlgorithmParameterGenerator(
```

```
                        AlgorithmParameterGeneratorSpi, Provider, String);

    // Class Methods
    public static final AlgorithmParameterGenerator
                                getInstance(String);
    public static final AlgorithmParameterGenerator
                                getInstance(String, String);

    // Instance Methods
    public final String getAlgorithm();
    public final Provider getProvider();
    public final void init(int);
    public final void init(int, SecureRandom);
    public final void init(AlgorithmParameterSpec);
    public final void init(AlgorithmParameterSpec, SecureRandom);
    public final AlgorithmParameters generateParameters();
}
```

See also: AlgorithmParameters

Class
java.security.AlgorithmParameterGeneratorSpi

This class is the Security Provider Interface for the algorithm parameter generator. If you want to implement your own algorithm parameter generator, you subclass this class and register your implementation with an appropriate security provider.

Class Definition

```
    public abstract class java.security.AlgorithmParameterGeneratorSpi {

    // Instance Methods
    protected abstract void engineInit(int, SecureRandom);
    protected abstract void engineInit(
                                AlgorithmParameterSpec, SecureRandom);
    protected abstract AlgorithmParameters engineGenerateParameters();
}
```

See also: AlgorithmParameterGenerator

Class java.security.AlgorithmParameters

This engine class is used to generate algorithm-specific parameter specifications, which may then be used to initialize other engine classes. In normal usage, those engines can be initialized directly via the same init() methods that exist in this class; hence, this class is little used.

Class Definition

```
public class java.security.AlgorithmParameters {

    // Class Methods
    public static final AlgorithmParameters getInstance(String);
    public static final AlgorithmParameters getInstance(
                                String, String);

    // Instance Methods
    protected AlgorithmParameters(AlgorithmParametersSpi,
                                Provider, String);
    public final String getAlgorithm();
    public final Provider getProvider();
    public final void init(AlgorithmParameterSpec);
    public final void init(byte[]);
    public final void init(byte[], String);
    public final AlgorithmParameterSpec getParameterSpec(Class);
    public final byte[] getEncoded();
    public final byte[] getEncoded(String);
    public final String toString();
}
```

See also: KeyPairGenerator

Class java.security.AlgorithmParametersSpi

This is the Security Provider Interface for algorithm parameters. If you want to implement your own algorithm parameters, you do so by subclassing this class and registering your implementation with an appropriate security provider.

Class Definition

```
public abstract class java.security.AlgorithmParametersSpi
        extends java.lang.Object {

    // Constructors
    public AlgorithmParametersSpi();

    // Protected Instance Methods
    protected abstract byte[] engineGetEncoded();
    protected abstract byte[] engineGetEncoded(String);
    protected abstract AlgorithmParameterSpec
                        engineGetParameterSpec(Class);
    protected abstract void engineInit(AlgorithmParameterSpec);
```

```
    protected abstract void engineInit(byte[]);
    protected abstract void engineInit(byte[], String);
    protected abstract String engineToString();
}
```

See also: AlgorithmParameters

Class java.security.AllPermission

This class represents permissions to perform any operation. This permission is typically granted to extension classes, which (like the core API) need to be able to perform any operation. Although it is a permission class, instances of this class have no name and no actions. The implies() method of this class always returns true.

Class Definition

```
    public final class java.security.AllPermission
        extends java.security.Permission {

        // Constructors
        public AllPermission();
        public AllPermission(String, String);

        // Instance Methods
        public boolean equals(Object);
        public String getActions();
        public int hashCode();
        public boolean implies(Permission);
        public PermissionCollection newPermissionCollection();
    }
```

See also: Permission

Class java.security.BasicPermission

A basic permission represents a binary permission—that is, a permission that you either have or do not have. Hence, the action string in a basic permission is unused. A basic permission follows the same naming convention as java properties: a series of period-separated words, like "exit" or "print.queueJob". The BasicPermission class is capable of wildcard matching if the last word in the permission is an asterisk. This class serves as the superclass for a number of default permission classes.

Class Definition

```
public abstract class java.security.BasicPermission
    extends java.security.Permission
    implements java.io.Serializable {

    // Constructors
    public BasicPermission(String);
    public BasicPermission(String, String);

    // Instance Methods
    public boolean equals(Object);
    public String getActions();
    public int hashCode();
    public boolean implies(Permission);
    public PermissionCollection newPermissionCollection();
}
```

See also: Permission, PermissionCollection

Class java.security.CodeSource

A code source encapsulates the location from which a particular class was loaded and the public keys (if any) that were used to sign the class. This information is used by a secure class loader to define a protection domain associated with the class; typically, the class loader is the only object that uses a code source.

Class Definition

```
public class java.security.CodeSource
    extends java.lang.Object
    implements java.io.Serializable {

    // Constructors
    public CodeSource(URL, PublicKey[]);

    // Instance Methods
    public boolean equals(Object);
    public final PublicKey[] getKeys();
    public final URL getLocation();
    public int hashCode();
    public String toString();
}
```

See also: SecureClassLoader, ProtectionDomain

Class java.security.DigestInputStream

A digest input stream is an input filter stream that is associated with a message digest object. As data is read from the input stream, it is automatically passed to its associated message digest object; once all the data has been read, the message digest object will return the hash of the input data. You must have an existing input stream and an initialized message digest object to construct this class; once the data has passed through the stream, call the methods of the message digest object explicitly to obtain the hash.

Class Definition

```
public class java.security.DigestInputStream
    extends java.io.FilterInputStream {

    // Variables
    protected MessageDigest digest;

    // Constructors
    public DigestInputStream(InputStream, MessageDigest);

    // Instance Methods
    public MessageDigest getMessageDigest();
    public void on(boolean);
    public int read();
    public int read(byte[], int, int);
    public void setMessageDigest(MessageDigest);
    public String toString();
}
```

See also: DigestOutputStream, MessageDigest

Class java.security.DigestOutputStream

A digest output stream is a filter output stream that is associated with a message digest object. When data is written to the output stream, it is also passed to the message digest object so that when the data has all been written to the output stream, the hash of that data may be obtained from the digest object. You must have an existing output stream and an initialized message digest object to use this class.

Class Definition

```
public classs java.security.DigestOutputStream
    extends java.io.FilterOutputStream {
```

```
        // Variables
        protected MessageDigest digest;

        // Constructors
        public DigestOutputStream(OutputStream, MessageDigest);

        // Instance Methods
        public MessageDigest getMessageDigest();
        public void on(boolean);
        public void setMessageDigest(MessageDigest);
        public String toString();
        public void write(int);
        public void write(byte[], int, int);
    }
```

See also: DigestInputStream, MessageDigest

Interface java.security.Guard

An object of a class that implements the Guard interface may be used to protect access to a resource. In typical usage, a guard is an object of the Permission class, so that access to the guarded resource is granted if and only if the current thread has been granted the given permission. This interface is used by the GuardedObject class to guard access to another object.

Interface Definition

```
    public abstract interface java.security.Guard {

        // Instance Methods
        public abstract void checkGuard(Object);
    }
```

See also: GuardedObject, Permission

Class java.security.GuardedObject

A guarded object is a container for another object. The contained object is guarded using an object that implements the Guard interface; in typical usage, that would be an instance of a Permission object. The guarded object stores a serialized version of the object it contains; the contained object will be deserialized and returned by the getObject() method only if the guard object allows access.

Class Definition

```
public class java.security.GuardedObject
    extends java.lang.Object
    implements java.io.Serializable {

    // Constructors
    public GuardedObject(Serializable, Guard);

    // Instance Methods
    public Object getObject();
}
```

See also: Guard

Class java.security.Identity

An identity encapsulates public knowledge about an entity (that is, a person or a corporation—or anything that could hold a public key). Identities have names and may hold a public key, along with a certificate chain to validate the public key. An identity may belong to an identity scope, but this feature is optional and is not typically used.

Class Definition

```
public class java.security.Identity
    extends java.lang.Object
    implements java.security.Principal, java.io.Serializable {

    // Constructors
    protected Identity();
    public Identity(String);
    public Identity(String, String, Certificate[], PublicKey);
    public Identity(String, IdentityScope);

    // Instance Methods
    public void addCertificate(Certificate);
    public final boolean equals(Object);
    public Certificate[] getCertificates();
    public String getInfo();
    public final String getName();
    public PublicKey getPublicKey();
    public final IdentityScope getScope();
    public int hashCode();
    public void removeCertificate(Certificate);
    public void setInfo(String);
    public void setPublicKey(PublicKey);
    public String toString();
```

```
        public String toString(boolean);

        // Protected Instance Methods
        protected boolean identityEquals(Identity);
    }
```

See also: Certificate, IdentityScope, Principal, PublicKey

Class java.security.IdentityScope

An identity scope is a collection of identities; an identity may belong to a single identity scope. The notion is that scope is recursive: an identity scope may itself belong to another identity scope (or it may be unscoped). This class is not often used in Java 1.2.

Class Definition

```
    public abstract class java.security.IdentityScope
        extends java.security.Identity {

        // Constructors
        protected IdentityScope();
        public IdentityScope(String);
        public IdentityScope(String, IdentityScope);

        // Class Methods
        public static IdentityScope getSystemScope();
        protected static void setSystemScope(IdentityScope);

        // Instance Methods
        public abstract void addIdentity(Identity);
        public abstract Identity getIdentity(String);
        public Identity getIdentity(Principal);
        public abstract Identity getIdentity(PublicKey);
        public abstract Enumeration identities();
        public abstract void removeIdentity(Identity);
        public abstract int size();
        public String toString();
    }
```

See also: Identity

Interface java.security.Key

A key is essentially a series of bytes that are used by a cryptographic algorithm. Depending on the type of the key, the key may be used only for particular operations and only for particular algorithms, and it may have certain mathematical properties (including a mathematical relationship to other keys). The series of bytes that comprise a key is the encoded format of the key.

Interface Definition

```
public abstract interface java.security.Key
    implements java.io.Serializable {

    // Instance Methods
    public abstract String getAlgorithm();
    public abstract byte[] getEncoded();
    public abstract String getFormat();
}
```

See also: PrivateKey, PublicKey, SecretKey

Class java.security.KeyFactory

A key factory is an engine class that is capable of translating between public or private key objects and their external format (and vice versa). Hence, key factories may be used to import or export keys, as well as to translate keys of one class (e.g., com.acme.DSAPublicKey) to another class (e.g., com.xyz.DSAPublicKeyImpl) as long as those classes share the same base class. Key factories operate in terms of key specifications; these specifications are the various external formats in which a key may be transmitted. Keys are imported via the generatePublic() and generatePrivate() methods, they are exported via the getKeySpec() method, and they are translated via the translateKey() method.

Class Definition

```
public class java.security.KeyFactory
    extends java.lang.Object {

    // Constructors
    protected KeyFactory(KeyFactorySpi, Provider, String);

    // Class Methods
    public static final KeyFactory getInstance(String);
    public static final KeyFactory getInstance(String, String);

    // Instance Methods
    public final PrivateKey generatePrivate(KeySpec);
    public final PublicKey generatePublic(KeySpec);
    public final String getAlgorithm();
    public final KeySpec getKeySpec(Key, Class);
```

```
    public final Provider getProvider();
    public final Key translateKey(Key);
}
```

See also: KeyFactorySpi, KeySpec

Class java.security.KeyFactorySpi

This is the Service Provider Interface for a key factory; if you want to implement your own key factory, you do so by extending this class and registering your implementation with an appropriate security provider. Instances of this class are expected to know how to create key objects from external key specifications and vice versa.

Class Definition

```
public abstract class java.security.KeyFactorySpi
    extends java.lang.Object {

    // Constructors
    public KeyFactorySpi();

    // Protected Instance Methods
    protected abstract PrivateKey engineGeneratePrivate(KeySpec);
    protected abstract PublicKey engineGeneratePublic(KeySpec);
    protected abstract KeySpec engineGetKeySpec(Key, Class);
    protected abstract Key engineTranslateKey(Key);
}
```

See also: KeyFactory, KeySpec

Class java.security.KeyPair

Public and private keys are mathematically related to each other and hence are generated together; this class provides an encapsulation of both the keys as a convenience to key generation.

Class Definition

```
public final class java.security.KeyPair
    extends java.lang.Object {

    // Constructors
    public KeyPair(PublicKey, PrivateKey);

    // Instance Methods
```

```
        public PrivateKey getPrivate();
        public PublicKey getPublic();
    }
```

See also: KeyPairGenerator, PrivateKey, PublicKey

Class KeyPairGenerator

This is an engine class that is capable of generating a public key and its related private key. Instances of this class will generate key pairs that are appropriate for a particular algorithm (DSA, RSA, etc.). A key pair generator may be initialized to return keys of a particular strength (which is usually the number of bits in the key), or it may be initialized in an algorithmic-specific way; the former case is the one implemented by most key generators. An instance of this class may be used to generate any number of key pairs.

Class Definition

```
    public abstract class java.security.KeyPairGenerator
        extends java.security.KeyPairGeneratorSpi {

        // Constructors
        protected KeyPairGenerator(String);

        // Class Methods
        public static KeyPairGenerator getInstance(String);
        public static KeyPairGenerator getInstance(String, String);

        // Instance Methods
        public final KeyPair genKeyPair();
        public String getAlgorithm();
        public final Provider getProvider();
        public void initialize(int);
        public void initialize(AlgorithmParameterSpec);
    }
```

See also: AlgorithmParameterSpec, KeyPair

Class KeyPairGeneratorSpi

This is the Service Provider Interface class for the key pair generation engine; if you want to implement your own key pair generator, you must extend this class and register your implementation with an appropriate security provider. Instances of this class must be prepared to generate key pairs of a particular strength (or length); they may optionally accept an algorithmic-specific set of initialization values.

Class Definition

```
public abstract class java.security.KeyPairGeneratorSpi
    extends java.lang.Object {

    // Constructors
    public KeyPairGeneratorSpi();

    // Instance Methods
    public abstract KeyPair generateKeyPair();
    public abstract void initialize(int, SecureRandom);
    public void initialize(AlgorithmParameterSpec, SecureRandom);
}
```

See also: AlgorithmParameterSpec, KeyPairGenerator, SecureRandom

Class java.security.KeyStore

This class is responsible for maintaining a set of keys and their related owners. In the default implementation, this class maintains the *.keystore* file held in the user's home directory, but you may provide an alternate implementation of this class that holds keys anywhere: in a database, on a remote filesystem, on a Java smart card, or any and all of the above. The class that is used to provide the default keystore implementation is specified by the keystore property in the *$JDKHOME/lib/java.security* file. The keystore may optionally require a passphrase for access to the entire keystore (via the load() method); this passphrase is often used only for sanity checking and is often not specified at all. On the other hand, private keys in the keystore should be protected (e.g., encrypted) by using a different passphrase for each private key.

Note that although the keystore associates entities with keys, it does not rely upon the Identity class itself.

Class Definition

```
public abstract class java.security.KeyStore
    extends java.lang.Object {

    // Constructors
    public KeyStore();

    // Class Methods
    public static final KeyStore getInstance();

    // Instance Methods
    public abstract Enumeration aliases();
    public abstract boolean containsAlias(String);
```

```
    public abstract void deleteEntry(String);
    public abstract Certificate getCertificate(String);
    public abstract String getCertificateAlias(Certificate);
    public abstract Certificate[] getCertificateChain(String);
    public abstract Date getCreationDate(String);
    public abstract PrivateKey getPrivateKey(String, String);
    public abstract boolean isCertificateEntry(String);
    public abstract boolean isKeyEntry(String);
    public abstract void load(InputStream, String);
    public abstract void setCertificateEntry(String, Certificate);
    public abstract void setKeyEntry(String, PrivateKey, String,
                          Certificate[]);
    public abstract void setKeyEntry(String, byte[], Certificate[]);
    public abstract int size();
    public abstract void store(OutputStream, String);
}
```

See also: Certificate, PublicKey

Class java.security.MessageDigest

The message digest class is an engine class that can produce a one-way hash value
for any arbitrary input. Message digests have two properties: they produce a
unique hash for each set of input data (subject to the number of bits that are
output), and the original input data is indiscernible from the hash output. The
hash value is variously called a digital fingerprint or a digest. Message digests are
components of digital signatures, but they are useful in their own right to verify
that a set of data has not been corrupted. Once a digest object is created, data
may be fed to it via the update() methods; the hash itself is returned via the
digest() method.

Class Definition

```
    public abstract class java.security.MessageDigest
        extends java.security.MessageDigestSpi {

        // Constructors
        protected MessageDigest(String);

        // Class Methods
        public static MessageDigest getInstance(String);
        public static MessageDigest getInstance(String, String);
        public static boolean isEqual(byte[], byte[]);

        // Instance Methods
        public Object clone();
        public byte[] digest();
```

```
        public byte[] digest(byte[]);
        public int digest(byte[], int, int);
        public final String getAlgorithm();
        public final int getDigestLength();
        public final Provider getProvider();
        public void reset();
        public String toString();
        public void update(byte);
        public void update(byte[]);
        public void update(byte[], int, int);
    }
```

Class java.security.MessageDigestSpi

This is the Service Provider Interface for the message digest engine; if you want to
implement your own message digest class, you do so by extending this class and
registering your implementation with an appropriate security provider. Since the
MessageDigest class itself extends this class, you may also extend the MessageDigest class directly. Implementations of this class are expected to accumulate a
hash value over data that is fed to it as a series of arbitrary bytes.

Class Definition

```
    public abstract class java.security.MessageDigestSpi
        extends java.lang.Object {

        // Constructors
        public MessageDigestSpi();

        // Instance Methods
        public Object clone();

        // Protected Instance Methods
        protected abstract byte[] engineDigest();
        protected int engineDigest(byte[], int, int);
        protected int engineGetDigestLength();
        protected abstract void engineReset();
        protected abstract void engineUpdate(byte);
        protected abstract void engineUpdate(byte[], int, int);
    }
```

See also: MessageDigest

Class java.security.Permission

This class forms the base class for all types of permissions that are used by the access controller. A permission object encapsulates a particular operation (e.g., reading the file */tmp/foo*). It does not, however, grant permission for that operation; rather, the permission object is constructed and passed to the access controller to see if that operation is one which the current security policy has defined as a permissible operation.

Permissions have names (e.g., the name of the file, or the name of the operation) and may optionally have actions (the semantics of which are dependent upon the type of permission). It is up to the implies() method to determine if one permission grants another; this allows you to specify wildcard-type permissions that imply specific permissions (e.g., the permission named "*" may imply the permission named "myfile").

Class Definition

```
public abstract class java.security.Permission
    extends java.lang.Object
    implements java.security.Guard, java.io.Serializable {

    // Constructors
    public Permission(String);

    // Instance Methods
    public void checkGuard(Object);
    public abstract boolean equals(Object);
    public abstract String getActions();
    public final String getName();
    public abstract int hashCode();
    public abstract boolean implies(Permission);
    public PermissionCollection newPermissionCollection();
    public String toString();
}
```

See also: AccessController, BasicPermission, PermissionCollection, Policy

Class java.security.PermissionCollection

As you might infer, a permission collection is a collection of permission objects. In theory, a permission collection can be a set of arbitrary, unrelated permission objects; however, that usage is best avoided and left to the Permissions class. Hence, a permission collection should be thought of as a collection of one type of permission: a set of file permissions, a set of socket permissions, etc. A permission collection is responsible for determining if an individual permission (passed as a parameter to the implies() method) is contained in the set of permissions in the object; presumably, it will do that more efficiently than by calling the implies() method on each permission in the collection. If you implement a new permission class that has wildcard semantics for its names, then you must implement a corresponding permission collection to aggregate instances of that class (if you don't need wildcard matching, the default implementation of the Permission class will provide an appropriate collection).

Class Definition

```
public abstract class java.security.PermissionCollection
    extends java.lang.Object
    implements java.io.Serializable {

    // Constructors
    public PermissionCollection();

    // Instance Methods
    public abstract void add(Permission);
    public abstract Enumeration elements();
    public abstract boolean implies(Permission);
    public String toString();
}
```

See also: Permission, Permissions

Class java.security.Permissions

This class is an aggregate of permission collections. Hence, it is an appropriate collection object for a group of unrelated permission, which is its typical use: the Policy class uses instances of this class to represent all the permissions associated with a particular protection domain.

Class Definition

```
public final class java.security.Permissions
    extends java.security.PermissionCollection
    implements java.io.Serializable {

    // Constructors
    public Permissions();

    // Instance Methods
    public void add(Permission);
    public Enumeration elements();
```

```
            public boolean implies(Permission);
            public boolean isReadOnly();
            public void setReadOnly();
        }
```

See also: Permission, PermissionCollection, Policy

Class java.security.Policy

The Policy class encapsulates all the specific permissions that the virtual machine knows about. This set of permissions is by default read from a series of URLs specified by policy.url properties in the *$JDKHOME/lib/security/java.security* file, although applications may specify their own policy objects by using the setPolicy() method of this class. Alternately, a different default implementation of the policy class may be specified by changing the policy.provider property in the *java.security* file.

Class Definition

```
        public abstract class java.security.Policy
            extends java.lang.Object {

            // Constructors
            public Policy();

            // Class Methods
            public static Policy getPolicy();
            public static void setPolicy(Policy);

            // Instance Methods
            public abstract Permissions evaluate(CodeSource);
            public abstract void refresh();
        }
```

See also: Permission, Permissions

Interface java.security.Principal

A principal is anything that has a name, such as an identity. The name in this case is often an X.500 distinguished name, but that is not a requirement.

Interface Definition

```
        public abstract interface java.security.Principal {

            // Instance Methods
            public abstract boolean equals(Object);
```

```
    public abstract String getName();
    public abstract int hashCode();
    public abstract String toString();
}
```

See also: Identity

Interface java.security.PrivateKey

A private key is a key with certain mathematical properties that allows it to perform inverse cryptographic operations with its matching public key. Classes implement this interface only for type identification.

Interface definition

```
public abstract interface java.security.PrivateKey
    implements java.security.Key {
}
```

See also: Key, PublicKey

Class java.security.ProtectionDomain

A protection domain encapsulates the location from which a class was loaded and the keys used to sign the class (that is, a CodeSource object) and the set of permissions that should be granted to that class. These protection domains are consulted by the access controller to determine if a particular operation should succeed; if the operation is in the set of permissions in each protection domain on the stack, then the operation will succeed. This class is typically only used within a class loader.

Class Definition

```
public class java.security.ProtectionDomain
    extends java.lang.Object {

    // Constructors
    public ProtectionDomain(CodeSource, Permissions);

    // Instance Methods
    public final CodeSource getCodeSource();
    public final Permissions getPermissions();
    public boolean implies(Permission);
    public String toString();
}
```

See also: AccessController, CodeSource, Permissions

Class java.security.Provider

An instance of the `Provider` class is responsible for mapping particular implementations to desired algorithm/engine pairs; instances of this class are consulted (indirectly) by the `getInstance()` methods of the engine classes to find a class that implements the desired operation. Instances of this class must be registered either with the `Security` class or by listing them in the *$JDKHOME/lib/security/java.security* file as a `security.provider` property.

Class Definition

```
public abstract class java.security.Provider
    extends java.util.Properties {

    // Constructors
    protected Provider(String, double, String);

    // Instance Methods
    public synchronized void clear();
    public String getInfo();
    public String getName();
    public double getVersion();
    public synchronized Object put(Object, Object);
    public synchronized Object remove(Object);
    public String toString();
}
```

See also: `Security`

Interface java.security.PublicKey

A public key is a key with certain mathematical properties that allows it to perform inverse cryptographic operations with its matching private key. Classes implement this interface only for type identification.

Interface Definition

```
public abstract interface java.security.PublicKey
    implements java.security.Key {
}
```

See also: `Key, PrivateKey`

Class java.security.SecureClassLoader

A secure class loader is a class loader that is able to associate code sources (and hence protection domains) with the classes that it loads (classes loaded by a traditional class loader have a default, null protection domain). All new class loaders are expected to extend this class.

Class Definition

```
public class java.security.SecureClassLoader
    extends java.lang.ClassLoader {

    // Constructors
    protected SecureClassLoader();
    protected SecureClassLoader(ClassLoader);

    // Protected Instance Methods
    protected final Class defineClass(String, byte[], int, int,
                          CodeSource, Object[]);
    protected final Class defineClass(String, byte[], int, int,
                          ProtectionDomain, Object[]);
    protected CodeSource getCodeSource(URL, Object[]);
}
```

See also: ClassLoader, CodeSource, ProtectionDomain

Class java.security.SecureRandom

This class generates random numbers. Unlike the standard random-number generator, numbers generated by this class are cryptographically secure—that is, they are less subject to pattern guessing and other attacks that can be made upon a traditional random-number generator.

Class Definition

```
public class java.security.SecureRandom
    extends java.util.Random {

    // Constructors
    public SecureRandom();
    public SecureRandom(byte[]);

    // Class Methods
    public static byte[] getSeed(int);

    // Instance Methods
    public synchronized void nextBytes(byte[]);
```

```
        public void setSeed(long);
        public synchronized void setSeed(byte[]);

        // Protected Instance Methods
        protected final int next(int);
    }
```

Class java.security.Security

This class manages the list of providers that have been installed into the virtual machine; this list of providers is consulted to find an appropriate class to provide the implementation of a particular operation when the getInstance() method of an engine class is called. The list of providers initially comes from the *$JDKHOME/lib/security/java.security* file, and applications may use methods of this class to add and remove providers from that list.

Class Definition

```
    public final class java.security.Security
        extends java.lang.Object {

        // Class Methods
        public static int addProvider(Provider);
        public static String getAlgorithmProperty(String, String);
        public static String getProperty(String);
        public static Provider getProvider(String);
        public static Provider[] getProviders();
        public static int insertProviderAt(Provider, int);
        public static void removeProvider(String);
        public static void setProperty(String, String);
    }
```

See also: Provider

Class java.security.SecurityPermission

This class represents permissions to interact with the methods of the java.security package. This permission is a basic permission; it does not support actions. Security permissions are checked by the Identity, Signer, and Provider classes.

Class Definition

```
    public final class java.security.SecurityPermission
        extends java.security.BasicPermission {

        // Constructors
        public SecurityPermission(String);
```

```
        public SecurityPermission(String, String);
    }
```

See also: BasicPermission

Class java.security.Signature

This engine class provides the ability to create or verify digital signatures by
employing different algorithms that have been registered with the Security class.
As with all engine classes, instances of this class are obtained via the getIn-
stance() method. The signature object must be initialized with the appropriate
private key (to sign) or public key (to verify), then data must be fed to the object
via the update() methods, and then the signature can be obtained (via the
sign() method) or verified (via the verify() method). Signature objects may
support algorithm-specific parameters, though this is not a common
implementation.

Class Definition

```
    public abstract class java.security.Signature
        extends java.security.SignatureSpi {

        // Constants
        protected static final int SIGN;
        protected static final int UNINITIALIZED;
        protected static final int VERIFY;

        // Variables
        protected int state;

        // Constructors
        protected Signature(String);

        // Class Methods
        public static Signature getInstance(String);
        public static Signature getInstance(String, String);

        // Instance Methods
        public Object clone();
        public final String getAlgorithm();
        public final Object getParameter(String);
        public final Provider getProvider();
        public final void initSign(PrivateKey);
        public final void initSign(PrivateKey, SecureRandom);
        public final void initVerify(PublicKey);
        public final void setParameter(String, Object);
        public final void setParameter(AlgorithmParameterSpec);
        public final byte[] sign();
```

```
        public String toString();
        public final void update(byte);
        public final void update(byte[]);
        public final void update(byte[], int, int);
        public final boolean verify(byte[]);
    }
```

See also: Provider

Class java.security.SignatureSpi

This is the Security Provider Interface for the signature engine. If you want to implement your own signature engine, you must extend this class and register your implementation with an appropriate security provider. Since the Signature class already extends this class, your implementation may extend the Signature class directly. Implementations of this class must be prepared both to sign and to verify data that is passed to the engineUpdate() method. Initialization of the engine may optionally support a set of algorithm-specific parameters.

Class Definition

```
    public abstract class java.security.SignatureSpi
        extends java.lang.Object {

        // Variables
        protected SecureRandom appRandom;

        // Constructors
        public SignatureSpi();

        // Instance Methods
        public Object clone();

        // Protected Instance Methods
        protected abstract Object engineGetParameter(String);
        protected abstract void engineInitSign(PrivateKey);
        protected void engineInitSign(PrivateKey, SecureRandom);
        protected abstract void engineInitVerify(PublicKey);
        protected abstract void engineSetParameter(String, Object);
        protected void engineSetParameter(AlgorithmParameterSpec);
        protected abstract byte[] engineSign();
        protected abstract void engineUpdate(byte);
        protected abstract void engineUpdate(byte[], int, int);
        protected abstract boolean engineVerify(byte[]);
    }
```

See also: Provider, Signature

Class java.security.SignedObject

A signed object is a container class for another (target) object; the signed object contains a serialized version of the target along with a digital signature of the data contained in the target object. You must provide a serializable object and a private key to create a signed object, after which you can remove the embedded object and verify the signature of the signed object by providing the appropriate public key.

Class Definition

```
public final class java.security.SignedObject
    extends java.lang.Object
    implements java.io.Serializable {

    // Constructors
    public SignedObject(Serializable, PrivateKey, Signature);

    // Instance Methods
    public String getAlgorithm();
    public Object getObject();
    public byte[] getSignature();
    public boolean verify(PublicKey, Signature);
}
```

See also: Signature

Class java.security.Signer

A signer abstracts the notion of a principal (that is, an individual or a corporation) that has a private key and a corresponding public key. Signers may optionally belong to an identity scope, but that usage is now rare.

Class Definition

```
public abstract class java.security.Signer
    extends java.security.Identity {

    // Constructors
    protected Signer();
    public Signer(String);
    public Signer(String, IdentityScope);

    // Instance Methods
    public PrivateKey getPrivateKey();
    public final void setKeyPair(KeyPair);
```

```
        public String toString();
    }
```

See also: Identity, Principal

Class java.security.UnresolvedPermission

An unresolved permission is one for which the implementing class has not been loaded. If you define a custom permission, the Policy class will represent that custom permission as an unresolved permission until it is time for the Policy class to actually load the class; if the class cannot be found, then it will remain an unresolved permission. By default, the implies() method of this class always returns false.

Class Definition

```
    public final class UnresolvedPermission extends Permission
        implements java.io.Serializable {

        // Constructors
        public UnresolvedPermission(String, String, String, PublicKey);

        // Instance methods
        public boolean equals(Object);
        public int hashCode();
        public boolean implies(Permission);
    }
```

See also: Permission

Package java.security.cert

Class java.security.cert.Certificate

This class represents any type of cryptographic certificate. A certificate contains a public key (see getPublicKey()) and other associated information. The certificate contains an internal signature that protects its integrity. You can verify the integrity of the certificate by calling one of the verify() methods with the public key of the certificate's issuer. (Note: don't confuse this class with the java.security.Certificate interface, which is deprecated.)

Class Definition

```
public abstract class java.security.cert.Certificate
    extends java.lang.Object {

    // Constructors
    public Certificate();

    // Instance Methods
    public boolean equals(Object);
    public abstract byte[] getEncoded();
    public abstract PublicKey getPublicKey();
    public int hashCode();
    public abstract String toString();
    public abstract void verify(PublicKey);
    public abstract void verify(PublicKey, String);
}
```

See also: PublicKey, X509Certificate

Class java.security.cert.RevokedCertificate

A revoked certificate represents a certificate whose contained key is no longer safe to use. Instances of this class are returned by X509CRL's getRevokedCertificate() method. You can examine the certificate's revocation date and X.509 extensions.

Class Definition

```
public abstract class java.security.cert.RevokedCertificate
    extends java.lang.Object
    implements java.security.cert.X509Extension {

    // Constructors
    public RevokedCertificate();

    // Instance Methods
    public abstract Set getCriticalExtensionOIDs();
    public abstract byte[] getExtensionValue(String);
    public abstract Set getNonCriticalExtensionOIDs();
    public abstract Date getRevocationDate();
    public abstract BigInteger getSerialNumber();
    public abstract boolean hasExtensions();
    public abstract String toString();
}
```

See also: Certificate, X509CRL, X509Extension

Class *java.security.cert.X509Certificate*

This class represents certificates as defined in the X.509 standard. Such certificates associate a public key with a subject, which is usually a person or organization. You can find out the certificate's subject by calling getSubjectDN(), while you can retrieve the subject's public key using getPublicKey(). The certificate's issuer is the person or organization that generated and signed the certificate (see getIssuerDN()). If you have a certificate file in the format described by RFC 1421, you can create an X509Certificate from that data by using one of the getInstance() methods.

Class Definition

```
public abstract class java.security.cert.X509Certificate
    extends java.security.cert.Certificate
    implements java.security.cert.X509Extension {

    // Constructors
    public X509Certificate();

    // Class Methods
    public static final X509Certificate getInstance(InputStream);
    public static final X509Certificate getInstance(byte[]);

    // Instance Methods
    public abstract void checkValidity();
    public abstract void checkValidity(Date);
    public abstract int getBasicConstraints();
    public abstract Set getCriticalExtensionOIDs();
    public abstract byte[] getExtensionValue(String);
    public abstract Principal getIssuerDN();
    public abstract boolean[] getIssuerUniqueID();
    public abstract boolean[] getKeyUsage();
    public abstract Set getNonCriticalExtensionOIDs();
    public abstract Date getNotAfter();
    public abstract Date getNotBefore();
    public abstract BigInteger getSerialNumber();
    public abstract String getSigAlgName();
    public abstract String getSigAlgOID();
    public abstract byte[] getSigAlgParams();
    public abstract byte[] getSignature();
    public abstract Principal getSubjectDN();
    public abstract boolean[] getSubjectUniqueID();
    public abstract byte[] getTBSCertificate();
    public abstract int getVersion();
}
```

See also: Principal, PublicKey, X509Extension

Class *java.security.cert.X509CRL*

A Certificate Revocation List (CRL) is a list of certificates whose keys are no longer valid. This class represents CRLs as defined in the X.509 standard. If you have a CRL file that you would like to examine, you can construct an X509CRL object from the file using one of the getInstance() methods. A CRL, just like a certificate, has an internal signature that protects its integrity. To verify the integrity of the CRL itself, call one of the verify() methods with the issuer's public key. To find out if a particular certificate is revoked, call the isRevoked() method with the certificate's serial number.

Class Definition

```
public abstract class java.security.cert.X509CRL
    extends java.lang.Object
    implements java.security.cert.X509Extension {

    // Constructors
    public X509CRL();

    // Class Methods
    public static final X509CRL getInstance(InputStream);
    public static final X509CRL getInstance(byte[]);

    // Instance Methods
    public boolean equals(Object);
    public abstract Set getCriticalExtensionOIDs();
    public abstract byte[] getEncoded();
    public abstract byte[] getExtensionValue(String);
    public abstract Principal getIssuerDN();
    public abstract Date getNextUpdate();
    public abstract Set getNonCriticalExtensionOIDs();
    public abstract RevokedCertificate
getRevokedCertificate(BigInteger);
    public abstract Set getRevokedCertificates();
    public abstract String getSigAlgName();
    public abstract String getSigAlgOID();
    public abstract byte[] getSigAlgParams();
    public abstract byte[] getSignature();
    public abstract byte[] getTBSCertList();
    public abstract Date getThisUpdate();
    public abstract int getVersion();
    public int hashCode();
    public abstract boolean isRevoked(BigInteger);
    public abstract String toString();
    public abstract void verify(PublicKey);
```

```
        public abstract void verify(PublicKey, String);
    }
```

See also: Certificate, PublicKey, RevokedCertificate, X509Extension

Interface java.security.cert.X509Extension

The X509Extension interface represents the certificate extensions defined by the X.509v3 standard. Extensions are additional bits of information contained in a certificate. Each extension is designated as critical or non-critical. An application that handles a certificate should either correctly interpret the critical extensions or produce some kind of error if they cannot be recognized.

Class Definition

```
    public abstract interface java.security.cert.X509Extension {

        // Instance Methods
        public abstract Set getCriticalExtensionOIDs();
        public abstract byte[] getExtensionValue(String);
        public abstract Set getNonCriticalExtensionOIDs();
    }
```

See also: RevokedCertificate, X509Certificate, X509CRL

Package java.security.interfaces

Interface java.security.interfaces.DSAKey

This interface represents public and private keys that are suitable for use in DSA signature algorithms. This interface allows you to retrieve DSA-specific information from a suitable DSA key.

Interface Definition

```
    public interface java.security.interfaces.DSAKey {

        // Instance Methods
        public DSAParams getParams();
    }
```

See also: PrivateKey, PublicKey

Interface java.security.interfaces.DSAKeyPairGenerator

This interface represents key generators that can be used to generate pairs of DSA keys. Key pair generators that implement this interface can be initialized with information specific to DSA key generation.

Interface Definition

```
public interface java.security.interfaces.DSAKeyPairGenerator {

    // Instance Methods
    public void initialize(DSAParams, SecureRandom);
    public void initialize(int, boolean, SecureRandom);
}
```

See also: KeyPairGenerator

Interface java.security.interfaces.DSAParams

Classes that implement this interface allow you to obtain the three variables that are common to both DSA public and private keys.

Interface Definition

```
public interface java.security.interfaces.DSAParams {

    // Instance Methods
    public BigInteger getP();
    public BigInteger getQ();
    public BigInteger getG();
}
```

See also: DSAPrivateKey, DSAPublicKey

Interface java.security.interfaces.DSAPrivateKey

Classes that implement this interface allow you to retrieve the private key parameter used to calculate a DSA private key.

Interface Definition

```
public interface java.security.interfaces.DSAPrivateKey {

    // Instance Methods
```

```
    public BigInteger getX();
}
```

See also: DSAParams, DSAPublicKey

Interface java.security.interfaces.DSAPublicKey

Classes that implement this interface allow you to retrieve the public key parameter used to calculate a DSA public key.

Interface Definition

```
public interface java.security.interfaces.DSAPublicKey {

    // Instance Methods
    public BigInteger getY();
}
```

See also: DSAParams, DSAPrivateKey

Package java.security.spec

Interface java.security.spec.AlgorithmParameterSpec

Algorithm parameter specifications are used to import and export keys via a key factory. This interface is used strictly for type identification; the specifics of the parameters are left to the implementing class.

Interface Definition

```
public interface java.security.spec.AlgorithmParameterSpec {
}
```

See also: DSAParameterSpec, KeyFactory

Class java.security.spec.DSAParameterSpec

This class provides the basis for DSA key generation via parameters; it encapsulates the three parameters that are common to DSA algorithms.

Class Definition

```
public class java.security.spec.DSAParameterSpec
    extends java.lang.Object
    implements java.security.spec.AlgorithmParameterSpec,
               java.security.interfaces.DSAParams {

    // Constructors
    public DSAParameterSpec(BigInteger, BigInteger, BigInteger);

    // Instance Methods
    public BigInteger getG();
    public BigInteger getP();
    public BigInteger getQ();
}
```

See also: AlgorithmParameterSpec, DSAParams, DSAPrivateKeySpec, DSAPublicKeySpec

---

Class java.security.spec.DSAPrivateKeySpec

This class provides the ability to calculate a DSA private key based upon the four parameters that comprise the key.

Class Definition

```
public class java.security.spec.DSAPrivateKeySpec
    extends java.lang.Object
    implements java.security.spec.KeySpec {

    // Constructors
    public DSAPrivateKeySpec(BigInteger, BigInteger,
                             BigInteger, BigInteger);

    // Instance Methods
    public BigInteger getG();
    public BigInteger getP();
    public BigInteger getQ();
    public BigInteger getX();
}
```

See also: DSAPublicKeySpec, KeyFactory

Class java.security.spec.DSAPublicKeySpec

This class provides the ability to calculate a DSA public key based upon the four parameters that comprise the key.

Class Definition

```
public class java.security.spec.DSAPublicKeySpec
    extends java.lang.Object
    implements java.security.spec.KeySpec {

    // Constructors
    public DSAPublicKeySpec(BigInteger, BigInteger,
                            BigInteger, BigInteger);

    // Instance Methods
    public BigInteger getG();
    public BigInteger getP();
    public BigInteger getQ();
    public BigInteger getY();
}
```

See also: DSAPrivateKeySpec, KeyFactory

Class java.security.spec.EncodedKeySpec

This class is used to translate between keys and their external encoded format. The encoded format is always simply a series of bytes, but the format of the encoding of the key information into those bytes may vary depending upon the algorithm used to generate the key.

Class Definition

```
public abstract class java.security.spec.EncodedKeySpec
    extends java.lang.Object
    implements java.security.spec.KeySpec {

    // Constructors
    public EncodedKeySpec();

    // Instance Methods
    public abstract byte[] getEncoded();
    public abstract String getFormat();
}
```

See also: KeyFactory, KeySpec, PKCS8EncodedKeySpec, X509EncodedKeySpec

Interface java.security.spec.KeySpec

A key specification is used to import and export keys via a key factory. This may be done either based upon the algorithm parameters used to generate the key or via

an encoded series of bytes that represent the key. Classes that deal with the latter
case implement this interface, which is used strictly for type identification.

Interface Definition

```
public abstract interface java.security.spec.KeySpec {
}
```

See also: AlgorithmParameterSpec, EncodedKeySpec, KeyFactory

Class java.security.spec.PKCS8EncodedKeySpec

This class represents the PKCS#8 encoding of a private key; the key is encoded in
DER format. This is the class that is typically used when dealing with DSA private
keys in a key factory.

Class Definition

```
public class java.security.spec.PKCS8EncodedKeySpec
    extends java.security.spec.EncodedKeySpec {

    // Constructors
    public PKCS8EncodedKeySpec(byte[]);

    // Instance Methods
    public byte[] getEncoded();
    public final String getFormat();
}
```

See also: EncodedKeySpec, X509EncodedKeySpec

Class java.security.spec.X509EncodedKeySpec

This class represents the X509 encoding of a public key. It may also be used for
private keys, although the PKCS#8 encoding is typically used for those keys.

Class Definition

```
public class java.security.spec.X509EncodedKeySpec
    extends java.security.spec.EncodedKeySpec {

    // Constructors
    public X509EncodedKeySpec(byte[]);

    // Instance Methods
    public byte[] getEncoded();
```

```
        public final String getFormat();
    }
```

See also: EncodedKeySpec, PKCS8EncodedKeySpec

Package javax.crypto

Class javax.crypto.Cipher

This engine class represents a cryptographic cipher, either symmetric or asymmetric. To get a cipher for a particular algorithm, call one of the getInstance() methods, specifying an algorithm name, a cipher mode, and a padding scheme. The cipher should be initialized for encryption or decryption using an init() method and an appropriate key (and, optionally, a set of algorithm-specific parameters, though these are typically unused). Then you can perform the encryption or decryption, using the update() and doFinal() methods.

Class Definition

```
    public class javax.crypto.Cipher
        extends java.lang.Object {

        // Constants
        public static final int DECRYPT_MODE;
        public static final int ENCRYPT_MODE;

        // Constructors
        protected Cipher(CipherSpi, Provider, String);

        // Class Methods
        public static final Cipher getInstance(String);
        public static final Cipher getInstance(String, String);

        // Instance Methods
        public final byte[] doFinal();
        public final byte[] doFinal(byte[]);
        public final int doFinal(byte[], int);
        public final byte[] doFinal(byte[], int, int);
        public final int doFinal(byte[], int, int, byte[]);
        public final int doFinal(byte[], int, int, byte[], int);
        public final int getBlockSize();
        public final byte[] getIV();
        public final int getOutputSize(int);
        public final Provider getProvider();
```

```
        public final void init(int, Key);
        public final void init(int, Key, SecureRandom);
        public final void init(int, Key, AlgorithmParameterSpec);
        public final void init(int, Key, AlgorithmParameterSpec,
                               SecureRandom);
        public final byte[] update(byte[]);
        public final byte[] update(byte[], int, int);
        public final int update(byte[], int, int, byte[]);
        public final int update(byte[], int, int, byte[], int);
    }
```

See also: AlgorithmParameterSpec, CipherSpi, Key, Provider, SecureRandom

---

Class javax.crypto.CipherInputStream

A cipher input stream is a filter stream that passes its data through a cipher. You can construct a cipher input stream by specifying an underlying stream and supplying an initialized cipher. For best results, use a byte-oriented cipher mode with this stream.

Class Definition

```
    public class javax.crypto.CipherInputStream
        extends java.io.FilterInputStream {

        // Constructors
        protected CipherInputStream(InputStream);
        public CipherInputStream(InputStream, Cipher);

        // Instance Methods
        public int available();
        public void close();
        public boolean markSupported();
        public int read();
        public int read(byte[]);
        public int read(byte[], int, int);
        public long skip(long);
    }
```

See also: Cipher

Class javax.crypto.CipherOutputStream

This class is a filter output stream that passes all its data through a cipher. You can construct a cipher output stream by specifying an underlying output stream and an initialized cipher. For best results, use a byte-oriented mode for the cipher.

Class Definition

```
public class javax.crypto.CipherOutputStream
    extends java.io.FilterOutputStream {

    // Constructors
    protected CipherOutputStream(OutputStream);
    public CipherOutputStream(OutputStream, Cipher);

    // Instance Methods
    public void close();
    public void flush();
    public void write(int);
    public void write(byte[]);
    public void write(byte[], int, int);
}
```

See also: Cipher

Class javax.crypto.CipherSpi

This class is the Security Provider Interface of the Cipher class. To implement a particular cipher algorithm, create a subclass of this class and register the class with an appropriate security provider. Like all SPI classes, the methods that begin with engine are called by their corresponding method (without engine) from the Cipher class.

Class Definition

```
public abstract class javax.crypto.CipherSpi
    extends java.lang.Object {

    // Constructors
    public CipherSpi();

    // Protected Instance Methods
    protected abstract byte[] engineDoFinal(byte[], int, int);
    protected abstract int engineDoFinal(byte[], int, int,
                                byte[], int);
    protected abstract int engineGetBlockSize();
    protected abstract byte[] engineGetIV();
```

```
        protected abstract int engineGetOutputSize(int);
        protected abstract void engineInit(int, Key, SecureRandom);
        protected abstract void engineInit(int, Key,
                    AlgorithmParameterSpec, SecureRandom);
        protected abstract void engineSetMode(String);
        protected abstract void engineSetPadding(String);
        protected abstract byte[] engineUpdate(byte[], int, int);
        protected abstract int engineUpdate(byte[], int, int, byte[], int);
    }
```

See also: AlgorithmParameterSpec, Cipher, Key, SecureRandom

Class javax.crypto.KeyAgreement

This engine class represents a key agreement protocol, which is an arrangement by which two parties can agree on a secret value. You can obtain an instance of this class by calling the getInstance() method. After initializing the object (see init()), you can step through the phases of the key agreement protocol using the doPhase() method. Once the phases are complete, the secret value (that is, the key) is returned from the generateSecret() method.

Class Definition

```
    public class javax.crypto.KeyAgreement
        extends java.lang.Object {

        // Constructors
        protected KeyAgreement(KeyAgreementSpi, Provider, String);

        // Class Methods
        public static final KeyAgreement getInstance(String);
        public static final KeyAgreement getInstance(String, String);

        // Instance Methods
        public final Key doPhase(int, Key);
        public final byte[] generateSecret();
        public final int generateSecret(byte[], int);
        public final String getAlgorithm();
        public final Provider getProvider();
        public final void init(SecureRandom);
        public final void init(AlgorithmParameterSpec);
        public final void init(AlgorithmParameterSpec, SecureRandom);
    }
```

See also: AlgorithmParameterSpec, Key, KeyAgreementSpi, Provider, SecureRandom

Class javax.crypto.KeyAgreementSpi

This is the Security Provider Interface class for the `KeyAgreement` class. If you want to implement a key agreement algorithm, create a subclass of this class and register it with an appropriate security provider.

Class Definition

```
public abstract class javax.crypto.KeyAgreementSpi
    extends java.lang.Object {

    // Constructors
    public KeyAgreementSpi();

    // Protected Instance Methods
    protected abstract Key engineDoPhase(int, Key);
    protected abstract byte[] engineGenerateSecret();
    protected abstract int engineGenerateSecret(byte[], int);
    protected abstract void engineInit(SecureRandom);
    protected abstract void engineInit(AlgorithmParameterSpec,
                                       SecureRandom);

}
```

See also: AlgorithmParameterSpec, Key, KeyAgreement, SecureRandom

---

Class javax.crypto.KeyGenerator

A key generator creates secret keys for use with symmetric ciphers. Key generators are obtained by calling the `getInstance()` method; they must then be initialized with an `init()` method. The key itself is then returned from the `generateSecret()` method.

Class Definition

```
public class javax.crypto.KeyGenerator
    extends java.lang.Object {

    // Constructors
    protected KeyGenerator(KeyGeneratorSpi, Provider, String);

    // Class Methods
    public static final KeyGenerator getInstance(String);
    public static final KeyGenerator getInstance(String, String);

    // Instance Methods
    public final SecretKey generateKey();
    public final String getAlgorithm();
    public final Provider getProvider();
```

```
        public final void init(SecureRandom);
        public final void init(AlgorithmParameterSpec);
        public final void init(AlgorithmParameterSpec, SecureRandom);
    }
```

See also: AlgorithmParameterSpec, KeyGeneratorSpi, Provider, SecretKey, SecureRandom

Class javax.crypto.KeyGeneratorSpi

This is the Security Provider Interface for the KeyGenerator class. To create an implementation of a key generation algorithm, make a subclass of this class and register the implementation with an appropriate security provider.

Class Definition

```
    public abstract class javax.crypto.KeyGeneratorSpi
        extends java.lang.Object {

        // Constructors
        public KeyGeneratorSpi();

        // Protected Instance Methods
        protected abstract SecretKey engineGenerateKey();
        protected abstract void engineInit(SecureRandom);
        protected abstract void engineInit(AlgorithmParameterSpec,
                                SecureRandom);
    }
```

See also: AlgorithmParameterSpec, KeyGenerator, SecretKey, SecureRandom

Class javax.crypto.NullCipher

As its name implies, null cipher is a cipher that does nothing. You can use it to test cryptographic programs. Since a null cipher performs no transformations, its ciphertext will be exactly the same as its plaintext.

Class Definition

```
    public class javax.crypto.NullCipher
        extends javax.crypto.Cipher {

        // Constructors
```

```
        public NullCipher();
    }
```

See also: Cipher

Class javax.crypto.SealedObject

A sealed object is a container for another object. The contained object is serialized and then encrypted using a cipher. You can construct a sealed object using any serializable object and a cipher that is initialized for encryption. To decrypt the contained object, call the getObject() method with a cipher that is initialized for decryption.

Class Definition

```
    public class javax.crypto.SealedObject
        extends java.lang.Object
        implements java.io.Serializable {

        // Constructors
        public SealedObject(Serializable, Cipher);

        // Instance Methods
        public final Object getObject(Cipher);
    }
```

See also: PublicKey, PrivateKey

Interface javax.crypto.SecretKey

A secret key represents a key that is used with a symmetric cipher. This interface is used strictly for type identification.

Interface Definition

```
    public abstract interface javax.crypto.SecretKey
        implements java.security.Key {
    }
```

See also: Key

Class javax.crypto.SecretKeyFactory

A secret key factory is used to convert between secret key data formats; like a key factory, this is typically used to import a key based on its external format or to export a key to its encoded format or algorithm parameters. Instances of this class are obtained by calling the getInstance() method. Keys may be exported by using the translateKey() method; they are imported by using the generate Secret() method.

Class Definition

```
public class javax.crypto.SecretKeyFactory
    extends java.lang.Object {

    // Constructors
    protected SecretKeyFactory(SecretKeyFactorySpi, Provider);

    // Class Methods
    public static final SecretKeyFactory getInstance(String);
    public static final SecretKeyFactory getInstance(String, String);

    // Instance Methods
    public final SecretKey generateSecret(KeySpec);
    public final KeySpec getKeySpec(SecretKey, Class);
    public final Provider getProvider();
    public final SecretKey translateKey(SecretKey);
}
```

See also: KeySpec, Provider, SecretKey, SecretKeyFactorySpi

Class javax.crypto.SecretKeyFactorySpi

This class is the Security Provider Interface for the SecretKeyFactory class. To create a secret key factory, make a subclass of this class and register your implementation with an appropriate provider.

Class Definition

```
public abstract class javax.crypto.SecretKeyFactorySpi
    extends java.lang.Object {

    // Constructors
    public SecretKeyFactorySpi();

    // Protected Instance Methods
    protected abstract SecretKey engineGenerateSecret(KeySpec);
    protected abstract KeySpec engineGetKeySpec(SecretKey, Class);
    protected abstract SecretKey engineTranslateKey(SecretKey);
}
```

See also: KeySpec, Provider, SecretKey, SecretKeyFactory

Package javax.crypto.interfaces

Interface javax.crypto.interfaces.DHKey

This interface represents a public or private key used the Diffie-Hellman key agreement implementation.

Interface Definition

```
public abstract interface javax.crypto.interfaces.DHKey {

    // Instance Methods
    public abstract DHParameterSpec getParams();
}
```

See also: DHPrivateKey, DHPublicKey

Interface javax.crypto.interfaces.DHPrivateKey

This interface represents a private key in a Diffie-Hellman key agreement protocol.

Interface Definition

```
public abstract interface javax.crypto.interfaces.DHPrivateKey
    implements javax.crypto.interfaces.DHKey, java.security.PrivateKey {

    // Instance Methods
    public abstract BigInteger getX();
}
```

See also: DHKey, DHPublicKey, PrivateKey

Interface javax.crypto.interfaces.DHPublicKey

This interface represents a public key in a Diffie-Hellman key agreement protocol.

Interface Definition

```
public abstract interface javax.crypto.interfaces.DHPublicKey
    implements javax.crypto.interfaces.DHKey, java.security.PublicKey {

    // Instance Methods
    public abstract BigInteger getY();
}
```

See also: DHKey, DHPrivateKey, PublicKey

Interface javax.crypto.interfaces.RSAPrivateKey

RSAPrivateKey represents a private key, suitable for use with RSA cryptographic operations. Use of this class requires a third-party security provider.

Interface Definition

```
public abstract interface javax.crypto.interfaces.RSAPrivateKey
    implements java.security.PrivateKey {

    // Instance Methods
    public abstract BigInteger getModulus();
    public abstract BigInteger getPrivateExponent();
}
```

See also: PrivateKey, RSAPublicKey

Interface javax.crypto.interfaces.RSAPrivateKeyCrt

This interface is an alternate representation of an RSA private key. It uses the Chinese Remainder Theorem (CRT) to represent the values of the private key. Use of this class requires a third-party security provider.

Interface Definition

```
public abstract interface javax.crypto.interfaces.RSAPrivateKeyCrt
    implements javax.crypto.interfaces.RSAPrivateKey {

    // Instance Methods
    public abstract BigInteger getCrtCoefficient();
    public abstract BigInteger getPrimeExponentP();
    public abstract BigInteger getPrimeExponentQ();
    public abstract BigInteger getPrimeP();
    public abstract BigInteger getPrimeQ();
    public abstract BigInteger getPublicExponent();
}
```

See also: PrivateKey, RSAPrivateKey, RSAPublicKey

Interface javax.crypto.interfaces.RSAPublicKey

This class represents an RSA public key, suitable for use with an RSA cryptographic algorithm. You must have a third-party security provider to use this class.

Interface Definition

```
public abstract interface javax.crypto.interfaces.RSAPublicKey
    implements java.security.PublicKey {

    // Instance Methods
    public abstract BigInteger getModulus();
    public abstract BigInteger getPublicExponent();
}
```

See also: PublicKey, RSAPrivateKey

Package javax.crypto.spec

Class javax.crypto.spec.DESKeySpec

This class represents a key specification for DES keys; this specification may be used with a secret key factory to import and export DES keys.

Class Definition

```
public class javax.crypto.spec.DESKeySpec
    extends java.lang.Object
    implements java.security.spec.KeySpec {

    // Constructors
    public DESKeySpec(byte[]);
    public DESKeySpec(byte[], int);

    // Class Methods
    public static boolean isParityAdjusted(byte[], int);

    // Instance Methods
    public byte[] getKey();
}
```

See also: SecretKeyFactory

Class javax.crypto.spec.DESParameterSpec

This class represents an IV (initialization vector) for a cipher that uses a feedback mode. Ciphers in CBC, PCBC, CFB, and OFB modes need to be initialized with an IV.

Class Definition

```
public class javax.crypto.spec.DESParameterSpec
    extends java.lang.Object
    implements java.security.spec.AlgorithmParameterSpec {

    // Constructors
    public DESParameterSpec(byte[]);
    public DESParameterSpec(byte[], int);

    // Instance Methods
    public byte[] getIV();
}
```

See also: AlgorithmParameterSpec, Cipher

Class javax.crypto.spec.DESedeKeySpec

This class represents a DESede key specification. It can be used with a secret key factory to import and export DESede keys.

Class Definition

```
public class javax.crypto.spec.DESedeKeySpec
    extends java.lang.Object
    implements java.security.spec.KeySpec {

    // Constructors
    public DESedeKeySpec(byte[]);
    public DESedeKeySpec(byte[], int);

    // Class Methods
    public static boolean isParityAdjusted(byte[], int);

    // Instance Methods
    public byte[] getKey();
}
```

See also: SecretKeyFactory

Class javax.crypto.spec.DHGenParameterSpec

Instances of this class may be used to supply the algorithm-specific initialization method for generating Diffie-Hellman keys.

Class Definition

```
public class javax.crypto.spec.DHGenParameterSpec
```

```
    extends java.lang.Object
    implements java.security.spec.AlgorithmParameterSpec {

    // Constructors
    public DHGenParameterSpec(int, int);

    // Instance Methods
    public int getExponentSize();
    public int getPrimeSize();
}
```

See also: AlgorithmParameterGenerator, AlgorithmParameterSpec

Class javax.crypto.spec.DHParameterSpec

This class encapsulates the public parameters used in the Diffie-Hellman key agreement protocol. Instances of this class can be passed to the algorithm-specific initialization methods of a key pair generator.

Class Definition

```
public class javax.crypto.spec.DHParameterSpec
    extends java.lang.Object
    implements java.security.spec.AlgorithmParameterSpec {

    // Constructors
    public DHParameterSpec(BigInteger, BigInteger);
    public DHParameterSpec(BigInteger, BigInteger, int);

    // Instance Methods
    public BigInteger getG();
    public int getL();
    public BigInteger getP();
}
```

See also: AlgorithmParameterSpec, KeyPairGenerator

Class javax.crypto.spec.DHPrivateKeySpec

This class represents a key specification for Diffie-Hellman private keys. It can be used with a key factory to import and export Diffie-Hellman keys.

Class Definition

```
public class javax.crypto.spec.DHPrivateKeySpec
    extends java.lang.Object
    implements java.security.spec.KeySpec {
```

```
    // Constructors
    public DHPrivateKeySpec(BigInteger, BigInteger, BigInteger);
    public DHPrivateKeySpec(BigInteger, BigInteger, BigInteger, int);

    // Instance Methods
    public BigInteger getG();
    public int getL();
    public BigInteger getP();
    public BigInteger getX();
}
```

See also: DHParameterSpec, DHPublicKeySpec, KeySpec

Class javax.crypto.spec.DHPublicKeySpec

This class represents a key specification for Diffie-Hellman public keys. It can be used with a key factory to import and export Diffie-Hellman keys.

Class Definition

```
public class javax.crypto.spec.DHPublicKeySpec
    extends java.lang.Object
    implements java.security.spec.KeySpec {

    // Constructors
    public DHPublicKeySpec(BigInteger, BigInteger, BigInteger);
    public DHPublicKeySpec(BigInteger, BigInteger, BigInteger, int);

    // Instance Methods
    public BigInteger getG();
    public int getL();
    public BigInteger getP();
    public BigInteger getY();
}
```

See also: DHParameterSpec, DHPrivateKeySpec, KeySpec

Class javax.crypto.spec.PBEKeySpec

This class represents a key specification for a key that is used with passphrase encryption.

Class Definition

```
public class javax.crypto.spec.PBEKeySpec
    extends java.lang.Object
```

```
    implements java.security.spec.KeySpec {

    // Constructors
    public PBEKeySpec(String);

    // Instance Methods
    public final String getPassword();
}
```

See also: PBEParameterSpec, SecretKey, SecretKeyFactory

Class javax.crypto.spec.PBEParameterSpec

This class encapsulates the salt and iteration count that are used in passphrase-based encryption.

Class Definition

```
    public class javax.crypto.spec.PBEParameterSpec
        extends java.lang.Object
        implements java.security.spec.AlgorithmParameterSpec {

        // Constructors
        public PBEParameterSpec(byte[], int);

        // Instance Methods
        public int getIterationCount();
        public byte[] getSalt();
    }
```

See also: AlgorithmParameterSpec, Cipher, PBEKeySpec

Class javax.crypto.spec.RSAPrivateKeyCrtSpec

This class represents a key specification for an RSA private key; this specification uses the Chinese Remainder Theorem (CRT). Instances of this class may be used with an appropriate key factory to generate private keys. Use of this class requires a third-party security provider.

Class Definition

```
    public class javax.crypto.spec.RSAPrivateKeyCrtSpec
        extends javax.crypto.spec.RSAPrivateKeySpec {

        // Constructors
        public RSAPrivateKeyCrtSpec(BigInteger, BigInteger, BigInteger,
            BigInteger, BigInteger, BigInteger, BigInteger, BigInteger);
```

```
    // Instance Methods
    public BigInteger getCrtCoefficient();
    public BigInteger getPrimeExponentP();
    public BigInteger getPrimeExponentQ();
    public BigInteger getPrimeP();
    public BigInteger getPrimeQ();
    public BigInteger getPublicExponent();
}
```

See also: KeyFactory, KeySpec, PrivateKey, RSAPrivateKeySpec

Class javax.crypto.spec.RSAPrivateKeySpec

This class represents a key specification for an RSA private key; this specification uses a modulus and a private exponent. Instances of this class may be used with an appropriate key factory to generate private keys. Use of this class requires a third-party security provider.

Class Definition

```
    public class javax.crypto.spec.RSAPrivateKeySpec
        extends java.lang.Object
        implements java.security.spec.KeySpec {

        // Constructors
        public RSAPrivateKeySpec(BigInteger, BigInteger);

        // Instance Methods
        public BigInteger getModulus();
        public BigInteger getPrivateExponent();
}
```

See also: KeyFactory, KeySpec, PrivateKey, RSAPrivateKeyCrtSpec

Class javax.crypto.spec.RSAPublicKeySpec

This class represents a key specification for an RSA public key. Instances of this class may be used with an appropriate key factory to generate public keys. Use of this class requires a third-party security provider.

Class Definition

```
    public class javax.crypto.spec.RSAPublicKeySpec
        extends java.lang.Object
        implements java.security.spec.KeySpec {
```

```
    // Constructors
    public RSAPublicKeySpec(BigInteger, BigInteger);

    // Instance Methods
    public BigInteger getModulus();
    public BigInteger getPublicExponent();
}
```

See also: KeyFactory, KeySpec, PublicKey

Miscellaneous Packages

This section lists security-related classes that appear in miscellaneous packages: permission classes, class loaders, and security managers.

Class java.awt.AWTPermission

This class represents permission to perform windowing operations, like opening a top-level window or examining the event queue. This is a basic permission, so it has no actions.

Class Definition

```
    public final class java.awt.AWTPermission
        extends java.security.BasicPermission {

        // Constructors
        public AWTPermission(String);
        public AWTPermission(String, String);
    }
```

See also: BasicPermission, Permission

Class java.io.FilePermission

This class represents permission to read, write, delete, or execute files. The name encapsulated in this permission is the name of the file; the string "<<ALL_ FILES>>" represents all files, while an asterisk represents all files in a directory and a hyphen represents all files that descend from a directory. The actions for this permission are read, write, execute, and delete.

Class Definition

```
    public final class java.io.FilePermission
```

```
    extends java.security.Permission
    implements java.io.Serializable {

    // Constructors
    public FilePermission(String, String);

    // Instance Methods
    public boolean equals(Object);
    public String getActions();
    public int hashCode();
    public boolean implies(Permission);
    public PermissionCollection newPermissionCollection();
}
```

See also: Permission

Class java.io.SerializablePermission

This class represents permission to perform specific operations during object seri-alization—specifically, whether or not object substitution may occur during serialization. As all basic permissions, there are no actions associated with this class, which has one valid name: enableSubstitution.

Class Definition

```
    public final class java.io.SerializablePermission
        extends java.security.BasicPermission {

    // Constructors
    public SerializablePermission(String);
    public SerializablePermission(String, String);
}
```

See also: BasicPermission, Permission

Class java.lang.ClassLoader

This class is the basis for loading a class dynamically in Java. For historical reasons, it appears in this package, but it is recommended that all new class loaders subclass the SecureClassLoader class in the java.security package instead of using this class. Loading a class explicitly may be done with the loadClass() method of this class (though classes are usually simply loaded as needed).

Class Definition

```
    public abstract class java.lang.ClassLoader
        extends java.lang.Object {
```

```
      // Constructors
      protected ClassLoader();
      protected ClassLoader(ClassLoader);

      // Class Methods
      public static URL getSystemResource(String);
      public static InputStream getSystemResourceAsStream(String);
      public static Enumeration getSystemResources(String);

      // Instance Methods
      public URL getLocalResource(String);
      public Enumeration getLocalResources(String);
      public ClassLoader getParent();
      public URL getResource(String);
      public InputStream getResourceAsStream(String);
      public final Enumeration getResources(String);
      public Class loadClass(String);

      // Protected Instance Methods
      protected void checkPackageAccess(String);
      protected final Class defineClass(String, byte[], int, int);
      protected final Class defineClass(byte[], int, int);
      protected Package definePackage(String, String, String, String,
                           String, String, String, URL);
      protected final Class findLoadedClass(String);
      protected Class findLocalClass(String);
      protected final Class findSystemClass(String);
      protected Package getPackage(String);
      protected Package[] getPackages();
      protected synchronized Class loadClass(String, boolean);
      protected final void resolveClass(Class);
      protected final void setSigners(Class, Object[]);
   }
```

See also: SecureClassLoader, URLClassLoader

Class java.lang.RuntimePermission

This class represents permission to perform certain runtime operations, such as executing other programs. Like all basic permissions, runtime permissions have no actions.

Class Definition

```
   public final class java.lang.RuntimePermission
      extends java.security.BasicPermission {

      // Constructors
```

```
    public RuntimePermission(String);
    public RuntimePermission(String, String);
}
```

See also: BasicPermission, Permission

Class java.lang.SecurityManager

This class forms the primary interface to the security model of the virtual machine; it is recommended for backwards compatibility that access to that model occur through this class rather than by calling the access controller directly. However, most of the methods of this class simply call the access controller.

Class Definition

```
    public class java.lang.SecurityManager
        extends java.lang.Object {

        // Variables
        protected boolean inCheck;

        // Constructors
        public SecurityManager();

        // Instance Methods
        public void checkAccept(String, int);
        public void checkAccess(Thread);
        public void checkAccess(ThreadGroup);
        public void checkAwtEventQueueAccess();
        public void checkConnect(String, int);
        public void checkConnect(String, int, Object);
        public void checkCreateClassLoader();
        public void checkDelete(String);
        public void checkExec(String);
        public void checkExit(int);
        public void checkLink(String);
        public void checkListen(int);
        public void checkMemberAccess(Class, int);
        public void checkMulticast(InetAddress);
        public void checkMulticast(InetAddress, byte);
        public void checkPackageAccess(String);
        public void checkPackageDefinition(String);
        public void checkPermission(Permission);
        public void checkPermission(Permission, Object);
        public void checkPrintJobAccess();
        public void checkPropertiesAccess();
        public void checkPropertyAccess(String);
        public void checkRead(FileDescriptor);
```

```
        public void checkRead(String);
        public void checkRead(String, Object);
        public void checkSecurityAccess(String);
        public void checkSetFactory();
        public void checkSystemClipboardAccess();
        public boolean checkTopLevelWindow(Object);
        public void checkWrite(FileDescriptor);
        public void checkWrite(String);
        public boolean getInCheck();
        public Object getSecurityContext();
        public ThreadGroup getThreadGroup();

        // Protected Instance Methods
        protected native int classDepth(String);
        protected native int classLoaderDepth();
        protected native ClassLoader currentClassLoader();
        protected Class currentLoadedClass();
        protected native Class[] getClassContext();
        protected boolean inClass(String);
        protected boolean inClassLoader();
    }
```

See also: AccessController

Class java.lang.reflect.ReflectPermission

This class represents the ability to obtain information via object reflections; specifically, whether private and protected variables and methods may be accessed through object reflection. As all basic permissions, this permission carries no actions; it has a single name: access.

Class Definition

```
    public final class java.lang.reflect.ReflectPermission
        extends java.security.BasicPermission {

        // Constructors
        public ReflectPermission(String);
        public ReflectPermission(String, String);
    }
```

See also: BasicPermission, Permission

Class java.net.NetPermission

This class represents the ability to work with multicast sockets and the ability to use the authenticator classes. As all basic permissions, this class carries no actions.

Class Definition

```
public final class java.net.NetPermission
    extends java.security.BasicPermission {

    // Constructors
    public NetPermission(String);
    public NetPermission(String, String);
}
```

See also: BasicPermission, Permission

Class java.net.SocketPermission

This class represents the ability to work with certain sockets. The name of this permission is constructed from the hostname or IP address of the machine on the other end of the socket and the port number; either portion of the name is subject to wildcard matching. Valid actions for this class include connect, accept, and listen.

Class Definition

```
public final class java.net.SocketPermission
    extends java.security.Permission
    implements java.io.Serializable {

    // Constructors
    public SocketPermission(String, String);

    // Instance Methods
    public boolean equals(Object);
    public String getActions();
    public int hashCode();
    public boolean implies(Permission);
    public PermissionCollection newPermissionCollection();
}
```

See also: Permission

Class java.net.URLClassLoader

This class provides a concrete class loader that may be used to load classes from one or more URLs (either http-based or file-based URLs). Since it is a secure class loader, classes loaded from a URL class loader will be fully integrated into the access controller's security model.

Class Definition

```
public class java.net.URLClassLoader
    extends java.security.SecureClassLoader {

    // Constructors
    public URLClassLoader(URL[], ClassLoader);

    // Class Methods
    public static URL fileToURL(File);
    public static URL[] pathToURLs(String);

    // Instance Methods
    public URL getLocalResource(String);
    public Enumeration getLocalResources(String);
    public void invokeClass(String, String[]);
    public void setListener(URLClassLoader$Listener);

    // Protected Instance Methods
    protected void checkPackageDefinition(String);
    protected Class defineClass(String, Resource);
    protected Package definePackage(String, Attributes, URL);
    protected Class findLocalClass(String);
}
```

See also: ClassLoader, SecureClassLoader

Class java.rmi.RMISecurityManager

The RMI security manager provides a security manager that is suitable for many RMI servers. It provides the ability for RMI applications to make socket-based connections to each other, and otherwise follows the default security manager implementation.

Class Definition

```
public class java.rmi.RMISecurityManager
    extends java.lang.SecurityManager {

    // Constructors
```

```
        public RMISecurityManager();

        // Instance Methods
        public synchronized void checkAccept(String, int);
        public synchronized void checkAccess(Thread);
        public synchronized void checkAccess(ThreadGroup);
        public synchronized void checkConnect(String, int);
        public void checkConnect(String, int, Object);
        public synchronized void checkPackageAccess(String);
        public synchronized void checkPackageDefinition(String);
        public synchronized void checkRead(String);
        public void checkRead(String, Object);
        public Object getSecurityContext();
        public ThreadGroup getThreadGroup();
    }
```

See also: SecurityManager

Class java.rmi.server.RMIClassLoader

While not a traditional class loader, this class allows classes to be loaded via the same mechanics as a class loader: the loadClass() method may be called to load a class explicitly, and this class will also be used to load all subsequent classes required by the target class. This class loader will only load classes from the URL specified by the java.rmi.server.codebase property. The internal class loader used by this class is a secure class loader, so the security model of the access controller will be used by classes loaded in this manner.

Class Definition

```
    public class java.rmi.server.RMIClassLoader
        extends java.lang.Object {

        // Class Methods
        public static Object getSecurityContext(ClassLoader);
        public static Class loadClass(String);
        public static Class loadClass(URL, String);
    }
```

See also: ClassLoader, SecureClassLoader

Class java.util.PropertyPermission

This class represents the ability to read or write properties. The name of a property permission is the name of the property itself; the action for a property permission is either set or get.

Class Definition

```
public final class java.util.PropertyPermission
    extends java.security.BasicPermission {

    // Constructors
    public PropertyPermission(String, String);

    // Instance Methods
    public boolean equals(Object);
    public String getActions();
    public int hashCode();
    public boolean implies(Permission);
    public PermissionCollection newPermissionCollection();
}
```

See also: Permission

Index

About the Author

Scott Oaks is a Java Technologist at Sun Microsystems, where he has worked since 1987. While at Sun, he has specialized in many disparate technologies, from the SunOS kernel to network programming and RPCs to the X Window System to threading. Since early 1995, he has primarily focused on Java and bringing Java technology to end users; he writes a monthly column on Java solutions for *The Java Report*. Around the Internet, Scott is best known as the author of olvwm, the OPEN LOOK window manager.

Scott holds a Bachelor of Science in mathematics and computer science from the University of Denver and a Master of Science in computer science from Brown University. Prior to joining Sun, he worked in the research division of Bear, Stearns.

In his other life, Scott enjoys music (he plays flute and piccolo with community groups in New York), cooking, theatre, and traveling with his husband James.

Colophon

Our look is the result of reader comments, our own experimentation, and feedback from distribution channels. Distinctive covers complement our distinctive approach to technical topics, breathing personality and life into potentially dry subjects.

Hanna Dyer designed the cover of *Java Security*, based on a series design by Edie Freedman. The image of a bird's nest was photographed by Kevin Thomas and manipulated in Adobe Photoshop by Michael Snow. The cover layout was produced with Quark XPress 3.3 using the Bodoni Black font from URW Software and Bodoni BT Bold Italic from Bitstream. The inside layout was designed by Nancy Priest. Text was prepared by Mike Sierra in FrameMaker 5.0. The heading font is Bodoni BT; the text font is New Baskerville. The illustrations that appear in the book were created in Macromedia Freehand 7.0 by Robert Romano.

Whenever possible, our books use RepKover™, a durable and flexible lay-flat binding. If the page count exceeds RepKover's limit, perfect binding is used.

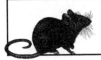

More Titles from O'Reilly

Java Programming

Java in a Nutshell, DELUXE EDITION

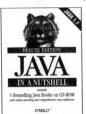

By David Flanagan, et al.
1st Edition June 1997
628 pages, includes CD-ROM and book
ISBN 1-56592-304-9

Java in a Nutshell, Deluxe Edition, is a Java programmer's dream come true in one small package. The heart of this Deluxe Edition is the Java Reference Library on CD-ROM, which brings together five volumes for Java developers and programmers, linking related info across books. It includes: *Exploring Java, 2nd Edition*; *Java Language Reference, 2nd Edition*; *Java Fundamental Classes Reference*; *Java AWT Reference*; and *Java in a Nutshell, 2nd Edition*, included both on the CD-ROM and in a companion desktop edition. *Java in a Nutshell, Deluxe Edition,* is an indispensable resource for anyone doing serious programming with Java 1.1.

The Java Reference Library alone is also available by subscription on the World Wide Web. Please see http://www.oreilly.com/catalog/javarlw/ for details. The electronic text on the Web and on the CD is fully searchable and includes a complete index to all five volumes as well as the sample code found in the print volumes. A web browser that supports HTML 3.2, Java, and Javascript, such as Netscape 3.0 or Internet Explorer 3.0, is required. (The CD-ROM is readable on all UNIX and Windows platforms. However, current implementations of the Java Virtual Machine for the Mac do not support the Java search applet in the CD-ROM.)

Java Cryptography

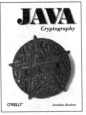

By Jonathan B. Knudsen
1st Edition May 1998 (est.)
250 pages (est.), ISBN 1-56592-402-9

Java 1.1 and Java 1.2 provide extensive support for cryptography with an elegant architecture, the Java Cryptography Architecture (JCA). Another set of classes, the Java Cryptography Extension (JCE), provides additional cryptographic functionality. This book covers the JCA and the JCE from top to bottom, describing how to use cryptographic classes as well as how they work.

The book is designed for moderately experienced Java programmers who want to learn how to build cryptography into their applications, and no prior knowledge of cryptography is assumed. It's peppered with useful examples, ranging from simple demonstrations in the first chapter to full-blown applications in later chapters.

Java Security

By Scott Oaks
1st Edition May 1998
472 pages, ISBN 1-56592-403-7

Java Security covers Java's security mechanisms and teaches you how to work with them. It discusses class loaders, security managers, access lists, digital signatures, and authentication and shows how to use these to create and enforce your own security policy. *Java Security* is essential reading for serious Java programmers. Covers Java 1.2.

Exploring Java, Second Edition

By Pat Niemeyer & Josh Peck
2nd Edition September 1997
614 pages, ISBN 1-56592-271-9

Whether you're just migrating to Java or working steadily in the forefront of Java development, this book, fully revised for Java 1.1, gives a clear, systematic overview of the language. It covers the essentials of hot topics like Beans and RMI, as well as writing applets and other applications, such as networking programs, content and protocol handlers, and security managers.

Java Virtual Machine

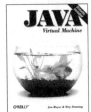

By Jon Meyer & Troy Downing
1st Edition March 1997
452 pages, includes diskette
ISBN 1-56592-194-1

This book is a comprehensive programming guide for the Java Virtual Machine (JVM). It gives readers a strong overview and·reference of the JVM so that they may create their own implementations of the JVM or write their own compilers that create Java object code. A Java assembler is provided with the book, so the examples can all be compiled and executed.

Java Programming

Java Examples in a Nutshell

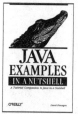

By David Flanagan
1st Edition September 1997
414 pages, ISBN 1-56592-371-5

From the author of *Java in a Nutshell*, this companion book is chock full of practical real-world programming examples to help novice Java programmers and experts alike explore what's possible with Java 1.1. If you learn best by example, this is the book for you.

Java Threads

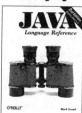

By Scott Oaks and Henry Wong
1st Edition January 1997
268 pages, ISBN 1-56592-216-6

With this book, you'll learn how to take full advantage of Java's thread facilities: where to use threads to increase efficiency, how to use them effectively, and how to avoid common mistakes like deadlock and race conditions. Covers Java 1.1.

Java Language Reference, Second Edition

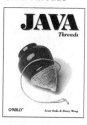

By Mark Grand
2nd Edition July 1997
492 pages, ISBN 1-56592-326-X

This book helps you understand the subtle nuances of Java—from the definition of data types to the syntax of expressions and control structures—so you can ensure your programs run exactly as expected. The second edition covers the new language features that have been added in Java 1.1, such as inner classes, class literals, and instance initializers.

Java Fundamental Classes Reference

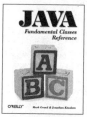

By Mark Grand & Jonathan Knudsen
1st Edition May 1997
1114 pages, ISBN 1-56592-241-7

The *Java Fundamental Classes Reference* provides complete reference documentation on the core Java 1.1 classes that comprise the *java.lang, java.io, java.net, java.util, java.text, java.math, java.lang.reflect*, and *java.util.zip* packages. Part of O'Reilly's Java documentation series, this edition describes Version 1.1 of the Java Development Kit. It includes easy-to-use reference material and provides lots of sample code to help you learn by example.

Netscape IFC in a Nutshell

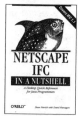

By Dean Petrich with David Flanagan
1st Edition August 1997
370 pages, ISBN 1-56592-343-X

This desktop quick reference and programmer's guide is all the documentation programmers need to start creating highly customizable graphical user interfaces with the Internet Foundation Classes (IFC), Version 1.1. The IFC is a Java class library freely available from Netscape. It is also bundled with Communicator, making it the preferred development environment for the Navigator 4.0 web browser. Master the IFC now for a head start on the forthcoming Java Foundation Classes (JFC).

Developing Java Beans

By Robert Englander
1st Edition June 1997
316 pages, ISBN 1-56592-289-1

Developing Java Beans is a complete introduction to Java's component architecture. It describes how to write Beans, which are software components that can be used in visual programming environments. This book discusses event adapters, serialization, introspection, property editors, and customizers, and shows how to use Beans within ActiveX controls.

Java Programming

Java Network Programming

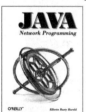

By Elliotte Rusty Harold
1st Edition February 1997
442 pages, ISBN 1-56592-227-1

The network is the soul of Java. Most of what is new and exciting about Java centers around the potential for new kinds of dynamic, networked applications. *Java Network Programming* teaches you to work with Sockets, write network clients and servers, and gives you an advanced look at the new areas like multicasting, using the server API, and RMI. Covers Java 1.1.

Java in a Nutshell, Second Edition

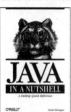

By David Flanagan
2nd Edition May 1997
628 pages, ISBN 1-56592-262-X

This second edition of the bestselling Java book describes all the classes in the Java 1.1 API, with the exception of the still-evolving Enterprise APIs. And it still has all the great features that have made this the Java book most often recommended on the Internet: practical real-world examples and compact reference information. It's the only quick reference you'll need.

Java Native Methods

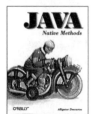

By Alligator Descartes
1st Edition August 1998 (est.)
300 pages (est.), ISBN 1-56592-345-6

Although Java offers the promise of platform-independent programming, there are situations where you may still need to use native C or C++code compiled for a particular platform. Maybe you have to tie some legacy code into a Java application. Or maybe you want to implement some computer-intensive methods for a performance-critical application in native code. *Java Native Methods* tells you everything you need to know to get your native code working with Java, using either Sun's Java Native Interface (JNI) or Microsoft's Raw Native Interface (RNI).

Database Programming with JDBC and Java

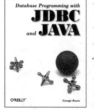

By George Reese
1st Edition June 1997
240 pages, ISBN 1-56592-270-0

Database Programming with JDBC and Java describes the standard Java interfaces that make portable, object-oriented access to relational databases possible and offers a robust model for writing applications that are easy to maintain. It introduces the JDBC and RMI packages and includes a set of patterns that separate the functions of the Java application and facilitate the growth and maintenance of your application.

Java AWT Reference

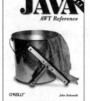

By John Zukowski
1st Edition April 1997
1074 pages, ISBN 1-56592-240-9

The *Java AWT Reference* provides complete reference documentation on the Abstract Window Toolkit (AWT), a large collection of classes for building graphical user interfaces in Java. Part of O'Reilly's Java documentation series, this edition describes both Version 1.0.2 and Version 1.1 of the Java Development Kit, includes easy-to-use reference material on every AWT class, and provides lots of sample code.

Java Distributed Computing

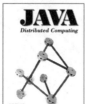

By Jim Farley
1st Edition January 1998
384 pages, ISBN 1-56592-206-9

Java Distributed Computing offers a general introduction to distributed computing, meaning programs that run on two or more systems. It focuses primarily on how to structure and write distributed applications and, therefore, discusses issues like designing protocols, security, working with databases, and dealing with low bandwidth situations.

How to stay in touch with O'Reilly

1. Visit Our Award-Winning Web Site
http://www.oreilly.com/

★ "Top 100 Sites on the Web" —*PC Magazine*
★ "Top 5% Web sites" —*Point Communications*
★ "3-Star site" —*The McKinley Group*

Our web site contains a library of comprehensiveproduct information (including book excerpts and tables of contents), downloadable software, background articles, interviews with technology leaders, links to relevant sites, book cover art, and more. File us in your Bookmarks or Hotlist!

2. Join Our Email Mailing Lists
New Product Releases
To receive automatic email with brief descriptions of all new O'Reilly products as they are released, send email to:
listproc@online.oreilly.com
Put the following information in the first line of your message (*not* in the Subject field):
subscribe oreilly-news

O'Reilly Events
If you'd also like us to send information about trade show events, special promotions, and other O'Reilly events, send email to:
listproc@online.oreilly.com
Put the following information in the first line of your message (*not* in the Subject field):
subscribe oreilly-events

3. Get Examples from Our Books via FTP
There are two ways to access an archive of example files from our books:

Regular FTP
- ftp to:
  ftp.oreilly.com
  (login: anonymous
  password: your email address)
- Point your web browser to:
  ftp://ftp.oreilly.com/

FTPMAIL
- Send an email message to:
  ftpmail@online.oreilly.com
  (Write "help" in the message body)

4. Contact Us via Email
order@oreilly.com
To place a book or software order online. Good for North American and international customers.

subscriptions@oreilly.com
To place an order for any of our newsletters or periodicals.

books@oreilly.com
General questions about any of our books.

software@oreilly.com
For general questions and product information about our software. Check out O'Reilly Software Online at **http://software.oreilly.com/** for software and technical support information. Registered O'Reilly software users send your questions to: **website-support@oreilly.com**

cs@oreilly.com
For answers to problems regarding your order or our products.

booktech@oreilly.com
For book content technical questions or corrections.

proposals@oreilly.com
To submit new book or software proposals to our editors and product managers.

international@oreilly.com
For information about our international distributors or translation queries. For a list of our distributors outside of North America check out:
http://www.oreilly.com/www/order/country.html

O'Reilly & Associates, Inc.
101 Morris Street, Sebastopol, CA 95472 USA
TEL   707-829-0515 or 800-998-9938
          (6am to 5pm PST)
FAX   707-829-0104

Titles from O'Reilly

WEB PROGRAMMING

Advanced Perl Programming
Apache: The Definitive Guide
Building Your Own Web Conferences
Building Your Own Website™
CGI Programming for the World Wide
Web
Designing for the Web
Dynamic HTML: The Complete
Reference
Frontier: The Definitive Guide
HTML: The Definitive Guide, 2nd
Edition
Information Architecture for the
World Wide Web
JavaScript: The Definitive Guide, 2nd
Edition
Learning Perl, 2nd Edition
Learning Perl for Win32 Systems
Mastering Regular Expressions
Netscape IFC in a Nutshell
Perl5 Desktop Reference
Perl Cookbook
Perl in a Nutshell
Perl Resource Kit—UNIX Edition
Perl Resource Kit—Win32 Edition
Programming Perl, 2nd Edition
WebMaster in a Nutshell
WebMaster in a Nutshell, Deluxe
Edition
Web Security & Commerce
Web Client Programming with Perl

GRAPHIC DESIGN

Director in a Nutshell
Photoshop in a Nutshell
QuarkXPress in a Nutshell

JAVA SERIES

Database Programming with JDBC and
Java
Developing Java Beans
Exploring Java, 2nd Edition
Java AWT Reference
Java Cryptography
Java Distributed Computing
Java Examples in a Nutshell
Java Fundamental Classes Reference
Java in a Nutshell, 2nd Edition
Java in a Nutshell, Deluxe Edition
Java Language Reference, 2nd Edition
Java Native Methods
Java Network Programming
Java Security
Java Threads
Java Virtual Machine

SONGLINE GUIDES

NetLaw   NetResearch
NetLearning   NetSuccess
NetLessons   NetTravel

SYSTEM ADMINISTRATION

Building Internet Firewalls
Computer Crime: A Crimefighter's
Handbook
Computer Security Basics
DNS and BIND, 2nd Edition
Essential System Administration, 2nd
Edition
Essential WindowsNT System
Administration
Getting Connected: The Internet at
56K and Up
Linux Network Administrator's Guide
Managing Internet Information
Services, 2nd Edition
Managing IP Networks with Cisco
Routers
Managing Mailing Lists
Managing NFS and NIS
Managing the WinNT Registry
Managing Usenet
MCSE: The Core Exams in a Nutshell
MCSE: The Electives in a Nutshell
Networking Personal Computers with
TCP/IP
Palm Pilot: The Ultimate Guide
Practical UNIX & Internet Security,2nd
Edition
PGP: Pretty Good Privacy
Protecting Networks with SATAN
sendmail, 2nd Edition
sendmail Desktop Reference
System Performance Tuning
TCP/IP Network Administration, 2nd
Edition
termcap & terminfo
Using & Managing PPP
Using & Managing UUCP
Virtual Private Networks
Volume 8: X Window System
Administrator's Guide
Web Security & Commerce
WindowsNT Backup & Restore
WindowsNT Desktop Reference
WindowsNT in a Nutshell
WindowsNT Server 4.0 for Netware
Administrators
WindowsNT SNMP
WindowsNT User Administration

WEB REVIEW STUDIO SERIES

Designing Sound for the Web
Designing with Animation
Designing with JavaScript
Gif Animation Studio
Photoshop for the Web
Shockwave Studio
Web Navigation: Designing the User
Experience

UNIX

Exploring Expect
Learning VBScript
Learning GNU Emacs, 2nd Edition
Learning the bash Shell, 2nd Edition
Learning the Korn Shell
Learning the UNIX Operating System,
4th Edition
Learning the vi Editor, 5th Edition
Linux Device Drivers
Linux in a Nutshell
Linux Multimedia Guide
Running Linux, 2nd Edition
SCO UNIX in a Nutshell
sed & awk, 2nd Edition
Tcl/Tk Tools
UNIX in a Nutshell, Deluxe Edition
UNIX in a Nutshell, System V Edition
UNIX Power Tools, 2nd Edition
Using csh & tsch
What You Need To Know: When You
Can't Find Your UNIX System
Administrator
Writing GNU Emacs Extensions

WINDOWS

Access Database Design and
Programming
Developing Windows Error Messages
Excel97 Annoyances
Inside the Windows 95 File System
Inside the Windows 95 Registry
Office97 Annoyances
VB/VBA in a Nutshell: The Languages
Win32 Multithreaded Programming
Windows95 in a Nutshell
Windows97 Annoyances
Windows NT File System Internals
Windows NT in a Nutshell
Word97 Annoyances

USING THE INTERNET

AOL in a Nutshell
Bandits on the Information
Superhighway
Internet in a Nutshell
Smileys
The Whole Internet for Windows95
The Whole Internet: The Next
Generation
The Whole Internet User's Guide &
Catalog

PROGRAMMING

Advanced Oracle PL/SQL
Programming with Packages
Applying RCS and SCCS
BE Developer's Guide
BE Advanced Topics
C++: The Core Language
Checking C Programs with lint
Encyclopedia of Graphics File
Formats, 2nd Edition
Guide to Writing DCE Applications
lex & yacc, 2nd Edition
Managing Projects with make
Mastering Oracle Power Objects
Oracle8 Design Tips
Oracle Built-in Packages
Oracle Design
Oracle Performance Tuning, 2nd
Edition
Oracle PL/SQL Programming, 2nd
Edition
Oracle Scripts
Porting UNIX Software
POSIX Programmer's Guide
POSIX.4: Programming for the Real
World
Power Programming with RPC
Practical C Programming, 3rd Edition
Practical C++ Programming
Programming Python
Programming with curses
Programming with GNU Software
Pthreads Programming
Software Portability with imake, 2nd
Edition
Understanding DCE
UNIX Systems Programming for SVR4

X PROGRAMMING

Vol. 0: X Protocol Reference Manual
Vol. 1: Xlib Programming Manual
Vol. 2: Xlib Reference Manual
Vol. 3M: X Window System User's
Guide, Motif Edition
Vol. 4M: X Toolkit Intrinsics
Programming Manual, Motif
Edition
Vol. 5: X Toolkit Intrinsics Reference
Manual
Vol. 6A: Motif Programming Manual
Vol. 6B: Motif Reference Manual
Vol. 8 : X Window System
Administrator's Guide

SOFTWARE

Building Your Own WebSite™
Building Your Own Web Conference
WebBoard™ 3.0
WebSite Professional™ 2.0
PolyForm™

O'REILLY™

TO ORDER: **800-998-9938** • **order@oreilly.com** • **http://www.oreilly.com/**
OUR PRODUCTS ARE AVAILABLE AT A BOOKSTORE OR SOFTWARE STORE NEAR YOU.
FOR INFORMATION: **800-998-9938** • **707-829-0515** • **info@oreilly.com**

International Distributors

UK, EUROPE, MIDDLE EAST AND NORTHERN AFRICA (EXCEPT FRANCE, GERMANY, SWITZERLAND, & AUSTRIA)

INQUIRIES

International Thomson Publishing Europe
Berkshire House
168-173 High Holborn
London WC1V 7AA
United Kingdom
Telephone: 44-171-497-1422
Fax: 44-171-497-1426
Email: itpint@itps.co.uk

ORDERS

International Thomson Publishing Services, Ltd.
Cheriton House, North Way
Andover, Hampshire SP10 5BE
United Kingdom
Telephone: 44-264-342-832 (UK)
Telephone: 44-264-342-806 (outside UK)
Fax: 44-264-364418 (UK)
Fax: 44-264-342761 (outside UK)
UK & Eire orders: itpuk@itps.co.uk
International orders: itpint@itps.co.uk

FRANCE

Editions Eyrolles
61 bd Saint-Germain
75240 Paris Cedex 05
France
Fax: 33-01-44-41-11-44

FRENCH LANGUAGE BOOKS

All countries except Canada
Telephone: 33-01-44-41-46-16
Email: geodif@eyrolles.com
English language books
Telephone: 33-01-44-41-11-87
Email: distribution@eyrolles.com

GERMANY, SWITZERLAND, AND AUSTRIA

INQUIRIES

O'Reilly Verlag
Balthasarstr. 81
D-50670 Köln
Germany
Telephone: 49-221-97-31-60-0
Fax: 49-221-97-31-60-8
Email: anfragen@oreilly.de

ORDERS

International Thomson Publishing
Königswinterer Straße 418
53227 Bonn, Germany
Telephone: 49-228-97024 0
Fax: 49-228-441342
Email: order@oreilly.de

JAPAN

O'Reilly Japan, Inc.
Kiyoshige Building 2F
12-Banchi, Sanei-cho
Shinjuku-ku
Tokyo 160-0008 Japan
Telephone: 81-3-3356-5227
Fax: 81-3-3356-5261
Email: kenji@oreilly.com

INDIA

Computer Bookshop (India) PVT. Ltd.
190 Dr. D.N. Road, Fort
Bombay 400 001 India
Telephone: 91-22-207-0989
Fax: 91-22-262-3551
Email: cbsbom@giasbm01.vsnl.net.in

HONG KONG

City Discount Subscription Service Ltd.
Unit D, 3rd Floor, Yan's Tower
27 Wong Chuk Hang Road
Aberdeen, Hong Kong
Telephone: 852-2580-3539
Fax: 852-2580-6463
Email: citydis@ppn.com.hk

KOREA

Hanbit Media, Inc.
Sonyoung Bldg. 202
Yeksam-dong 736-36
Kangnam-ku
Seoul, Korea
Telephone: 822-554-9610
Fax: 822-556-0363
Email: hant93@chollian.dacom.co.kr

SINGAPORE, MALAYSIA, AND THAILAND

Addison Wesley Longman Singapore PTE Ltd.
25 First Lok Yang Road
Singapore 629734
Telephone: 65-268-2666
Fax: 65-268-7023
Email: daniel@longman.com.sg

PHILIPPINES

Mutual Books, Inc.
429-D Shaw Boulevard
Mandaluyong City, Metro
Manila, Philippines
Telephone: 632-725-7538
Fax: 632-721-3056
Email: mbikikog@mnl.sequel.net

CHINA

Ron's DataCom Co., Ltd.
79 Dongwu Avenue
Dongxihu District
Wuhan 430040
China
Telephone: 86-27-3892568
Fax: 86-27-3222108
Email: hongfeng@public.wh.hb.cn

ALL OTHER ASIAN COUNTRIES

O'Reilly & Associates, Inc.
101 Morris Street
Sebastopol, CA 95472 USA
Telephone: 707-829-0515
Fax: 707-829-0104
Email: order@oreilly.com

AUSTRALIA

WoodsLane Pty. Ltd.
7/5 Vuko Place, Warriewood NSW 2102
P.O. Box 935
Mona Vale NSW 2103
Australia
Telephone: 61-2-9970-5111
Fax: 61-2-9970-5002
Email: info@woodslane.com.au

NEW ZEALAND

Woodslane New Zealand Ltd.
21 Cooks Street (P.O. Box 575)
Waganui, New Zealand
Telephone: 64-6-347-6543
Fax: 64-6-345-4840
Email: info@woodslane.com.au

THE AMERICAS

McGraw-Hill Interamericana Editores,
S.A. de C.V.
Cedro No. 512
Col. Atlampa 06450
Mexico, D.F.
Telephone: 52-5-541-3155
Fax: 52-5-541-4913
Email: mcgraw-hill@infosel.net.mx

SOUTH AFRICA

International Thomson Publishing
South Africa
Building 18, Constantia Park
138 Sixteenth Road
P.O. Box 2459
Halfway House, 1685 South Africa
Telephone: 27-11-805-4819
Fax: 27-11-805-3648

O'REILLY™

TO ORDER: **800-998-9938** • **order@oreilly.com** • **http://www.oreilly.com/**

OUR PRODUCTS ARE AVAILABLE AT A BOOKSTORE OR SOFTWARE STORE NEAR YOU.

FOR INFORMATION: **800-998-9938** • **707-829-0515** • **info@oreilly.com**

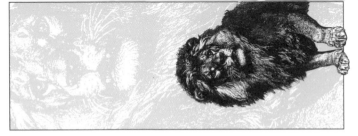

O'REILLY™

O'Reilly & Associates, Inc.
101 Morris Street
Sebastopol, CA 95472-9902
1-800-998-9938

Visit us online at:
http://www.ora.com/
orders@ora.com

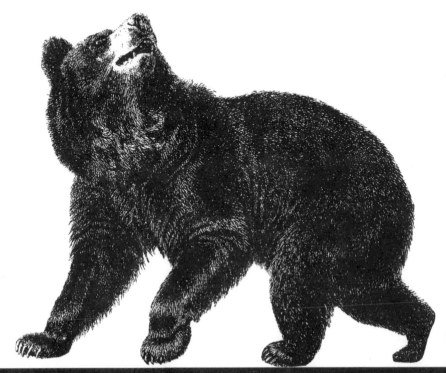

O'REILLY WOULD LIKE TO HEAR FROM YOU

Which book did this card come from?

_____

Where did you buy this book?
❏ Bookstore   ❏ Computer Store
❏ Direct from O'Reilly   ❏ Class/seminar
❏ Bundled with hardware/software
❏ Other _____

What operating system do you use?
❏ UNIX   ❏ Macintosh
❏ Windows NT   ❏ PC(Windows/DOS)
❏ Other _____

What is your job description?
❏ System Administrator   ❏ Programmer
❏ Network Administrator   ❏ Educator/Teacher
❏ Web Developer
❏ Other _____

❏ Please send me O'Reilly's catalog, containing
a complete listing of O'Reilly books and
software.

_____
Name   Company/Organization

_____
Address

_____
City   State   Zip/Postal Code   Country

_____
Telephone   Internet or other email address (specify network)

Nineteenth century wood engraving
of a bear from the O'Reilly &
Associates Nutshell Handbook®
Using & Managing UUCP.

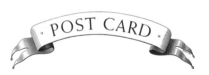

BUSINESS REPLY MAIL

FIRST CLASS MAIL   PERMIT NO. 80   SEBASTOPOL, CA

Postage will be paid by addressee

O'Reilly & Associates, Inc.
101 Morris Street
Sebastopol, CA 95472-9902

||l||u||l||l||u||l||ul||l|u||l|u||l||l||l|l||l||l||l|l||l|l||l||l||u||u||l||l|u||l||l|l||l|